Massachusetts General Hospital
Psychopharmacology and Neurotherapeutics

First Edition

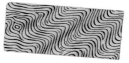

Massachusetts General Hospital
Psychopharmacology and Neurotherapeutics

First Edition

Massachusetts General Hospital
Psychopharmacology and Neurotherapeutics

First Edition

Created with content from:
Massachusetts General Hospital Comprehensive Clinical Psychiatry, Second Edition
ISBN: 978-0-323-29507-9

Editors

THEODORE A. STERN MD
Chief, Avery D. Weisman Psychiatry Consultation Service
Massachusetts General Hospital
Director, Office for Clinical Careers Massachusetts General Hospital
Ned H. Cassem Professor of Psychiatry in the field of Psychosomatic Medicine/Consultation
Harvard Medical School
Boston, MA, USA

MAURIZIO FAVA MD
Director, Clinical Research Program
Executive Vice-Chair, Department of Psychiatry
Executive Director, Clinical Trials Network and Institute, Massachusetts General Hospital
Slater Family Professor of Psychiatry, Harvard Medical School
Boston, MA, USA

TIMOTHY E. WILENS MD
Senior Staff, Child Psychiatry and Pediatric Psychopharmacology
Director of the Center for Addiction Medicine
Massachusetts General Hospital
Associate Professor of Psychiatry
Harvard Medical School
Boston, MA, USA

JERROLD F. ROSENBAUM MD
Psychiatrist-in-Chief, Massachusetts General Hospital
Chair, Executive Committee on Research
Massachusetts General Hospital
Stanley Cobb Professor of Psychiatry
Harvard Medical School
Boston, MA, USA

ELSEVIER   London, New York, Oxford, Philadelphia, St Louis, Sydney, Toronto

ELSEVIER

ISBN: 978-0-323-35764-7
eISBN: 978-0-323-41323-7

Content Strategist: Lotta Kryhl
Content Development Specialist: Alexandra Mortimer
Content Coordinator: Sam Crowe
Project Manager: Andrew Riley
eProject Manager: Denise Roslonski
Design Direction: Christian Bilbow
Illustration Manager: Amy Naylor
Illustrator: MacPS
Marketing Manager: Deborah Davis.

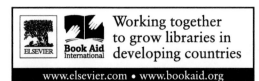

Contents

Preface

The field of Psychiatry continues to evolve, and it has become readily apparent that more than just psychiatrists need to know about psychopharmacologic and somatic treatments for psychiatric and neurologic conditions. Nurses, psychologists, and internists, to name just a few types of practitioners, care for patients with a wide range of disorders with psychiatric symptoms, many of which will benefit from the practical, clinically relevant, timely, accessible, and authoritative knowledge that we have compiled. Our faculty at the Massachusetts General Hospital collaborated enthusiastically and efficiently to create this compendium of psychopharmacological and somatic interventions, bolstered by knowledge of differential diagnosis, pathophysiology, strategies for evaluation, and treatment. We are incredibly appreciative of the countless hours spent conceptualizing, creating, and refining information in each chapter.

With the assistance of the watchful eyes of the staff at Elsevier (led by Charlotta Kryhl, Alexandra Mortimer, Andrew Riley, and Sam Crowe) our journey was completed within two years, ensuring up-to-date information on key topics essential for psychiatric treatment. In addition, Naomi Plasky (at the Massachusetts General Hospital) helped shepherd us through thousands of emails and packages for the completion of this text.

On behalf of the patients we service, we hope this collection facilitates the conceptualization, diagnosis, understanding, and treatment of psychiatric problems and brings much needed relief.

T.A.S.

M.F.

T.E.W.

J.F.R.

List of Contributors

Menekse Alpay, MD
Clinical Assistant
Department of Psychiatry
Massachusetts General Hospital
Instructor
Department of Psychiatry
Harvard Medical School
Boston, MA, USA

Jonathan E. Alpert, MD, PhD
Associate Chief of Psychiatry for
    Clinical Services
Director, Depression Clinical and
    Research Program
Massachusetts General Hospital
Joyce R. Tedlow Associate Professor of
    Psychiatry
Harvard Medical School
Boston, MA, USA

Ji Hyun Baek, MD
Research Fellow
Massachusetts General Hospital
Boston, MA, USA

Scott R. Beach, MD
Associate Training Director
MGH/McLean Adult Psychiatry
    Residency Program
Assistant Psychiatrist
Acute Psychiatric and Consultation-
    Liaison Services
Massachusetts General Hospital
Assistant Professor of Psychiatry
Harvard Medical School
Boston, MA, USA

Joseph Biederman, MD
Director of the Joint Program in
    Pediatric Psychopharmacology
McLean and Massachusetts General
    Hospital
Professor of Psychiatry
Harvard Medical School
Boston, MA, USA

Megan Moore Brennan, MD
Attending Psychiatrist
Bassett Medical Center
Assistant Clinical Professor, Columbia
    University College of Physicians and
    Surgeons
Cooperstown, NY, USA

Eric Bui, MD, PhD
Center for Anxiety and Traumatic Stress
    Disorders
Massachusetts General Hospital/
Harvard Medical School
Boston, MA, USA

Joan A. Camprodon, MP, MPH, PhD
Director, Laboratory for
    Neuropsychiatry and
    Neuromodulation
Director, Transcranial Magnetic
    Stimulation Clinical Service
Massachusetts General Hospital
Instructor of Psychiatry
Harvard Medical School
Boston, MA

Hannah Delong, BA
Research Coordinator
Massachusetts General Hospital
Boston, MA, USA

Darin D. Dougherty, MD, MSc
Director, Division of Neurotherapeutics
Massachusetts General Hospital
Associate Professor of Psychiatry
Harvard Medical School
Boston, MA, USA

William E. Falk, MD
Director, Geriatric Psychiatry
Department of Psychiatry
Massachusetts General Hospital
Assistant Professor in Psychiatry
Harvard Medical School
Boston, MA, USA

Maurizio Fava, MD
Director, Clinical Research Program
Executive Vice-Chair, Department of
    Psychiatry
Executive Director, Clinical Trials
    Network and Institute
Massachusetts General Hospital
Slater Family Professor of Psychiatry,
    Harvard Medical School
Boston, MA, USA

Oliver Freudenreich, MD
Medical Director, Massachusetts
    General Hospital Schizophrenia
    Program
Associate Professor of Psychiatry
Harvard Medical School
Boston, MA, USA

Jennifer R. Gatchel, MD PhD
Chief Resident in Psychopharmacology
Massachusetts General Hospital and
    McLean Hospital Adult Psychiatry
    Residency Program, Harvard Medical
    School
Boston, MA, USA

Donald C. Goff, MD
Director, Nathan Kline Institute for
    Psychiatric Research
Vice Chair of Psychiatry
NYU Langone Medical Center
Marvin Stern Professor of Psychiatry
NYU School of Medicine
New York City, NY, USA

David C. Henderson, MD
Director, Schizophrenia Clinical and
    Research Program
Director, Chester M. Pierce, M.D.
    Division of Global Psychiatry
Associate Professor of Psychiatry
Massachusetts General Hospital
Harvard Medical School
Boston, MA, USA

John B. Herman, MD
Associate Chief of Psychiatry
Massachusetts General Hospital
Associate Professor of Psychiatry
Harvard Medical School
Boston, MA, USA

Honor Hsin, MD, PhD
Resident in Psychiatry
Department of Psychiatry and
    Behavioral Sciences
Stanford University School of Medicine
Stanford, CA, USA

Jeff C. Huffman, MD
Director, Cardiac Psych Inpatient
    Program, MGH
Medical Director, Inpatient Psychiatry
Massachusetts General Hospital
Associate Professor of Psychiatry,
    Harvard Medical School
Boston, MA, USA

Navneet Kaur, BS
Clinical Research Coordinator
Laboratory for Neuropsychiatry and
    Neuromodulation
Division of Neurotherapeutics
Massachusetts General Hospital
Boston, MA, USA

John F. Kelly, PhD
Program Director, Addiction Recovery
  Management Service
Massachusetts General Hospital
Elizabeth R. Spallin Associate Professor
  of Psychiatry in Addiction Medicine
Harvard Medical School
Boston, MA, USA

Gustavo Kinrys, MD
Associate Medical Director
Clinical Trials Network and Institute
  (CTNI)
Bipolar Clinic and Research Program
  (BCRP)
Massachusetts General Hospital
Assistant Professor of Psychiatry
Boston, MA, USA

David Mischoulon, MD, PhD
Director of Research, Depression
  Clinical and Research Program
Department of Psychiatry
Massachusetts General Hospital
Associate Professor of Psychiatry
Harvard Medical School
Boston, MA, USA

Shamim H. Nejad, MD
Director, Adult Burns and Trauma
  Psychiatry
Division of Psychiatry and Medicine
  Psychiatry Consultation Service
Massachusetts General Hospital
Assistant Professor of Psychiatry
Harvard Medical School
Boston, MA, USA

Andrew A. Nierenberg, MD
Associate Director, Depression Clinical
  and Research Program
Director, Bipolar Clinic and Research
  Program
Director, Clinical Research Support
  Office
Massachusetts General Hospital
Professor of Psychiatry
Harvard Medical School
Boston, MA, USA

Michael J. Ostacher, MD, MPH, MMSc
Associate Director, Bipolar Disorder and
  Depression Research Program,
VAPAHCS Director, MIRECC Fellowship
  Program,
VAPAHCS Associate Professor of
  Psychiatry,
Department of Psychiatry and
Behavioral Sciences
Stanford University School of Medicine
Palo Alto, CA, USA

George I. Papakostas, MD
Scientific Director
Clinical Trials Network and Institute
Massachusetts General Hospital
Associate Professor of Psychiatry
Harvard Medical School
Boston, MA, USA

Roy H. Perlis, MD, MSc
Medical Director, Bipolar Clinic and
  Research Program
Massachusetts General Hospital
Associate Professor of Psychiatry
Harvard Medical School
Boston, MA, USA

Mark H. Pollack, MD
Department of Psychiatry
Rush University Medical Center
  Chicago, IL, USA

Jefferson B. Prince, MD
Director of Child Psychiatry
Massachusetts General for Children at
  North Shore Medical Center and Staff
Pediatric Psychopharmacology Clinic
Massachusetts General Hospital
Instructor in Psychiatry
Harvard Medical School
Yawkey Center for Outpatient Care
Boston, MA, USA

Scott L. Rauch, MD
President and Psychiatrist in Chief
McLean Hospital
Belmont, MA, USA
Chair, Partners Psychiatry and Mental
  Health
Professor of Psychiatry
Harvard Medical School
Belmont, MA, USA

John A. Renner, Jr., MD
Associate Professor
Department of Psychiatry
Boston University School of Medicine
Clinical Instructor
Department of Psychiatry
Harvard Medical School
Associate Chief
Department of Psychiatry
Boston VA Healthcare System
Boston, MA, USA

Joshua L. Roffman, MD, MMSc
Department of Psychiatry
Massachusetts General Hospital
Assistant Professor of Psychiatry
Harvard Medical School
Boston, MA, USA

Naomi M. Simon, MD, MSc
Center for Anxiety and Traumatic Stress
  Disorders
Massachusetts General Hospital
Chief Medical Officer
Red Sox Foundation and MGH Home
  Base Program
Associate Professor of Psychiatry,
  Harvard Medical School Director
Boston, MA, USA

Felicia A. Smith, MD
Program Director, MGH/McLean Adult
  Psychiatry Residency
Associate Director, MGH Division of
  Psychiatry and Medicine
Assistant Professor of Psychiatry
Harvard Medical School
Boston, MA, USA

Thomas J. Spencer, MD
Associate Director
Pediatric Psychopharmacology Clinic
Massachusetts General Hospital
Associate Professor of Psychiatry
Harvard Medical School
Boston, MA, USA

Theodore A. Stern, MD
Chief, Avery D. Weisman Psychiatry
  Consultation Service
Director, Office for Clinical Careers
Massachusetts General Hospital
Ned H. Cassem Professor of Psychiatry
  in the Field of Psychosomatic
Medicine/Consultation
Harvard Medical School
Boston, MA, USA

Lara Traeger, PhD
Psychologist
Massachusetts General Hospital
Assistant Professor in Psychiatry
Harvard Medical School
Boston, MA, USA

Nhi-Ha Trinh, MD, MPH
Director of Multicultural Studies,
  Depression Clinical and Research
  Program
Massachusetts General Hospital
Assistant Professor in Psychiatry
Harvard Medical School
Boston, MA, USA

Débora Vasconcelos e Sá, BA, MSc
Research Coordinator
Cambridge Hospital
Harvard Medical School
Cambridge, MA, USA

E. Nalan Ward, MD
Clinical Assistant in Psychiatry
Medical Director
West End Clinic
Outpatient Addiction Services
Massachusetts General Hospital
Instructor in Psychiatry
Harvard Medical School
Boston, MA, USA

Ajay D. Wasan, MD, MSc
Visiting Professor of Anesthesiology
  and Psychiatry
University of Pittsburgh
Vice Chair for Pain Medicine,
  Department of Anesthesiology
UPMC Pain Medicine
Pittsburgh, PA, USA

Charles A. Welch, MD
Psychiatrist
McLean Hospital
Belmont, MA, USA
Assistant Professor of Psychiatry
Harvard Medical School
Boston, MA, USA

Timothy E. Wilens, MD,
Senior Staff in Child Psychiatry and
    Pediatric Psychopharmacology
Director of the Center for Addiction
    Medicine
Massachusetts General Hospital
Associate Professor of Psychiatry
Harvard Medical School
Boston, MA, USA

Christopher I. Wright, MD PhD
Associate Neurologist
Division of Behavioral and Cognitive
    Neurology
Department of Neurology
Brigham and Women's Hospital
Boston, MA, USA

1

Psychiatric Neuroscience: Incorporating Pathophysiology into Clinical Case Formulation

Joan A. Camprodon, MD, MPH, PhD, and Joshua L. Roffman, MD, MMSc

KEY POINTS

- One can approach the study of the brain and its pathophysiology from various perspectives with different levels of resolution: molecular, genetic, cellular, synaptic, systems, and behavioral.
- Pathological processes and therapeutic interventions can target one or more of these levels, leading to a cascade of events that changes each of them.
- Affect, behavior, and cognition are processed in specific brain circuits, and their altered function leads to the signs, symptoms, and syndromes that clinicians identify.
- Neurobiological knowledge often provides mechanistic insight, explanation for behavior, and rationale for treatment, which are important to patients and families, as well as to providers.
- Clinical presentation reflects an interaction of static and dynamic factors, including genetic and environmental ones, often mediated by adaptive or maladaptive plastic changes.

OVERVIEW

People with major mental illness suffer as a result of abnormal brain function. This is the fundamental premise of psychiatric neuroscience, which seeks to identify biological mechanisms underlying mental illness and the effects of psychiatric treatments. An essential goal is to characterize these mechanisms at the different levels of biological resolution that exist in the brain (from ions, to proteins, to DNA, to genes and chromosomes [that encode the structure and function of cells], to synapses, and finally to brain circuits that process affect, behavior, and cognition). This approach does not negate the critical role of psychological, social, and environmental factors; to the contrary, it provides a framework for understanding how these higher levels of resolution affect, and are affected by, neural function. A deeper understanding of brain mechanisms will provide better explanations for patients and families and lead to improvements in diagnosis, treatment, and prognosis.

Psychiatric neuroscience is one of the most interesting and challenging endeavors in all of medicine.[1-5] While a great deal is already known, a wide gap remains between the clinical phenomena of affect, behavior, and cognition and neuroscientific explanations. The brain is extraordinarily complex and less physically accessible than other organ systems, posing great challenges to researchers. However, recent advances, particularly in neuroimaging and genetics, have provided important tools for tackling these problems. Although progress is difficult, the high prevalence, morbidity, and mortality rates of mental illness make progress essential. Mental health practitioners will need to incorporate the lessons learned from

psychiatric neuroscience into everyday practice, and communicate them to patients, families, and members of the general public.

One might ask if the term "psychiatric neuroscience" is still valid. While it has traditionally related to neuroscience research with clinical relevance to disorders embedded within the limits of psychiatry, as opposed to neurology, these boundaries are becoming more porous as knowledge progresses and clinical practice adapts. The unclear limits between the two subspecialties have been defined historically by amorphous criteria, such as differences in clinical attitude (diagnostic vs. therapeutic) or brain function of interest (motor and sensory vs. affective and behavioral, with cognition always occupying an unclear frontier). Neurology once focused mainly on pathologies that resulted in major structural changes that one could observe in an autopsy or under a microscope. Though the label "functional" is at times still casually and inappropriately attached to neurological deficits of presumed "psychological" etiology, a neurobiological re-acquaintance with the original medical meaning of the word emphasizes physiological (functional) over anatomical (structural) pathophysiological mechanisms. This shift led to two very distinct clinical paradigms, one focused on finding the focal lesion and the other on identifying signs and symptoms that present in established syndromal patterns that can then be physiologically investigated.

As new generations of clinician scientists emerge who did not train in psychiatric or neurological neuroscience, but in systems neuroscience, translational efforts are highlighting the common principles of structure, function, pathology, and therapeutics. From this effort, new models are emerging with a clinical focus on brain circuits, as opposed to focal lesions or clinical syndromes. For scientists and clinicians alike it is, and will become increasingly, important to have an understanding of the different levels of biological resolution and how they influence each other in health, in disease, and in therapy.[6] For clinicians treating disorders of affect, behavior, and cognition, it will be particularly important to understand the circuit level, as this is where mental states, including the pathological affective, behavioral, and cognitive states that we treat, are computed.

An important goal of this chapter will therefore be to explain the different levels of biological resolution that determine brain structure and function. A second goal will be to offer a framework with which the biological components of clinical cases may be formulated. This chapter provides an approach to conceptually organizing the biological component of our work with patients, from the dual vantage points of pathophysiology and mechanisms of treatment.

HISTORY OF PSYCHIATRIC NEUROSCIENCE

Psychiatry has a strong neuroscientific tradition. Describing all of the important contributions to brain science made by psychiatric researchers could fill many chapters; here we will cite only a few illustrative examples. Early in the last century, the German psychiatrist and neuropathologist Alois Alzheimer discovered plaques and tangles in the brain of his amnestic patient Mrs. Auguste D. and provided the first description of the clinical syndrome that now bears his name.[7] Together with his colleague and renowned psychiatrist Emil Kraepelin, Alzheimer also described abnormalities in the cortical neurons of patients with dementia praecox, likely representing the first neuropathological studies of schizophrenia.[8] Their discoveries have been extended to the molecular level in modern studies identifying abnormalities in γ-aminobutyric acid (GABA)–ergic neurons of the prefrontal cortex.[9,10] While Alzheimer's passion was neuropathology, he also spent many years caring for patients with mental illness. Reflecting on his life's work, he reportedly said that he "wanted to help psychiatry with the microscope."[11]

Another historical landmark in psychiatric neuroscience was the demonstration of genetic predispositions to major mental illness.[12] Danish adoption studies in the 1960s reported a much greater incidence of schizophrenia in biological as opposed to adoptive relatives of people with schizophrenia, providing key evidence for a significant etiological role of genetics in a psychiatric illness. Other landmark contributions include the work of Julius Axelrod, Ulf von Euler, and Bernard Katz on neurotransmitters and their mechanisms of release, reuptake, and metabolism; their discoveries, recognized with a Nobel Prize in 1970, provide a foundation for much of the content of this chapter.[13] In the 1970s, the discovery that antipsychotic medications targeted brain dopamine receptors led to the influential dopamine hypothesis of schizophrenia.[14,15] Later, converging work characterizing information processing in the brain at a molecular level earned Arvid Carlsson, Paul Greengard, and Eric Kandel the 2000 Nobel Prize at the end of the decade of the brain.[16] These brief highlights emphasize the great progress already attributable to psychiatric neuroscience, and illustrate the great potential for important discoveries in the future.

PSYCHIATRIC DIAGNOSIS: BIOMARKERS AND BIOLOGICAL VALIDITY

In the context of psychiatric neuroscience, the recent diagnostic system (DSM-IV-TR)[17] has both strengths and weaknesses. A major advance of the post-1980s DSM was the development of diagnostic categories of psychiatric illness with good inter-rater reliability, largely based on observation and data collection. This provided a firm starting point for scientific investigation, in contrast to previous diagnostic systems based on unproven etiological theories and associated ill-defined terminology. However, the intentional avoidance of etiological theories in generating DSM diagnoses also makes their biological validity uncertain; the extent to which specific DSM diagnoses correspond to specific pathological neural processes is unknown. Unlike most medical illnesses, the vast majority of psychiatric illnesses have so far not been tightly linked to specific biological markers. The descriptive criteria demarcating current diagnoses are likely several steps removed from core pathological processes.

These diagnostic difficulties can be illustrated by comparing the diagnosis of schizophrenia to that of methicillin-resistant streptococcal pneumonia, a medical diagnosis with obvious biological validity. While pneumonia has a collection of clinical signs and symptoms that may be non-specific and variable (e.g., fever, productive cough, and shortness of breath), it implies a distinct pathophysiology (infection of lung tissue leading to an inflammatory reaction). Subdividing the diagnosis by the infectious agent links it to a specific biological etiology, with tremendous value in guiding prognosis and treatment. In contrast, the diagnosis of schizophrenia, while it has a high level of inter-rater reliability, is not based at present on known biomarkers or pathophysiological mechanisms. It is therefore confined to the syndromic level, comprising a cluster of variable and non-specific clinical features. It can be further divided into more specific clinical subtypes, but these suffer from the same shortcomings. Just as pneumonia may have various specific etiologies, schizophrenia may also have diverse causes; most likely it does not reflect a single "disease." Recent advances in genetics reinforce this conclusion. While schizophrenia is highly heritable, linkage and association studies indicate in the majority of cases that it is a disorder of complex genetics, in which multiple genes of modest effect interact with environmental risk factors to cause the phenotype. In light of these issues, one of the major goals of psychiatric neuroscience is to identify specific biomarkers and pathophysiological mechanisms for each disorder.

METHODS IN PSYCHIATRIC NEUROSCIENCE

Researchers have adopted a variety of methods for studying the neural mechanisms of mental illness and behavior (Box 1-1). Each of these methods has particular strengths and weakness.

Brain Lesions and Behavior

There is a strong tradition within classical neuropsychology and behavioral neurology of understanding neuroanatomical circuitry by studying the emergent or lost behaviors in patients with focal brain lesions.[18] These studies have provided us with a rich view of various brain regions and their relationship to behavior. Perhaps the most famous case is that of Phineas Gage, the Vermont railway worker who suffered a traumatic lesion bilaterally to the medial frontal lobes and developed personality changes.[19] Another famous patient (known by his initials) is H. M., who underwent bilateral medial temporal lobe resection for intractable epilepsy and as a result lost the ability to form new declarative memories.[20] While striking and informative, findings from these rare cases may be difficult to extrapolate to the pathophysiology of common psychiatric illnesses, which generally do not involve focal lesions. Traditionally, biological psychiatry has relied more on biometrics and quantitative methods; these population-based approaches risk losing insights available from rare cases but are more likely to produce broadly generalizable findings.

Neuropsychology and Endophenotypes

An increasingly important approach in psychiatric neuroscience is to identify and study intermediate phenotypes. These are quantitative phenotypes that are closely associated with the clinical syndrome of interest, but which are less complex and easier to link to the function of specific neural circuits. They can also be used to identify biologically relevant

---

BOX 1-1 Methods in Psychiatric Neuroscience

Animal models
Brain lesion cases
Brain stimulation and neuromodulation
Genetics and molecular biology
Neuroimaging
Neuropathology
Neurophysiology
Neuropsychology/endophenotypes
Psychopharmacology

subtypes within a diagnostic category, reducing heterogeneity that may limit the power of scientific investigations. Endophenotypes are intermediate phenotypes that are present both in affected individuals and in their unaffected relatives, therefore reflecting genetic risk independent of actual disease. Neuropsychological tests of cognitive function are commonly used to identify endophenotypes. For example, impairment of working memory, which is closely related to the function of dorsolateral prefrontal cortex, is found within a subgroup of patients with schizophrenia.[21] Endophenotypes thus help bridge the gap between brain circuits, which are amenable to study at the molecular and cellular level, and clinical syndromes, which are less tractable. This approach becomes especially powerful when combined with other methods, such as neuroimaging or genetics.[22]

Neuroimaging

Neuroimaging has provided one of the best modern tools for examining the pathophysiology of mental illness in the living brain. Neuroimaging can provide many different quantitative measures (including morphometry, metabolism, and functional activity). Neuroimaging research using groups of subjects can determine whether mental illness is associated with changes in the size or shape of specific brain regions, the functional activity within these regions, or their concentration of particular neurotransmitters, receptors, or key metabolites.[23] Although neuroimaging methods can be used to measure cellular and molecular phenomena, the currently achievable spatial resolution still represents an important limitation in examining the microscopic pathological changes implicated in psychiatric illness.

Neurophysiology

There is a strong tradition within psychiatric neuroscience of studying the electrical activity of the brain and its relation to function. These methods include electroencephalography (EEG), event-related potentials (ERPs), and, most recently, magnetoencephalography (MEG), and transcranial magnetic stimulation (TMS). Like functional neuroimaging, these modalities provide information about the living, functioning brain. At present, electrophysiological techniques cannot provide anatomical resolution at the level of neurochemistry or synaptic physiology, and are limited to the study of cortical phenomena; however, they can provide excellent temporal and spatial resolution and are invaluable in studying the coordinated function of widely distributed neural circuits. Abnormalities in the timing of oscillations in neural circuit activity have been associated with psychiatric illnesses, and this is an area of intense research activity. For example, the reduction of gamma frequency (30 to 80 Hz) oscillations in schizophrenia has been ascribed to impaired N-methyl-D-aspartate (NMDA) receptor activity on GABA-ergic interneurons.[24] These noninvasive methods are particularly heavily used in studies of brain development and function in children.[25]

Brain Stimulation and Neuromodulation

Brain stimulation and neuromodulation techniques encompass a variety of device-based methodologies able to generate focal electrical currents in pre-selected brain regions. These currents are able to increase or decrease the excitability of the target neurons, and modulate the networks they belong to by acting as a neural pacemaker.[26]

Brain stimulation can be divided among invasive and noninvasive approaches. Invasive techniques require the surgical implantation of stimulating electrodes in the brain, and are therefore exclusively used in therapeutic settings where the risk/benefit analysis is favorable. They include deep brain stimulation (DBS) and vagus nerve stimulation (VNS). Noninvasive methods do not require surgery or anesthesia, are very safe, and alter brain function in ways that are transient and reversible. The better-known and most commonly used methods are transcranial magnetic stimulation (TMS) and transcranial direct current stimulation (tDCS).[27] Chapter 18 describes these methods and their therapeutic applications in detail.

TMS has been used since the mid 1980s as a tool to study brain structure and function. Event-related paradigms using single pulses time-locked to a given stimulus or task have been used to determine the chronometry of the computations in a given brain region with great temporal resolution (in the order of milliseconds).[28] Repetitive TMS (rTMS) can increase or decrease the excitability of a given area beyond the time of stimulation, creating a "virtual lesion" that lasts 15–60 minutes after the stimulation. This virtual lesion approach has been used, following the tradition of classical lesion studies, to understand the functional role of discrete brain regions.[29]

Although neuroimaging and electrophysiological techniques are defined by their spatial and temporal resolution, what sets brain stimulation methods apart is their *causal resolution*. Neuroimaging and electrophysiological methods are observational; they measure patterns of brain activity (the dependent variable) in the context of a given task or disease state (independent variable). Such a design is able to establish correlations among these measures, but can never determine that a given pattern of brain activity is *causing* a mental state (or vice versa). On the other hand, brain stimulation techniques are interventional. They modify the system by changing brain activity (now the independent variable) and measure the behavioral, cognitive or affective changes that follow. This design offers causal explanatory power, which makes it a useful tool to answer a number of questions.[30]

Neuropathology

Many researchers examine post-mortem neural tissue from those who suffered from psychiatric illness during their lifetime. Post-mortem analysis reaches a level of molecular and cellular resolution currently unachievable *in vivo*; however, it is commonly limited by confounds (such as age, effects of chronic medication, and non-specific effects of chronic psychiatric illness).

Neuropathology was clearly in fashion in the late 1800s and early 1900s, when Alzheimer first described plaques in the brain of his patient with dementia,[7] and identified frontal cortex abnormalities in schizophrenia.[8] While some skeptics have described schizophrenia as the "graveyard of neuropathologists,"[31] recent studies have actually provided reproducible descriptions of deficits (such as those in parvalbumin-expressing GABA-ergic interneurons in deep layers 3 and 4, akin to Alzheimer's findings) in the cortex. These neuropathological findings have provided one of the strongest etiological hypotheses for schizophrenia.[9,10]

Psychopharmacology

More than any other methodology in psychiatric neuroscience, pharmacology has been used to understand the neurochemical basis of behavior and to develop hypotheses regarding psychopathological mechanisms. Famous examples include the dopamine[32] and glutamate hypotheses of schizophrenia,[33] the catecholamine depletion hypothesis of depression,[34] and the dopaminergic models of attention-deficit/hyperactivity disorder (ADHD) and substance abuse. In relating pharmacological effects to potential disease mechanisms, it is important to note that the effects of drugs on clinical symptoms may reflect mechanisms that are downstream of the core pathophysiology, or even unrelated to core disease mechanisms. By analogy, diuretics can improve the symptoms of congestive heart failure while providing less direct insight into its core pathophysiology. Nonetheless, by clearly connecting cellular and synaptic mechanisms with clinical symptoms, pharmacology provides mechanistic tools and information with enormous clinical and scientific utility.

Animal Experiments

In the authors' opinion, the value of animal experiments has received too little emphasis in psychiatric neuroscience. Clearly, complex psychiatric symptoms (such as delusions) cannot be modeled well in animals, and anthropomorphic interpretations of animal behavior should be taken with due skepticism. Despite these caveats, animal behaviors with known neuroanatomical correlates have been critical in elucidating the neurocircuitry and neurochemistry underlying many psychiatric phenomena. For example, anxiety- and fear-related behaviors have been very productively modeled in animals, leading to a detailed understanding of the role of the amygdala in these behaviors.[35] Of course, animal studies also permit a wider range of experimental perturbations than possible with human investigations. Independent of their value as behavioral models, animal models therefore offer the opportunity to explore cellular and molecular pathophysiology in ways that are ethically or technically impossible in human subjects. For example, the fragile X knock-out mouse is an excellent model for fragile X syndrome, the most common form of inherited cognitive impairment. Studying these mice has led to a deep understanding of relevant defects in dendrite formation and neurophysiology.[36]

Human Genetics and Molecular Biology

Adoption, twin, and familial segregation studies have proven that many psychiatric conditions are highly heritable (i.e., caused in large part by the additive effect of genes).[37] Genetic endeavors in psychiatric neuroscience may be broken up into two broad categories: "forward genetics," or genome-wide attempts to identify genetic loci (genes or their regulatory elements) that underlie susceptibility or contribute to pathophysiology; and "genotype-phenotype" studies, whereby candidate genes are chosen based on *a priori* biological hypotheses and the degree to which a gene plays a role in a given phenotype is assessed. Such phenotypes may be clinical diagnoses, or endophenotypes from neuropsychology or neuroimaging. The promise for human genetics in psychiatry is tremendous,[37] especially for forward genetics, wherein researchers may be led to the core pathophysiology without requiring any *a priori* hypotheses. Yet human genetics research is exceedingly challenging for various reasons that are beyond the scope of the current discussion. In brief, the genetic architecture of neuropsychiatric conditions is heterogeneous and complex. That is, the majority of psychiatric illnesses likely reflect complex interactions of multiple genes, as well as their interaction with environmental factors that are difficult to assess. Despite these difficulties, there have already been a few notable examples of success.

Analysis of rare, large families with early-onset dementia led to the discovery of mutations in amyloid precursor protein (APP) and presenilins in Alzheimer's disease (AD).[38] In these rare families, these mutations are statistically "linked" to disease and considered "highly penetrant." However, the vast majority of AD patients do not have mutations in these genes. Indeed, in psychiatry examples of highly penetrant, simple dominant or recessive gene mutations are rare. That is, examples in neuropsychiatry of a particular gene mutation "causing" a specific condition are exceedingly rare and somewhat controversial, and the generalizability of these findings to the common conditions with more complex inheritance is usually unclear. Nonetheless, the APP pathway has provided an important target for drug development, which may lead to a medicine that stalls the progress of disease.

Genetic association studies through population genetics represent another approach to identifying susceptibility genes in "forward genetics." In this approach, a common variation in the genome, such as single nucleotide polymorphisms (SNPs), is assessed for a statistically significant association with illness. This approach is based on the so-called common disease–common variant hypothesis. That is, psychiatric disorders may be in part due to a disadvantageous combination of a number of common forms of genetic variation as opposed to frank deleterious mutations. Again, a successful example of a gene association in neuropsychiatry comes from the field of AD wherein there is a fairly robust association at the level of population genetics or epidemiology between a common polymorphism in *ApoE4* and susceptibility to AD. However, sometimes even when genetic associations are robust, the amount of the phenotype (i.e., the variance) that is explained by the given gene may be small and therefore the role in causation may be indirect or unclear. In addition, association studies have often used small sample sizes and thereby risked false-positive findings or problems of reproducibility. Now, appropriately-powered association studies (involving thousands of subjects) are underway; many of these use new and more powerful high-density genotype methods, namely "SNP chips" or microarrays. Even still, critical insights into the causative roles of genes in some psychiatric illness may only come from studies of gene–gene or gene–environmental interaction, or by using endophenotypes (such as neuroimaging) that may be closer to the action of the gene.

Methodologies in molecular genetics and molecular neuroscience also promise improved understanding of gene function in the brain. These methods include the following: comparison of gene sequences in human to non-human primate and other animals[39]; a deeper understanding of how non-coding elements within the genome may regulate important brain genes[40] and thereby play a role in psychiatry; the study of gene expression using microarrays[41]; the study of gene function in mice in which specific genes have been modified by recombinant methods (e.g., "knock-out" or "knock-in" studies)[42]; and studies examining how experience and the environment alter gene expression.[43] In summary, genomics and molecular genetics hold great promise for identifying genes and thus biological mechanisms at the core of psychiatric pathophysiology.

BIOLOGICAL CASE FORMULATION: NEUROSCIENTIFIC CONTENT AND PROCESS

Clinical case formulation in psychiatry is structured around the bio-psycho-social model. In this chapter, we offer a framework for formulating the biological aspects of this model. Specifically, neuroscientific explanations may be organized in two broad conceptual areas: process and content. Process refers to dynamic brain mechanisms that lead to illness, while content refers to the brain properties including neural circuits,

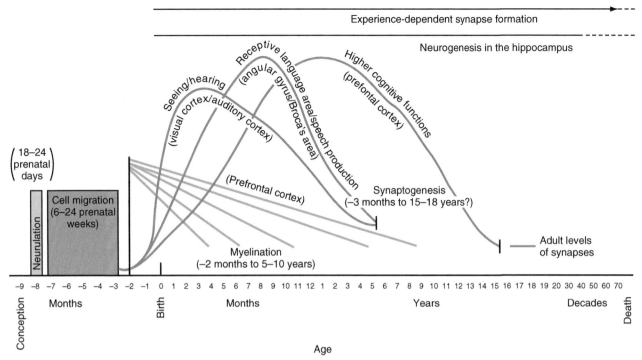

Figure 1-1. A depiction of the processes of brain development, including intrauterine neuronal patterning, neurogenesis, cortical migration, gliogenesis, myelination, and experience-dependent synapse modification. *(From Thompson RA, Nelson CA. Developmental science and the media. Early brain development,* Am Psychol 56[1]:5–15, 2001.)

brain regions, synapses, cells, and molecules that form the substrate for these changes.

Process

A key concept in basic neuroscience and its clinical specialties is neuroplasticity. Although it is defined in different ways and can be studied at various levels of resolution (e.g., circuits, synapses), this term generally refers to the capacity of the neural system to change in response to external or internal stimuli following predetermined rules. Neuroplasticity provides a great deal of flexibility and adaptive capacity to the brain, permitting variable computational strategies and patterns of connectivity in a changing environment.[44] Despite the significant potential for reactive (and adaptive) change, this happens around an exquisitely regulated homeostatic equilibrium point. Nevertheless, when the plastic changes are restricted, excessive, or occur around an altered equilibrium state, pathology develops. Luckily, the brain remains plastic, and any intervention (e.g., medications, psychotherapy or brain stimulation) that is effective in changing pathological cognition, behavior or affect induces adaptive plasticity. That is, a pathological mental state is sustained by a given pattern of brain activity, and changing this mental state will require changing its associated neural computational algorithm.[45] Therefore, neuroplasticity is a key dynamic property of the brain that allows adaptive change (including learning and memory), but it is also an important source of pathology, and a necessary mechanism of action of effective neuropsychiatric treatments.

Although the specific pathophysiological mechanisms that lead to neuropsychiatric disease are many, we will consider two relevant examples: neurodevelopment, and neurodegeneration. Under neurodevelopment we include related processes that continue into adulthood (such as neurogenesis).

Previously underestimated, adult neurogenesis is now known to continue in select regions of the human brain, most notably the olfactory bulb and the hippocampus. Although the role of adult neurogenesis in humans remains largely unknown, some evidence has connected altered hippocampal neurogenesis to mood disorders.[46]

Neurodevelopmental processes shaping brain circuits have life-long effects on patterns of affect, behavior, and cognition with direct relevance to mental health. The effects of childhood experience have always been central to psychiatric understanding; psychiatric neuroscience has also attempted to provide a biological grounding for this understanding.[43,47] Thus, neurodevelopmental processes include the interacting effects of genes and environment on brain and behavior. Figure 1-1 shows the processes of brain development, including intrauterine neuronal patterning, neurogenesis, cortical migration, gliogenesis, myelination, and experience-dependent synapse modification.[48,49] In the first years and decade of life, the brain undergoes a process of synapse formation and pruning.[50] Initially, neurons form an over-abundance of synapses that are then strengthened and pruned possibly based on experience, learning, or aging (Figure 1-2).

Specific psychiatric disorders may be framed in terms of one or more of these three mechanisms. Autism or attention deficit hyperactivity disorder are examples in which a process of brain development goes awry. At the other end of life, neurodegenerative processes dominate, and can lead to dementias (e.g., Alzheimer's or frontotemporal lobar degeneration) or movement disorders (such as Parkinson's disease). Substance use disorders may reflect a combination of both processes modulated by maladaptive plasticity. Patients with substance dependence may have a susceptibility based on neurodevelopment, including a predisposition to risk-taking behaviors.[51] Substance abuse also causes neuroplastic changes at the level of the synapse.[52] Finally, chronic use of substances can cause neurodegeneration and dementia.[53]

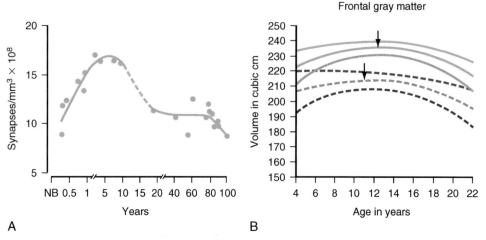

Figure 1-2. (A) A depiction of the number of synapse counts in layer 3 of the middle frontal gyrus as a function of age. (B) A graph of the volume, in cubic centimeters, of frontal gray matter with respect to age in years. Males represented by solid lines and females by dashed lines with 95% confidence intervals, respectively. Arrows indicate peak volume. (*A, Data from Huttenlocher PR. Synaptic density in human frontal cortex: developmental changes and effects of aging*, Brain Res 163[2]:195–205, 1979. B, Data from Lenroot RK, Giedd JN. Brain development in children and adolescents: insights from anatomical magnetic resonance imaging, Neurosci Biobehav Rev 30[6]:718–729, 2006.)

Content

The "content" of a psychiatric illness comprises the different structural and functional levels of biological resolution that form the nervous system: ions, proteins, genes, cells, synapses, circuits, behaviors, and mental states. These can all be the target of pathological changes leading to diseases and clinical syndromes. This is the subject of the remaining sections of this chapter. For most conditions, our knowledge of content is incomplete, but this should not lead us to ignore the large amount of information that *is* available for many conditions. Characterizing neuropsychiatric conditions in terms of both biological processes and substrates (content) can provide a framework to facilitate understanding of etiology, loci of intervention, and potential treatments.

OVERVIEW OF THE STRUCTURE OF THE CENTRAL NERVOUS SYSTEM

The structural organization of the central nervous system (CNS) is shown in Figure 1-3A. The human brain is organized into the cerebral cortex, brainstem, subcortical structures (e.g., basal ganglia, brainstem, thalamus, hypothalamus, pituitary), and cerebellum.[3,54,55] These anatomical structures are made of inter-connected elements that create distributed and highly inter-connected circuits. It is in these circuits where cognition, behavior, and affect are processed. This section will provide an overview of neuroanatomy with a structural focus.

The cerebral cortex is the outermost layer of the cerebrum. The cerebral cortex consists of a foliated structure, encompassing gyri and sulci. Within the most highly evolved cortical regions (isocortex), a six-cell layered structure orchestrates complex brain functions (including perceptual awareness, thought, language, planning, memory, attention, and consciousness). Cortical anatomy can be subdivided in myriad ways, including into anatomical regions (such as the occipital, parietal, temporal, insular, limbic, and frontal lobes) (Figure 1-3B, C, and D). The limbic "lobe" is a ring (limbus) of phylogenetically older cortex surrounding the upper brainstem and includes the hippocampus, amygdala, hypothalamus, parahippocampal gyrus, and cingulate cortex (see Figure 1-3D). Structures within the medial temporal lobe are especially important in psychiatry; the hippocampus plays a

critical role in memory, and the amygdala is an important element of fear circuitry and for assigning emotional valence to stimuli.

Functionally, the cortex may be divided into primary sensory or motor (unimodal) regions, and association (multimodal) regions that receive inputs from multiple areas.[54] Association cortex may be subdivided into three areas: frontal (involved in a wide variety of higher functions, such as planning, attention, abstract thought, problem-solving, judgment, initiative, and inhibition of impulses); limbic (involved in emotion and memory); and sensory (e.g., parietal, occipital, temporal), involved in integrating sensory information.

The cortical systems can also be represented in a hierarchical fashion.[54] For example, within sensorimotor sequencing, we see reception of somatosensory, visual, or auditory stimuli in primary sensory cortex; interpretation or representation of the combined sensory modalities in the heteromodal association cortex; integration of this information with the other association cortices (i.e., limbic and frontal); and output via the motor or language system.

In addition to the cerebral cortex, many other brain regions are of critical importance to psychiatry. The cerebellum (see Figure 1-3A and B), traditionally known for its role in motor coordination and learning, has more recently been implicated in cognitive and affective processes as well.[56] The thalamus is a major relay station for incoming sensory information and other critical circuitry, including connections between association cortices (via the mediodorsal nucleus) and outputs regulating motor activity. Interestingly, the mediodorsal nucleus, a critical relay station between association cortices, is a region of the thalamus found to be smaller in some neuropathological studies of patients with schizophrenia.[57,58] Figure 1-3C shows the parts of the basal ganglia, which comprise the striatum (i.e., caudate, putamen, and nucleus accumbens) and globus pallidus rostrally, and the subthalamic nucleus and substantia nigra caudally. The basal ganglia orchestrate multiple functions[59]; the dorsal striatum plays an important role in motor control, and the ventral striatum (in particular, the nucleus accumbens) plays key roles in emotion and learning via connections with the hippocampus, amygdala, and prefrontal cortex. The hypothalamus plays a critical role in neuroendocrine regulation of the internal milieu.[60] Via its effects on pituitary hormone release and connections to other regions

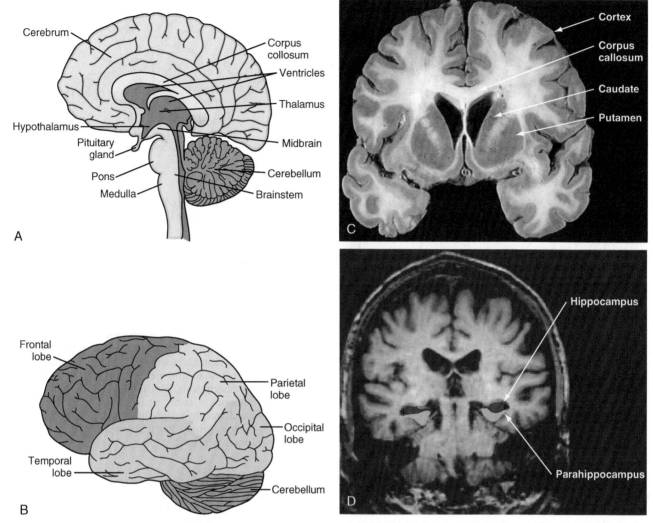

Figure 1-3. (A) Schematic of the human brain organized into the cerebral cortex, brainstem, subcortical structures (e.g., basal ganglia, brainstem, thalamus, hypothalamus, and pituitary), and cerebellum. (B) Depiction of cortical anatomy divided into anatomical regions (such as the occipital, parietal, temporal, insular, limbic, and frontal lobes). (C) Brain cut demonstrating the limbic "lobe" as a ring (limbus) of phylogenetically older cortex surrounding the upper brainstem. (D) Brain cut highlighting the hippocampus, amygdala, hypothalamus, parahippocampal gyrus, and cingulate cortex. *(C, From http://library.med.utah.edu/WebPath/HISTHTML/NEURANAT/CNS213A.html. D, From Dickerson BC, Salat DH, Bates JF, et al. Medial temporal lobe function and structure in mild cognitive impairment, Ann Neurol 56[1]:27–35, 2004.)*

of the brain, the hypothalamus exerts homeostatic effects on numerous psychiatrically-relevant factors, including mood, motivation, sexual drive, hunger, temperature, and sleep. Finally, a number of discrete nuclei in the brainstem synthesize key modulatory neurotransmitters, exerting major effects on brain function via their widespread projections to striatal and corticolimbic regions of the brain.[5] These neuromodulatory nuclei include the dopaminergic ventral tegmental area (VTA) in the midbrain, serotonergic raphe nuclei in the brainstem, noradrenergic locus coeruleus neurons in the pons, and cholinergic neurons of the basal forebrain and brainstem.

CELLULAR DIVERSITY IN THE BRAIN: NEURONS AND GLIA

The cellular diversity of the primate nervous system is truly fantastic. There are two broad classes of cells in the brain: neurons and glia. The Spanish neuroanatomist Santiago Ramon y Cajal prolifically and painstakingly documented the cellular diversity of the nervous system (Figure 1-4).[61] Images made with modern fluorescent staining techniques also

convey the exquisite beauty of the cells of the CNS (Figure 1-5). Based on his observations, Ramon y Cajal proposed that neurons act as physically discrete functional units within the brain, communicating with each other through specialized junctions. This theory became known as the "neuron doctrine," and Ramon y Cajal's enormous contributions were recognized with a Nobel Prize in 1906.[62]

Neurons

There are approximately 100 billion neurons in the human brain, and each neuron makes up to 10,000 synaptic connections. At the peak of synapse formation in the third year of life, the total number of brain synapses is estimated at 10,000 trillion, thereafter declining and stabilizing in adulthood to between 1,000 trillion and 5,000 trillion synapses.

Consistent with their functional diversity, neurons come in a wide variety of shapes and sizes. Nonetheless, all neurons share several characteristic features (Figure 1-6), including the cell soma (housing the nucleus with its genomic DNA), the axon, the pre-synaptic axon terminal, and the dendritic field

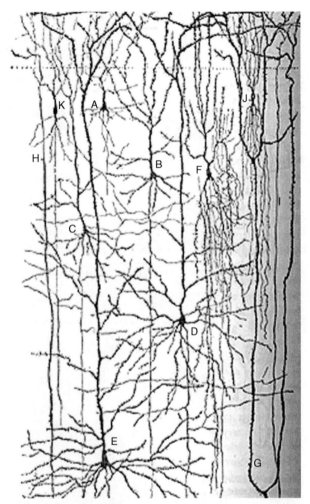

Figure 1-4. Ramon y Cajal's drawing from his classic "Histologie du Système Nerveux de l'Homme et des Vertébrés" showing the cellular diversity of the nervous system. *(From Ramon y Cajal S. Histologie du système nerveux de l'homme et des vertébrés, Paris, 1909, A Maloine.)*

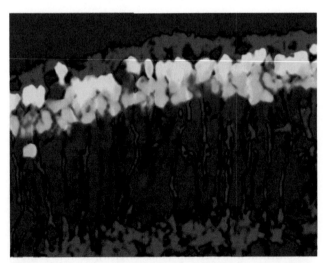

Figure 1-5. Images made with modern fluorescent staining techniques also convey the exquisite beauty of the cells of the CNS. *(From Morrow, et al, unpublished.)*

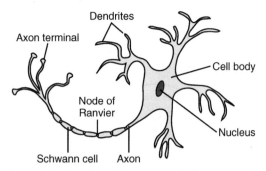

Figure 1-6. Depiction of the neuron with its components.

(the receptive component of the neuron containing post-synaptic dendritic structures). Axon length is highly variable; short axons are found on inhibitory inter-neurons, which make only local connections, while axons many inches long are found on cortical projection neurons, which must reach to the contralateral hemisphere or down to the spinal cord. Motor and sensory neurons have axons that may be several feet long.

There are many ways to classify neurons: by structure (i.e., projection neuron or local inter-neuron); by histology (i.e., bipolar, multipolar, or unipolar); by function (i.e., excitatory, inhibitory, or modulatory); by electrophysiology (i.e., tonic, phasic, or fast-spiking); or by neurotransmitter type.[3] For the purposes of this chapter, classifications using a combination of structural, functional, and neurotransmitter type provide the most useful descriptions. For example, it is useful to appreciate that the major excitatory neurotransmitter is glutamate (commonly used by projection neurons), while the major inhibitory neurotransmitter in the brain is GABA (commonly used by local inter-neurons).

Glia

Although neurons have captured the lion's share of attention since the time of Ramon y Cajal, there are up to 10-fold more glial cells in the brain than neurons. The word "glia" means "glue," aptly summarizing the structural and supportive role traditionally attributed to them. Indeed, glia do support neuronal function in many ways, by supplying nutrition, maintaining homeostasis, stabilizing synapses, and myelinating axons. They also play important roles in synaptic transmission. In the CNS there are two large categories of glia: microglia and macroglia. Microglia are small, phagocytic cells related to peripheral macrophages. Macroglia can be further classified into two types: astrocytes maintain the synaptic milieu, and oligodendrocytes myelinate axons. Astrocytes play an active and critical role in glutamatergic neurotransmission, releasing co-agonists required for glutamate receptor function and transporting glutamate to terminate its synaptic action. New functions of glia continue to be discovered, and belated appreciation of their importance to psychiatric neuroscience continues to grow. Mood disorders are associated with a reduction in the number of glia in select brain regions.[63] In adult-onset metachromatic leukodystrophy, a genetic enzyme deficiency produces diffuse myelin destruction; the illness may manifest in mid-adolescence with neuropsychiatric symptoms resembling schizophrenia.[64] Furthermore, studies looking for genes whose expression is altered in schizophrenia have identified prominent changes in myelin-related genes.[65]

THE STRUCTURE OF THE SYNAPSE

The previous section described how inter-cellular communication serves as an organizing feature of neuroanatomy. Neurons and glia are elegantly situated within the brain to facilitate signaling between adjacent cells, and between cells in distinct brain regions. Depending on the specific neurotransmitters released pre-synaptically, and the specific receptors located post-synaptically, the transmitted signal may have excitatory, inhibitory, or other modulatory effects on the post-synaptic neuron. Detailed knowledge of the neurochemical anatomy of the brain is therefore a prerequisite to the optimal use of psychotropic medicines in psychiatry. Important aspects of neurochemical anatomy include how neurotransmitters are distributed within brain circuits; how these neurotransmitter systems function; and how these systems are altered either by disease or by our treatments.

Neurotransmitters

Neurotransmitters are defined by four essential characteristics (Figure 1-7 and Box 1-2): they are synthesized within the pre-synaptic neuron; they are released with depolarization from the pre-synaptic neuron to exert a discrete action on the post-synaptic neuron; their action on the post-synaptic neuron can be replicated by administering the transmitter exogenously (as a drug); and their action in the synaptic cleft is terminated by a specific mechanism.[3] However, they otherwise differ considerably in structure, distribution, and function. Their chemical make-up (including small molecules [such as amino acids, biogenic amines, and nitrous oxide] as well as larger peptides [such as opioids and substance P]) varies substantially. Certain neurotransmitters are found ubiquitously throughout the cortex, whereas others act in more select locations. Moreover, while certain neurotransmitters are always excitatory (e.g., glutamate) or inhibitory (e.g., GABA in the adult brain), others can exert variable downstream effects based on where they are located and to which receptors they bind.

Nearly 100 neurotransmitters have been identified within the mammalian brain. However, we will focus on several well-characterized neurotransmitter systems with major relevance to neuropsychiatric phenomena (Box 1-3). Each of these neurotransmitters plays an important role in normal brain function; thus, abnormal activity in any of these neurotransmitter systems may contribute to neuropsychiatric dysfunction. We will consider the normal "life cycle" for each neurotransmitter system—including synthesis, synaptic release, receptor binding, neurotransmitter degradation, post-synaptic signaling through ion channels or second messengers, and activity-dependent changes in gene expression and subsequent neuronal activity (see Box 1-2). We will focus particularly on the various points in this cycle that are amenable to pharmacological intervention.

For example, consider the hypothetical synapse in Figure 1-8. Suppose a particular psychiatric symptom was related to abnormally high synaptic concentrations of a specific

---

BOX 1-2 Schema of Neurochemical Systems

Neurotransmitter biosynthesis
Neurotransmitter storage and synaptic vesicle release
Neurotransmitter receptors:
- Post-synaptic
- Pre-synaptic autoreceptors

Post-synaptic ion channels
Post-synaptic second messenger systems
Activity-dependent gene regulation
Neurotransmitter degradation
Neurotransmitter reuptake
Functional neurochemical anatomy

BOX 1-3 Major Neurotransmitter Systems in the Brain

AMINO ACIDS
Glutamate
γ-Aminobutyric acid (GABA)

MONOAMINES
Dopamine
Norepinephrine (noradrenaline)
Epinephrine (adrenaline)
Serotonin
Histamine

SMALL MOLECULE NEUROTRANSMITTER
Acetylcholine

PEPTIDES
Opioids (enkephalins, endorphin, dynorphin)
Hypothalamic factors (CRH, orexins/hypocretins, and others)
Pituitary hormones (ACTH, TSH, oxytocin, vasopressin, and others)
Neuroactive CNS peptides also expressed in the GI system (substance P, VIP, and others)
Others (leptin and others)

ACTH, Adrenocorticotropic hormone; CNS, central nervous system; CRH, corticotropin-releasing hormone; GI, gastrointestinal; TSH, thyroid-stimulating hormone; VIP, vasoactive intestinal polypeptide.

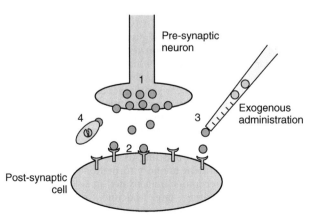

Figure 1-7. Essential characteristics of neurotransmitters.

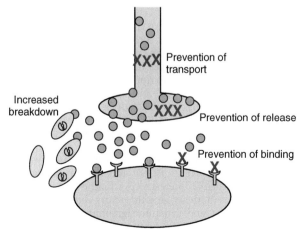

Figure 1-8. Psychopharmacology and the synapse.

neurotransmitter. The diversity of biochemical steps involved in the neurotransmitter cycle provides many targets for pharmacological intervention[5]: one could inhibit neurotransmitter synthesis; interfere with neurotransmitter transport, vesicle formation, or release; block post-synaptic receptor effects; or increase the clearance rate from the synapse by degradation or transport. We will re-visit this model as we consider each of the neurotransmitter systems and their relation to normal and abnormal brain function below.

Synaptic Transmission, Second Messenger Systems, and Activity-Dependent Gene Expression

Neurotransmitter signals alter post-synaptic neuron function via a complex collection of receptors and second messenger systems.[66] These signals ultimately result in changes in neuronal activity, often associated with changes in gene expression. While neurotransmitter receptors are the classic targets of pharmacological intervention, it has become apparent that second messenger systems may also provide important targets for existing and novel therapies.[67,68]

In general, neurotransmitter receptors trigger either rapid or slow effector systems. Rapid-effect neurotransmitter receptors are either themselves ion channels (e.g., NMDA glutamate receptors), or are coupled to ion channels. Ion flux through these transmitter-activated channels rapidly alters membrane potential and neuronal activity. Other neurotransmitter receptors, including the large family of G-protein–coupled receptors (GPCRs), work via slower second messenger systems.[69,70] Such second messenger systems usually involve sequential multi-enzyme cascades. Post-translational modifications, such as protein phosphorylation (introduced by kinase proteins and removed by phosphatase proteins), can act as on–off switches to propagate or terminate the signal at specific branch points. Second messenger systems convert receptor signals into a coordinated set of cellular effects by altering the function of multiple target proteins. These targets include ion channels that control neuronal firing, synaptic proteins that regulate synaptic efficacy, and cytoskeletal elements that determine cellular morphology. While there are over 500 different kinases in the human genome, several that have been heavily studied in psychiatry are worthy of special mention, such as the cyclic AMP (cAMP)–dependent kinase (also known as protein kinase A [PKA]) and calcium/calmodulin-dependent protein kinase (CAMK), which both play critical roles in memory formation.[71] Another second messenger pathway, involving glycogen synthase kinase (GSK), has been proposed to mediate at least some of the therapeutic efficacy of lithium salts in bipolar disorder.[72]

Transcription factors are also critical downstream targets of neurotransmitter signals and second messenger systems. By modifying gene expression in the nucleus, transcription factors can produce persistent changes in neural function. The most widely studied neuronal transcription factors include immediate early genes *c-Jun*, *c-Fos*, and cAMP response element binding protein (CREB), whose activity is quickly regulated by neurotransmitter signals.[73] CREB has been shown to be up-regulated and phosphorylated in neurons in response to antipsychotic medication, as well as drugs of abuse,[74-76] and in response to neurotrophic factors, such as brain-derived neurotrophic factor (BDNF).[77] BDNF and related neurotrophic factors are of particular interest to psychiatric neuroscience, as they exert effects both as growth factors during embryonic neurodevelopment and synaptic signaling in adults. BDNF signaling modulates CREB activity and gene expression; both factors play important roles in neural plasticity, and have

been heavily studied in genetic association studies in psychiatric disorders.[78-81]

A REVIEW OF CLINICALLY RELEVANT NEUROTRANSMITTER SYSTEMS

In this section we review the major neurotransmitter systems, all of which have clinical importance in psychiatry. In each subsection, emphasis will be placed on the "content" of neuropsychiatric explanation.

Glutamate

As the major excitatory neurotransmitter in the CNS, glutamate is found ubiquitously throughout the brain. A nonessential amino acid, glutamate does not cross the blood–brain barrier; thus, synthesis of the glutamate neurotransmitter pool relies entirely on conversion from its precursors (glutamine or aspartate) within nerve terminals (Figure 1-9). Aspartate is converted to glutamine via transamination, while glutamine is converted to glutamate within mitochondria via glutaminase. Glutamate is packaged within synaptic vesicles, and, when released into the synapse, binds post-synaptic glutamate receptors. Unable to diffuse across cell membranes, glutamate is cleared from the synapse primarily by sodium (Na^+)–dependent uptake into astrocytic processes that ensheath the glutamatergic synapse ("tripartite synapse"), where it is converted back to glutamine (which is then transported back to the pre-synaptic glutamatergic terminal).

Glutamate receptors are varied in structure and function, capable of imparting either rapid or gradual change in the function of the post-synaptic neuron. The ionotropic family of glutamate receptors, which includes NMDA, α-amino-3-hydroxy-5-methyl-4-isoxazolepropionic acid (AMPA), and kainate (KA) receptors, act rapidly by opening channels for Na^+ and (to a variable degree) calcium (Ca^{2+}) influx. This influx causes post-synaptic depolarization, which, if present in sufficient force, causes the neuron to fire. The metabotropic glutamate receptors (mGluRs) effect gradual change in neuronal function. These seven membrane-spanning G-protein–coupled receptors (GPCRs) are linked to cytoplasmic enzymes via G proteins embedded within the cell membrane. Once activated, these enzymes can induce second messenger cascades that can influence intra-cellular processes, including gene transcription.

The *N*-methyl-D-aspartate Receptor and the Role of Glutamate in Neuropsychiatric Illness

The NMDA receptor deserves special attention due to its role in normal and abnormal cognitive processes. When activated, the NMDA receptor serves as a channel for the influx of Ca^{2+} into the neuron (Figure 1-10). This process relies on both the binding of ligands (such as glutamate and a co-agonist, glycine) to the receptor and on recent depolarization of the post-synaptic cell membrane, which displaces a magnesium (Mg^{2+}) ion that normally blocks the channel. NMDA receptor signaling thus requires near-simultaneous activity of the pre-synaptic and post-synaptic neurons; this provides a molecular mechanism for associating two temporally linked inputs, a key ingredient in basic forms of learning. Indeed, NMDA receptors, along with AMPA receptors, mediate long-term potentiation in the hippocampus, a process critical for hippocampal-dependent memory formation.

When NMDA receptors are activated in sufficient number, however, the resulting large calcium influx can result in cell death, a process known as excitotoxicity (see Figure 1-10). Excitotoxicity is thought to contribute to

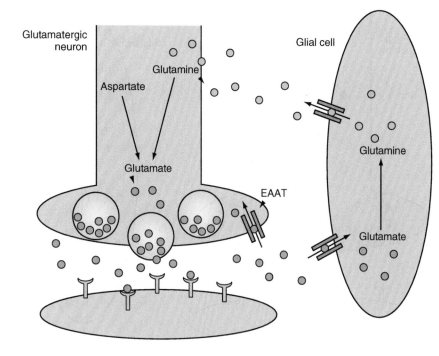

Figure 1-9. The glutamate life cycle.

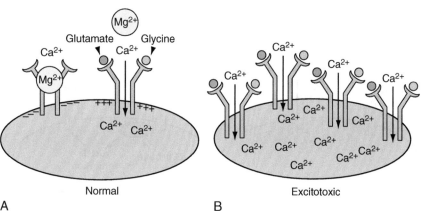

Figure 1-10. *N*-methyl-D-aspartate receptors and excitotoxicity. (A) Normal. (B) Excitotoxic.

Normal   A   Excitotoxic   B

neurodegenerative disorders (such as Alzheimer's disease, Huntington's disease, and amyotrophic lateral sclerosis).[82] Memantine, an NMDA antagonist, is used for the treatment of Alzheimer's Dementia Memantine is hypothesized to slow disease progression by dampening excitotoxic injury.[83]

While overactive NMDA receptors may contribute to neurodegeneration and attendant memory loss in dementia, blockade of these receptors can also cause profound cognitive disruption. NMDA antagonists (such as ketamine and phencyclidine [PCP]) produce psychotic symptoms (e.g., disorganization, dissociation, hallucinations, delusions) in healthy people, and exacerbate psychosis in patients with schizophrenia. This pattern, in concert with observed alterations in glutamate-related proteins, has spurred the "glutamate hypothesis" of schizophrenia.[33] The glutamate system thus represents a promising target for the development of new antipsychotic medications. The NMDA receptor, in addition to its binding site for glutamate, also has a co-regulatory site for the amino acids glycine or D-serine, which must be occupied for glutamate to open the channel. Based on the hypothesis of a hypoactive glutamatergic system in schizophrenia, these amino acids, and the related D-cycloserine, are being actively studied as potential augmentation strategies for antipsychotic treatment.

GABA

Another amino acid, γ-aminobutyric acid (GABA), serves as the major inhibitory transmitter in the CNS. When bound to membrane receptors, GABA causes hyperpolarization either directly, by causing chloride channels to open, or indirectly, through second messenger systems. Although found throughout the CNS, GABA is concentrated specifically in both cortical and spinal interneurons, and plays a major role in dampening excitatory signals. As such, GABA receptors have been of considerable interest to researchers concerned about the normal and abnormal function of neural networks.

GABA is synthesized primarily from glucose, which is converted via the Krebs cycle into α-ketoglutarate and then to glutamate (Figure 1-11). Conversion from glutamate to GABA occurs through the action of glutamic acid decarboxylase (GAD). Because GAD is found only in GABA-producing neurons, antibodies to the enzyme have been used to identify GABA-ergic neurons with high specificity. Following depolarization of the pre-synaptic neuron, vesicles containing GABA discharge it into the synapse, where binding to post-synaptic receptors occurs. GABA is then cleared from the synapse and transported into pre-synaptic terminals and surrounding glia. It is then broken down by GABA α-oxoglutarate transaminase

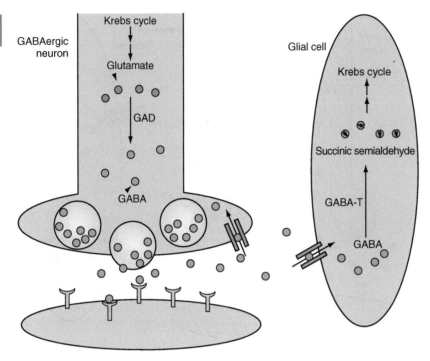

Figure 1-11. The GABA life cycle.

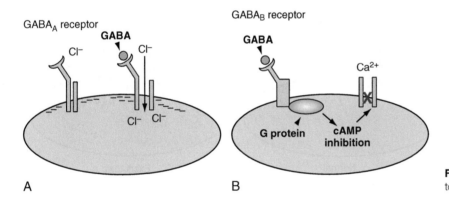

Figure 1-12. GABA receptors. (A) GABA$_A$ receptor. (B) GABA$_B$ receptor.

(GABA-T), and downstream products are returned to the Krebs cycle. GABA synthesis and metabolism are thus referred to as the GABA shunt reaction.

GABA Receptors

There are two major classes of GABA receptors: GABA$_A$ and GABA$_B$ receptors. Binding of GABA to the GABA$_A$ receptor causes a chloride channel to open, which, under most circumstances, renders the post-synaptic membrane potential more negative (Figure 1-12). Of note, several other agents bind allosterically to the GABA$_A$ receptor, including alcohol, barbiturates, and benzodiazepines, and render it more sensitive to GABA. The anticonvulsant activity of benzodiazepines and barbiturates is thought to reflect neural inhibition mediated through the GABA$_A$ receptor.[84]

GABA$_B$ receptors, akin to the metabotropic glutamate receptors, are G-protein–coupled receptors rather than ion channels. Activation of GABA$_B$ causes downstream changes in potassium (K$^+$) and Ca^{2+} channels, largely via G-protein–mediated inhibition of cAMP. Specific interactions between GABA$_B$ receptors and Ca^{2+} channel activity may be linked to absence seizures.[85]

GABA in Neuropsychiatric Illness

Altered GABA activity may contribute significantly to psychiatric disorders. In schizophrenia, reduced GABA synthesis in a select population of inter-neurons within the dorsolateral prefrontal cortex is thought to affect inhibition of pyramidal neurons in this region. Reduced inter-neuron input may thus disrupt synchronized neuronal activity, which, in turn, may underlie working memory deficits in schizophrenia.[9] Further, although the exact mechanism remains uncertain, the chronic action of alcohol, benzodiazepines, and barbiturates on specific GABA$_A$ receptor subunits is hypothesized to underlie such clinical phenomena as tolerance and withdrawal. GABA-ergic dysfunction has also been posited to contribute to panic disorder.

Dopamine

While glutamate and GABA are found throughout the brain, other neurotransmitter systems are localized to specific neural pathways. The monoamines (e.g., norepinephrine, serotonin, dopamine) and acetylcholine are synthesized in several discrete brainstem nuclei, yet project widely, affecting a majority of brain systems. Dopamine, a catecholamine neurotransmitter, affects many brain regions that are consistently implicated in psychiatric disorders. It is hardly surprising, then, that a host of psychopharmacological interventions target the dopamine system.

Dopamine Pathways and Relevance to Neuropsychiatry

There are four major dopamine projections (Figure 1-13), each with great relevance to neuropsychiatric phenomena. The name of each projection indicates the location of the dopaminergic cell bodies, as well as the region targeted by their axons; for example, the nigrostriatal system consists of dopamine cell bodies in the substantia nigra, with axons projecting to the striatum. Degeneration of the nigrostriatal pathway leads to extrapyramidal motor symptoms (such as tremor, bradykinesia, and rigidity), as seen in Parkinson's disease. An analogous mechanism underlies extrapyramidal symptoms (EPS) associated with antipsychotic medications, which block dopamine receptors in the striatum.

Dopamine neurons in the mesolimbic pathway project from the ventral tegmental area (VTA), also in the mid-brain, to limbic and paralimbic structures, including the nucleus accumbens, amygdala, hippocampus, septum, anterior cingulate cortex, and orbitofrontal cortex. Given the importance of these downstream structures to emotion, sensory perception, and memory, it has been speculated that altered activity in the mesolimbic pathway may underlie the perceptual disturbances common to positive symptoms of schizophrenia, hallucinogen use, and even temporal lobe seizures. The mesolimbic pathway is also implicated in the addictive actions of drugs of abuse, which share the common feature of enhancing dopamine release in the nucleus accumbens. In addition, loss of mid-brain nigrostriatal dopaminergic neurons in Parkinson's disease may spread to VTA neurons, and this may underlie the depressive symptoms commonly seen in Parkinson's disease.

Mesocortical dopamine neurons also have their cell bodies in the VTA, but project to the neocortex, primarily prefrontal cortex. Release of dopamine in the prefrontal cortex is believed to affect the efficiency of information processing, attention, and wakefulness. The relationship between prefrontal dopamine and frontal lobe function does not appear to be linear, but rather reflects an "inverted-U" shape (Figure 1-14).[86] For example, brain activation during working memory tasks, largely mediated by prefrontal activation, is inefficient under conditions of either low or high prefrontal dopamine release. Altered availability of prefrontal dopamine may underlie cognitive impairment in schizophrenia, ADHD, Parkinson's disease, and other neuropsychiatric conditions.

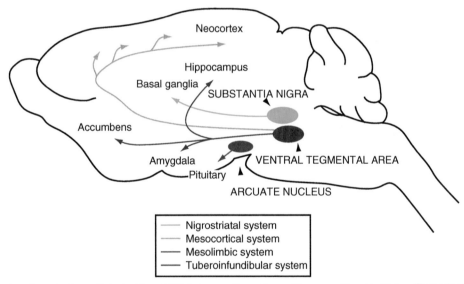

Figure 1-13. Dopaminergic projections. *(Adapted from NIAAA at www.niaaa.nih.gov/Resources/GraphicsGallery/EndocrineReproductiveSystem/LengthwiseView.htm.)*

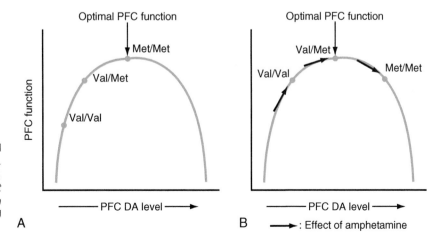

Figure 1-14. (A and B) Dopamine and prefrontal function. PFC, prefrontal cortex; DA, dopamine. *(Adapted from Mattay VS, Goldberg TE, Fera F, et al. Catechol O-methyltransferase val158-met genotype and individual variation in the brain response to amphetamine,* Proc Natl Acad Sci U S A *100:6186–6191, 2003.)*

The tuberoinfundibular dopamine system projects from the arcuate nucleus of the hypothalamus to the stalk of the pituitary gland. When released in the pituitary, dopamine inhibits the secretion of prolactin. Individuals who take dopamine-blocking medications (including some antipsychotics) are therefore at risk for hyperprolactinemia, which can in turn cause menstrual cycle abnormalities, galactorrhea, gynecomastia, and sexual dysfunction.

Dopamine Synthesis, Binding, and Inactivation and More Clinical Correlates

The catecholamines (dopamine, norepinephrine, and epinephrine) are synthesized sequentially in the same biosynthetic pathway. First, dopamine is synthesized from tyrosine through the actions of tyrosine hydroxylase (TH, the rate-limiting enzyme for catecholamine synthesis) and 3,4-dihydroxy-L-phenylalanine (Dopa) decarboxylase (Figure 1-15). The dopamine precursor, L-Dopa, crosses the blood–brain barrier and is given systemically to ameliorate symptoms of Parkinson's disease. Dopamine is packaged and stored in synaptic vesicles by the vesicular monoamine transporter (VMAT), and when released binds to post-synaptic dopamine receptors.

Although numerous classes of dopamine receptors have been described, they each affect intra-cellular signaling through second messenger systems. Dopamine receptors fall into one of two families: D_1-like or D_2-like receptors. D_1-like receptors (which include D_1 and D_5) activate adenylyl cyclase, while D_2-like receptors (including D_2, D_3, and D_4) inhibit cAMP production. D_1 and D_2 receptors significantly outnumber other dopamine receptor types. Most typical antipsychotics were developed as D_2 antagonists, while atypical antipsychotics usually have less activity at D_2 receptors (clozapine, for example, has a high affinity for the D_4 receptor).

There are several mechanisms for inactivating dopamine. Within the neuron, extra-vesicular dopamine may be catabolized by the mitochondrial enzymes monoamine oxidase-A or -B (MAO-A or MAO-B). MAO-A metabolizes norepinephrine, serotonin, and dopamine; inhibitors of this enzyme, such as clorgyline and tranylcypromine, are used to treat depression and anxiety. MAO is also present in the liver and gastrointestinal tract, where it degrades dietary amines (such as tyramine and phenylethylamine), thereby preventing their access to the general circulation. Phenylethylamine can cause hypertension when systemically absorbed; thus, patients receiving MAO inhibitors are at risk of hypertensive crisis if they ingest food products containing these amines. MAO-B targets dopamine most specifically, and therefore agents that inhibit this enzyme are used in Parkinson's disease.

Two other molecules, catechol-O-methyltransferase (COMT) and the dopamine transporter (DAT), have the ability to clear dopamine from the synaptic cleft. In the mid-brain and striatum, DAT plays a more substantial role than COMT, while in the prefrontal cortex, COMT predominates. A common, functional polymorphism in the *COMT* gene, Val 108/158 Met, has been identified: individuals with one or more copies of the Met allele have significantly reduced COMT activity. Thus, these individuals presumably have greater concentrations of prefrontal dopamine (see Figure 1-14). In humans, in the setting of a challenging working memory task, healthy individuals homozygous for the Met allele (Met/Met) may exhibit more efficient brain activation than Val/Val or Val/Met subjects. However, if given amphetamine, which blocks dopamine reuptake and increases synaptic dopamine, Val/Val individuals are shifted to a more optimal position in the curve, while those with Met/Met are shifted to the less efficient downward slope of the curve.[87] Among individuals with altered prefrontal dopamine levels, such as patients with schizophrenia and Parkinson's disease, variation in *COMT* genotype may play a significant role in determining prefrontal efficiency, and hence performance on tasks involving planning, sequencing, and working memory. Similarly, patients with velo-cardio-facial syndrome (VCFS) often have psychotic symptoms that may relate to altered COMT function. VCFS is caused by a 3

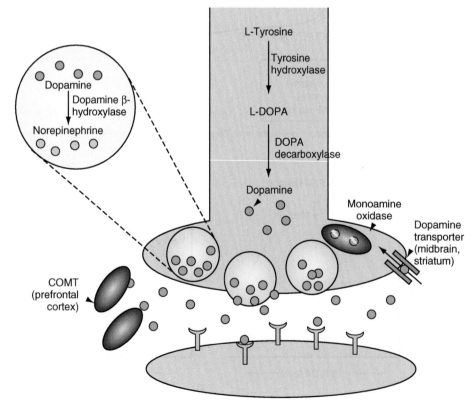

Figure 1-15. The dopamine life cycle.

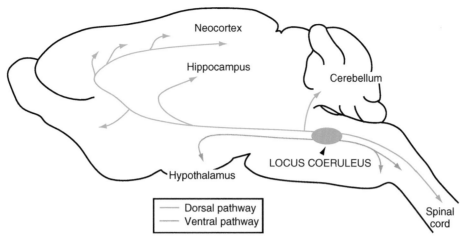

Figure 1-16. Noradrenergic projections. *(Adapted from NIAAA at www.niaaa.nih.gov/Resources/GraphicsGallery/EndocrineReproductiveSystem/ LengthwiseView.htm; and from Siegel GJ, Agranoff BW, Albers RW, et al.* Basic neurochemistry, *ed 6, Philadelphia, 1999, Lippincott-Raven, p. 252.)*

Mb (million base pairs) deletion of the genome on chromosome 22q11.2, which results in the complete loss of one parental copy of approximately 30 genes, one of which is *COMT*. These patients, who exhibit a somewhat variable phenotype (which may also include abnormalities of the heart, thymus, parathyroid, and palate), also have an increased risk for psychotic disorders. Almost 30% of VCFS patients have a psychiatric condition akin to bipolar disorder or schizophrenia.[88]

Norepinephrine

Like dopamine, norepinephrine (noradrenaline [NE]) is a catecholamine neurotransmitter that is present in discrete neural projections. NE cell bodies are concentrated in the locus coeruleus, which is located in the pons near the fourth ventricle (Figure 1-16). This dorsal collection of noradrenergic neurons innervates the cerebral cortex, hippocampus, cerebellum, and spinal cord, while a ventral collection projects to the hypothalamus and other CNS sites.

NE overlaps substantially with dopamine with regard to synthesis and degradation pathways; in fact, dopamine is the immediate precursor to NE, which is produced within synaptic vesicles by dopamine β-hydroxylase (see Figure 1-15). Like dopamine, NE is also degraded by COMT and MAO.

There are three families of noradrenergic receptors: α_1, α_2, and β. Like the dopamine receptors, NE receptors are all coupled to G proteins and thus modify intra-cellular signaling pathways. The α_1 receptors augment protein kinase C activity through the release of inositol 1,4,5-triphosphate and diacylglycerol. While activated α_2 receptors decrease cAMP through inhibition of adenylyl cyclase, β receptors do the opposite, stimulating cAMP production. In this sense, α_2 receptors are somewhat akin to D_2, and β receptors to D_1. In the CNS, α_2 receptors frequently act as "autoreceptors" present pre-synaptically on noradrenergic neurons themselves, providing negative-feedback regulation of noradrenergic output.

Norepinephrine in Opiate Withdrawal

Clonidine, a drug commonly used to treat hypertension, activates CNS α_2 autoreceptors and thereby dampens noradrenergic tone. Use of clonidine in the treatment of opiate withdrawal provides a wonderful example of a case where psychiatric neuroscience has successfully characterized the links between a clinical disorder, therapeutic drug effects, and mechanisms at the molecular, cellular, and neural circuit levels. Acutely,

opiates act through G-protein–coupled receptors to inhibit the cAMP system and reduce the activity of locus coeruleus neurons; this partly mediates their calming and sedating effects. With chronic opiate administration, tolerance develops, in part due to homeostatic up-regulation in the activity of cAMP pathway elements (such as PKA and CREB). In opiate withdrawal, this adaptive up-regulation is no longer balanced by the opiate inhibition. Rebound hyperactivity of the locus coeruleus then occurs, with a great increase in NE release from its widespread projections. This in turn leads to the autonomic and psychological hyperarousal seen during withdrawal; these symptoms are greatly dampened by clonidine.[89]

Serotonin

The serotonin system is involved in many processes in psychiatry, including most prominently mood, sleep, and psychosis.[60,90,91] Serotonin (5-hydroxytryptamine [5-HT]), a monoamine and indolamine, is synthesized from the amino acid tryptophan by tryptophan hydroxylase (TPH) (Figure 1-17). Serotonin is synthesized in mid-line neurons of the brainstem, known as the raphe nuclei.[92] Serotonergic neurons project diffusely to numerous targets (including cerebral cortex, thalamus, basal ganglia, mid-brain dopaminergic nuclei, hippocampus, and amygdala) (Figure 1-18).

Like the catecholamines, serotonin is transported into vesicles by VMAT. Serotonin is subsequently released into the synaptic cleft, and after receptor binding, is inactivated either by pre-synaptic reuptake via the serotonin transporter or degradation via MAO. The serotonin transporter is a critical molecule in neuropsychopharmacology. Drugs that block the serotonin transporter (SERT) prolong serotonin's action; these agents include the selective serotonin reuptake inhibitors (SSRIs) commonly used in treating depression and anxiety disorders. Like the norepinephrine transporter (NET) and dopamine transporter (DAT), SERT is also a common target of drugs of abuse. For example, both cocaine and amphetamine prolong the action of serotonin by inhibiting SERT. Similarly, the club drug ecstasy (MDMA) is a fast-acting SERT inhibitor; MDMA may also be neurotoxic to serotonergic neurons in the dorsal raphe.[93]

The discovery of a common genetic variant in the promoter of the *SERT* gene has had a major impact on psychiatric neuroscience. The "long" form or L-variant (which contains an additional 44-bp sequence) generates more mRNA, and

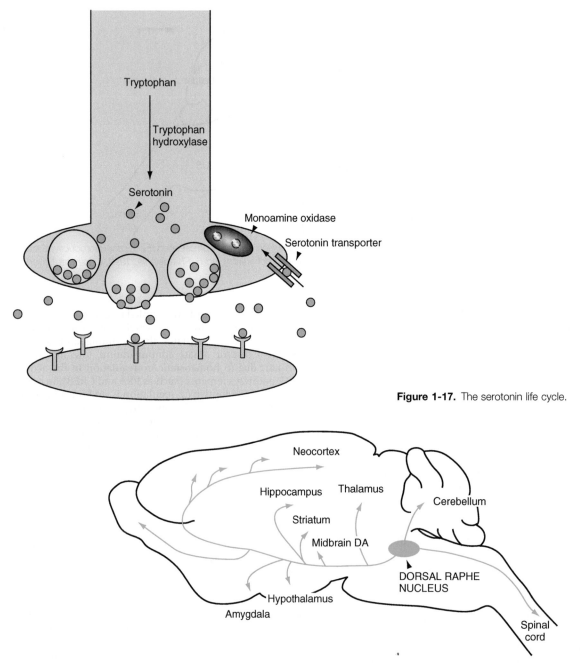

Figure 1-17. The serotonin life cycle.

Figure 1-18. Serotonergic projections. *(Adapted from NIAAA at www.niaaa.nih.gov/Resources/GraphicsGallery/EndocrineReproductiveSystem/ LengthwiseView.htm.)*

thereby protein, than the "short" or S-variant (which lacks this 44-bp sequence). The L-variant thus enhances transporter activity in the synaptic cleft, reducing the duration and intensity of serotonin neurotransmission, while the S-variant leads to lower transporter activity and prolonged serotonin signaling. The S-variant has been implicated in the etiology of depression and anxiety disorders.[94,95]

Seven classes of serotonin receptors exhibit distinct patterns of expression in CNS and peripheral tissues and activate distinct second messenger systems. For example, 5-HT$_{1A}$ receptors are GPCRs that are inhibitory and thereby decrease cAMP; agonists at this receptor (e.g., buspirone) have anxiolytic properties. 5-HT$_2$ receptors (which have three subtypes, A to C) act through a different G protein to activate inositol triphosphate (IP$_3$) and diacylglycerol (DAG) second messenger systems.[96]

5-HT$_2$ signaling is particularly relevant to psychosis: the hallucinogen LSD activates 5-HT$_2$receptors, while many atypical antipsychotics inhibit them.[91]

Acetylcholine

The first neurotransmitter to be discovered, acetylcholine (ACh) was initially characterized by Otto Loewi as *Vagusstoff*, the mediator of vagal parasympathetic outflow to the heart. As we now know, of course, ACh plays important roles in central as well as peripheral neurophysiology, and cholinergic transmission underlies a host of normal cognitive functions. In recent years, the cholinergic system has become an important target in the psychopharmacology of dementia and movement disorders.

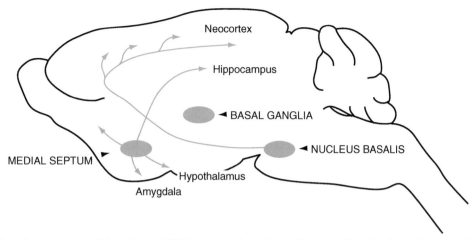

Figure 1-19. Cholinergic projections. *(Adapted from NIAAA at www.niaaa.nih.gov/Resources/GraphicsGallery/EndocrineReproductiveSystem/ LengthwiseView.htm.)*

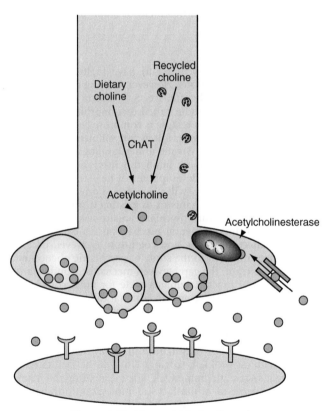

Figure 1-20. The acetylcholine life cycle.

In the periphery, ACh is the neurotransmitter for the neuromuscular junction, for pre-ganglionic neurons in the autonomic nervous system, and for parasympathetic post-ganglionic neurons. In the CNS, cholinergic neurons are concentrated in the nucleus basalis of Meynert in the basal forebrain, and project diffusely to the neocortex (Figure 1-19). There are also cholinergic projections from the septum and diagonal band of Broca to the hippocampus. Cholinergic inter-neurons are found in the basal ganglia.

ACh is formed in nerve terminals through the action of choline acetyltransferase (ChAT; Figure 1-20). Its precursor,

choline, is supplied through both breakdown of dietary phosphatidylcholine, and recycling of synaptic ACh (which is catabolized by acetylcholinesterase to choline and actively transported back into the pre-synaptic terminal).

There are two classes of ACh receptors: muscarinic and nicotinic. While muscarinic receptors are G-protein–coupled, nicotinic receptors are ion channels, which allows for rapid influx of Na^+ and Ca^{2+} into the post-synaptic neuron. Both receptor types are abundant in brain tissue.

Acetylcholine and Cognition

Anticholinergic medications affect the balance of dopamine and ACh in the basal ganglia, which can improve EPS in patients with movement disorders (either primary or secondary to antipsychotic use). However, alterations in cholinergic transmission, due to medications or to underlying disease, can profoundly affect cognition. Anticholinergic medications, such as diphenhydramine, are a common source of delirium in elderly or medically ill patients. Many antipsychotic and tricyclic antidepressant drugs have some anticholinergic activity, which can affect cognition (and also produce significant peripheral side effects, including dry mouth, urinary retention, constipation, and tachycardia). The degeneration of cholinergic neurons in Alzheimer's disease contributes strongly to cognitive decline; acetylcholinesterase inhibitors may slow this effect somewhat, but do not reverse the degeneration process.[97] Nicotine, acting through nicotinic ACh receptors, may produce significant cognitive effects (as well as addictive rewarding effects).

Histamine

Like ACh and NE, histamine serves important functions both in the CNS and peripherally. Histamine is best known for its roles outside the brain in activating immune and inflammatory responses and in stimulating gastric acid secretion. Within the brain, it acts both as a classical neurotransmitter and as a neuromodulator, potentiating the excitability of other neurotransmitter systems.

Histaminergic neurons are concentrated within the hypothalamus, in the tuberomammillary nucleus. They project diffusely to cortical and subcortical targets, as well as to the brainstem and spinal cord. Histamine is derived from its precursor, L-histidine, through the action of L-histidine decarboxylase. Histamine can be broken down either through oxidation (via diamine oxidase) or methylation (via histamine *N*-methyltransferase and, subsequently, MAO).

Three classes of histamine receptors, H_1, H_2, and H_3, have been found both within brain tissue and in the periphery. Each affects second messenger systems through coupling to G proteins. H_3 may also function as an inhibitory autoreceptor. More recently, a fourth class of histamine receptor (H_4) has also been described, but apparently is not expressed in human brain.

Histamine stimulates wakefulness, suppresses appetite, and may enhance cognition through its excitatory effects on brainstem, hypothalamic, and cortical neurons. Drugs with antihistaminic properties can cause significant disruptions of these processes, producing the therapeutic effects of sleep medications, as well as side effects (sedation and weight gain) of some atypical antipsychotics and, in particular, the antidepressant mirtazapine.[98] Animal research shows that histamine depletion adversely affects short-term memory, while H_3 autoreceptor antagonists may have the opposite effect; these findings have fueled the development of H_3 antagonists as a potential treatment for memory disorders.

Other Neurotransmitters, and Interactions among Neurotransmitters

Many additional neurotransmitters mediate important effects in the brain; some with particular relevance to psychiatry include neuropeptides (e.g., endogenous opioids), neurohormones (e.g., corticotropin-releasing hormone), and steroids, cannabinoids, and short-acting gases (such as nitric oxide). And while we have focused on one neurotransmitter at a time, numerous and complex interactions occur among neurotransmitter systems. Although discussion of these other neurotransmitters and neurotransmitter interactions is beyond the scope of this chapter, they are of great importance to psychiatric neuroscience and the subject of intensive research.

GENES, ENVIRONMENT, AND EPIGENETICS

At the outset of this chapter, we stated that major mental illness reflects abnormal brain function, and we have described many genes that could contribute to such dysfunction. However, while neuropsychiatric conditions are frequently highly heritable, the emergence of psychopathology likely requires a complex interaction of a genetic susceptibility and exposure to environmental risk factors. Note that the "environment" must be understood broadly, and includes the prenatal uterine environment as well as peri-natal and post-natal events into childhood, adolescence, and adulthood. Epidemiological studies relating gene–environment interactions to the development of psychiatric conditions have already contributed significantly to psychiatric neuroscience.[99] For example, in a prospective longitudinal study, Caspi and colleagues[100] discovered that genetic variations in the serotonin transporter (*SERT*) promoter interacted with stressful life events to influence depression risk. Individuals with one or two copies of the short S-variant allele (the hypoactive form of the gene) exhibited more depression and suicidality in relation to stressful life events than those carrying two copies of the long L-variant allele. This remarkable study demonstrated that even when genetic susceptibility and environmental exposure do not independently produce a strong increase in risk for psychopathology, in combination they may impressively increase this risk.[100]

Finally, the mechanisms by which experience may interact with genes are various, but one recent study in the field of "epigenetics" merits attention. Epigenetics has various definitions, but includes the idea that a gene function may be changed without a specific alteration in the code, and that this change in gene function also may be heritable.[101] Frequently, this may occur by a change in the structure of the DNA molecule: for example, chromatin, around a gene, which alters gene expression. An important animal model may have shed light on the biological effects of child abuse.[43,102] While it has been widely noted in psychiatry that child abuse or mistreatment can have long-term effects on cognition and behavior, a model system of rodent maternal care has also demonstrated that rodent pups mistreated during development will have long-standing dysfunctional programming of their hypothalamic–pituitary–adrenal axis, and thereby response to stress. Investigators have further demonstrated that these occur due to specific changes in chromatin structure and subsequent gene expression, and have also shown that these changes and downstream effects may be heritable. These effects may be treatable or even reversible with novel medicines that affect chromatic structure,[103] and, indeed, some of our older medicines, most notably valproic acid,[104] may act in part through such mechanisms. This is an important example of how a detailed mechanistic understanding of gene–environment interactions may truly make vast contributions to the understanding and treatment of major mental illness.

CONCLUSION

We are fortunate in psychiatry to have multiple treatment choices for most conditions. However, existing treatments are frequently only partially effective. Side effects may interfere with compliance and produce their own morbidity, and even after successful treatment relapse is common. Despite 50 years of progress in psychopharmacology, we still need better treatments for mental illness. Greater understanding of the biological mechanisms underlying brain function and dysfunction will be essential in the development of new and better remedies. Important insights will also come from clarifying the specific therapeutic mechanisms of existing treatments.

Over the past century psychiatric neuroscience has made great strides in linking neural mechanisms to conditions of abnormal affect, behavior, and cognition. However, because of challenges inherent to the study of psychiatric phenomena and brain function, the gap between mechanistic understanding and clinical practice remains wide for most conditions. Genetics and neuroimaging have dramatically enhanced our ability to bridge these gaps, and the accelerating development of these fields provides great hope.

While our biological knowledge is incomplete, there is already a great deal of information that may be incorporated into our clinical problem-solving. This will be facilitated by applying a systematic framework when evaluating the neuroscientific aspects of clinical cases. Biological formulations should involve consideration of two broad domains: process (the dynamic mechanisms of neurodevelopment, neurotransmission, and neurodegeneration) and content (key regional, cellular, and molecular neural substrates). These biological components of major mental illness, identified through decades of research, are extremely valuable in our explanations to patients and families.

Acknowledgments

The authors would like to thank Stephan Heckers in particular for his rigor and commitment to teaching psychiatric neuroscience at Harvard. This teaching has contributed greatly to the framing of this chapter. We would also like to thank Nicholas Kontos for critical comments of this manuscript.

Access the complete reference list and multiple choice questions (MCQs) online at https://expertconsult.inkling.com

KEY REFERENCES

3. Kandel ER, Schwartz JH, Jessell TM, et al. *Principles of neural science*, ed 5, New York, 2013, McGraw-Hill.
6. Price BH, Adams RD, Coyle JT. Neurology and psychiatry: closing the great divide. *Neurology* 54(1):8–14, 2000.
7. Alzheimer A, Stelzmann RA, Schnitzlein HN, et al. An English translation of Alzheimer's 1907 paper, "Uber eine eigenartige Erkankung der Hirnrinde." *Clin Anat* 8(6):429–431, 1995.
10. Benes FM. Emerging principles of altered neural circuitry in schizophrenia. *Brain Res Brain Res Rev* 31(2–3):251–269, 2000.
13. Snyder SH. Turning off neurotransmitters. *Cell* 125(1):13–15, 2006.
18. Geschwind N. Mechanisms of change after brain lesions. *Ann N Y Acad Sci* 457:1–11, 1985.
19. Fleischman J. *Phineas Gage: a gruesome but true story about brain science*, Boston, 2002, Houghton Mifflin.
20. Corkin S. What's new with the amnesic patient H.M.? *Nat Rev* 3(2):153–160, 2002.
22. Hariri AR, Weinberger DR. Imaging genomics. *Br Med Bull* 65:259–270, 2003.
23. Dougherty DD, Rauch SL, Rosenbaum JF. *Essentials of neuroimaging for clinical practice*, Washington, DC, 2004, American Psychiatric Publishing.
26. Haber SN, Rauch SL. Neurocircuitry: a window into the networks underlying neuropsychiatric disease. *Neuropsychopharmacology* 35(1):1–3, 2010. [Epub 2009/12/17].
29. Pascual-Leone A, Walsh V, Rothwell J. Transcranial magnetic stimulation in cognitive neuroscience—virtual lesion, chronometry, and functional connectivity. *Curr Opin Neurobiol* 10(2):232–237, 2000.
34. Schildkraut JJ. The catecholamine hypothesis of affective disorders. A review of supporting evidence. *Int J Psychiatry* 4(3):203–217, 1967.
35. LeDoux J. The emotional brain, fear, and the amygdala. *Cell Mol Neurobiol* 23(4–5):727–738, 2003.
37. Cowan WM, Kopnisky KL, Hyman SE. The human genome project and its impact on psychiatry. *Annu Rev Neurosci* 25:1–50, 2002.
38. Tanzi RE, Bertram L. Twenty years of the Alzheimer's disease amyloid hypothesis: a genetic perspective. *Cell* 120(4):545–555, 2005.
46. Warner-Schmidt JL, Duman RS. Hippocampal neurogenesis: opposing effects of stress and antidepressant treatment. *Hippocampus* 16(3):239–249, 2006.
47. Rapoport JL, Castellanos FX, Gogate N, et al. Imaging normal and abnormal brain development: new perspectives for child psychiatry. *Aust N Z J Psychiatry* 35(3):272–281, 2001.
52. Hyman SE, Malenka RC, Nestler EJ. Neural mechanisms of addiction: the role of reward-related learning and memory. *Annu Rev Neurosci* 29:565–598, 2006.
54. Mesulam MM. *Principles of behavioral and cognitive neurology*, ed 2, New York, 2000, Oxford University Press.
56. Schmahmann JD. An emerging concept. The cerebellar contribution to higher function. *Arch Neurol* 48(11):1178–1187, 1991.
59. Graybiel AM. The basal ganglia: learning new tricks and loving it. *Curr Opin Neurobiol* 15(6):638–644, 2005.
61. Ramon y Cajal S. *Histology of the nervous system of man and vertebrates*, New York, 1995, Oxford University Press.
63. Ongur D, Drevets WC, Price JL. Glial reduction in the subgenual prefrontal cortex in mood disorders. *Proc Natl Acad Sci U S A* 95(22):13290–13295, 1998.
82. Bossy-Wetzel E, Schwarzenbacher R, Lipton SA. Molecular pathways to neurodegeneration. *Nat Med* 10(Suppl.):S2–S9, 2004.
84. Rowlett JK, Cook JM, Duke AN, et al. Selective antagonism of $GABA_A$ receptor subtypes: an in vivo approach to exploring the therapeutic and side effects of benzodiazepine-type drugs. *CNS Spectr* 10(1):40–48, 2005.
86. Goldman-Rakic PS. The cortical dopamine system: role in memory and cognition. *Adv Pharmacol* 42:707–711, 1998.
90. Arango V, Underwood MD, Mann JJ. Serotonin brain circuits involved in major depression and suicide. *Prog Brain Res* 136:443–453, 2002.
99. Caspi A, Moffitt TE. Gene-environment interactions in psychiatry: joining forces with neuroscience. *Nat Rev* 7(7):583–590, 2006.
101. Petronis A, Gottesman II, Crow TJ, et al. Psychiatric epigenetics: a new focus for the new century. *Mol Psychiatry* 5(4):342–346, 2000.

2 Treatment Adherence

Lara Traeger, PhD, Megan Moore Brennan, MD, and John B. Herman, MD

KEY POINTS

Background

- Among patients with a psychiatric illness, treatment adherence is associated with better treatment outcomes, a lower risk of relapse and hospitalization, and better adherence to treatments for co-morbid medical illnesses. However, barriers to adherence are common and rates of suboptimal adherence remain critically high.

History

- Over the past several decades, approaches have evolved to help patients continue treatment for chronic health problems. The term "adherence," promoted by the World Health Organization, reflects that optimal health outcomes require multi-level efforts to reduce treatment barriers encountered by patients.

Clinical and Research Challenges

- Patient adherence is a necessary component of treatment response and remission. Standardized definitions and measures of adherence are needed to support comparisons of risk factors and intervention outcomes across studies and translation to clinical work. More research also is needed to establish effective, cost-efficient ways to improve adherence in clinical settings. Adherence curricula should be included in mental health professional training and continuing education programs.

Practical Pointers

- Practitioners are encouraged to collaborate actively with patients to select and monitor psychiatric treatment regimens. Optimal patient adherence requires a complex series of behaviors. Routine assessment of both modifiable and non-modifiable barriers to adherence throughout the course of treatment will enable practitioners to tailor treatment approaches and adherence interventions for individual patients. Patient education can enhance adherence by incorporating cognitive and behavioral strategies into care plans.

OVERVIEW

Poor adherence to psychiatric treatments is a widespread clinical problem that negatively impacts rates of treatment response and remission.[1,2] While empirically-supported treatments are available for many psychiatric disorders,[3] these treatments are not universally effective. Patients commonly face difficulties in taking prescribed psychotropic medications or attending psychotherapy sessions as recommended, and therefore may not achieve optimal outcomes.[1,4] Moreover, some patients who adhere to treatment recommendations may not experience a clinically significant response, and this often leads them to remain in care and to tolerate treatment plan modifications.[5]

The World Health Organization has defined adherence as the extent to which patients' health behaviors are consistent with recommendations that they have agreed to with their practitioners.[6] This definition emphasizes that practitioners must collaborate with their patients in making decisions throughout treatment. However, researchers frequently evaluate patient adherence to psychiatric regimens in ways which do not capture the dynamics among patients, practitioners, and health care systems.[7] Common measures include the extent to which patients take their medications at the prescribed dose and timing, attend scheduled clinic appointments, and remain in care. These broad measures are discussed in this chapter (summarizing findings on the prevalence of, and the barriers to, psychiatric treatment adherence). This chapter also highlights the fact that optimal adherence is a moving target that involves complex patient behaviors and multi-factorial challenges, and may be enhanced by targeted strategies for patients, practitioners, and systems.

EPIDEMIOLOGY OF ADHERENCE

The estimated prevalence of patient adherence to the use of psychotropic medications has varied widely, due to differences in study populations, diagnoses, medication classes, and the definition of adherence. However, evidence strongly supports the notion that poor adherence is common across groups. Substantial proportions of community-dwelling patients take less than their prescribed daily doses of antipsychotics (34.6%), sedative-hypnotics (34.7%), anxiolytics (38.1%), mood stabilizers (44.9%) and antidepressants (45.9%).[8] In a retrospective study of managed care patients, approximately 57% of patients who had started a selective serotonin re-uptake inhibitor (SSRI) for depression and/or anxiety were not adherent to the medication.[7] In fact, many patients with depression (19%–28%) also do not show for scheduled clinic appointments.[9]

Reports of adherence to taking psychotropic medications further reflect problems with premature treatment discontinuation. Moreover, many patients do not inform their physician about having stopped their medication. Across studies of treatment trials for anxiety disorders (generally lasting 10–12 weeks), 18%–30% of patients discontinued their treatment prematurely.[4] Among patients with depression who were taking an SSRI, almost half (47%) had stopped filling their prescription within 2 months of treatment initiation.[10] Similarly, a pooled analysis of 1,627 patients with psychosis treated with atypical antipsychotics revealed that about half (53%) of the patients discontinued their medication soon after treatment began.[11] Researchers in the Clinical Antipsychotic Trials of Intervention Effectiveness (CATIE) reported that almost three-fourths (74%) of patients with chronic schizophrenia discontinued treatment within 4 months of its initiation.[12]

Some studies have shown that adults with depression prefer psychotherapy over antidepressants.[13] Yet, in a sample of primary care patients with depression, 74% endorsed that barriers to care made it very difficult or impossible to attend regular psychotherapy sessions.[14] Meta-analyses of cognitive-behavioral therapy (CBT) trials for anxiety disorders indicated that for patients who started CBT, between 9% and 21% discontinued the treatment early.[4]

CLINICAL AND ECONOMIC IMPACT OF NON-ADHERENCE

Poor adherence to psychiatric treatments leads to worse clinical outcomes and to excess health care utilization; these factors contribute, in turn, to the economic burden of mental illness.[1,15,16] Among patients with depression, non-adherence to antidepressants is associated with higher medical costs[7] and accounts for 5%–40% of hospital readmissions.[9] Medication non-adherence also is the most powerful predictor of relapse after a first episode of schizophrenia, independent of gender, age of onset, premorbid function, patient insight, or other key factors.[2,17] Moreover, non-adherent patients with schizophrenia are at greater risk for substance use, violence, and victimization, as well as worse overall quality of life.[18] Although little studied, patient non-adherence also may increase the risk of burnout and fatigue among psychiatric practitioners. Findings emphasize that intervening at multiple levels to enhance adherence has the potential to improve population health and well-being and to reduce excess health care utilization, beyond individual improvements in specific treatments.[6]

RISK FACTORS FOR NON-ADHERENCE

Risk factors for non-adherence are complex and varied, and remain incompletely understood. Findings are typically drawn from secondary analyses or exit interviews from randomized controlled trials (RCTs), which employ strict eligibility criteria and rigorous patient monitoring.[4] In clinical settings, practitioners must consider and address multi-factorial challenges to optimal patient adherence (Table 2-1). Key risk factors are summarized below.

Clinical Factors

Mood

Mood symptoms can increase patients' perceptions of barriers to psychiatric care and can adversely affect treatment adherence.[14] Dysphoria and hopelessness may reduce intrinsic motivation for treatment. Patients who experience psychomotor slowing, decreased energy, and poor concentration also may have difficulty engaging in self-care, attending appointments, completing cognitive-behavioral therapy (CBT) assignments, and/or taking their medications appropriately. In comparison, when patients enter a manic episode, they may experience elevated mood and energy as positive and may not want to take their medications that slow them down. Moreover, when insight and judgment are impaired, patients may not believe that they have an illness that requires treatment.

Anxiety

Anxiety disorders are associated with hyper-vigilance to internal and/or external stimuli, which may affect a patient's adherence to treatment recommendations in several ways. Some patients become too anxious to leave their home and to attend scheduled clinic appointments. Anxiety also may interfere with the optimal upward titration or tapering of medications, as patients may attribute transient physical symptoms to changes in medication dose. Among patients with obsessive-compulsive disorder (OCD), counting rituals and fears of contamination may preclude adherence to both medication and psychotherapy regimens.

Psychosis

Most reports on adherence to psychiatric treatment regimens have focused on psychotic disorders, including schizophrenia.

TABLE 2-1 Multi-factorial Influences on Treatment Adherence

Factors	Examples
Clinical	Psychiatric symptoms that may interfere with adherence
	Substance misuse
	Cognitive impairment
Treatment-related	Treatment efficacy
	Side effects
	Dose timing and frequency
	Psychotherapy modality
Patient-level	Knowledge about psychiatric symptoms and their treatments
	Attitudes, beliefs, and concerns about psychiatric symptoms/treatments
	Attitudes, beliefs, and concerns about health care systems
Practitioner-level	Knowledge, attitudes, and beliefs about psychiatric symptoms/treatments
	Knowledge, attitudes, and beliefs about barriers to patient adherence
	Use of adherence assessments and interventions throughout treatment
	Facilitation of therapeutic alliance
	Collaboration with patient in treatment decision-making
Systems-level	Mental health care coverage
	Fragmentation of patient care
	Distance from patient home to clinic/availability of care
	Financial barriers (transportation, co-payments, child care)
	Barriers to mental health care among racial/ethnic minorities
Sociocultural	Attitudes and beliefs about psychiatric symptoms/treatments within the patient's identified communities (e.g., family, cultural, and religious)
	Mental health stigma within communities
Interactions among factors	Practitioner–patient therapeutic alliance
	Match between the patient's preferences/values and treatments
	Match between the patient's resources/needs and prescribed treatments
	Level of a patient's trust in practitioner and health care systems
	The patient's access to/use of support for navigating barriers to adherence

Problems related to both the disorders and their treatments present significant barriers to adherence. Factors (such as positive symptoms, emotional distress, and treatment side effects [e.g., akathisia]) have predicted poor adherence.[19-23] Among patients treated with atypical antipsychotics, early discontinuation of treatment has been attributed to perceptions of poor response, to worsening of symptoms, and to an inability to tolerate the medications.[11] Notably, patients who need to change or augment their current treatment are at higher risk for its discontinuation.[24]

Substance Misuse

Misuse of substances is an important risk factor for non-adherence in patients with a variety of psychiatric disorders.[25,26] Patients who believe that mixing alcohol or illicit drugs with prescribed medications can be dangerous may eschew use of their medication in favor of alcohol or drugs. Drug intoxication and withdrawal also affect a patient's attention, memory, and mood state, which in turn, can interfere with adherence.

The financial burden of substances may also negatively affect a patients' ability to make co-payments for medications and clinic appointments.

Patient Factors: Knowledge, Attitudes, and Beliefs

Across different psychiatric diagnoses, patients' perceptions of their disorder and its treatment consistently predict adherence or the lack thereof. Patients are more likely to adhere to their medication regimen if they believe that their need for the medication is high and that risk of adverse effects related to the medication is low.[4,27,28] On the other hand, mental health stigma, denial of one's diagnosis, and lack of insight all increase the risk for treatment non-adherence.[19,20,22,23,29] Patients also may stop treatment if they believe it is unhelpful once an acute illness phase has resolved.[30] In a study of patients with bipolar I disorder, more than half were non-adherent to their medications 4 months after an episode of acute mania.[31] With regard to psychotherapy, trials of CBT for anxiety have shown that patients with a low motivation for treatment, little readiness for change, and/or low confidence in CBT in comparison to other treatments have an elevated risk for early treatment discontinuation.

Economic and Racial/Ethnic Disparities

Structural and financial barriers to taking medications and attending appointments (e.g., a lack of resources for child care, transportation, or co-payments) are important risk factors for non-adherence.[4,14] U.S. health insurance providers historically have restricted mental health services more than other medical services. Some patients may be more likely to forego psychiatric medications if they are balancing medication costs for multiple health conditions.

Racial/ethnic disparities in access to quality psychiatric care are well-documented.[32,33] However, among patients who do initiate medication or psychotherapy, evidence for differences in treatment adequacy or retention in care is more equivocal.[34] Some studies of schizophrenia and mood disorders suggests that black and Latino patients have poorer adherence to psychiatric medications, relative to white patients.[24,26,31,35] A combination of factors, such as access to psychiatric care; differences in medication metabolism, response, and side effects; and patients' beliefs and concerns about treatment, may underlie these disparities.[31] Practitioners should consider these factors during treatment selection, titration, and management.

Clinical Encounters

Poor practitioner–patient therapeutic alliances and a lack of follow-up increase the risk for treatment non-response and attrition.[4,36] Adherence and medication effects need to be monitored on an ongoing basis. Practitioners can help patients manage expectations by discussing with patients that certain treatments may cause side effects or require adjustments before they confer benefits on psychiatric symptoms and quality of life. The following sections summarize suggestions for assessing adherence and integrating adherence into all phases of treatment.

ASSESSING ADHERENCE

Currently, there is no "gold standard" measure of treatment adherence or a consensus on the adequate or optimal level of adherence among patients. Available tools for assessing patient adherence to psychotropic medications include self-report measures, daily diaries, electronic pill containers, prescription refill records, pill counts, laboratory assays, directly-observed therapy, and collateral information.[37] Practitioners should consider strengths and limitations of each method in the context of available resources and the intended purpose of assessment. Self-report measures[38] and daily diaries are inexpensive to administer, yet may be subject to the impact of social desirability or forgetting. Electronic pill containers yield detailed adherence data but may be impractical when tracking multiple medications. Having free samples and left-over pills from other prescriptions reduces the accuracy of pill-counts. Laboratory assays may identify the presence of medication classes or individual agents but cannot confirm daily administration. When appropriate, multiple measures can be used to support a more complete view of adherence.

INTEGRATING ADHERENCE INTO THE TREATMENT COURSE
Initial Consultation

Practitioners commonly underestimate patient barriers to treatment adherence.[39] Adherence must be an explicit, core element of treatment, starting with the initial consultation (Table 2-2). The practitioner begins to facilitate a therapeutic alliance early-on by transmitting a warm, non-judgmental

TABLE 2-2 Incorporation of Adherence-related Inquiries into Initial Consultation

Components	Areas of Inquiry
History of present illness	What are the patient's beliefs about symptoms and acceptable treatments?
	To what extent are barriers to adherence related to present symptoms?
	How may present symptoms affect adherence behaviors?
Past psychiatric history	To what extent were barriers to adherence related to prior psychiatric risk?
	What were the patient's attitudes about medication versus psychotherapy?
Substance abuse	Is the patient actively using alcohol or illicit drugs?
Medical history	What are the patient's beliefs about medical conditions and treatments?
Medications	What are the patient's attitudes, beliefs, and concerns about current medications?
	How does the patient cope with current medication side effects?
	What types of barriers to adherence does the patient experience?
Family history	What are familial attitudes, beliefs, and coping with psychiatric symptoms?
Social history	What are attitudes and beliefs about psychiatric symptoms and treatments within the patient's identified cultural and religious communities?
	How may non-modifiable financial concerns or living situations influence the ability to obtain, store, and take certain medications or to attend clinic?
	What role should the family play in treatment decision-making and monitoring?
Mental status examination	To what extent may insight, judgment, and/or cognitive impairments influence treatment adherence?

TABLE 2-3 Patterns of Poor Medication Adherence and Corresponding Concerns to Explore

Adherence Pattern	Potential Concerns to Explore
Takes higher dose than recommended	Are treatment recommendations understood and/or acceptable? Are symptoms inadequately managed at the lower dose? Is the patient abusing the medication?
Takes lower dose than recommended	Are treatment recommendations understood and/or acceptable? Are side effects too bothersome? Has the desired effect been achieved at the lower dose? Is the patient concerned about medication tolerance or dependence? Is the patient misusing the remaining medication?
Misses one dose per week	Are treatment recommendations understood and/or acceptable? Is the patient facing particular barriers on days in which the dose is missed? Is the patient skipping the dose or doubling the next dose?
Takes pills every other day	Are treatment recommendations understood and/or acceptable? Is the patient facing particular barriers on days in which the dose is missed? Is the patient facing difficulty with medication expenses?
Takes medications sporadically	Are treatment recommendations understood and/or acceptable? Does the patient have sufficient understanding or acceptance of the illness being treated or the treatment's mechanism of action?

stance and by demonstrating support and commitment to the patient's well-being.[40,41] Key tasks include exploring a patient's values and perspectives about symptoms and their acceptable treatment. By evaluating modifiable barriers (e.g., misinformation about medications), the practitioner may identify opportunities for intervention. The practitioner should also assess non-modifiable barriers to adherence (e.g., the patient lives far from the clinic) in order to recommend feasible treatment options.

Treatment Planning

Active collaboration will help the practitioner and the patient develop an appropriate, acceptable, and feasible treatment plan. The practitioner may present pros and cons of available treatment options to arrive at treatment recommendations. Following treatment selection, the practitioner may express belief in the treatment and thereby promote optimism that the treatment will result in positive change. As mentioned earlier, however, practitioners also should manage patients' expectations by stating that medications may require adjustments before they confer benefits. Patients are told that treatments can be discontinued if they are ineffective, cause intolerable side effects, or create other issues that are personally important. Notably, the best way for some patients to commit to a particular plan is to enhance their sense of agency to otherwise say "no".

Introduction to Adherence

As early as possible, the practitioner should explicate the role of adherence in facilitating treatment goals. This includes normalizing adherence challenges, preparing the patient for regular adherence assessments, and adopting a non-judgmental attitude toward risk of adherence lapses. Depending on a patient's barriers to adherence, practitioners may integrate specific strategies into the treatment plan, such as increasing the frequency of clinic visits,[42] using a depot injection of an antipsychotic medication,[43,44] limiting the number of daily doses,[45] and selecting medications based on tolerable side effects.[46] Authors of the 2009 Expert Consensus Guideline Series on adherence among patients with serious mental illness also emphasized the importance of services, when available, to reduce logistical barriers to care.[47]

Ongoing Assessment

Adherence can change over time, with drug over-utilization being more common during the early stages of treatment and under-utilization during its later stages.[48] The patient's initial evaluation, evolving symptom profile, and barriers to adherence will guide the nature and extent of follow-up adherence assessments (Table 2-3). Regular discussions will help the practitioner foster a treatment relationship in which a patient feels comfortable discussing adherence challenges.

The practitioner should also ask about adherence in an empathic, non-judgmental manner, using a tone of genuine curiosity (*How is it going with taking your medications?*). After introducing the topic, the practitioner may ask patients which medications they are taking and how they are taking them. Open-ended questions will identify when patients are taking medications incorrectly (with or without realizing it). Disarming inquiries are less likely to appear shaming or punitive (*Many people find it difficult to take medication—have you ever forgotten to take yours?*).

PROBLEM-SOLVING BARRIERS TO ADHERENCE

Most patients will face barriers to optimal adherence during the course of treatment. The practitioner should invest time during clinic appointments to explore non-adherence and tailor adherence strategies accordingly. A foundational approach focuses on developing and maintaining a strong therapeutic alliance with the patient. The following sections and Table 2-4 provide examples of more targeted strategies.

Education

Patients will benefit from building knowledge and insight about their condition and its treatment. Education should be provided in multiple formats (e.g., oral, written, graphic), to illustrate the rationale for the treatment dose and timing and the reason for the expected treatment duration. However, patients commonly face multiple complex challenges to managing their medication regimens. Interventions that combine patient education with cognitive and behavioral strategies are more effective than the use of education strategies alone. Across diverse health conditions, multi-component approaches have led to moderate improvements in both adherence and

TABLE 2-4 Components of Patient-focused Interventions to Enhance Adherence

Components	Sample Strategies
Education	Education on target symptoms, their treatments, and treatment side effects
	Information in multiple formats (oral, written, visual)
Motivation	Development of strong practitioner–patient therapeutic alliance
	Identification of intrinsic motivation for adherence (e.g., life goals)
	Other rewards and reinforcements for adherence
	Peer mentoring
Skills	**PROBLEM-SOLVING**
	Identification of steps involved in optimal adherence and potential barriers
	Generation and testing of potential solutions to barriers
	Use of incremental goals to reach desired level of adherence
	ADAPTIVE THINKING
	Socratic questioning to guide the patient in the discovery of problematic patterns about adherence (e.g., depressive hopelessness)
	Cognitive re-structuring to generate more realistic and helpful thoughts
	USE OF CUES
	Daily alarm (mobile phone or wrist watch)
	Pill box or electronic pill container
	Mobile phone app for adherence
	Written reminders or stickers in key areas of a patient's home
	Reminders from an informal caregiver
	Tailoring of medication schedule to daily life schedule and activities
	Telephone- or computer-based reminders for pill-taking, appointments, and/or refills
	SUPPORT
	Patient counseling/education on support-seeking skills
	Family or group-based interventions
Logistics	Case management or financial counseling to increase access to care
	Simplified dose schedule
	Adherence monitoring via diary or electronic pill cap

BOX 2-1 Adherence-related Tasks for Patients on Psychiatric Medications

- Describe psychiatric symptoms (frequency, severity, characteristics)
- Comprehend information about recommended medications
- Collaborate with the practitioner to make treatment decisions
- Obtain prescribed medications
- Safely store medications
- Follow the regimen's dose and timing (and/or make decisions about taking PRN medications)
- Identify, manage, and cope with side effects
- Obtain informal caregiver support as needed
- Attend regular follow-up clinic appointments
- Identify and raise concerns about medications
- Continue collaborating to titrate and modify the regimen as needed

improve adherence to their prescribed regimen.[51] Adherence comprises a complex series of tasks. Practitioners may use Box 2-1 as a starting point to help a patient break adherence into practical steps and to identify potential barriers at each step—such as obtaining medication (e.g., difficulty with co-payments), storing medication (e.g., unstable housing or desire to conceal one's psychiatric diagnosis from a housemate), taking medications on time (e.g., problems with forgetting or a co-morbid attention deficit disorder), or raising concerns with the practitioner (e.g., desire to avoid being a "bad" patient). Socratic questioning may help a patient further uncover problematic thought or behavior patterns that interfere with adherence.

Once barriers are identified, the practitioner may work with the patient to generate and test solutions for reducing them. Forgetting is one of the most common reasons that patients cite for missing or delaying use of psychiatric medications.[8] Based on an adherence intervention for patients with co-morbid depression and medical conditions,[54] patients are encouraged to identify both a plan (e.g., set up a daily alarm) and a back-up plan (e.g., stick a written reminder on one's bathroom mirror) to address each specific barrier. Moreover, the practitioner may help review the patient's daily schedule and revise medication times to match specific activities that the patient never forgets (e.g., brushing one's teeth or filling a coffee pot in the morning). Finally, patients may benefit from learning adaptive thinking strategies, such as cognitive re-structuring, to reduce severe interfering thoughts (e.g., *My need for medication is a sign that I am a weak person*). The practitioner and patient will review the success of the patient's strategies at each visit, revising them as needed and setting incremental goals for achieving optimal adherence.

Patients also may benefit from communication skills to increase social support for adherence within their family or community. Occasionally, a patient's loved ones may have concerns about the treatment or may have high expressed-emotion at home, which in turn may impede adherence. The practitioner and patient may plan to initiate an open discussion of these issues directly with loved ones, to engage them in the collaborative relationship and invite them to "walk the treatment path" with the patient. Family interventions may be needed to address problems with high expressed-emotion.[4]

clinical outcomes.[49-51] When available, some patients also may benefit from CBT or other problem-focused therapies for more intensive adherence intervention.

Motivation

Based on the transtheoretical model, readiness-to-change may fluctuate across five stages, from *pre-contemplation* (not yet committed to the need for psychiatric treatment) to *maintenance* (already adhering to treatment).[52] The practitioner should explore patients' motivations for treatment on an ongoing basis. Motivational interviewing (MI) techniques can be used as-needed to elicit intrinsic motivation and resolve ambivalence toward treatment.[53] Patients who are mandated or urged by others to start treatment are at higher risk for non-adherence relative to patients who are ready for change.[4]

Skills

Even with knowledge and motivation for treatment, many patients need to enhance their problem-solving skills to

Logistics

As mentioned earlier, many non-modifiable barriers, such as limitations in mental health insurance coverage and limited resources or mobility to attend clinic appointments, reduce a patient's access to care. Moreover, problems such as depression exacerbate hopelessness in navigating these types of barriers.[55] Patients with limited resources need specific, practical support to problem-solve ideas and gain access to available services. Practitioners may consider lower-cost alternatives, explore how patients pay for other medications, and refer patients to resource specialists when available.

FUTURE DIRECTIONS
Research

Standardized terminology and measures for treatment adherence are needed to compare study outcomes and translate this information into clinical practice. Prospective studies of non-adherence, including *a priori* measures of potential risk factors, multiple adherence measures, and longer follow-up periods, will increase our understanding of adherence and our ability to identify patients at risk for non-adherence or treatment attrition over time. These findings, in turn, will help researchers and clinicians to target modifiable risk factors in patients who need more intensive adherence interventions.

More research is also needed to establish effective, cost-efficient ways to improve adherence—particularly among patients who are medically complex and/or lower functioning. In stepped or collaborative care models, care managers provide patients with support in consultation with a supervising psychiatrist and each patient's primary medical provider.[56] Telephone-based care represents another model for maintaining patient engagement in care and monitoring treatment response.[57,58] Quantitative economic studies will provide leverage with privatized managed care and government agencies, by allowing researchers to demonstrate that interventions to improve adherence result in cost benefits—such as decreasing emergency department visits and hospitalizations.

Education

There are critical gaps in training for psychiatric practitioners on the assessment and management of treatment adherence. Residency training programs can provide opportunities to teach about the integration of adherence into routine clinical care. The following curricular components have been recommended: defining adherence; identifying the relationship between adherence and treatment efficacy; assessing adherence; intervening to enhance adherence; and maintaining the therapeutic alliance.[59] National conferences and continuing medical education (CME) programs provide further opportunities to disseminate state-of-the-art interventions and outcomes research.

CONCLUSION

The importance of treatment adherence among patients with psychiatric disorders cannot be over-stated. Adherence increases the likelihood that patients will experience treatment response and remission, thereby reducing the burden of mental illness for patients and health care systems. Improving adherence requires strategies that target multi-factorial barriers. In the clinic setting, practitioners should utilize a collaborative approach with patients and integrate adherence assessment and interventions into all phases of treatment. Brief strategies can be tailored to help patients increase knowledge, motivation, skills, and support for treatment adherence. Practitioner training and CME programs need to increase attention to adherence as an integral part of clinical care and an opportunity to improve patient quality-of-life and optimize health care utilization.[60]

Access the complete reference list and multiple choice questions (MCQs) online at https://expertconsult.inkling.com

KEY REFERENCES

1. Akerblad A-C, Bengtsson F, von Knorring L, et al. Response, remission and relapse in relation to adherence in primary care treatment of depression: a 2-year outcome study. *Int Clin Psychopharmacol* 21:117–124, 2006.
2. Caseiro O, Pérez-Iglesias R, Mata I, et al. Predicting relapse after a first episode of non-affective psychosis: a three-year follow-up study. *J Psychiatr Res* 46:1099–1105, 2012.
4. Taylor S, Abramowitz JS, McKay D. Non-adherence and non-response in the treatment of anxiety disorders. *J Anxiety Disord* 26:583–589, 2012.
5. Gaynes BN, Warden D, Trivedi MH, et al. What did STAR✷D teach us? Results from a large-scale, practical, clinical trial for patients with depression. *FOCUS J Lifelong Learn Psychiatry* 10:510–517, 2012.
6. World Health Organization. Adherence to long-term therapies: evidence for action. Available from: <http://www.who.int/chp/knowledge/publications/adherence_report/en/>; [Cited 2013 Jul 27].
7. Cantrell CR, Eaddy MT, Shah MB, et al. Methods for evaluating patient adherence to antidepressant therapy: a real-world comparison of adherence and economic outcomes. *Med Care* 44:300–303, 2006.
8. Bulloch AGM, Patten SB. Non-adherence with psychotropic medications in the general population. *Soc Psychiatry Psychiatr Epidemiol* 45:47–56, 2010.
11. Liu-Seifert H, Adams DH, Kinon BJ. Discontinuation of treatment of schizophrenic patients is driven by poor symptom response: a pooled post-hoc analysis of four atypical antipsychotic drugs. *BMC Med* 3:21, 2005.
14. Mohr DC, Hart SL, Howard I, et al. Barriers to psychotherapy among depressed and nondepressed primary care patients. *Ann Behav Med Publ Soc Behav Med* 32:254–258, 2006.
16. Katon W, Cantrell CR, Sokol MC, et al. Impact of antidepressant drug adherence on comorbid medication use and resource utilization. *Arch Intern Med* 165:2497–2503, 2005.
17. Alvarez-Jimenez M, Priede A, Hetrick SE, et al. Risk factors for relapse following treatment for first episode psychosis: a systematic review and meta-analysis of longitudinal studies. *Schizophr Res* 139:116–128, 2012.
19. Perkins DO, Johnson JL, Hamer RM, et al. Predictors of antipsychotic medication adherence in patients recovering from a first psychotic episode. *Schizophr Res* 83:53–63, 2006.
24. Ahn J, McCombs JS, Jung C, et al. Classifying patients by antipsychotic adherence patterns using latent class analysis: characteristics of nonadherent groups in the California Medicaid (Medi-Cal) program. *Value Heal J Int Soc Pharmacoeconomics Outcomes Res* 11:48–56, 2008.
25. Jónsdóttir H, Opjordsmoen S, Birkenaes AB, et al. Predictors of medication adherence in patients with schizophrenia and bipolar disorder. *Acta Psychiatr Scand* 127:23–33, 2013.
26. Perkins DO, Gu H, Weiden PJ, et al. Predictors of treatment discontinuation and medication nonadherence in patients recovering from a first episode of schizophrenia, schizophreniform disorder, or schizoaffective disorder: a randomized, double-blind, flexible-dose, multicenter study. *J Clin Psychiatry* 69:106–113, 2008.
30. Byrne N, Regan C, Livingston G. Adherence to treatment in mood disorders. *Curr Opin Psychiatry* 19:44–49, 2006.
34. Teh CF, Sorbero MJ, Mihalyo MJ, et al. Predictors of adequate depression treatment among Medicaid-enrolled adults. *Health Serv Res* 45:302–315, 2010.
36. Wang PS, Schneeweiss S, Brookhart MA, et al. Suboptimal antidepressant use in the elderly. *J Clin Psychopharmacol* 25:118–126, 2005.

47. Velligan DI, Weiden PJ, Sajatovic M, et al. Strategies for addressing adherence problems in patients with serious and persistent mental illness: recommendations from the expert consensus guidelines. *J Psychiatr Pr* 16:306–324, 2010.

50. Vergouwen ACM, Bakker A, Katon WJ, et al. Improving adherence to antidepressants: a systematic review of interventions. *J Clin Psychiatry* 64:1415–1420, 2003.

53. Miller WR, Rollnick S. *Motivational interviewing: helping people change*, New York, 2013, Guilford Press.

54. Safren S, Gonzalez J, Soroudi N. *Coping with chronic illness: a cognitive-behavioral approach for adherence and depression therapist guide*, ed 1, New York, 2007, Oxford University Press.

55. Mohr DC, Ho J, Duffecy J, et al. Perceived barriers to psychological treatments and their relationship to depression. *J Clin Psychol* 66:394–409, 2010.

57. Mohr DC, Ho J, Duffecy J, et al. Effect of telephone-administered vs face-to-face cognitive behavioral therapy on adherence to therapy and depression outcomes among primary care patients: a randomized trial. *JAMA* 307:2278–2285, 2012.

58. Cook PF, Emiliozzi S, Waters C, et al. Effects of telephone counseling on antipsychotic adherence and emergency department utilization. *Am J Manag Care* 14:841–846, 2008.

3

Antidepressants

Maurizio Fava, MD, and George I. Papakostas, MD

KEY POINTS

- The immediate mechanism of action of modern antidepressants ("immediate effects") involves influencing the function of one or more monoamine neurotransmitter systems (serotonin, norepinephrine [noradrenaline], or dopamine).
- Influencing monoaminergic function has been shown to result in several changes in second-messenger systems and gene expression/regulation ("downstream effects").
- "Downstream effects" may explain the delayed onset of antidepressant response seen with all contemporary agents (most patients improve following at least 3 weeks of treatment).
- For the most part, all contemporary antidepressants are equally effective when treating major depressive disorder.
- There are significant differences in the relative tolerability and safety of contemporary antidepressants.

OVERVIEW

A large number of compounds have been developed to treat depression. Traditionally, these compounds have been called "antidepressants," even though most of these drugs are also effective in the treatment of a number of anxiety disorders (such as panic and obsessive-compulsive disorder [OCD]) and a variety of other conditions (Box 3-1). The precursors of two of the major contemporary antidepressant families, the monoamine oxidase inhibitors (MAOIs) and the tricyclic antidepressants (TCAs), were discovered by serendipity in the 1950s.

Specifically, the administration of iproniazid, an antimycobacterial agent, was first noted to possess antidepressant effects in depressed patients suffering from tuberculosis.[1] Shortly thereafter, iproniazid was found to inhibit MAO, which is involved in the catabolism of serotonin, norepinephrine (noradrenaline), and dopamine.

In parallel, imipramine was initially developed as an antihistamine, but Kuhn[2] discovered that of some 500 imipramine-treated patients with various psychiatric disorders, only those with endogenous depression with mental and motor retardation showed a remarkable improvement during 1 to 6 weeks of daily imipramine therapy. The same compound was also found to inhibit the re-uptake of serotonin and norepinephrine.[3,4] Thus, it was the discovery of the antidepressant effects of iproniazid and imipramine that led to the development of the MAOIs and TCAs, and this discovery was instrumental in the formulation of the monoamine theory of depression. In turn, guided by this theory, the subsequent development of compounds selective for the re-uptake of either serotonin or norepinephrine or both was designed, rather than accidental. As a result, over the last few decades, chemical alterations of these first antidepressants have resulted in the creation of a wide variety of monoamine-based antidepressants with a variety of mechanisms of action. The antidepressant drugs are a

heterogeneous group of compounds that have been traditionally subdivided into major groups according to their chemical structure or, more commonly, according to their effects on monoamine neurotransmitter systems: selective serotonin re-uptake inhibitors (SSRIs); TCAs and the related cyclic antidepressants (i.e., amoxapine and maprotiline); MAOIs; serotonin norepinephrine re-uptake inhibitors (SNRIs); norepinephrine re-uptake inhibitors (NRIs); norepinephrine/dopamine re-uptake inhibitors (NDRIs); serotonin receptor antagonists/agonists; and alpha$_2$-adrenergic receptor antagonists. Because they overlap, the mechanisms of action and the indications for use for the antidepressants are discussed together, but separate sections are provided for their method of administration and their side effects.

MECHANISM OF ACTION

The precise mechanisms by which the antidepressant drugs exert their therapeutic effects remain unknown, although much is known about their immediate actions within the nervous system. All of the currently marketed antidepressants interact with the monoamine neurotransmitter systems in the brain, particularly the norepinephrine and serotonin systems, and to a lesser extent the dopamine system. Essentially all currently marketed antidepressants have as their molecular targets components of monoamine synapses, including the re-uptake transporters (that terminate the action of norepinephrine, serotonin, or dopamine in synapses), monoamine receptors, or enzymes that serve to metabolize monoamines. What remains unknown is how these initial interactions produce a therapeutic response.[5] The search for the molecular events that convert altered monoamine neurotransmitter function into the lifting of depressive symptoms remains a matter of very active research.

Since TCAs and MAOIs were the first antidepressants to be discovered and introduced, this was initially interpreted as suggesting that antidepressants work by increasing noradrenergic or serotonergic neurotransmission, thus compensating for a postulated state of relative monoamine "deficiency." However, this simple theory could not fully explain the action of antidepressant drugs for a number of reasons. The most important of these include the lack of convincing evidence that depression is characterized by a state of inadequate or "deficient" monoamine neurotransmission. In fact, the results of studies testing the monoamine depletion hypothesis in depression have yielded inconsistent results.[5] Moreover, blockade of monoamine re-uptake or inhibition of monoamine degradation occurs rapidly (within hours) following monoamine re-uptake inhibitor or MAOI administration, respectively. However, treatment with antidepressants for less than 2 weeks is unlikely to result in a significant lifting of depression; it has been consistently observed and reported that remission of depression often requires 4 weeks of treatment or more. These considerations have led to the idea that inhibition of monoamine re-uptake or inhibition of MAO by antidepressants represents an initiating event. The actual therapeutic actions of antidepressants, however, result from slower adaptive responses within neurons to these initial biochemical perturbations ("downstream events").[6] Although research geared toward understanding the therapeutic actions of antidepressants has been challenging, receptor studies have been useful in

BOX 3-1 Possible Indications for Antidepressants

- Major depressive disorder and other unipolar depressive disorders
- Bipolar depression
- Panic disorder
- Social anxiety disorder
- Generalized anxiety disorder
- Post-traumatic stress disorder
- Obsessive-compulsive disorder (e.g., clomipramine and SSRIs)
- Depression with psychotic features (in combination with an antipsychotic drug)
- Bulimia nervosa
- Neuropathic pain (tricyclic drugs and SNRIs)
- Insomnia (e.g., trazodone, amitriptyline)
- Enuresis (imipramine best studied)
- Atypical depression (e.g., monoamine oxidase inhibitors)
- Attention-deficit/hyperactivity disorder (e.g., desipramine, bupropion)

SNRIs, Serotonin norepinephrine re-uptake inhibitors; SSRIs, selective serotonin re-uptake inhibitors.

by catechol O-methyltransferase (COMT), an enzyme that acts extracellularly.

The classification of antidepressant drugs has perhaps focused too narrowly on synaptic pharmacology (i.e., "immediate effects"), and has certainly failed to take into account molecular and cellular changes in neural function that are brought about by the chronic administration of these agents.[5] For example, it has been postulated that changes in post-receptor signal transduction may account for the aforementioned characteristic lag-time between the time a drug is administered and the drug-induced resolution of a depressive episode. In fact, studies have shown that hippocampal neurogenesis occurs following chronic antidepressant treatment in animal models.[8] In parallel, rapid activation of the TrkB neurotrophin receptor and PLC gamma-1 signaling has been described with almost all antidepressant drugs, a possible mechanism by which the process of neuronal neurogenesis observed following chronic administration of antidepressants may occur.[9] Alternatively, one could postulate that this lag phase in antidepressant action may be related to a re-organization of neuronal networks, postulated as a potential "final common pathway" for antidepressant effects to occur.[5] Nevertheless, further research is urgently needed in order to help us understand the specific effects of the antidepressants and what constitutes illness and recovery in depression.

Mechanism of Action of Selective Serotonin Re-uptake Inhibitors

At therapeutically relevant doses, the SSRIs exhibit significant effects primarily on serotonin re-uptake in the human brain.[10] Some SSRIs also appear to have effects on other monoamine transporters, with sertraline demonstrating modest dopamine re-uptake inhibition, and paroxetine and fluoxetine demonstrating modest norepinephrine re-uptake inhibition.[10] In addition, fluoxetine, particularly the R-isomer, has mild 5-HT$_{2A}$ and 5-HT$_{2C}$ antagonist activity. Non-monoaminergic effects have also been described for some of the SSRIs, including moderate and selective effects on glutamate receptor expression and editing.[11] The SSRIs have minimal or no affinity for muscarinic cholinergic, histaminergic, and adrenergic receptors, with the exception of paroxetine (which is a weak cholinergic receptor antagonist), citalopram (which is a weak antagonist of the histamine H$_1$ receptor), and sertraline (which has weak affinity for the alpha$_1$ receptors).[10] Overall, the affinity of these agents for these specific receptors is lower than those of the TCAs, resulting in a milder side-effect profile. Similarly, the lack of significant action for the remaining SSRIs on these receptors is also thought to contribute to the milder side-effect profile of these agents compared with the TCAs.

Mechanism of Action of Serotonin Norepinephrine Re-uptake Inhibitors

Unlike the TCAs, SNRIs inhibit the re-uptake of serotonin more potently than the re-uptake of norepinephrine.[10] Similar to most SSRIs, the SNRIs have minimal or no affinity for muscarinic cholinergic, histaminergic, and adrenergic receptors.[10] Interestingly enough, administration of these drugs has been shown to prevent a decrease in cell proliferation and BDNF expression in rat hippocampus observed with chronic stress, in a study that offers further insights into the "downstream effects" of these agents.[12] In parallel, studies suggest that chronic treatment with the SNRI duloxetine not only produces a marked up-regulation of BDNF mRNA and protein but may also affect the sub-cellular re-distribution of neurotrophin, potentially improving synaptic plasticity.[13]

understanding and predicting some of the side effects of contemporary antidepressants. For example, the binding affinity of antidepressants at muscarinic cholinergic receptors generally parallels the prevalence of certain side effects during treatment (e.g., dry mouth, constipation, urinary hesitancy, poor concentration). Similarly, treatment with agents that have high affinities for histamine H$_1$ receptors (e.g., doxepin and amitriptyline) appears to be more likely to result in sedation, and increased appetite. Such information is very useful to clinicians and patients when making treatment decisions or to researchers when attempting to develop new antidepressants.

The architecture of the monoamine neurotransmitter systems in the central nervous system (CNS) is based on the synthesis of the neurotransmitter within a restricted number of nuclei within the brainstem, with neurons projecting widely throughout the brain and, for norepinephrine and serotonin, the spinal cord as well.[5] Norepinephrine is synthesized within a series of nuclei in the medulla and pons, of which the largest is the nucleus locus coeruleus. Serotonin is synthesized in the brainstem raphe nuclei. Dopamine is synthesized in the substantia nigra and the ventral tegmental area of the midbrain. Through extensive projection networks, these neurotransmitters influence a large number of target neurons in the cerebral cortex, basal forebrain, striatum, limbic system, and brainstem, where they interact with multiple receptor types to regulate arousal, vigilance, attention, sensory processing, emotion, and cognition (including memory).[7]

Norepinephrine, serotonin, and dopamine are removed from synapses after release by re-uptake, mostly into pre-synaptic neurons.[5] This mechanism of terminating neurotransmitter action is mediated by specific norepinephrine, serotonin, and dopamine re-uptake transporter proteins. After re-uptake, norepinephrine, serotonin, and dopamine are either re-loaded into vesicles for subsequent release or broken down by MAO. MAO is present in two forms (MAO$_A$ and MAO$_B$), which differ in their substrate preferences, inhibitor specificities, tissue expression, and cell distribution. MAO$_A$ preferentially oxidizes serotonin and is irreversibly inactivated by low concentrations of the acetylenic inhibitor clorgyline. MAO$_B$ preferentially oxidizes phenylethylamine (PEA) and benzylamine and is irreversibly inactivated by low concentrations of pargyline and deprenyl.[5] Dopamine, tyramine, and tryptamine are substrates for both forms of MAO. Catecholamines are also broken down

Mechanism of Action of Norepinephrine Re-uptake Inhibitors

At therapeutically relevant doses, the NRIs have significant effects primarily on norepinephrine re-uptake, although the NRI atomoxetine is also a weak inhibitor of serotonin uptake.[14] NRIs also appear to have several non-monoaminergic properties. Specifically, the NRI reboxetine also appears to functionally inhibit nicotinic acetylcholine receptors.[15] In addition, in rats, atomoxetine has been shown to increase *in vivo* extracellular levels of acetylcholine (ACh) in cortical but not subcortical brain regions, with a mechanism dependent on norepinephrine alpha$_1$ and/or dopamine D$_1$ receptor activation.[16] Furthermore, the major human metabolite of atomoxetine (4-hydroxyatomoxetine) is a partial agonist of the kappa-opioid receptor.[17] Finally, reboxetine has also been found to be the antidepressant that affects glutamate receptors (GluR) most, with a decrease of GluR3 expression.[11]

Mechanism of Action of Serotonin Receptor Agonist/Antagonists

Both trazodone and nefazodone are relatively weak inhibitors of serotonin and norepinephrine uptake, and they primarily block serotonin 5-HT$_{2A}$ receptors (in some cases, demonstrating partial agonist properties as well).[18–21] They also share a metabolite, m-chlorophenylpiperazine (mCPP), which acts as a serotonin 5-HT$_{2C}$ agonist and appears to be able to release serotonin pre-synaptically.[22] Trazodone also appears to stimulate the mu$_1$- and mu$_2$-opioid receptors[23] and is a potent agonist of the serotonin 5-HT$_{2C}$ receptors, which, when activated,[24,25] may inhibit NMDA-induced cyclic GMP elevation. Since trazodone is also a weak inhibitor of serotonin re-uptake as well, the overall effect of trazodone appears to be an increase in extracellular levels of serotonin in the brain.[26] This effect explains the fact that trazodone treatment has been associated with the occurrence of a serotonin syndrome.[27] Both trazodone and (although to a lesser degree) nefazodone are potent blockers of the alpha$_1$-adrenergic receptor.

Agomelatine, available in Europe as an antidepressant, is a selective 5-HT$_{2C}$ antagonist and acts as a melatonin MT$_1$ and MT$_2$ receptor agonist. The 5-HT$_{2C}$ antagonism properties of agomelatine have been thought to be responsible for increases in frontocortical dopaminergic and adrenergic activity in animals during administration of agomelatine.[28]

Buspirone and gepirone act as full agonists at serotonin 5-HT$_{1A}$ autoreceptors and are generally, but not exclusively, partial agonists at post-synaptic serotonin 5-HT$_{1A}$ receptors.[29] Neither buspirone or gepirone are approved for depression, but buspirone is FDA-approved for the treatment of anxiety. Buspirone and gepirone show weak alpha$_1$-adrenoceptor affinity, but significant and selective alpha$_1$-adrenoceptor intrinsic efficacy, which was expressed in a tissue- and species-dependent manner.[30] Buspirone also shows binding with high affinity to recombinant human D$_3$ and D$_4$ receptors (~98 and ~29 nm respectively).[31] Buspirone and gepirone are thought to lead to excitation of noradrenergic cell firing,[32] antagonizing primarily pre-synaptic inhibitory dopamine D$_2$ autoreceptors at dopaminergic neurons.[33] Buspirone also has potent alpha$_2$-adrenoceptor antagonist properties via its principal metabolite, 1-(2-pyrimidinyl)-piperazine.[34,35] Vilazodone is a serotonin 5-HT$_{1A}$ receptor partial agonist and a selective serotonin re-uptake inhibitor that induces maximal serotonin levels that are similar in the medial and the lateral cortex and are up to six-fold higher than those induced by SSRIs tested in parallel, when serotonin levels are measured in two sub-regions of the rat prefrontal cortex by microdialysis.[36] It

appears that the net effect of vilazodone at release-regulating 5-HT$_{1A}$ autoreceptors is inhibitory, leading to markedly increased serotonin output.

Vortioxetine is a recently-approved antidepressant with multi-modal activity that functions as a serotonin 5-HT$_3$, 5-HT$_7$ and 5-HT$_{1D}$ receptor antagonist, serotonin 5-HT$_{1B}$ receptor partial agonist, serotonin 5-HT$_{1A}$ receptor agonist and inhibitor of the serotonin transporter *in vitro*.[37] Vortioxetine has shown to be able to increase extracellular serotonin, dopamine, and norepinephrine in the medial prefrontal cortex and ventral hippocampus,[38] and to significantly increase cell proliferation and cell survival and stimulate maturation of immature granule cells in the sub-granular zone of the dentate gyrus of the hippocampus after 21 days of treatment.[37]

Mechanism of Action of Norepinephrine/ Dopamine Re-uptake Inhibitors

The NDRIs primarily block the re-uptake of dopamine and norepinephrine and have minimal or no affinity for pre-synaptic or post-synaptic monoamine receptors. The mechanism of action of bupropion has not been fully elucidated, although it appears to primarily block the re-uptake of both dopamine and norepinephrine.[39] Bupropion and its metabolites have been shown to be able to inhibit striatal uptake of the selective dopamine transporter (DAT)-binding radioligand (11)C-betaCIT-FE *in vivo*,[40] and to have mild affinity for the norepinephrine transporter,[41] although some researchers have argued that the effect of bupropion on norepinephrine is primarily through an increase in pre-synaptic norepinephrine release.[42] Whatever the exact mechanism may be, it appears that the overall effect of bupropion is a dose-dependent increase in brain extracellular dopamine and norepinephrine concentrations.[43] It also appears that bupropion acts as an antagonist at alpha$_3$beta$_2$ and alpha$_3$beta$_4$ nAChRs in rat striatum and hippocampus, respectively, across the same concentration range that inhibits DAT and norepinephrine transporter (NET) function.[44]

Mechanism of Action of Alpha$_2$-Adrenergic Receptor Antagonists

The alpha$_2$-adrenergic receptor antagonists (e.g., mirtazapine and mianserin) appear to enhance the release of both serotonin and norepinephrine by blocking auto- and hetero-alpha$_2$ receptors.[45] Since mirtazapine appears to be a blocker of serotonin 5-HT$_2$ and 5-HT$_3$ receptors as well, it is thought to enhance the release of norepinephrine and also enhance 5-HT$_{1A}$–mediated serotonergic transmission.[46] Mirtazapine was the first alpha$_2$-adrenergic receptor antagonist to be approved by the Food and Drug Administration (FDA) for depression. Mirtazapine is also a potent histaminergic H$_1$-receptor antagonist.[10] Mianserin, also an alpha$_2$-noradrenergic receptor antagonist and a serotonin 5-HT$_2$ antagonist, is available in Europe and is not FDA-approved.

Mechanism of Action of Tricyclic Antidepressants

TCAs, referred to as such because they share a chemical structure with two joined benzene rings, have been in use for almost half a century for the treatment of depression. With the exception of clomipramine, and in contrast with the SNRIs, the TCAs inhibit the re-uptake of norepinephrine more potently than the re-uptake of serotonin. Recent studies have also shown that five of the TCAs bind to the S1S2 domain of the GluR2 subunit of the AMPA receptor, suggesting an effect of TCAs on the glutamergic system.[47] In addition, doxepin, amitriptyline, and nortriptyline also inhibit glycine uptake by blocking the glycine transporter 1b ($GLYT_{1b}$) and glycine transporter 2a ($GLYT_{2a}$) to a similar extent.[48] Amoxapine displays a selective inhibition of $GLYT_{2a}$ behaving as a 10-fold more efficient inhibitor of this isoform than of $GLYT_{1b}$[48] and is also a dopamine D_2 receptor antagonist.[49] Interestingly, *in vitro* data suggest that trimipramine and clomipramine have comparable affinity for the dopamine D_2 receptor.[50] The TCAs, to varying degrees, are also fairly potent blockers of histamine H_1 receptors, serotonin 5-HT_2 receptors, muscarinic acetylcholine receptors, and alpha$_1$-adrenergic receptors.[10,50]

Mechanism of Action of Monoamine Oxidase Inhibitors

MAOIs act by inhibiting MAO, an enzyme found on the outer membrane of mitochondria, where it catabolizes (degrades) a number of monoamines including dopamine, norepinephrine, and serotonin. Specifically, following their re-uptake from the synapse into the pre-synaptic neuron, norepinephrine, serotonin, and dopamine are either loaded into vesicles for subsequent re-release or broken down by MAO. MAO is present in two forms (MAO_A and MAO_B), which differ in their substrate preferences, inhibitor specificities, tissue expression, and cell distribution. MAO_A preferentially oxidizes serotonin and is irreversibly inactivated by low concentrations of the acetylenic inhibitor clorgyline. MAO_B preferentially oxidizes phenylethylamine (PEA) and benzylamine and is irreversibly inactivated by low concentrations of pargyline and deprenyl. Dopamine and the dietary (exogenous) amines, tyramine and tryptamine, are substrates for *both* forms of MAO.[51] In the gastrointestinal (GI) tract and the liver, MAO catabolizes a number of dietary pressor amines (such as dopamine, tyramine, tryptamine, and phenylethylamine).[52] For this reason, consumption of certain foods (that contain high levels of dietary amines) while on an MAOI may precipitate a hypertensive crisis, characterized by hypertension, hyperpyrexia, tachycardia, tremulousness, and cardiac arrhythmias.[53] The same reaction may also occur during co-administration of dopaminergic agents and MAOIs, while the co-administration of MAOIs with other antidepressants that potentiate serotonin could result in serotonin syndromes due to toxic CNS serotonin levels. The serotonin syndrome is characterized by alterations in cognition (e.g., disorientation and confusion), behavior (e.g., agitation and restlessness), autonomic nervous system function (e.g., fever, shivering, diaphoresis, and diarrhea), and neuromuscular activity (e.g., ataxia, hyperreflexia, and myoclonus).[54-56] Since MAO enzymatic activity requires approximately 14 days to be fully restored, such food or medications should be avoided for 2 weeks following the discontinuation of an irreversible MAOI ("MAOI washout period"). Serotonergic and dopaminergic antidepressants are typically discontinued 2 weeks before the initiation of an MAOI, with the exception of fluoxetine, which needs to be discontinued 5 weeks in advance because of its much longer half-life.

Older MAOIs, including phenelzine, tranylcypromine, and isocarboxazid, irreversibly inhibit the enzymatic activity of both MAO_A and MAO_B, while newer ones are relatively selective (brofaromine and moclobemide preferentially inhibit MAO_A; oral selegiline selectively inhibits MAO_B). Reversible MAO_A-selective inhibitors are designed to minimize the risk of hypertensive crises, and patients on conventional doses of moclobemide do not need to strictly adhere to the low-tyramine diet, although, at very high doses (e.g., 900 mg/day of moclobemide), inhibition of MAO_B also occurs.[57] All MAOIs available in the US are irreversible inhibitors of MAO_A and MAO_B activity.

More recently, additional pharmacological properties for the MAOIs have been revealed. MAOIs, for instance, also appear to inhibit the binding of [3H] quinpirole, a dopamine agonist with high affinity for D_2 and D_3 dopamine receptors.[58,59] To complicate the pharmacology of MAOIs further, two of the MAOIs, selegiline and tranylcypromine, have methamphetamine and amphetamine as metabolites.[60,61] In addition, phenelzine also elevates brain gamma-aminobutyric acid (GABA) levels, and as yet unidentified metabolites of phenelzine may be responsible for this effect.[61] R(−)- but not S(+)- selegiline also appears to induce dopamine release by directly modulating ATP-sensitive potassium channels.[62] Finally, (+)-tranylcypromine (TCP) has been shown to be more potent than (−)-TCP as an inhibitor of 5-HT uptake, whereas (−)-TCP has been shown to be more potent than (+)-TCP as an inhibitor of dopamine and norepinephrine uptake.[63]

Although the risk for serotonin syndromes may be lower than with the older MAOIs, and a number of studies suggested the safety of combining moclobemide with SSRIs,[64-66] there have been a number of non-fatal[67,68] and fatal serotonin syndromes involving the co-administration of moclobemide and SSRIs.[69-74] For these reasons, the concomitant use of moclobemide and serotonergic agents should be avoided. In addition, the co-ingestion of moclobemide and SSRIs in overdose may result in death, which needs to be taken into account for patients at risk for suicide.[70]

CLINICAL USES OF ANTIDEPRESSANTS

Since the introduction of fluoxetine, the SSRIs and the SNRIs have become the most often prescribed initial pharmacological treatment for major depressive disorder (MDD). The success of these newer agents in displacing TCAs as first-choice agents is not based on established differences in efficacy, but rather on a generally more favorable side-effect profile (such as a lack of anticholinergic and cardiac side effects, and a high therapeutic index, i.e., the ratio of lethal dose to therapeutic dose), combined with ease of administration. Furthermore, with certain co-morbidities of depression (such as OCD), SSRIs offer advantages in efficacy over the TCAs. Nonetheless, the TCAs remain useful alternatives for the treatment of some patients with depression. In contrast, because of their inferior safety profile, the traditional MAOIs are a class of drugs reserved for patients in whom other treatments have failed. Clearly, the newer antidepressants (SSRIs, SNRIs, NRIs, NDRIs, and serotonin receptor antagonists) all have major safety or tolerability advantages over the TCAs and MAOIs. The recently-approved serotonin receptor antagonist vortioxetine may have the additional advantage of distinctive pro-cognitive effects.

Continuation and Maintenance of Antidepressant Treatment

Originally, based on studies with TCAs, patients with unipolar depressive disorders were observed to be at high risk for relapse when treatment was discontinued within the first 16 weeks of therapy. Therefore, in treatment-responders, most experts favor a continuation of antidepressant therapy for a minimum of 6 months following the achievement of remission. The value of continuation therapy for several months to prevent relapse into the original episode has also been established for virtually all of the newer agents.[75] Risk of recurrence after this 6- to 8-month continuation period (i.e., the development of a new episode after recovery from the index episode) is particularly elevated in patients with a chronic course before recovery, residual symptoms, and multiple prior episodes (three or more).[76] For these individuals, the optimal duration of maintenance treatment is unknown, but is assumed to be much longer (measured in years). In fact, based on research to date, prophylactic efficacy of an antidepressant has been observed for as long as 5 years with clear benefit.[77] In contrast to the initial expectation that maintenance therapy would be effective at dosages lower than that required for acute treatment, the current consensus is that full-dose therapy is required for effective prophylaxis.[78] About 20% to 30% of patients who are treated with each of the classes of antidepressants will experience a return of depressive symptoms despite continued treatment. In such patients, a dose increase of the antidepressant is typically the first-line approach.[79]

Suicide Risk

Unlike the SSRIs and other newer agents, the MAOIs, TCAs, and related cyclic antidepressants (maprotiline and amoxapine) are potentially lethal in overdose. Thus, a careful evaluation of impulsiveness and suicide risk influences not only the decision as to the need for hospitalizing a person with depression but also the choice of an antidepressant. For potentially suicidal or highly impulsive patients, the SSRIs and the other newer agents would be a better initial choice than a cyclic compound or an MAOI. Patients at elevated suicide risk who cannot tolerate these safer compounds or who do not respond to them should not receive large quantities or refillable prescriptions for TCAs or MAOIs. Generally, patients who are new to treatment or those at more than minimal risk for suicide or whose therapeutic relationship is unstable should receive a limited supply of any medication. Evaluation for suicide risk must continue even after the initiation of treatment. Although suicidal thoughts are often among the first symptoms to improve with antidepressant treatment, they may also be slow to respond to treatment, and patients may become demoralized before therapeutic efficacy is evident. Side effects (such as agitation and restlessness) and, most important, inter-current life events may exacerbate suicidal thoughts before a full therapeutic response. Thus, rarely, for a variety of reasons, patients may temporarily become more suicidal following the initiation of treatment. Should such worsening occur, appropriate interventions may include management of side effects, more frequent monitoring, discontinuation of the initial treatment, or hospitalization. In 2004, the FDA asked manufacturers of almost all the newer antidepressant drugs to include in their labeling a warning statement that recommends close observation of adult and pediatric patients treated with these drugs for worsening depression or the emergence of suicidality. This warning was based on the analyses of clinical trials data that compared the relative risk of emergence of suicidal ideation on these drugs compared to placebo following initiation of treatment. The difference was small, but statistically significant. This finding underscores the need for good practice, which includes education of patients (and families if the patient is a child) about side effects of drugs (including the possible emergence of suicidal thoughts and behaviors), close monitoring (especially early in treatment), and the availability of a clinician in case suicidality emerges or worsens. A general consensus remains, however, that the risks associated with withholding antidepressant treatment from patients, including pediatric patients, with serious depression vastly outweighs the risks associated with the drugs by many orders of magnitude.

CHOICE OF AN ANTIDEPRESSANT

A large number of antidepressants are available (Table 3-1), including SSRIs, SNRIs, NRIs, NDRIs, serotonin receptor antagonists/agonists, the alpha2-adrenergic receptor antagonists, TCAs and related compounds, and MAOIs. The available formulations and their typical dosages are listed in Table 3-1, and aspects of their successful use are listed in Box 3-2.

Selective Serotonin Re-uptake Inhibitors

The overall efficacy of the SSRIs in the treatment of depression is equivalent to that of older agents, including the TCAs and the MAOIs moclobemide[80] and phenelzine,[81] while all SSRIs appear to be equally effective in the treatment of depression.[82] However, there is some evidence suggesting that that the SSRI escitalopram may be more effective than the remaining five SSRIs in the treatment of MDD,[83] although this evidence remains controversial.

Because of their favorable side-effect profile, the SSRIs are used as first-line treatment in the overwhelming majority of cases, with more than 90% of clinicians in one survey indicating that SSRIs were their first-line treatment.[84] Despite the tolerability and the widespread efficacy of the SSRIs, there is mounting evidence to suggest that depressed patients with certain characteristics (including co-morbid anxiety disorders[85] and a greater number of somatic symptoms [such as pain, headaches, and fatigue][86]) respond less well to SSRIs than those without such characteristics.

TABLE 3-1A Available Preparations of Antidepressants: Selective Serotonin Re-uptake Inhibitors (SSRIs)

Drug	Therapeutic Dosage Forms	Usual Daily Dose (mg/day)	Extreme Dosage (mg/day)	Plasma Levels (ng/ml)
Fluoxetine (Prozac and generics)	C: 10, 20, 40 mg LC: 20 mg/5 ml Weekly: 90 mg	20–40	5–80	
Fluvoxamine (Luvox and generics)*	T: 50, 100 mg	50–150	50–300	
Paroxetine (Paxil and generics)	T: 10, 20, 30, 40 mg LC: 10 mg/5 ml CR: 12.5, 25, 37.5 mg	20–40 25–50	10–50 12.5–50	
Sertraline (Zoloft and generics)	T: 25, 50, 100 mg LC: 20 mg/ml	50–150	25–300	
Citalopram (Celexa and generics)	T: 10, 20, 40 mg LC: 10 mg/5 ml	20–40	10–60	
Escitalopram (Lexapro and generics)	T: 10, 20 mg	10–20	10–30	

*Not marketed for depression in the US.
C, Capsules; CR, controlled release; LC, liquid concentrate or solution; T, tablets.

TABLE 3-1B Available Preparations of Antidepressants: Serotonin Norepinephrine Re-uptake Inhibitors (SNRIs)

Drug	Therapeutic Dosage Forms	Usual Daily Dose (mg/day)	Extreme Dosage (mg/day)	Plasma Levels (ng/ml)
Venlafaxine (Effexor and generics)	T: 25, 37.5, 50, 75, 100 mg XR: 37.5, 75, 150 mg	75–300	75–450	
Duloxetine (Cymbalta and generics)	C: 20, 30, 60 mg	60–120	30–180	
Desvenlafaxine (Pristiq)	T: 50, 100 mg	50–100	25–200	
Levomilnacipran ER (Fetzima)	C: 20, 40, 80, 120 mg	40–120	20–240	

C, Capsules; T, tablets; XR, extended-release.

TABLE 3-1C Available Preparations of Antidepressants: Norepinephrine Re-uptake Inhibitors (NRIs)

Drug	Therapeutic Dosage Forms	Usual Daily Dose (mg/day)	Extreme Dosage (mg/day)	Plasma Levels (ng/ml)
Reboxetine*	T: 4 mg	4–10	4–12	
Atomoxetine (Strattera)	T: 10, 18, 25, 40, 60 mg	40–80	40–120	

*Not marketed for depression in the US.
T, tablets.

TABLE 3-1D Available Preparations of Antidepressants: Serotonin Receptor Antagonists/Agonists

Drug	Therapeutic Dosage Forms	Usual Daily Dose (mg/day)	Extreme Dosage (mg/day)	Plasma Levels (ng/ml)
Trazodone (Desyrel and generics)	T: 50, 100, 150, 300 mg	200–400	100–600	
Trazodone Extended Release (Oleptro)	T: 150, 300 mg	150–300	75–600	
Nefazodone (Serzone and generics)	T: 50, 100, 150, 200, 250 mg	200–400	100–600	
Vilazodone (Viibryd)	T: 10, 20, 40 mg	40–80	20–160	
Vortioxetine (Brintellix)	T: 5, 10, 20 mg	10–20	5–40	

T, tablets.

TABLE 3-1E Available Preparations of Antidepressants: Norepinephrine Dopamine Re-uptake Inhibitors (NDRIs)

Drug	Therapeutic Dosage Forms	Usual Daily Dose (mg/day)	Extreme Dosage (mg/day)	Plasma Levels (ng/ml)
Bupropion (Wellbutrin and generics)	T: 75, 100 mg XR: 100, 150, 200 mg XL: 150, 300 mg Soltabs: 15, 30, 45 mg	200–300	100–450	

Soltabs, orally disintegrating tablet; T, tablets; XL, extended-release; XR, extended-release.

TABLE 3-1F Available Preparations of Antidepressants: Alpha$_2$-receptor Antagonists

Drug	Therapeutic Dosage Forms	Usual Daily Dose (mg/day)	Extreme Dosage (mg/day)	Plasma Levels (ng/ml)
Mirtazapine (Remeron and generics)	T: 15, 30, 45 mg Soltabs: 15, 30, 45 mg	15–45	7.5–90	

Soltabs, orally disintegrating tablet; T, tablets.

Dosage

Because of their relatively low side-effect burden, the starting dose of SSRIs is often the minimally effective daily dose: 10 mg for escitalopram (Lexapro); 20 mg for fluoxetine (Prozac), paroxetine (Paxil), and citalopram (Celexa); 50 mg for sertraline (Zoloft); 25 mg for paroxetine CR (Paxil CR); and 100 mg for fluvoxamine (Luvox). Starting at lower doses and increasing the dose shortly thereafter (i.e., after 1 to 2 weeks) may further improve tolerability. Maximum therapeutic doses for SSRIs are typically one-fold to four-fold greater than the starting dose. The dosages and formulations of the SSRIs marketed in the US are listed in Table 3-1. Only one of the SSRIs, fluvoxamine, is not approved for the treatment

TABLE 3-1G Available Preparations of Antidepressants: Tricyclic Antidepressants (TCAs) and Other Cyclic Compounds

Drug	Therapeutic Dosage Forms	Usual Daily Dose (mg/day)	Extreme Dosage (mg/day)	Plasma Levels (ng/ml)
Imipramine (Tofranil and generics)	T: 10, 25, 50 mg C: 75, 100, 125, 150 mg INJ: 25 mg/2 ml	150–200	50–300	>225*
Desipramine (Norpramin and generics)	T: 10, 25, 50, 75, 100, 150 mg C: 25, 50 mg	150–200	50–300	>125
Amitriptyline (Elavil and generics)	T: 10, 25, 50, 75, 100, 150 mg INJ: 10 mg/ml	150–200	50–300	>120†
Nortriptyline (Pamelor and generics)	C: 10, 25, 50, 75 mg LC: 10 mg/5 ml	75–100	25–150	50–150
Doxepin (Adapin, Sinequan, and generics)	C: 10, 25, 50, 75, 100, 150 mg LC: 10 mg/ml	150–200	25–300	100–250
Trimipramine (Surmontil and generics)	C: 25, 50, 100 mg	150–200	50–300	
Protriptyline (Vivactil and generics)	T: 5, 10 mg	10–40	10–60	
Maprotiline (Ludiomil and generics)	T: 25, 50, 75 mg	100–150	50–200	
Amoxapine (Asendin and generics)	T: 25, 50, 100, 150 mg	150–200	50–300	
Clomipramine (Anafranil and generics)	C: 25, 50, 75 mg	150–200	50–250	

*Sum of imipramine plus desipramine.
†Sum of amitriptyline plus nortriptyline.
C, Capsules; INJ, injectable form; LC, liquid concentrate or solution; T, tablets.

TABLE 3-1H Available Preparations of Antidepressants: Monoamine Oxidase Inhibitors (MAOIs)

Drug	Therapeutic Dosage Forms	Usual Daily Dose (mg/day)	Extreme Dosage (mg/day)	Plasma Levels (ng/ml)
Phenelzine (Nardil and generics)	T: 15 mg	45–60	15–90	
Tranylcypromine (Parnate and generics)	T: 10 mg	30–50	10–90	
Isocarboxazid (Marplan and generics)	T: 10 mg	30–50	30–90	
Selegiline Transdermal System (patch) (Emsam)	P: 6, 9, 12/day	6–12	6–18	

T, tablets.

BOX 3-2 Requirements for Successful Use of Antidepressants

1. Good patient selection as determined by a thorough and comprehensive diagnostic evaluation. In particular, attention should be paid to co-morbid psychiatric and medical disorders.
2. Choice of a drug with an acceptable side-effect profile for the given patient.
3. Adequate dosage. In the absence of side effects and response, dose escalations within the recommended range should be pursued aggressively.
4. Use of the antidepressant for at least 6–12 weeks to determine whether it is helping or not.
5. Consideration of drug side effects. Although there are some differences in efficacy across the class of antidepressants for sutypes of depression, the major clinically significant differences among the antidepressants are in their side effects.
6. Use of a drug that was clearly effective in the past if it was well tolerated by the patient.
7. Selection of an appropriate agent for patients with initial insomnia, for example, a sedating secondary amine TCA (e.g., nortriptyline) given at bedtime (a strategy used by some clinicians), avoidance of agents with anticholinergic and cardiovascular side effects (therefore, the sleep-enhancing, alpha$_2$-adrenergic receptor antagonist mirtazapine would be preferred, with the expectation that daytime sedation will abate over time with these medications). An alternative to prescribing a sedating antidepressant is the temporary use of a short-acting benzodiazepine or other hypnotic combined with an SSRI or another non-sedating newer antidepressant, with the expectation of tapering and discontinuing the hypnotic when the depression has improved. Trazodone at lower doses (50–300 mg at bedtime) has been used in place of benzodiazepines or other hypnotics to treat insomnia, particularly middle to late insomnia, in patients treated for depression with an SSRI.
8. Consideration of effects on sexual function. In particular, decreased libido, delayed orgasm or anorgasmia, arousal difficulties, and erectile dysfunction have been reported with almost all of the classes of antidepressants.
9. Awareness of co-morbid conditions. The co-morbid disorder should influence initial treatment selection in choosing an agent thought to be efficacious for the co-morbid condition, as well as the depression, as with SSRIs and OCD or the NDRI bupropion and attention-deficit disorder.
10. Consideration of metabolic effects on drug levels and elimination half-life. The elderly may have alterations in hepatic metabolic pathways, especially so-called phase I reactions, which include demethylation and hydroxylation, which are involved in the metabolism of both SSRIs and cyclic antidepressants. In addition, renal function may be decreased, and there may be increased end-organ sensitivity to the effects of antidepressant compounds. Because the elimination half-life of antidepressants can be expected to be significantly greater than what it is in younger patients, accumulation of active drug will be greater and occur more slowly. Clinically this means that the elderly should be started on lower doses, that dosage increases should be slower, and that the ultimate therapeutic dose may be lower than in younger patients.

NDRI, Norepinephrine/dopamine re-uptake inhibitor; OCD, obsessive-compulsive disorder; SSRI, selective serotonin re-uptake inhibitor.

of depression in the US, as it is approved only for the treatment of OCD, although several placebo-controlled trials have demonstrated the efficacy of fluvoxamine in MDD.[87,88]

Side-effect Profile

The most common side effects of the SSRIs are nausea, tremor, excessive sweating, flushing, headache, insomnia, activation or sedation, jitteriness, dizziness, rash, and dry mouth.[89] Sedation does not appear to occur more often with any particular SSRI, while the SSRIs appear to be equally well tolerated and effective in the treatment of depressed patients, regardless of whether they cause insomnia, activation, or sedation.[82] The use of SSRIs is also associated with the emergence of sexual dysfunction (including decreased libido, delayed ejaculation, impotence, and anorgasmia), or the worsening of pre-existing sexual dysfunction in depression.[90] These side effects tend to improve rapidly after temporary ("drug holiday") discontinuation of the SSRIs, particularly those SSRIs with a shorter half-life,[91] although prolonging such drug holidays carries a risk of withdrawal effects and of depressive relapse. Some patients treated with SSRIs may also experience cognitive symptoms (such as mental slowing and worsened attention), psychological symptoms (such as apathy and emotional blunting),[92] and motor symptoms (such as bruxism and akathisia).[93,94] Other, less common, adverse events associated with SSRI treatment include diarrhea, tremor, bruxism, rash, hyponatremia, hair loss, and the syndrome of inappropriate antidiuretic hormone (SIADH) secretion. There are also case reports of the SSRIs worsening motor symptoms in patients with Parkinson's disease,[95–97] as well as creating increased requirements for levodopa in Parkinson's patients following initiation of an SSRI for depression.[98] SSRIs have been associated with abnormal bleeding (e.g., bruising and epistaxis) in children and adults who have unremarkable routine hematological laboratory results, except for abnormal bleeding time or platelet counts.[99] A systematic study of this issue has failed to reveal abnormalities in platelet aggregation, hematopoiesis, or coagulation profile in SSRI-treated patients.[100] Although many patients may also experience reduced appetite and weight loss during the acute phase of treatment with SSRIs,[101,102] any beneficial effects of the SSRIs with respect to weight loss do not seem to be sustained during the continuation and maintenance phases of treatment,[101,102] while one study reveals a greater risk for significant weight gain during long-term treatment with paroxetine, but not fluoxetine or sertraline.[103] Although SSRI-induced side effects appear to be well tolerated by most patients,[104] for depressed patients who are unable to tolerate one SSRI, switching to another SSRI has been effective and well tolerated in most cases.[105–108] For patients complaining of GI side effects with paroxetine, the continued-release formulation (Paxil CR), reported to have a lower incidence of nausea, may be used in place of the standard formulation.[109] As with other antidepressants, the potential adverse neuroendocrine and skeletal effects of the SSRIs have yet to be systematically explored.[110] However, a study from our group has shown that 4.5% of men and 22.2% of women with MDD developed new-onset hyperprolactinemia following SSRI treatment,[111] and daily SSRI use in adults 50 years and older was associated with a two-fold increased risk of fractures after adjustment for potential co-variates.[112] The SSRIs also appear to possess extremely low toxicity in overdose.[113] Finally, of all antidepressants, fluoxetine has the most extensive literature supporting its reproductive safety.[114]

Selective Serotonin Re-uptake Inhibitors Discontinuation Syndrome

A number of reports also describe discontinuation-emergent adverse events after abrupt cessation of SSRIs, including dizziness, insomnia, nervousness, irritability, nausea, and agitation.[115,116] The risk of such adverse events occurring seems to be inversely related to the half-life of the SSRI, with fluoxetine reported as having a significantly lower risk than paroxetine in two studies.[115,117] For more severe discontinuation-related adverse events, re-institution of the SSRI and slow taper may be necessary to alleviate these symptoms.[118]

Drug Interactions

With the exception perhaps of citalopram, and its stereoisomer escitalopram,[119] SSRIs may inhibit cytochrome P (CYP) 450 isoenzymes to varying degrees, potentially causing substrate levels to rise, or reducing conversion of a substrate into its active form. Concern about drug interactions, however, is pertinent to patients who take medications with narrow therapeutic margins that are metabolized by isoenzymes inhibited by an SSRI and if the prescriber is unfamiliar with or unable to determine the appropriate dose adjustment. Given their vast availability, reports of clinically significant interactions with the SSRIs are remarkably rare. Among the SSRIs, fluvoxamine is a potent CYP 1A2 and CYP 2C19 inhibitor, and a moderate CYP 2C9, CYP 2D6, and CYP 3A4 inhibitor, while fluoxetine and paroxetine are potent CYP 2D6 inhibitors, and fluoxetine's main metabolite, norfluoxetine, has a moderate inhibitory effect on CYP 3A4.[119] Sertraline is a moderate CYP 2D6 inhibitor, while citalopram and escitalopram appear to have little effect on the major CYP isoforms.[119] However, for all of the SSRIs, some vigilance is reasonable concerning the possibility of increased therapeutic or toxic effects of other co-prescribed drugs metabolized by P450 2D6. In particular, if combining a TCA with an SSRI, the TCA should be initiated with low doses, and plasma levels should be monitored. Given the high capacity of the CYP 450 3A3/3A4 system, inhibition of this isoenzyme is not a major concern for the SSRIs, although fluvoxamine, and less so fluoxetine, can inhibit it to some extent. Of little importance to drug interactions is the high rate of protein-binding of the SSRIs because, if other drugs are displaced from carrier proteins, the result is simply an increase in the rate and amount of free drug being metabolized. The augmentation and combination of SSRIs with other serotonergic agents, tryptophan, 5-HT, or MAOIs may also result in the serotonin syndrome; SSRIs should never be used concomitantly with MAOIs, because there have been a number of reports of fatal cases of serotonin syndrome due to the simultaneous use of these classes of drugs or to the inadequate washout period between the two.[54–56]

Use of Selective Serotonin Re-uptake Inhibitors in Pregnancy and the Post-partum Period

There is accumulating information about the use of SSRIs in pregnancy, although the bulk of the available data are on fluoxetine. One prospective study of 128 pregnant women who took fluoxetine,[120] 10 to 80 mg/day (mean 25.8 mg), during their first trimester did not find elevated rates of major malformations compared with matched groups of women taking TCAs or drugs thought not to be teratogenic. There was a higher, albeit not statistically significant, rate of miscarriages in the fluoxetine (13.5%) and TCA (12.2%) groups compared with the women exposed to known non-teratogenic drugs (6.8%). Whether this increased rate of miscarriages is biologically significant and, if so, whether it relates to the drugs or to the depressive disorder could not be determined from this study. Decisions on continuing antidepressant drugs during pregnancy must be individualized, but it must be recalled that the effects of severe untreated depression on maternal and fetal health may be far worse than the unknown risks of fluoxetine or tricyclic drugs. A large registry of fluoxetine exposure during pregnancy is consistent with generally reassuring data from the TCA era that antidepressant agents are not evidently teratogens.

On the other hand, infants exposed to SSRIs during late pregnancy may be at increased risk for serotonergic CNS adverse effects, although the incidence of these events has not been well established. Recently, the FDA has issued a warning for all SSRIs, reporting an increased risk for neonatal toxicity and recommending cessation of treatment before delivery. However, in clinical practice, the risk of post-partum depression often warrants continued treatment and close monitoring of the newborn.

Whenever possible, unnecessary exposure to any drug should be minimized, and thoughtful pre-pregnancy treatment planning and consideration of alternative interventions, such as psychotherapies (e.g., cognitive-behavioral therapy [CBT]), are to be recommended.

SSRIs are secreted in breast milk. Because their effects on normal growth and development are unknown, breast-feeding should be discouraged for mothers who are on SSRIs.

Serotonin Norepinephrine Re-uptake Inhibitors

Venlafaxine, duloxetine, desvenlafaxine, and levomilnacipran share the property of being relatively potent re-uptake inhibitors of serotonin and norepinephrine and are therefore considered SNRIs. They are all approved for the treatment of depression in the US.

Venlafaxine and Desvenlafaxine

Venlafaxine (Effexor) was the first SNRI to gain FDA approval for the treatment of depression. At daily doses greater than 150 mg,[121] venlafaxine inhibits the re-uptake of both serotonin and norepinephrine, while mostly inhibiting the re-uptake of serotonin at lower doses.[122,123] The augmentation and combination of venlafaxine with other serotonergic agents, tryptophan, 5-HT, or MAOIs may also result in the serotonin syndrome. Venlafaxine lacks significant cholinergic, antihistaminergic, and alpha₁-adrenergic–blocking effects. Venlafaxine is metabolized by CYP 450 2D6, of which it is also a very weak inhibitor. The half-lives of venlafaxine and its active metabolite O-desmethylvenlafaxine are about 5 and 11 hours, respectively. The drug and this metabolite reach steady state in plasma within 3 days in healthy adults. Venlafaxine is generally effective at daily doses at or above 150 mg, and is often started at 75 mg or even 37.5 mg, typically in its extended-release (XR) formulation.[124] Several meta-analyses suggest venlafaxine to be more effective than the SSRIs in the treatment of MDD,[125-127] with the exception of escitalopram, whose relative efficacy appears to be comparable.[83]

Venlafaxine, along with the SSRIs and bupropion, is also commonly chosen as a first-line treatment for depression.[84] Venlafaxine is also used in treatment-refractory depression as a "next-step" strategy,[128-135] reported as the most popular switch strategy for refractory depression in one large survey of clinicians.[136]

Common side effects of venlafaxine include nausea, insomnia, sedation, sexual dysfunction, headache, tremor, palpitations, and dizziness,[137] as well as excessive sweating, tachycardia, and palpitations. There are also reports of bruxism.[138,139] Venlafaxine's potential for sexual dysfunction appears to be comparable to that of the SSRIs.[140,141] The incidence of GI side effects and dizziness appears to be lower with the use of the XR formulation than the immediate-release formulation.[142] Between 2% and 6% of patients also experience an increase in diastolic blood pressure,[143] which appears to be dose-related.[144] The abrupt discontinuation of venlafaxine, given its short half-life, also carries a risk of discontinuation-related adverse events similar to those described for the SSRIs.[145] Finally, in one uncontrolled study, 4 of 13 patients treated with venlafaxine during electroconvulsive therapy (ECT) experienced asystole.[146] Although the authors noted that this serious adverse event only occurred in patients on daily doses of venlafaxine greater than 300 mg and in patients anesthetized with propofol, in the absence of further data the use of venlafaxine in patients requiring ECT and perhaps even general anesthesia should be avoided.

Desvenlafaxine (Pristiq) is a major active metabolite of venlafaxine and an SNRI with little affinity for muscarinic, histaminic, or adrenergic receptors. Desvenlafaxine is metabolized by CYP 450 3A4 and it is a very weak inhibitor of 2D6. The half-life of desvenlafaxine is about 10 hours. The augmentation and combination of desvenlafaxine with other serotonergic agents, tryptophan, 5-HT, or MAOIs may also result in the serotonin syndrome. Desvenlafaxine was found to be more effective than placebo in the treatment of MDD in two separate randomized, double-blind clinical trials. Side effects reported in those studies included nausea, dry mouth, sweating, somnolence, anorexia, constipation, asthenia, vomiting, tremor, nervousness, abnormal vision, and sexual dysfunction. There have been reports of increases in diastolic blood pressure, and the abrupt discontinuation of desvenlafaxine also carries a risk of discontinuation-related adverse events similar to those described for the SSRIs. There are also reports of an increase in liver enzymes among patients treated with desvenlafaxine. Desvenlafaxine is commonly used at doses between 50 and 100 mg daily in a single administration.

Duloxetine

Duloxetine (Cymbalta) also inhibits the re-uptake of both serotonin and norepinephrine.[147] Duloxetine appears to be as effective as the SSRIs in the treatment of MDD, although in more severe depression there may be some advantages.[148]

Duloxetine lacks significant cholinergic, antihistaminergic, and alpha₁-adrenergic blocking effects. Duloxetine is extensively metabolized to numerous metabolites that are primarily excreted into the urine in the conjugated form. The major metabolites in plasma are glucuronide conjugates of 4-hydroxy duloxetine (M6), 6-hydroxy-5-methoxy duloxetine (M10), 4,6-dihydroxy duloxetine (M9), and a sulfate conjugate of 5-hydroxy-6-methoxy duloxetine (M7). Duloxetine is metabolized by CYP 450 2D6, of which it is also a moderate inhibitor, intermediate between paroxetine and sertraline. Drugs that inhibit this enzyme may increase duloxetine concentrations. The half-life of duloxetine is about 12.5 hours. Abrupt discontinuation of duloxetine is associated with a discontinuation-emergent adverse event profile similar to that seen with SSRIs and SNRI antidepressants.[149] Therefore, duloxetine's discontinuation should be accomplished with a gradual taper (over at least 2 weeks) to reduce the risk of discontinuation-emergent adverse events. Duloxetine is commonly used at daily doses of 60 to 120 mg, often started at 30 mg. Duloxetine also appears to be effective in the treatment of somatic symptoms of depression, such as pain.[150,151] Common side effects associated with duloxetine include dry mouth, headache, nausea, somnolence, sweating, insomnia, and fatigue.[152] Duloxetine does not appear to cause hypertension.[152]

Levomilnacipran and Milnacipran

Levomilnacipran (Fetzima) is an SNRI and is the 1S-2R enantiomer of milnacipram, an SRNI approved for depression in Europe (brand names: Dalcipran, Ixel). Levomilnacipran is metabolized by CYP 450 3A4 and it is not an inhibitor of CYP 450 systems. Its half-life is about 12 hours. The augmentation and combination of milnacipran or levomilnacipran with other serotonergic agents, tryptophan, 5-HT, or MAOIs may also result in the serotonin syndrome. A number of studies had demonstrated that the SNRI milnacipran[153] is equivalent to the SSRIs[154-157] and the TCAs[158-162] and superior to placebo in the treatment of depression.[163,164] Similarly, several studies have shown that the norepinephrine and serotonin re-uptake inhibitor levomilnacipran is superior to placebo in the treatment of depression.[165-167] Because of the potent norepinephrine re-uptake inhibition, levomilnacipran appears to be particularly effective in treating fatigue in depression. Common side effects reported during treatment with milnacipran include headaches, dry mouth, dysuria, tremor, tachycardia, weight gain, and sedation, although the incidence of weight gain and sedation with milnacipran is lower than with the TCAs.[162] Levomilnacipran's frequently reported adverse events (≥ 5% in levomilnacipran ER and twice the rate of placebo) are nausea, dizziness, constipation, tachycardia, urinary hesitation, hyperhidrosis, insomnia, vomiting, and elevated blood pressure. Daily doses of milnacipran range from 50 to 200 mg, often divided in twice-daily dosing, whereas the usual dose of levomilnacipran ER is 40–120 mg once/daily

Norepinephrine Re-uptake Inhibitors
Reboxetine

Reboxetine[168] acts by selectively inhibiting the norepinephrine transporter, thereby increasing synaptic norepinephrine levels. Reboxetine, a morpholine compound, is chemically unrelated to the other antidepressants. It is highly protein-bound and has a plasma half-life of about 13 hours. The drug does not appear to be a meaningful inhibitor of the CYP 450 system and is metabolized itself by CYP 450 3A4 isozyme with two inactive metabolites. Increased blood pressure has been reported to be a problem for some patients, particularly those with a genetic variant of the norepinephrine transporter (SCL6A2). Reboxetine has not received FDA approval for the treatment of depression, but is available in Europe for the treatment of depression (brand name: Edronax). Double-blind, placebo-controlled trials suggest reboxetine to be more effective than placebo[169-172] and as effective as fluoxetine[170] in the treatment of MDD. The starting daily dose is usually 8 mg but can be as low as 4 mg, with effective daily doses ranging from 8 to 10 mg given in divided doses (twice a day). Common side effects include insomnia, headache, dry mouth, diaphoresis, and constipation,[170] as well as urinary hesitancy. The incidence of nausea, headache, fatigue,[170] and sexual dysfunction[173] appears to be more common during treatment with the SSRIs than with reboxetine. The urinary hesitancy and constipation do not appear to reflect anticholinergic, but rather noradrenergic, effects.

Atomoxetine

Atomoxetine also selectively inhibits the re-uptake of norepinephrine.[174] *In vitro*, *ex vivo*, and *in vivo* studies have shown that atomoxetine is a highly selective antagonist of the pre-synaptic norepinephrine transporter, with little or no affinity for other noradrenergic receptors or other neurotransmitter transporters or receptors, with the exception of a weak affinity for the serotonin transporter. Atomoxetine is rapidly absorbed, with peak plasma concentrations occurring 1 to 2 hours after dosing, and its half-life hovers around 3 to 4 hours. While atomoxetine is an FDA-approved treatment for attention-deficit/hyperactivity disorder (ADHD) (brand name: Strattera), there is a single open trial of atomoxetine in depression involving 10 patients, with daily doses ranging from 40 to 70 mg.[175] Common side effects reported so far include decreased appetite, insomnia, and increased blood pressure.[176]

Atomoxetine has also been associated with mild increases in blood pressure and pulse that plateau during treatment and resolve after discontinuation. There have been no effects seen on the QT interval. It is a substrate of CYP 2D6 and its biotransformation involves aromatic ring hydroxylation, benzylic oxidation, and N-demethylation. At high therapeutic doses, atomoxetine inhibits CYP 2D6 and CYP 3A activity, although *in vivo* studies clearly indicate that atomoxetine administration with substrates of CYP 2D6 and CYP 3A does not result in clinically significant drug interactions.

Norepinephrine/Dopamine Re-uptake Inhibitors
Bupropion

The NDRI bupropion appears to be as effective as the SSRIs in the treatment of depressive[177,178] and anxiety symptoms in depression,[179] and more effective than the SSRIs in the treatment of sleepiness and fatigue in depression.[180] Interestingly, bupropion has been shown to be as effective as the SNRI venlafaxine in the treatment of MDD.[181]

Bupropion is a phenethylamine compound that is effective for the treatment of MDD. Bupropion is structurally related to amphetamine and the sympathomimetic diethylpropion, and it primarily blocks the re-uptake of dopamine and norepinephrine and has minimal or no affinity for post-synaptic receptors. Although some researchers have argued that the NDRI bupropion's effect on norepinephrine is primarily through an increase in pre-synaptic release, there is still convincing evidence for binding of both norepinephrine and dopamine transporters. Bupropion is rapidly absorbed after oral administration and demonstrates biphasic elimination, with an elimination half-life of 11 to 14 hours. It is converted to three active metabolites, hydroxybupropion, threohydrobupropion, and erythrohydrobupropion, all of which have been demonstrated to have antidepressant activity in animal models. Bupropion lacks anticholinergic properties and does not cause postural hypotension or alter cardiac conduction in a clinically significant manner. It is a substrate of CYP 450 2B6 and appears to have CYP 450 2D6 inhibition potential, which suggests that, when it is combined with fluoxetine or paroxetine, both 2D6 substrates, levels of the SSRI may increase. One advantage of treatment with bupropion compared to the SSRIs is the lower risk of sexual dysfunction.[140,141,182-187] Treatment with bupropion is also associated with a lower incidence of GI side effects (e.g., nausea and diarrhea)[185,186] and sedation[177,179,185] than the SSRIs. Although a difference in terms of weight changes in bupropion and SSRI-treated depressed patients is not immediately apparent during the acute phase of treatment in randomized trials,[183,185,186,188-190] there is evidence to suggest that any beneficial effects of SSRIs in terms of weight reduction during the acute phase are not sustained during the continuation and maintenance phases.[101,102] In fact, long-term treatment with some SSRIs may also result in long-term weight gain.[103] In contrast, long-term (44 weeks) bupropion treatment appears to result in weight changes no different than those of placebo in MDD.[191] Thus, long-term treatment with bupropion may carry a lower risk of weight gain than long-term treatment with the SSRIs.

The dose range for the sustained-release (SR) formulation of bupropion (Wellbutrin SR) is 150 to 450 mg in twice a day or three times a day dosing, with 100 or 150 mg being a common starting dose. A once-daily dose formulation (Wellbutrin XL), available in 150 and 300 mg doses, was subsequently introduced. Common side effects include agitation, insomnia, weight loss, dry mouth, headache, constipation, and tremor.[189] The major medically important adverse event associated with bupropion is seizure. With the immediate-release formulation the rate is 0.4% (4 per 1,000) at doses up to 450 mg/day, whereas with bupropion SR the rate is of 0.1% (1 per 1,000) at doses up to the target antidepressant dose of 300 mg/day (Wellbutrin SR Prescribing Information).[192] SSRI antidepressants are also associated with seizures at a similar rate of approximately 0.1% (Wellbutrin SR Prescribing Information). Patients should only be administered bupropion with extreme caution if a predisposition to seizure is present. For this reason, the maximum daily dose for bupropion SR and bupropion XL is 450 mg, with no single dose above 200 mg for the SR formulation. In addition, bupropion may be more likely to induce seizures in patients with bulimia nervosa and histories of head trauma and it should not be used in these patients. Since the risk of seizure appears to be dose-related and related to the peak plasma concentrations, the SR and XL formulations are thought to be associated with a somewhat lower seizure risk, estimated at 0.1% for daily doses lower than 450 mg.[192]

Serotonin Receptor Antagonists/Agonists

Trazodone

Although the serotonin receptor antagonists trazodone (Desyrel) and nefazodone (Serzone) have been shown to be as effective as the SSRIs in the treatment of depression,[193] they are used extremely infrequently as monotherapy for depression.[84] Trazodone is rapidly absorbed following oral administration, achieving peak levels in 1 to 2 hours. It has a relatively short elimination half-life of 3 to 9 hours and is excreted mainly in urine (75%); its metabolite mCPP has a similar pharmacokinetic profile. Despite the short half-life, once-daily dosing at bedtime is the usual route of administration because of its sedating properties. When used as monotherapy for the treatment of depression, a patient is typically started on 100 to 150 mg daily either in divided doses or in a single bedtime dose and gradually increased to 200 to 300 mg/day. An extended-release formulation of trazodone (Oleptro) is available. The dose range for the extended-release is between 150 and 300 mg qHS. For optimal benefit, doses in the range of 400 to 600 mg may be needed for either formulation. Low-dose trazodone (25 to 150 mg at bedtime) is commonly used in the treatment of insomnia secondary to antidepressant use,[194] a strategy that may also result in an improvement in depressive symptoms.[195] The most common side effects of trazodone are sedation, orthostatic hypotension, and headaches. Trazodone lacks the quinidine-like properties of the cyclic antidepressants but has been associated in rare cases with cardiac arrhythmias, which may be related to trazodone's ability to inhibit potassium channels. Thus, trazodone should be used with caution in patients with known cardiac disease. A rare but serious side effect of trazodone is priapism of both the penis and clitoris,[196,197] which requires immediate medical attention. Priapism has been attributed to the alpha-adrenoceptor blocking properties of trazodone by interference with the sympathetic control of penile detumescence.[198] Rare cases of hepatotoxicity have been associated with the use of trazodone,[199] and fatal cases of trazodone overdose have also been reported.[200] In one review, trazodone was reported to carry one of the lowest risks for seizure of all antidepressants examined.[201] The minimal effective dose for trazodone is usually 300 mg daily.

Nefazodone

Nefazodone has less affinity for the alpha$_1$-adrenergic receptor and is therefore less sedating. The half-life of nefazodone is approximately 5 hours. The usual starting dosage is 50 mg/day given at bedtime or twice a day, titrated up in the absence of daytime sedation as rapidly as tolerated to achieve a usually effective antidepressant dosage in the 450 to 600 mg/day range in divided doses. Slower dose titration is recommended in the elderly. Nefazodone has been found to inhibit CYP 3A4 and to result in serotonin syndrome when combined with SSRIs. Common side effects include somnolence, dizziness, dry mouth, nausea, constipation, headache, amblyopia, and blurred vision.[202] An unusual but occasional adverse effect is irritability (possibly related to its mCPP metabolite, which may occur in higher levels in the presence of a CYP 450 2D6 inhibitor). Treatment with nefazodone has the advantage of a lower risk of long-term weight gain than the SSRIs or TCAs,[97] perhaps because of the appetite-reducing effects of mCPP.[203] Nefazodone also has the advantage of a lower risk of sexual side effects than the SSRIs.[140,141,204] A rare but serious side effect of nefazodone is priapism of both the penis and clitoris,[205,206] which requires immediate medical attention. In addition, an increasing number of reports suggest that treatment with nefazodone is associated with an increase risk of hepatotoxicity (approximately 29 cases per 100,000 patient years),[207] often severe (more than 80% of cases), and often appearing during the first 6 months of treatment.[208] To date, there has even been one reported death due to such hepatotoxicity.[209] Therefore, this agent should be avoided in patients with current or a history of liver abnormalities; liver enzymes should be checked periodically in patients on nefazodone. The minimal effective doses for nefazodone are usually 300 mg daily, with 600 mg daily being the optimal dose.

Vilazodone

Vilazodone (Vibryd) is a serotonin 5-HT$_{1A}$ receptor partial agonist and a selective serotonin re-uptake inhibitor. Studies have shown its superiority over placebo in the treatment of depression.[210] The augmentation and combination of vilazodone with other serotonergic agents, tryptophan, 5-HT, or MAOIs may also result in the serotonin syndrome. Vilazodone lacks significant cholinergic, antihistaminergic, and alpha$_1$-adrenergic–blocking effects. Vilazodone is metabolized primarily by CYP 450 3A4 and is a moderate inhibitor of 2C19 and 2D6. The terminal half-life of vilazodone is about 25 hours. Vilazodone therapy is typically initiated at a dosage of 10 mg once daily and incrementally adjusted over 14 days to the recommended target daily dose of 40 mg; for optimal bioavailability and effectiveness, it should be taken after a light or high-fat meal. The adverse effects most commonly reported in clinical trials of vilazodone were diarrhea, nausea, vomiting, dizziness, insomnia and dry mouth. Treatment-related sexual side effects may be less likely than with SSRIs: in three placebo-controlled studies, 8.0% of vilazodone-treated patients and 0.9% of placebo-treated patients reported ≥ 1 sexual-function-related treatment-emergent adverse event ($P < 0.001$)).[211] Vilazodone was not associated with clinically-relevant weight change in the short-term trials. In an open-label 1-year study of vilazodone, mean weight increased by 1.7 kg among the observed cases.[212]

Vortioxetine

Vortioxetine (Brintellix) is a recently-approved antidepressant with multi-modal activity that functions as a serotonin 5-HT$_3$, 5-HT$_7$ and 5-HT$_{1D}$ receptor antagonist, serotonin 5-HT$_{1B}$ receptor partial agonist, serotonin 5-HT$_{1A}$ receptor agonist and inhibitor of the serotonin transporter *in vitro*. Vortioxetine has shown to be able to increase extracellular serotonin, dopamine, and norepinephrine levels in the medial prefrontal cortex and ventral hippocampus. The augmentation and combination of vortioxetine with other serotonergic agents, tryptophan, 5-HT, or MAOIs may result in the serotonin syndrome. Vortioxetine lacks significant cholinergic, anti-histaminergic, and alpha$_1$-adrenergic–blocking effects. Vortioxetine is metabolized primarily by CYP 450 2D6. The terminal half-life of vortioxetine is about 66 hours. Vortioxetine therapy is typically initiated at a dosage of 10 mg once daily and incrementally adjusted 20 mg once daily, if necessary; the dose can be lowered to 5 mg daily, if necessary based on tolerability issues. Nausea, dry mouth, diarrhea, nasopharyngitis, headache, dizziness, somnolence, vomiting, dyspepsia, constipation and fatigue were reported in $\geq$ 5% of patients receiving vortioxetine.[213] Rates of treatment-emergent sexual dysfunction (TESD) in the vortioxetine dosing groups were similar to placebo.[213] In a 52-week open-label extension study, vortioxetine was associated with minimal weight gain.[214] Recently presented data suggest that vortioxetine may have the additional advantage of distinctive pro-cognitive effects.

Ritanserin

Ritanserin, a serotonin 5-HT$_{2A}$ and 5-HT$_{2C}$ antagonist, is not FDA-approved, but is available in Europe. One placebo-controlled study revealed ritanserin to be effective in the treatment of dysthymic disorder,[215] while a separate study found ritanserin to be as effective as amitriptyline in patients with depression and chronic headaches.[216] Ritanserin appears to be effective for depression at doses above 5 mg.

Agomelatine

Agomelatine, a newer agent, is a selective 5-HT$_{2C}$ antagonist and acts as a melatonin MT$_1$ and MT$_2$ receptor agonist. To date, at least two placebo-controlled trials have found agomelatine (25 mg) to be more effective than placebo and as effective as the SSRIs in the treatment of MDD,[217-219] and as effective as the SSRI paroxetine in MDD.[217] Agomelatine is approved for the treatment of depression in Europe, but not in the US.

Buspirone and Gepirone

Buspirone (BuSpar) and gepirone (Ariza) act as full agonists at serotonin 5-HT$_{1A}$ autoreceptors and are generally, but not exclusively, partial agonists at post-synaptic serotonin 5-HT$_{1A}$ receptors.[29] Buspirone is FDA-approved as a treatment for anxiety and not for depression, while gepirone has not been FDA-approved. Nevertheless, a number of double-blind trials report buspirone[220-223] and gepirone[224-228] to be more effective than placebo in the treatment of MDD. One advantage of gepirone and perhaps buspirone is that their use does not appear to be related to a greater incidence of weight gain or sexual side effects than placebo, at least during the acute phase of treatment of depression.[228] Effective doses for buspirone and gepirone for depression range between 30 and 90 mg and 20 and 80 mg, respectively. Side effects are similar for these two agents and include headache, dizziness, light-headedness, nausea, and insomnia.[222,229]

Alpha$_2$-Adrenergic Receptor Antagonists
Mirtazapine

Mirtazapine is as effective as the SSRIs[230] and venlafaxine[231,232] in the treatment of MDD. Mirtazapine shows linear pharmacokinetics over a dose range of 15 to 80 mg and its elimination half-life ranges from 20 to 40 hours, consistent with its time to reach steady state (4 to 6 days). Biotransformation is mainly mediated by the CYP 2D6 and CYP 3A4 isoenzymes. Inhibitors of these isoenzymes, such as paroxetine and fluoxetine, cause modestly increased mirtazapine plasma concentrations, while mirtazapine has little inhibitory effects on CYP isoenzymes; therefore, the pharmacokinetics of co-administered drugs are hardly affected by mirtazapine. Mirtazapine is associated with more sedation and weight gain than the SSRIs.[233-236] The widespread use of mirtazapine as a first-line agent in depression has been primarily limited by its sedative effects and weight gain.[237] In addition to sedation and weight gain, common side effects associated with mirtazapine include dizziness, dry mouth, constipation, and orthostatic hypotension. Due to blockade of 5-HT$_2$ and 5-HT$_3$ receptors, mirtazapine is associated with a lower risk of headaches[233] and nausea[233-235,238,239] than the SSRIs. Treatment with mirtazapine is also associated with a lower incidence of sexual dysfunction than the SSRIs.[141,234] In addition, switching to mirtazapine may alleviate SSRI induced sexual dysfunction in SSRI-remitters.[240] Severe neutropenia has been rarely reported (1 in 1,000) with an uncertain relationship to the drug, but as with other psychotropics, the onset of infection and fever should prompt the patient to contact his or her physician. The drug is most efficacious at doses of 30 to 45 mg (although 60 mg/day has been used in refractory cases) usually given in a single bedtime dose. Available in 15, 30, and 45 mg scored tablets and in an orally soluble tablet formulation (Soltab) at 15, 30, and 45 mg, the lower dose may be sub-optimal, and compared with 15 mg, the 30 mg dose also may be less or at least not more sedating, possibly as a consequence of the noradrenergic effects being recruited at that dose. The starting daily dose can be as low as 7.5 mg in the elderly.

Mianserin

Mianserin is approved for depression in Europe (brand name: Lantanon) and is not FDA-approved. Double-blind studies report the efficacy of mianserin in the treatment of MDD to be equivalent to the TCAs.[241-243] The most common side effects include somnolence, weight gain, dry mouth, sleep problems, tremor, and headaches.[244] Effective daily doses for mianserin range from 30 to 60 mg, usually given at bedtime.

Tricyclic and Related Cyclic Antidepressants

Oral preparations of TCAs and related drugs are rapidly and completely absorbed from the GI tract; a high percentage of an oral dose is metabolized by the liver as it passes through the portal circulation (first-pass effect). The TCAs are metabolized by the microsomal enzymes of the liver; the tertiary amines are first monodemethylated to yield compounds that are still active. Indeed, the desmethyl metabolites of amitriptyline and imipramine are nortriptyline and desipramine, respectively, and are marketed as antidepressants. Other major metabolic pathways include hydroxylation (which may yield partially active compounds) and conjugation with glucuronic acid to produce inactive compounds. TCAs are highly lipophilic, meaning the free fraction passes easily into the brain and other tissues. They are also largely bound to plasma proteins. Given their lipophilicity and protein-binding, they are not removed effectively by hemodialysis in cases of overdose. The time course of metabolism and elimination is biphasic, with approximately half of a dose removed over 48 to 72 hours and the remainder, strongly bound to tissues and plasma proteins, slowly excreted over several weeks. There is considerable variation among individuals in their metabolic rate for cyclic antidepressants based on genetic factors, age, and concomitantly taken drugs. In fact, when metabolic differences are combined with variation in the degree of protein-binding, as much as a 300-fold difference in effective drug levels may be found among individuals.

Although TCAs' overall efficacy in treating depression is equivalent to that of the SSRIs,[245] they tend to have considerably more side effects and, due to their ability to block the aforementioned receptors, as well as the sodium channel,[246] TCAs are often arrythmogenic[247] and epileptogenic[248] when taken in very large (supra-therapeutic) quantities. As a result, they are rarely chosen as first-line agents in the treatment of depression.[84] Furthermore, several studies also suggest that TCAs may be more effective than the SSRIs in the treatment of melancholic depression, or in the treatment of depressed patients with certain co-morbid medical conditions.[249-253] In addition, perhaps due to their ability to inhibit the re-uptake of both serotonin and norepinephrine, as well as their ability to block sodium channels, TCAs appear to be more effective in treating neuropathic pain than the SSRIs.[254] In fact, the results of a separate meta-analysis reveal that the TCAs are superior to the SSRIs in the treatment of a number of somatic/pain disorders (including headaches, fibromyalgia, irritable bowel disorder, idiopathic pain, tinnitus, and chronic fatigue) often diagnosed in patients with chronic depression.[255] The TCAs may be sub-divided into tertiary amines and secondary amines (their demethylated secondary amine derivatives). In addition, maprotiline (Ludiomil), which is classified as a tetracyclic antidepressant, is commonly grouped with the TCAs, due to similarities in dosing, mechanism of action, and side effects. Tertiary amine TCAs include amitriptyline (Elavil, Adepril), imipramine (Tofranil, Antidepril), trimipramine (Surmontil, Herphonal), clomipramine (Anafranil, Clopress), and doxepin (Sinequan, Deptran). Secondary amine TCAs are nortriptyline (Pamelor, Aventyl), desipramine (Norpramin, Metylyl), protriptyline (Vivactil, Concordin), and amoxapine (Ascendin, Defanyl).

Side-effect Profile

In general, the side effects of the TCAs and related cyclic antidepressants are more difficult for patients to tolerate than are the side effects of the newer drugs (Table 3-2) and they probably account for higher drop-out rates than are associated with the SSRIs.[256] Thus, treatment is typically initiated at lower doses (e.g., 10 mg/day for imipramine) in order to minimize the risk of adverse events and premature treatment discontinuation. The side-effect profile of the TCAs can be sub-categorized in terms of their relative affinity for a number of monoamine receptors and transporters. Overall, secondary amine TCAs tend to cause fewer anticholinergic, antihistaminergic, and anti-alpha$_1$–related side effects than tertiary amine TCAs.

Amoxapine is the only TCA with documented, significant dopamine D$_2$ receptor antagonism.[49] Therefore, there have been case reports of tardive dystonia and dyskinesia associated with amoxapine treatment,[257,258] and amoxapine should be avoided in patients with co-morbid depression and Parkinson's disease.[259]

Anticholinergic-related side effects result from the affinity of TCAs for muscarinic cholinergic receptors and typically include dry mouth, blurred vision, constipation, urinary hesitancy, tachycardia, memory difficulties, and ejaculatory difficulties. Finally, due to their anticholinergic effects, TCAs should be avoided in patients with narrow-angle glaucoma and prostatic hypertrophy, as symptoms related to these conditions may worsen because of such anticholinergic effects.

Antihistaminergic-related side effects result from histaminergic H$_1$-receptor blockade and typically include increased appetite, weight gain, sedation, and fatigue. Weight gain with TCAs can be substantial, averaging 1 to 3 lb per month of treatment.[260] As a result, TCAs may complicate the management of diabetes and worsen glycemic control, and should be avoided whenever possible in diabetics.[261] TCAs may also have hyperlipidemic effects, thus complicating their long-term use in patients with hyperlipidemia.[262] Xerostomia secondary to anticholinergic and antihistaminergic effects may also increase the risk of oral pathology, particularly dental caries.[263]

Orthostatic hypotension and reflex tachycardia may result from alpha$_1$-adrenergic receptor antagonism. Nortriptyline is generally thought to be less likely to cause orthostatic hypotension than tertiary amine TCAs, such as imipramine[264,265]; however, nortriptyline's affinity for the alpha$_1$-adrenergic receptor, although less than the affinity of most TCAs, is actually much greater (e.g., by a factor of two) than the affinity of desipramine and protriptyline.[50] In addition, homozygosity for 3435T alleles of *ABCB1*, the multi-drug resistance gene that encodes a P-glycoprotein (P-gp) regulating the passage of many substances across the blood–brain barrier, appears to be a risk factor for occurrence of nortriptyline-induced postural hypotension.[266] Antidepressant-induced postural hypotension in the elderly may, in turn, increase the risk of falls and fractures (e.g., hip fractures).[267] Although less likely to suffer a fall or fracture, the sedative potential of various TCA antidepressants is also a serious consideration in younger depressed patients as well, as this effect may increase the mortality risk from

TABLE 3-2 Tricyclic Antidepressants and Monoamine Oxidase Inhibitors Side-effect Profile

Category and Drug	Sedative Potency	Anticholinergic Potency	Orthostatic Hypotensive Potency	Usual Adult Daily Dose (mg/day)	Dosage (mg/day)
*Tricyclic and Related Cyclic Compounds**					
Amitriptyline	High	Very high	High	150–200	75–300
Amoxapine	Low	Moderate	Moderate	150–200	75–300
Clomipramine	High	High	High	150–200	75–250
Desipramine	Low	Moderate (lowest of the tricyclics)	Moderate	150–200	75–300
Doxepin	High	High	Moderate	150–200	75–300
Imipramine	Moderate	High	High	150–200	75–300
Maprotiline	Moderate	Low	Moderate	150–200	75–225
Nortriptyline	Moderate	Moderate	Lowest of the tricyclics	75–100	40–150
Protriptyline	Low	High	Low	30	10–60
Trimipramine	High	Moderate	Moderate	150–200	75–300
Monoamine Oxidase Inhibitors					
Isocarboxazid	—	Very low	High	30	20–60
Phenelzine	Low	Very low	High	60–75	30–90
Tranylcypromine	—	Very low	High	30	20–90

*All of the tricyclic and related cyclic compounds have well-established cardiac arrhythmogenic potential.
(From Rosenbaum JF, Arana GW, Hyman SE, et al., editors: Handbook of psychiatric drug therapy, ed 5, Philadelphia, 2005, Lippincott Williams & Wilkins.)

automobile accidents. In fact, in a recent review,[268] sedating antidepressants (dothiepin, amitriptyline, imipramine, doxepin, and mianserin) were found to result in driving impairments on a standardized road test comparable to impairments found in drivers with a blood alcohol level of 0.8 mg/ml, whereas non-sedating antidepressants (moclobemide, fluoxetine, paroxetine, venlafaxine, and nefazodone) were not found to adversely affect driving performance. TCAs may also cause sexual dysfunction and excessive sweating.

The ability of TCAs to inhibit the sodium channel may also result in electrocardiographic changes in susceptible individuals (e.g., in post–myocardial infarction patients, as well as in patients with bifascicular heart block, left bundle branch block, or a prolonged QT interval), even at therapeutic doses,[269] and, given that contemporary psychopharmacologists have access to a multitude of alternative treatment options, TCAs should be avoided in these patients. Due to the inhibition of sodium channels and cholinergic receptors, the TCAs also carry a risk of seizure. Maprotiline and clomipramine are considered the TCAs with the greatest risk of seizures.[270] This combined risk of seizure and arrhythmia renders the TCAs as the least safe during overdose.[271]

Prescribing Tricyclic and Related Cyclic Antidepressants

Aside from the electrocardiogram (ECG), no other tests are generally indicated in healthy adults before starting a TCA. TCAs are started at a low dose followed by gradual increases until the therapeutic range is achieved. Finding the right TCA dose for a patient often involves a process of trial and error. The most common error leading to treatment failure is inadequate dosage. In healthy adults, the typical starting dose is 25 to 50 mg of imipramine or its TCA equivalent. Nortriptyline is about twice as potent; thus, its starting dose is 10 to 25 mg. In some clinical situations, especially in the elderly and patients with panic disorder, it may be necessary to start with lower doses (as low as 10 mg of imipramine or the equivalent) because of intolerance to side effects. Generally, TCAs are administered once a day at bedtime to help with compliance and, when the sedating compounds are used, to help with sleep. Divided doses are used if patients have side effects due to high peak levels. The dosage can be increased by 50 mg every 3 to 4 days, as side effects allow, up to a dose of 150 to 200 mg of imipramine or its equivalent at bedtime (see Table 3-1). If there is no therapeutic response in 3 to 4 weeks, the dosage should be slowly increased, again as side effects allow. The maximum dosage of most TCAs is the equivalent of 300 mg/day of imipramine, although uncommonly, patients who metabolize the drug rapidly may do well on higher dosages. Of the currently available cyclic antidepressants, only four drugs (imipramine, desipramine, amitriptyline, and nortriptyline) have been studied well enough to make generalizations about the value of their blood levels in treatment of depression. Serum levels of the other cyclic antidepressants have not been investigated well enough to be clinically meaningful, although they can confirm presence of the drug or document extremely high serum levels. There is a wide range of effective doses for TCAs. Typical antidepressant doses are 100 to 300 mg/day for imipramine. There is evidence to suggest a relationship between serum levels of TCAs and clinical response. Perry and colleagues[272] pooled and analyzed all available studies examining the relationship between TCA blood levels and clinical response with the use of receiver operating-characteristics curves. The relationship between clinical response and blood levels for desipramine was linear, with the threshold concentration in plasma for therapeutic response being greater than or equal to 116 ng/ml (response rates: 51% versus 15% for patients with levels above or below that threshold, respectively). The

remaining TCAs exhibited a curvilinear (inverse "U"–shaped curve) relationship between blood level and clinical response. The optimal ranges for nortriptyline, "total" imipramine (imipramine plus desipramine), and "total" amitriptyline (amitriptyline plus nortriptyline) (with their corresponding response rates within versus outside the level range) were 58 to 148 ng/ml (66% versus 26%), 175 to 350 ng/ml (67% versus 39%), and 93 to 140 ng/ml (50% versus 30%), respectively.

Nortriptyline levels have been the best studied of the antidepressants. Some researchers believe that such studies reveal a more complex pattern than with imipramine or desipramine—an inverted U-shape correlation with clinical improvement, which is sometimes referred to as a therapeutic window. Clinical improvement correlates with levels of 50 to 150 ng/ml. The reason for the poorer response with doses above 150 ng/ml is not known, but it does not appear to relate to any measurable toxicity. On the other hand, the number of subjects in well-designed studies that indicate a window is small, so not all researchers believe there is adequate evidence in favor of a therapeutic window. Studies of amitriptyline levels have resulted in disagreement about the utility of levels, with linear, curvilinear, and lack of relationship reported by different investigators. When used, blood levels should be drawn when the drug has achieved steady-state levels (at least 5 days after a dosage change in healthy adults; longer in the elderly) and 10 to 14 hours after the last oral dose. Abrupt discontinuation symptoms may emerge with TCAs and in part represent cholinergic rebound, and include GI distress, malaise, chills, coryza, and muscle aches.

Use of Tricyclic and Related Cyclic Antidepressants during Pregnancy and the Post-partum Period

There are limited data on the use of TCAs during pregnancy. There have been reports of congenital malformations in association with TCA use, but there is no convincing causal association. Overall, the TCAs may be safe, but given the lack of proven safety, the drugs should be avoided during pregnancy, unless the indications are compelling. Pregnant women who are at risk for serious depression might be maintained on TCA therapy. This decision should always be made very carefully and with extensive discussion of the risk–benefit factors. Due to more clinical experience, older agents, such as imipramine, may be preferred to newer drugs during pregnancy. TCAs appear to be secreted in breast milk. Because their effects on normal growth and development are unknown, breast-feeding should be discouraged for mothers who are on tricyclics.

Overdoses with Tricyclic and Related Cyclic Antidepressants

Acute doses of more than 1 g of TCAs are often toxic and may be fatal. Death may result from cardiac arrhythmias, hypotension, or uncontrollable seizures. Serum levels should be obtained when overdose is suspected, both because of distorted information that may be given by patients or families and because oral bioavailability with very large doses of these compounds is poorly understood. Nonetheless, serum levels of the parent compound and its active metabolites provide less specific information about the severity of the overdose than one might hope. Serum levels of greater than 1,000 ng/ml are associated with serious overdose, as are increases in the QRS duration of the ECG to 0.10 second or greater. However, serious consequences of a TCA overdose may occur with serum levels under 1,000 ng/ml and with a QRS duration of less than 0.10 second. In acute overdose, almost all symptoms develop within 12 hours.

BOX 3-3 Drug Interactions with Cyclic Antidepressants

WORSEN SEDATION

Alcohol
Antihistamines
Antipsychotics
Barbiturates, chloral hydrate, and other sedatives

WORSEN HYPOTENSION

α-Methyldopa (Aldomet)
β-Adrenergic blockers (e.g., propranolol)
Clonidine
Diuretics
Low-potency antipsychotics

ADDITIVE CARDIOTOXICITY

Quinidine and other type 1 antiarrhythmics
Thioridazine, mesoridazine, pimozide, ziprasidone

ADDITIVE ANTICHOLINERGIC TOXICITY

Anti-histamines (diphenhydramine and others)
Anti-parkinsonians (benztropine and others)
Low-potency antipsychotics, especially thioridazine
Over-the-counter sleeping medications
Gastrointestinal antispasmodics and anti-diarrheals (Lomotil and others)

OTHER

Tricyclics may increase the effects of warfarin
Tricyclics may block the effects of guanethidine

(From Rosenbaum JF, Arana GW, Hyman SE, et al., editors: Handbook of psychiatric drug therapy, *ed 5, Philadelphia, 2005, Lippincott Williams & Wilkins.)*

Anti-muscarinic effects are prominent, including dry mucous membranes, warm dry skin, mydriasis, blurred vision, decreased bowel motility, and, often, urinary retention. Either CNS depression (ranging from drowsiness to coma) or an agitated delirium may occur. The CNS depressant effects of cyclic antidepressants are potentiated by concomitantly ingested alcohol, benzodiazepines, and other sedative-hypnotics. Seizures may occur, and in severe overdoses, respiratory arrest may occur. Cardiovascular toxicity presents a particular danger (Box 3-3). Hypotension often occurs, even with the patient supine.

A variety of arrhythmias may develop, including supraventricular tachycardia, ventricular tachycardia, or fibrillation, and varying degrees of heart block, including complete heart block.

Drug Interactions

The cyclic antidepressants have a variety of important pharmacodynamic and pharmacokinetic drug–drug interactions that may worsen the toxicity of other drugs (see Box 3-3).

Monoamine Oxidase Inhibitors

The MAOIs are well absorbed after oral administration. A transdermal form of selegiline (Emsam) is also available and approved by the FDA for the treatment of depression. Since MAOIs irreversibly inhibit the enzymes, return of enzyme function after discontinuation may require 2 weeks (the time it takes for *de novo* synthesis of the enzyme). The metabolism of MAOIs is not well understood. Selegiline and tranylcypromine have meta-amphetamine and amphetamine as

metabolites. There is controversy as to whether phenelzine is cleaved and acetylated in the liver. It is known that a sizable number of people are slow acetylators (a high percentage of Asians and about 50% of whites and blacks), but there is little evidence that the rate of acetylation is clinically significant for this class of drugs. Of clinical importance is the observation that metabolism of MAOIs does not seem to be affected by use of anticonvulsants.

Although the overall efficacy of MAOIs does not differ from that of other commonly used antidepressants in the treatment of MDD, their use is considerably limited by the risk of potentially lethal adverse events, such as hypertensive crises and serotonin syndromes, and by the strict dietary restrictions required to minimize such risks. As a result, they are rarely chosen as first-line agents in the treatment of depression[84]; their use is mainly limited to the treatment of treatment-refractory depression, either as a "next-step" strategy in TCA-resistant depression,[273-279] or even depression resistant to a number of antidepressants.[280-284] High doses of the MAOI tranylcypromine (90 to 170 mg daily) may also be effective in depressed patients who do not experience sufficient improvement during treatment with lower doses.[285] In addition, perhaps due to their ability to inhibit the re-uptake of dopamine in addition to serotonin and norepinephrine, MAOIs appear to be more effective than TCAs[286] in the treatment of atypical depression (characterized by mood reactivity in addition to symptoms such as hypersomnia, hyperphagia, extreme fatigue, and rejection sensitivity). In parallel, while the MAOIs also seem to be effective in the treatment of fatigue in fibromyalgia or chronic fatigue syndrome,[287-291] four of five studies do not show any effect of the SSRIs on fatigue.[292-296] Although, to date, there are no double-blind studies that compare the relative efficacy of MAOIs versus the SSRIs or TCAs in the treatment of fatigue in depression, these studies suggest a potential advantage for MAOIs over SSRIs.

In the GI tract and the liver, MAO catabolizes a number of dietary pressor amines (such as dopamine, tyramine, tryptamine, and phenylethylamine).[52] For this reason, consumption of foods containing high levels of dietary amines while on an MAOI may precipitate a hypertensive crisis, characterized by hypertension, hyperpyrexia, tachycardia, tremulousness, and cardiac arrhythmias.[53] The same reaction may also occur during co-administration of dopaminergic agents and MAOIs, while the co-administration of MAOIs with other antidepressants that potentiate serotonin could result in serotonin syndromes due to toxic CNS serotonin levels. The serotonin syndrome is characterized by alterations in cognition (disorientation, confusion), behavior (agitation, restlessness), autonomic nervous system function (fever, shivering, diaphoresis, diarrhea), and neuromuscular activity (ataxia, hyperreflexia, and myoclonus).[54-56] Since MAO enzymatic activity requires approximately 14 days to be restored, such food or medications should be avoided for 2 weeks after the discontinuation of an irreversible MAOI ("MAOI washout period"). Serotonergic and dopaminergic antidepressants are typically discontinued 2 weeks before the initiation of an MAOI, with the exception of fluoxetine, which needs to be discontinued 5 weeks in advance due to its relatively longer half-life. In addition to its oral formulation, selegiline is also available in a transdermal form (patch), designed to minimize the inhibition of the MAO enzymes found in the lining of the GI tract. Treating MDD with transdermal selegiline appears to be effective[297,298] and also safe, even in the absence of a tyramine-restricted diet.[298] Although rare, serotonin syndrome may occur when oral selegiline is combined with serotonergic agents, particularly the SSRIs.[299] The risk of such drug interactions with the transdermal formulation of selegiline has not been studied.

Side-effect Profile

The most common side effects of MAOIs include postural hypotension, insomnia, agitation, sedation, and sexual dysfunction, although the incidence of sexual dysfunction is lower than with the SSRIs.[300] Other side effects include weight change, dry mouth, constipation, and urinary hesitancy.[51] Peripheral neuropathies have been reported, and may be prevented by concomitant therapy with pyridoxine.[301] A list of side effects with MAOIs is reported in Table 3-2. Elderly patients may develop constipation or urinary retention. Alternatively, nausea and diarrhea have been reported by some patients. Sweating, flushing, or chills may occur. Rarely, hepatotoxicity (which may be serious) may occur with phenelzine. Peripheral edema likely reflecting effects of the drug on small vessels may prove difficult to manage. Finally, some patients complain of muscle twitching or electric shock–like sensations.

Dietary Restrictions and Drug Interactions

As discussed previously, treatment with MAOIs carries a risk of hypertensive crisis. To minimize this risk, patients on MAOIs need to adhere to a strict dietary regimen that excludes foods and beverages that have a high content of dietary amines, including all aged cheeses; sour cream; yogurt; fermented or dried meats (sausages, basderma, pastrami, pepperoni, louza, lingiça, chorizo); offal (liver, sweetbread, kidney, tripe, brains); fava and broad bean pods (lima, lentils, snow-peas); marmite yeast extract; sauerkraut; soy sauce and other soy products; over-ripe bananas and avocado; eggplant; spinach; pickled, dried, or salted fish; caviar; fish roe (tarama); and foods containing monosodium glutamate (MSG). Patients should also avoid consumption of caffeinated drinks, and most alcoholic beverages, especially tap beer and red wine, but also certain white wines, including those that are resinated (retsina), botrytized (sauternes, cadillac, loupiac, monbazillac, coteaux du layon, Alsace vendage tardive, tokaji aszú, trockenbeerenausle), aged (sherry), and others (Riesling, vermouth). Sympathomimetics, both prescribed and over-the-counter (pseudoephedrine, ephedrine, oxymetazoline, dextroamphetamine, and methylphenidate), potent noradrenergic and dopaminergic antidepressants, dextromethorphan, and meperidine (Demerol) may also precipitate a hypertensive crisis. In addition, as mentioned previously, combining MAOIs with potent serotonergic agents (such as the TCAs, SSRIs, and others) carries a risk of serotonergic syndrome. MAOIs must be used with caution in patients with diabetes (due to possible potentiation of oral hypoglycemics and worsened hypoglycemia).

Dosage

The optimal dosages for MAOIs vary from agent to agent. Initially, MAOIs are administered at low doses, with gradual increases as side effects allow. Some tolerance may develop to side effects, including postural hypotension. Phenelzine is usually started at 15 mg twice daily (7.5 to 15 mg/day in the elderly), isocarboxazid at 10 mg twice daily, and tranylcypromine at 10 mg twice daily (5 to 10 mg/day in the elderly). Dosages can be increased by 15 mg weekly for phenelzine and 10 mg weekly for isocarboxazid and tranylcypromine (as side effects allow) to 45 to 60 mg/day for phenelzine (30 to 60 mg/day in the elderly) and 30 to 40 mg/day for the others. Dosages as high as 90 mg/day of these drugs may be required, although these exceed the manufacturer's recommendations. Once depressive symptoms remit, full therapeutic doses are protective against relapse, although in managing patients on MAOIs, dose adjustments over time to manage side effects or clinical response are common. For transdermal selegiline, the minimal effective dose reported is 6 mg/day. It is prudent to taper MAOIs over 2 weeks or more when discontinuing them because discontinuation reactions have been reported with abrupt discontinuation. There is little experience with the use of MAOIs in pregnancy. For this reason, their use should be avoided.

Patients have reported weight gain on all MAOIs and occasionally weight loss (more commonly on tranylcypromine). Anticholinergic-like side effects occur, although they are not due to muscarinic antagonism. These side effects are less severe than those seen with TCAs, although patients on phenelzine may experience dry mouth. Elderly patients may develop constipation or urinary retention. Nausea and diarrhea have been reported by some patients. Sweating, flushing, or chills also may occur. Rarely, hepatotoxicity may occur with phenelzine, which may be serious. Peripheral edema likely reflecting effects of the drug on small vessels may prove difficult to manage. Finally, some patients complain of muscle twitching or electric shock–like sensations. The latter may respond to clonazepam, although the emergence of neurological or neuropathic symptoms may reflect interference with absorption of vitamin B6 that should improve with dietary supplementation of pyridoxine (vitamin B6) 50 to 100 mg/day.

TABLE 3-3 Interactions of Monoamine Oxidase Inhibitors with Other Drugs*

Drug	Effect
Sympathomimetics (e.g., amphetamines, dopamine, ephedrine, epinephrine [adrenaline], isoproterenol [Isuprel], metaraminol, methylphenidate, oxymetazoline [Afrin], norepinephrine, phenylephrine [Neo-Synephrine], phenylpropanolamine, pseudoephedrine [Sudafed])	Hypertensive crisis
Meperidine (Demerol and others)	Fever, delirium, hypertension, hypotension, neuromuscular excitability, death
Oral hypoglycemics	Further lowering of serum glucose
L-dopa	Hypertensive crisis
Tricyclic antidepressants,† duloxetine, venlafaxine, SSRIs, clomipramine, tryptophan	Fever, seizures, delirium
	Nausea, confusion, anxiety, shivering, hyperthermia, rigidity, diaphoresis, hyperreflexia, tachycardia, hypotension, coma, death
Bupropion	Hypertensive crisis

*This may include selegiline even at low doses.
†Tricyclics and MAOIs are occasionally used together.
SSRIs, Selective serotonin re-uptake inhibitors.
(From Rosenbaum JF, Arana GW, Hyman SE, et al., editors: Handbook of psychiatric drug therapy, ed 5, Philadelphia, 2005, Lippincott Williams & Wilkins.)

Overdose

MAOIs are extremely dangerous in overdose. Because they circulate at very low concentrations in serum and are difficult to assay, there are no good data on therapeutic or toxic serum levels. Manifestations of toxicity may appear slowly, often taking up to 12 hours to appear and 24 hours to reach their peak; thus, even if patients appear clinically well in the emergency department, they should be admitted for observation after any significant overdose. After an asymptomatic period, a serotonin syndrome may occur, including hyperpyrexia and autonomic excitation. Neuromuscular excitability may be severe enough to produce rhabdomyolysis, which may cause renal failure. This phase of excitation may be followed by CNS depression and cardiovascular collapse. Death may occur early due to seizures or arrhythmias, or later due to asystole, arrhythmias, hypotension, or renal failure. Hemolysis and a coagulopathy also may occur and contribute to morbidity and mortality risk.

Drug Interactions

Important drug interactions with MAOIs are listed in Table 3-3.

Access the complete reference list and multiple choice questions (MCQs) online at https://expertconsult.inkling.com

KEY REFERENCES

5. Fava M, Kendler KS. Major depressive disorder. *Neuron* 28(2):335–341, 2000.
51. Fava M, Rosenbaum JF. Pharmacotherapy and somatic therapies. In Beckham EE, Leber WR, editors: *Handbook of depression*, New York, 1995, Guilford.
76. Thase ME. Preventing relapse and recurrence of depression: a brief review of therapeutic options. *CNS Spectr* 11(12 Suppl. 15):12–21, 2006.
78. Papakostas GI, Perlis RH, Seifert C, et al. Antidepressant dose-reduction and the risk of relapse in major depressive disorder. *Psychother Psychosom* 76(5):266–270, 2007.
79. Fava M, Detke MJ, Balestrieri M. Management of depression relapse: re-initiation of duloxetine treatment or dose increase. *J Psychiatr Res* 40(4):328–336, 2006.
80. Papakostas GI, Fava M. A meta-analysis of clinical trials comparing moclobemide with selective serotonin reuptake inhibitors for the treatment of major depressive disorder. *Can J Psychiatry* 51(12):783–790, 2006.
82. Fava M, Hoog SL, Judge RA, et al. Acute efficacy of fluoxetine versus sertraline and paroxetine in major depressive disorder including effects of baseline insomnia. *J Clin Psychopharmacol* 22(2):137–147, 2002.
85. Fava M, Uebelacker LA, Alpert JE, et al. Major depressive subtypes and treatment response. *Biol Psychiatry* 42(7):568–576, 1997.
90. Fava M, Rankin M. Sexual functioning and SSRIs. *J Clin Psychiatry* 63(Suppl. 5):13–16, discussion 23–25, 2002.
92. Fava M, Graves LM, Benazzi F, et al. A cross-sectional study of the prevalence of cognitive and physical symptoms during long-term antidepressant treatment. *J Clin Psychiatry* 67(11):1754–1759, 2006.

103. Fava M, Judge R, Hoog SL, et al. Fluoxetine versus sertraline and paroxetine in major depressive disorder: changes in weight with long-term treatment. *J Clin Psychiatry* 61(11):863–867, 2000.
106. Thase ME, Ferguson JM, Lydiard RB, et al. Citalopram treatment of paroxetine-intolerant depressed patients. *Depress Anxiety* 16(3):128–133, 2002.
107. Thase ME, Blomgren SL, Birkett MA, et al. Fluoxetine treatment of patients with major depressive disorder who failed initial treatment with sertraline. *J Clin Psychiatry* 58(1):16–21, 1997.
116. Fava M. Prospective studies of adverse events related to antidepressant discontinuation. *J Clin Psychiatry* 67(Suppl. 4):14–21, 2006.
125. Thase ME, Entsuah AR, Rudolph RL. Remission rates during treatment with venlafaxine or selective serotonin reuptake inhibitors. *Br J Psychiatry* 178:234, 2001.
140. Clayton AH, Pradko JF, Croft HA, et al. Prevalence of sexual dysfunction among newer antidepressants. *J Clin Psychiatry* 63(4):357–366, 2002.
144. Thase ME. Effects of venlafaxine on blood pressure: a meta-analysis of original data from 3744 depressed patients. *J Clin Psychiatry* 59(10):502–508, 1998.
145. Fava M, Mulroy R, Alpert J, et al. Emergence of adverse events following discontinuation of treatment with extended-release venlafaxine. *Am J Psychiatry* 154(12):1760–1762, 1997.
157. Papakostas GI, Fava M. A meta-analysis of clinical trials comparing milnacipran, a serotonin-norepinephrine reuptake inhibitor, with a selective serotonin reuptake inhibitor for the treatment of major depressive disorder. *Eur Neuropsychopharmacol* 17(1):32–36, 2007.
178. Papakostas GI. Dopaminergic-based pharmacotherapies for depression. *Eur Neuropsychopharmacol* 16(6):391–402, 2006.
179. Trivedi MH, Rush AJ, Carmody TJ, et al. Do bupropion SR and sertraline differ in their effects on anxiety in depressed patients? *J Clin Psychiatry* 62(10):776–781, 2001.
180. Papakostas GI, Nutt DJ, Hallett LA, et al. Resolution of sleepiness and fatigue in major depressive disorder: a comparison of bupropion and the selective serotonin reuptake inhibitors. *Biol Psychiatry* 60(12):1350–1355, 2006.
193. Papakostas GI, Fava M. A meta-analysis of clinical trials comparing the serotonin (5HT)-2 receptor antagonists trazodone and nefazodone with a selective serotonin reuptake inhibitor for the treatment of major depressive disorder. *Eur Psychiatry* 22(7):444–447, 2007.
230. Papakostas GI, Homberger CH, Fava M. A meta-analysis of clinical trials comparing mirtazapine with a selective serotonin reuptake inhibitor for the treatment of major depressive disorder. *J Psychopharmacol* 22(8):843–848, 2008.
237. Schatzberg AF, Kremer C, Rodrigues HE, et al. Mirtazapine vs. Paroxetine Study Group: Double-blind, randomized comparison of mirtazapine and paroxetine in elderly depressed patients. *Am J Geriatr Psychiatry* 10(5):541–550, 2002.
260. Fava M. Weight gain and antidepressants. *J Clin Psychiatry* 61(Suppl. 11):37–41, 2000.
274. McGrath PJ, Stewart JW, Nunes EV, et al. A double-blind cross-over trial of imipramine and phenelzine for outpatients with treatment-refractory depression. *Am J Psychiatry* 150(1):118–123, 1993.
279. McGrath PJ, Stewart JW, Harrison W, et al. Treatment of tricyclic refractory depression with a monoamine oxidase inhibitor antidepressant. *Psychopharmacol Bull* 23(1):169–172, 1987.
286. Thase ME, Trivedi MH, Rush AJ. MAOIs in the contemporary treatment of depression. *Neuropsychopharmacology* 12(3):185–219, 1995.

4 Pharmacological Approaches to Treatment-Resistant Depression

Ji Hyun Baek, MD, Andrew A. Nierenberg, MD, and Maurizio Fava, MD

KEY POINTS

Background

- Treatment-resistant depression (TRD) refers to an inadequate response to at least one antidepressant given in sufficient doses and for an appropriate duration.

History

- Despite the recent advances in treatment of depression, only 30%–40% of patients achieve remission following initial treatment.

Clinical and Research Challenges

- Inadequate response usually means failure to achieve remission. However, the, importance of functional recovery in treatment has also been emphasized.
- Staging methods to include the types and numbers of failed antidepressant trials might help clinicians and researchers to plan treatment strategies.
- Various strategies including switching antidepressant, combining two different antidepressants, augmentation, and non-pharmacological approaches, can be applied to TRD. However, the standard approach for TRD has not been established mainly due to lack of comprehensive investigations.
- Biomarkers to identify the predicting factors of TRD can help clinicians determine an appropriate treatment plan.

Practical Pointers

- Many patients with TRD are either inadequately treated or misdiagnosed. Clinicians need to systematically re-evaluate the primary diagnosis of depression as well as search for medical and psychiatric co-morbidities.
- Switching antidepressants, combining two antidepressants and applying augmentation strategies are the most commonly used approaches.
- More rigorous studies on definition, clinical trials, and biomarkers of TRD are necessary.

OVERVIEW

Treatment-resistant depression (TRD) refers to an inadequate response to adequate antidepressant treatment. TRD is common in clinical settings. In the Sequenced Treatment Alternatives to Relieve Depression (STAR*D), only 36.8% of patients with major depressive disorder (MDD) who were initially treated with citalopram achieved remission.[1] A recent meta-analytic study reviewed 91 antidepressant monotherapy randomized controlled trials and showed an average remission rate of 44%.[2]

TRD leads to poorer psychosocial functioning[3,4] and raises the risk of suicide,[5] which increases the disease burden of MDD. Cases of TRD tend to be highly recurrent, with up to 80% of patients requiring multiple treatments. The clinical outcomes of patients who fail to remit are usually worse than those of first-episode patients.[6]

DEFINITION OF TREATMENT-RESISTANT DEPRESSION

Although it appears simple, defining "inadequate response" and "adequate antidepressant treatment" remains controversial.

Inadequate response typically means failure to achieve remission; patients who improve but who fail to remit with initial treatment are more likely to have a recurrence. In clinical trials, remission is usually defined by scores on depression symptom severity scales (e.g., a Hamilton Depression Rating Scale-17 $\leq$ 7). Several researchers have suggested that functional recovery also needs to be taken into consideration when defining adequate response.[7]

At least one trial with an antidepressant with established efficacy in MDD (with sufficient duration and doses) is considered to be "adequate antidepressant treatment." However, defining sufficient duration and dose is difficult. Sufficient dose is either the minimum dosage that will produce the expected effect or the maximum dosage that the patient can tolerate until the expected effect is achieved. Typically, sufficient duration of an antidepressant is considered to be long enough to produce a robust therapeutic effect.[8] In clinical trials 4–6 weeks has been used as the threshold for sufficient duration, but some researchers suggest using a longer period, up to 8–12 weeks.[9] In STAR*D, many patients who initially failed to achieve remission or response, eventually achieved remission or a response by 14 weeks.[10]

STAGING MODELS OF TREATMENT-RESISTANT DEPRESSION

Another important characteristic of TRD is the number of failed trials. As previously mentioned, most clinical studies use a definition of TRD as failure to remit to at least one antidepressant. In other words, those with TRD can fail a number of antidepressant trials. Although there is no clear method of defining the severity of TRD, it is generally thought that as the number of failed trials increases, the chance of remission will diminish. In STAR*D, 30.6% of patients achieved remission at Level 2 and about 13% of subjects achieved remission at Level 3.[1]

Several staging models have been suggested involving the number of non-response to adequate treatment strategies and the types of antidepressants used.[8,11] However, several factors have not been fully studied. In the staging models, non-response to two agents of different classes has been thought to be more difficult to treat than non-response to two agents of the same class. In addition, there is an implicit hierarchy of antidepressant treatments, with monoamine oxidase inhibitors (MAOIs) being considered as superior to tricyclic antidepressants (TCAs) and SSRIs, and TCAs being considered as more effective than SSRIs in some populations. These two concepts have never been fully investigated.[8] A recent study showed no significant difference in remission rates between venlafaxine-treated and sertraline-treated patients who had not responded to other SSRIs.[12] Similarly, a meta-analysis of antidepressants and a cross-over trial of imipramine[13] and setraline[14] did not prove superior to TCAs.

CLINICAL FEATURES ASSOCIATED WITH TREATMENT-RESISTANT DEPRESSION

Several clinical conditions (e.g., substance abuse and co-morbid anxiety disorder) have been associated with TRD.[10,15] Co-morbid personality disorders, subtypes of depression (including atypical depression, melancholic depression, and chronic depression) have also been associated with worse response to antidepressants; however, the studies have had mixed results.[15] Co-morbid personality disorders also have been associated with poorer outcome, but not all studies support these findings.[8] Medical co-morbidities also contribute to a poorer response to antidepressants.

CLINICAL APPROACH TO TREATMENT-RESISTANT DEPRESSION

Pseudo-resistance refers to non-response associated with inadequate treatment.[16] When patients with MDD show an inadequate response (i.e., not achieving remission) with adequate antidepressant treatment, clinicians should consider the possibility of pseudo-resistance.

Misdiagnosis of mood disorders is a relatively common problem in clinical practice. This may involve recall bias associated with retrospective evaluations. When remission does not occur, we recommend that clinicians re-do the diagnostic evaluation using a structured clinical interview. Psychiatric co-morbid conditions also need to be examined thoroughly.

It is also important to assess whether a patient actually receives an "adequate antidepressant treatment." Clinicians need to evaluate whether an antidepressant was used in an adequate dose for a sufficient amount of time and whether the patient actually took medication as prescribed. Medical co-morbidities (including hypothyroidism, fibromyalgia, and neurologic conditions) can also confound the treatment response. Conducting routine blood work and a physical examination can provide additional clues. Also, co-administered medication can affect antidepressant metabolism (via inducing cytochrome P450 enzymes). In some cases, a patient might be a rapid metabolizer of a drug and result in a lower blood level.

COMMON TREATMENT STRATEGIES FOR TREATMENT-RESISTANT DEPRESSION

Once TRD is confirmed, more rigorous treatment is necessary. Various strategies have been investigated, although the best sequence of treatment has not been established. In general, switching antidepressants, combining two antidepressants, and using augmenting strategies are the most reasonable for TRD. However, the optimal method has not been determined. A retrospective analysis from STAR*D showed no significant differences (in terms of remission rate, response rate, time to remission, and time to response) between switching and augmentation strategies.[17]

Switching an Antidepressant

One of the most common strategies is switching antidepressants; however, the superiority of switching to a different class (e.g., from a SSRI to a SNRI) or switching within the same class has not been proven. In STAR*D, switching treatments in Level 2 (i.e., those who had unsatisfactory results or intoler-ance of citalopram) involved use of sertraline, venlafaxine XR, or bupropion sustained-release (SR). No significant difference was observed in terms of remission rates (24.8% for venlafaxine XR, 21.3% for bupropion SR, and 18.1% for sertraline).[1] In addition, the ARGOS study did not find significant differences (in terms of remission rates) between venlafaxine XR and other second-generation-antidepressants (mostly SSRIs) (59.3% for venlafaxine XR, 51.5% for another antidepressant).[18] On the contrary, two of four randomized controlled trials (RCTs) demonstrated that switching from a SSRI to venlafaxine was superior to the switching to a second SSRI.[19] One RCT compared the efficacy of mirtazapine, venlafaxine, and paroxetine after failure of two antidepressant trials did not find statistically significant differences in remission rates.[20] A meta-analysis of four clinical trials found only modest, but statistically significant increases after switching to a non-SSRI in patients with SSRI-resistant depression.[21]

Combining Two Antidepressants with Different Mechanisms of Action

Combining two antidepressants with different mechanisms of action is an attractive approach for managing TRD. Combination of an SSRI or an SNRI with a norepinephrine-dopamine re-uptake inhibitor (bupropion) or a serotonin-norepinephrine antagonist (mirtazapine or mianserin) is a commonly used combination, with expected synergistic effects of their pharmacodynamic properties.

A double blind placebo-controlled study found significant benefit using mirtazapine for augmentation after failing to respond to an antidepressant. Blier et al.[22] conducted a RCT of mirtazapine in combination with fluoxetine, venlafaxine, or bupropion compared with fluoxetine monotherapy and found that combination therapies were associated with approximately twice the remission rate of fluoxetine monotherapy. In contrast, in single-blind studies, no significant differences in remission rates were found with escitalopram plus placebo, bupropion SR plus escitalopram, or venlafaxine ER plus mirtazapine.[19]

When using combination treatments, clinicians should be mindful of pharmacokinetic and phamacodynamic interactions. Serotonin syndrome or the effects associated with increased drug levels (due to cytochrome P450 enzyme inhibition, e.g., CYP2D6 inhibition by fluoxetine or paroxetine) might develop.

Augmentation

Lithium

Lithium is one of the most common augmenting agents in TRD. A minimum daily dose of 900 mg is generally recommended. The efficacy of lithium augmentation (with either a TCA or an SSRI) has been supported by randomized, placebo-controlled double-blind studies. In a meta-analysis, lithium augmentation was found to be significantly more effective than placebo (OR = 3.1; 95% confidence interval [CI] 1.8–5.4).[23]

Triiodothyronine (T_3)

A meta-analysis of T_3 augmentation of TCA (8 clinical trials, n = 292),[24] showed that T_3 augmentation almost doubled the response rate. Limited data on the effect of T_3 augmentation of SSRIs is available. A recent double-blind, RCT[25] compared the effects of T_3 plus sertraline and sertraline plus placebo in MDD at treatment initiation. No significant difference was noted in remission rates, response rates, or time-to-response between two groups. In the STAR*D study, T_3 and lithium augmentation was used in patients who failed to achieve remission after two trials. Although no statistical significant difference was observed (remission rate of T_3 was 24.7% and that of lithium was 15.9%), use of T_3 had superior tolerability and adherence. While T_3 augmentation appears safe, there is a limited evidence to guide its long-term adjunctive use. More controlled trials are needed to determine the efficacy of T_3 as an adjunctive medication.[26]

Atypical Antipsychotics

Recently, use of atypical antipsychotics as adjunctive agents has been increasing. A meta-analysis by Nelson and Papakostas[27] of the adjunctive use of olanzapine, quetiapine, aripiprazole, and risperidone (16 trials, n = 3480) demonstrated that use of adjunctive atypical antipsychotics was significantly more effective than use of placebo (remission: odds ratio = 2.00 95% CI = 2.68–5.72). Aripiprazole, quetiapine, and olanzapine-fluoxetine combinations are appropriate for use in TRD in the US. Newer atypical antipsychotics, i.e., ziprasidone, paliperidone, asenapine, and iloperidone, have not been examined for their efficacy in controlled trials.

Atypical antipsychotics are apt to induce adverse effects, including extrapyramidal symptoms, tardive dyskinesia, and metabolic syndrome. Discontinuation rates due to such adverse effects are also high. Use of newer atypical antipsychotics with fewer metabolic concerns might be reasonable, although limited evidence is available.

Buspirone

Buspirone is a serotonin$_{1A}$ receptor partial agonist. In the STAR*D study, adjunctive use of buspirone showed a similar remission rate to that of adjunctive bupropion SR in citalopram non-responders (30.1% vs. 29.7%). While there have been positive data from open-label studies, two randomized placebo-controlled trials have failed to find a significant benefit from buspirone.[28]

L-Methylfolate

Folate is an essential co-factor involved in methylation reactions, which are crucial for monoamine synthesis and homocysteine regulation. Abnormal folate metabolism has long been associated with mood disorders. L-Methylfolate is a biologically-active form of dietary folate. In a recent study Papakostas et al.[29] examined use of L-Methylfolate as an augmentation strategy for poor responder to SSRIs. The response rate was 32.3% compared to 14.6% for placebo over the course of two trials. Since L-Methylfolate is a neutraceutical, it is safe and has few (minor) side effects. Considering its safety and tolerabililty, it may be a promising candidate as an augmentation agent for TRD.

S-adenosyl-L-methionine

S-adenosyl-L-methionine (SAMe) is the major donor for methyl group in synthesis of neurotransmitters. Along with folic acid, SAMe also has received attention as a promising complementary alternative medicine for the treatment of depression. In a 6-week, double-blind, randomized trial of adjunctive SAMe with SSRI non-responders, remission rates were significantly higher for patients treated with SAMe than with placebo (25.8% vs. 11.7%).[30] It is also safe and has few adverse effects.

Novel Therapeutic Agents

New drugs with mechanisms that fall outside of those associated with the classical monoamine receptor hypothesis of depression offer great promise for the treatment of TRD.[19]

Ketamine, an NMDA receptor antagonist, has shown rapid antidepressant effects. Recently, several open-label studies[31,32] with repeated intravenous ketamine infusions have shown promising results. Inflammation is thought to be associated with treatment response in depression. In this context, anti-inflammatory agents may be effective. Aspirin, celecoxib, infliximab, N-acetylcysteine have all been studied; however, no definite answer has been reached about their benefits.[19]

Non-pharmacological Interventions

Adjunctive psychotherapy can be helpful in TRD. In the STAR*D study, cognitive therapy was included in Level 2. No significant difference was observed in remission rates between the cognitive therapy group and the medication-only group. A randomized trial investigating the effects of cognitive-behavioral therapy (CBT) in women with TRD (n = 469), adding CBT to usual care, significantly increased treatment response compared with usual care at 6 months (46% vs. 22%). However, the efficacy of other types of psychotherapy has not been investigated in TRD.

Brain stimulation focuses on the direct or indirect alteration of brain function by electrical or magnetic methods. Electroconvulsive therapy (ECT), the oldest brain stimulation methods, has long been viewed as an effective treatment for severe depression.[33] Cognitive impairment is its most common side effect. Vagus nerve stimulation (VNS) therapy stimulates the left vagus nerve repetitively using small electrical pulse from an neurostimulator implanted on patients' neck. In an open study with patients afflicted with chronic MDD who had failed to respond to more than four adequate antidepressant treatments, the response rate to VNS was approximately 30%. Recently, it has been approved as an adjunctive treatment for TRD in the US. Side effects (such as voice alteration, dyspnea, and neck pain) of VNS are generally mild. However, it requires an invasive procedure, and most of the studies done so far had relatively small sample sizes. Deep brain stimulation (DBS) was initially developed for the treatment of Parkinson's disease. DBS therapy stimulates targeted brain region via electrodes which are permanently implanted. Subcallosal cingulate white matter, the ventral caudate, the ventral striatum, and the subcallosal cingulate white matter are commonly targeted. Several small open studies have shown promise.[34]

In severe TRD, psychosurgery also has been tried. Subcaudate tractomy, anterior cingulatomy, limbic leucotomy, and anterior capsulotomy are the most common methods. Its efficacy has been established, but its use is still limited.

RESEARCH CHALLENGES

As previously mentioned, a precise definition of TRD is necessary. Staging models to identify the degree of TRD also need to be conducted.

Several antidepressant combination strategies have not been confirmed through placebo-controlled RCTs. Newer antidepressants with novel mechanisms of action may be promising. Innovative treatment strategies need to be evaluated through more collaborative, multi-center, controlled trials.

Predictive factors to identify which patients are likely to respond well to treatment remain elusive. Biomarkers can help to predict responses to certain treatments. Several studies have suggested that BDNF, inflammatory markers, and abnormalities in default mode network may be potential biomarkers for antidepressant response, but definitive answers are lacking.

CONCLUSIONS

TRD is common, although its definition is not exactly clear. Since some cases of TRD could actually be pseudo-resistance, or non-response due to suboptimal treatment, clinicians should re-do diagnostic evaluations and check patients' drug compliance when remission does not develop. Optimal treatment strategies for TRD are not well established. In order to develop efficacious treatment guidelines for TRD, more rigorous studies with collaborative, multi-center, controlled trials need to be done with a variety of promising agents. Identifying mechanisms and predicting factors of poor response to antidepressants will be important. Further studies on biomarkers for TRD are warranted.

Access a list of MCQs for this chapter at https://expertconsult .inkling.com

REFERENCES

1. Rush AJ, Trivedi MH, Wisniewski SR, et al. Acute and longer-term outcomes in depressed outpatients requiring one or several treatment steps: a STAR*D report. *Am J Psychiatry* 163:1905–1917, 2006.
2. Sinyor M, Schaffer A, Smart KA, et al. Sponsorship, antidepressant dose, and outcome in major depressive disorder: meta-analysis of randomized controlled trials. *J Clin Psychiatry* 73:e277–e287, 2012.
3. Ansseau M, Demyttenaere K, Heyrman J, et al. Objective: remission of depression in primary care The Oreon Study. *Eur Neuropsychopharmacol* 19:169–176, 2009.
4. Fekadu A, Wooderson SC, Markopoulo K, et al. What happens to patients with treatment-resistant depression? A systematic review of medium to long term outcome studies. *J Affect Disord* 116:4–11, 2009.
5. Kiloh LG, Andrews G, Neilson M. The long-term outcome of depressive illness. *Br J Psychiatry* 153:752–757, 1988.
6. Demyttenaere K, Adelin A, Patrick M, et al. Six-month compliance with antidepressant medication in the treatment of major depressive disorder. *Int Clin Psychopharmacol* 23:36–42, 2008.
7. Zimmerman M, McGlinchey JB, Posternak MA, et al. How should remission from depression be defined? The depressed patient's perspective. *Am J Psychiatry* 163:148–150, 2006.
8. Fava M. Diagnosis and definition of treatment-resistant depression. *Biol Psychiatry* 53:649–659, 2003.
9. Donovan SJ, Quitkin FM, Stewart JW, et al. Duration of antidepressant trials: clinical and research implications. *J Clin Psychopharmacol* 14:64–66, 1994.
10. Trivedi MH, Rush AJ, Wisniewski SR, et al. Evaluation of outcomes with citalopram for depression using measurement-based care in STAR*D: implications for clinical practice. *Am J Psychiatry* 163:28–40, 2006.
11. Thase ME, Rush AJ. When at first you don't succeed: sequential strategies for antidepressant nonresponders. *J Clin Psychiatry* 58(Suppl. 13):23–29, 1997.
12. Lenox-Smith AJ, Jiang Q. Venlafaxine extended release versus citalopram in patients with depression unresponsive to a selective serotonin reuptake inhibitor. *Int Clin Psychopharmacol* 23:113–119, 2008.
13. Mace S, Taylor D. Selective serotonin reuptake inhibitors: a review of efficacy and tolerability in depression. *Expert Opin Pharmacother* 1:917–933, 2000.
14. Thase ME, Rush AJ, Howland RH, et al. Double-blind switch study of imipramine or sertraline treatment of antidepressant-resistant chronic depression. *Arch Gen Psychiatry* 59:233–239, 2002.
15. Souery D, Oswald P, Massat I, et al. Clinical factors associated with treatment resistance in major depressive disorder: results from a European multicenter study. *J Clin Psychiatry* 68:1062–1070, 2007.
16. Nierenberg AA, Amsterdam JD. Treatment-resistant depression: definition and treatment approaches. *J Clin Psychiatry* 51(Suppl.): 39–47, discussion 48–50, 1990.
17. Gaynes BN, Dusetzina SB, Ellis AR, et al. Treating depression after initial treatment failure: directly comparing switch and augmenting strategies in STAR*D. *J Clin Psychopharmacol* 32:114–119, 2012.
18. Baldomero EB, Ubago JG, Cercos CL, et al. Venlafaxine extended release versus conventional antidepressants in the remission of depressive disorders after previous antidepressant failure: ARGOS study. *Depress Anxiety* 22:68–76, 2005.
19. Carvalho AF, Berk M, Hyphantis TN, et al. The integrative management of treatment-resistant depression: a comprehensive review and perspectives. *Psychother Psychosom* 83:70–88, 2014.
20. Fang Y, Yuan C, Xu Y, et al. Comparisons of the efficacy and tolerability of extended-release venlafaxine, mirtazapine, and paroxetine in treatment-resistant depression: a double-blind, randomized pilot study in a Chinese population. *J Clin Psychopharmacol* 30:357–364, 2010.
21. Papakostas GI, Fava M, Thase ME. Treatment of SSRI-resistant depression: a meta-analysis comparing within- versus across-class switches. *Biol Psychiatry* 63:699–704, 2008.
22. Blier P, Ward HE, Tremblay P, et al. Combination of antidepressant medications from treatment initiation for major depressive disorder: a double-blind randomized study. *Am J Psychiatry* 167:281–288, 2010.
23. Crossley NA, Bauer M. Acceleration and augmentation of antidepressants with lithium for depressive disorders: two meta-analyses of randomized, placebo-controlled trials. *J Clin Psychiatry* 68:935–940, 2007.
24. Aronson R, Offman HJ, Joffe RT, et al. Triiodothyronine augmentation in the treatment of refractory depression. A meta-analysis. *Arch Gen Psychiatry* 53:842–848, 1996.
25. Garlow SJ, Dunlop BW, Ninan PT, et al. The combination of triiodothyronine (T3) and sertraline is not superior to sertraline monotherapy in the treatment of major depressive disorder. *J Psychiatr Res* 46:1406–1413, 2012.
26. Rosenthal LJ, Goldner WS, O'Reardon JP. T3 augmentation in major depressive disorder: safety considerations. *Am J Psychiatry* 168:1035–1040, 2011.
27. Nelson JC, Papakostas GI. Atypical antipsychotic augmentation in major depressive disorder: a meta-analysis of placebo-controlled randomized trials. *Am J Psychiatry* 166:980–991, 2009.
28. Connolly KR, Thase ME. If at first you don't succeed: a review of the evidence for antidepressant augmentation, combination and switching strategies. *Drugs* 71:43–64, 2011.
29. Papakostas GI, Shelton RC, Zajecka JM, et al. L-methylfolate as adjunctive therapy for SSRI-resistant major depression: results of two randomized, double-blind, parallel-sequential trials. *Am J Psychiatry* 169:1267–1274, 2012.
30. Papakostas GI, Mischoulon D, Shyu I, et al. S-adenosyl methionine (SAMe) augmentation of serotonin reuptake inhibitors for antidepressant nonresponders with major depressive disorder: a double-blind, randomized clinical trial. *Am J Psychiatry* 167:942–948, 2010.
31. Haile CN, Murrough JW, Iosifescu DV, et al. Plasma brain derived neurotrophic factor (BDNF) and response to ketamine in treatment-resistant depression. *Int J Neuropsychopharmacol* 17: 331–336, 2014.
32. Shiroma PR, Johns B, Kuskowski M, et al. Augmentation of response and remission to serial intravenous subanesthetic ketamine in treatment resistant depression. *J Affect Disord* 155:123–129, 2014.
33. Kellner CH, Greenberg RM, Murrough JW, et al. ECT in treatment-resistant depression. *Am J Psychiatry* 169:1238–1244, 2012.
34. Gaynes BN, Lux LJ, Lloyd SW, et al. Nonpharmacologic interventions for treatment-resistant depression in adults. Rockville MD 2011.

5 Bipolar Disorder

Roy H. Perlis, MD, MSc, and Michael J. Ostacher, MD, MPH, MMSc

KEY POINTS

Incidence

- The lifetime prevalence of bipolar disorders is approximately 2%.

Epidemiology

- Bipolar disorder is associated with significant morbidity, including functional impairment, as well as significant risk for suicide.

Clinical Findings

- Diagnosis of bipolar disorder rests on establishing current or prior manic, hypomanic, mixed, or depressive episodes.

Treatment Options

- Treatments with evidence of efficacy for prevention of recurrence of mood episodes in bipolar disorder include use of lithium, valproate, lamotrigine, and some atypical antipsychotics, as well as psychosocial interventions.

Complications

- Depressive episodes, as well as inter-episode sub-threshold depressive symptoms, contribute substantially to the morbidity of bipolar disorder.

OVERVIEW

Bipolar disorder (BPD) is a group of brain diseases characterized by periods of depressed or elevated/irritable mood that last for weeks to years. Sometimes referred to as manic-depressive illness or manic-depressive disorder, it is traditionally considered a recurrent illness, although a growing body of evidence suggests that symptoms are chronic in many patients. The defining features of BPD are manic or hypomanic episodes; however, depressive symptoms contribute to much of the disability associated with this illness.

EPIDEMIOLOGY AND RISK FACTORS

The National Co-morbidity Survey—Replication (NCS-R) study, in which a random population-based sample of about 9,000 adults was contacted and screened using *Diagnostic and Statistical Manual of Mental Disorders*, ed 4 (DSM-IV)–based questions, estimated a lifetime prevalence of 1% for bipolar I disorder and 1.1% for bipolar II disorder.[1] A previous population-based survey using a validated self-report questionnaire estimated the prevalence of BPD at 3.4% to 3.7%.[2] In the NCS-R, the prevalence of "sub-threshold" BPD—that is, two or more core features of hypomania, without meeting criteria for BPD—was estimated at 2.4%. With this broader definition, the prevalence of all "bipolar spectrum" disorders reaches 4.4%.

The prevalence of BPD is similar for men and women[3] though gender differences may exist in illness features.[4] The risk for BPD also appears to be similar across racial groups and geographical regions. For example, epidemiological studies indicate a lifetime prevalence between 0.3% in Taiwan and 1.5% in New Zealand.[3] Past studies have also suggested that BPD might be under-recognized among non-Caucasians, because of a tendency instead to diagnose these individuals with schizophrenia. However, the NCS-R survey found no differences in the prevalence of BPD by race/ethnicity or by socio-economic status (defined by family income).[1]

The strongest established risk factor for BPD is a family history of BPD. Individuals with a first-degree relative (a parent or sibling) with BPD have a risk approximately 5 to 10 times that of those in the general population (see the section on genetics, later in this chapter). Importantly, however, their risk for major depressive disorder (MDD) is also increased more than twofold; given the greater prevalence of MDD; this means that family members of bipolar individuals are at greater risk for MDD than BPD, though some authors argue that many of those diagnosed with MDD simply have unrecognized BPD.

A number of putative environmental risks have been described for BPD[5]; these include pregnancy and obstetrical complications, season of birth (winter or spring birth, perhaps indicating maternal exposure to infection), stressful life events, traumatic brain injuries, and multiple sclerosis (MS). In MS, for example, the prevalence of BPD is roughly doubled[6]; this increase does not appear to result from adverse effects of pharmacotherapy. The prevalence may also be increased among individuals with certain neurological disorders, including epilepsy. Another intriguing finding is the association between dietary omega-3 fatty acid consumption and risk of mood disorders. Most such studies focus broadly on depressed mood, although one study reporting on data from 18 countries found greater seafood consumption to be associated with a lower risk for BPD.[7,8]

HISTORICAL CONTEXT

The concept of mood disorders dates back at least to the observations of the ancient Greeks, who recognized melancholia (depression) and mania. Beginning with the Greeks, and continuing through the nineteenth century, multiple authors independently connected the two mood states.[9,10] For example, the French physician Jules Baillarger referred to "la folie a double-forme," the alternation of manic and depressive episodes. Indeed, the concept of a dichotomy between MDD and BPD did not re-emerge until the 1960s, and remains a subject of controversy (see the section on bipolar spectrum illness, later in this chapter).

The modern concept of BPD is attributed to Emil Kraepelin, whose text described the principle of opposing mood states, and more broadly distinguished primary affective disorders from primary psychotic disorders, a distinction that still stands, despite increasing evidence that this distinction is not absolute (see the section on genetics, later in this chapter). Kraepelin's description of phenomenology, based on careful longitudinal evaluation, is instantly recognizable to many modern clinicians. However, some of the nuance of Kraepelin's descriptions has not been transmitted in modern definitions. To cite but one example, the description (by Kraepelin's student Weygandt) of multiple categories of mixed states actually presages modern debates about the overlap between rapid mood cycling, mixed manic and depressive

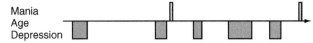

Figure 5-1. Typical bipolar course.

presentations, sub-threshold mood symptoms, and co-morbid anxiety and psychosis.[11]

CLINICAL FEATURES AND PHENOMENOLOGY

BPD is characterized by the presence of mood episodes—that is, periods of change in mood with associated symptoms. These mood episodes are described as depressive, hypomanic, manic, or mixed depending on the predominant mood and the nature of associated symptoms. Criteria for each mood state are included in the DSM-5. Mood episodes are not in and of themselves diagnoses, but rather they form the building blocks for the diagnosis of mood disorders. The key feature for the diagnosis of BPD is the presence of at least one period of mood elevation or significant irritability meeting criteria for a manic, mixed, or hypomanic episode. These episodes typically recur over time; see Figure 5-1 for a graphical illustration of the course of illness in one patient.

A manic episode is identified when a patient experiences an elevated or irritable mood for at least 1 week, along with at least three associated symptoms (described in Box 5-1). An important change in DSM-5 requires the presence of increased activity or energy as a core, or A, criterion, in an effort to improve diagnostic specificity. If the predominant affect is irritable, four rather than three associated symptoms are required. If the symptoms result in hospitalization at any point, the 1-week criterion is not required—for example, a patient hospitalized after 3 days of manic symptoms is still considered to have experienced a manic episode. As with episodes of major depression, DSM-5 criteria also require that symptoms be sufficient to markedly impair occupational or social function, or be associated with psychotic symptoms. The reliability of diagnosis for bipolar I was modest in DSM-5 field trials, with a kappa of 0.56. Hypomanic symptoms are generally similar to, but less severe and impairing than, manic symptoms. DSM-5 criteria require at least 4 days of mood elevation or irritability, along with associated symptoms; as with mania, required core symptoms now include increase in energy or activity. There are three important, but often overlooked, aspects of these criteria that bear highlighting. First, symptoms must be observable by others—that is, a purely subjective report of hypomania is not sufficient for a diagnosis. Second, symptoms represent a change from the individual's baseline; those who are "always" cheerful, impulsive, and talkative are not considered chronically hypomanic (though see the section on hyperthymia, later in this chapter). Third, symptoms by definition do not cause significant functional impairment—hypomanic-like symptoms that lead to loss of a job, for example, could be considered mania. As these criteria may be difficult to operationalize, it is not surprising that inter-rater reliability of hypomania criteria in DSM-5 field trials is somewhat lower.[12]

A major depressive episode is defined exactly as it is in MDD: the presence of depressed mood or loss of interest, most of the day, more days than not, with additional symptoms that include changes in sleep or appetite, poor self-esteem, feelings of guilt, fatigue, poor concentration, psychomotor agitation or slowing, and thoughts of suicide. In DSM-IV when criteria were met for both a major depressive and a manic episode nearly every day for at least 1 week, an episode would be characterized as a mixed state. In DSM-5, this mood state is omitted, but a modifier—"with mixed

---

BOX 5-1 DSM-5 Criteria: Manic Episode

A. A distinct period of abnormally and persistently elevated, expansive, or irritable mood and abnormally and persistently increased goal-directed activity or energy, lasting at least 1 week and present most of the day, nearly every day (or any duration if hospitalization is necessary).

B. During the period of mood disturbance and increased energy or activity, three (or more) of the following symptoms (four if the mood is only irritable) are present to a significant degree and represent a noticeable change from usual behaviour:
   1. Inflated self-esteem or grandiosity
   2. Decreased need for sleep (e.g., feels rested after only 3 hours of sleep)
   3. More talkative than usual or pressure to keep talking
   4. Flight of ideas or subjective experience that thoughts are racing
   5. Distractibility (i.e., attention too easily drawn to unimportant or irrelevant external stimuli)
   6. Increase in goal-directed activity (either socially, at work or school, or sexually) or psychomotor agitation
   7. Excessive involvement in pleasurable activities that have a high potential for painful consequences (e.g., engaging in unrestrained buying sprees, sexual indiscretions, or foolish business investments).

C. The mood disturbance is sufficiently severe to cause marked impairment in social or occupational functioning or to necessitate hospitalization to prevent harm to self or others, or there are psychotic features.

D. The episode is not attributable to the physiological effects of a substance (e.g., a drug of abuse, a medication, other treatment) or a general medical condition (e.g., hyperthyroidism).

Note: A full manic episode that emerges during antidepressant treatment (e.g., medication, electroconvulsive therapy) but persists at a fully syndromal level beyond the physiological effect of that treatment is sufficient evidence for a manic episode and, therefore, a bipolar I diagnosis.

Note: Criteria A–D constitute a manic episode. At least one lifetime manic episode is required for the diagnosis of bipolar I disorder.

Reprinted with permission from the Diagnostic and statistical manual of mental disorders, *ed 5, (Copyright 2013). American Psychiatric Association.*

TABLE 5-1 Diagnostic Features of Mood Disorders

	Mania/Mixed	Depression
Bipolar I	Yes	Typical but not required
Bipolar II	Hypomania only	Yes
MDD	Never	Yes
Cyclothymia	Never (but periods of elevation)	Symptoms but not full episode within first 2 years

MDD, Major depressive disorder.

---

features"—recognizes the common co-occurrence of manic and depressive features, setting a lower threshold than full syndromal criteria for each episode type.

Having identified the presence and type of current and past mood episodes, the clinician may then categorize the type of mood disorder and make a diagnosis. These diagnostic features are summarized in Table 5-1. Individuals with at least one manic episode are considered to have bipolar I disorder. Those with at least one hypomanic and one depressive episode, but never a manic episode, are considered to have bipolar II disorder. Individuals who have never experienced a period of hypomania, mania, or a mixed state do not have BPD (see the section on bipolar spectrum illness, later in this chapter). Note that individuals with episodes of hypomania but never manic/mixed states must also have had at least one depressive episode to meet criteria for BPD. In practice, the prevalence of hypomania without a single depressive episode is quite rare.

Two additional diagnoses are considered part of the bipolar spectrum in the DSM-5. Individuals with persistent mood instability who never meet full criteria for BPD or MDD are considered to have cyclothymia, a heterogeneous diagnosis whose relationship to other diagnostic categories is poorly understood. Specific criteria include at least 2 years marked by periods of hypomania, as well as periods of depressed mood and no more than 2 months without symptoms. Other specified bipolar and related disorder may be diagnosed in individuals with features of BPD (including mood elevation or depression) who do not meet criteria for another bipolar diagnosis (for example, where too few symptoms of hypomania are present).

ASSOCIATED ILLNESS FEATURES
Bipolar I versus II

The distinction between bipolar I and II disorder formally entered the American diagnostic system in the DSM-IV and continued in DSM-5, though it was initially described in 1976,[13] based on apparent stable differences in course of illness. Indeed, modern studies suggest that transition from bipolar II to bipolar I among adult patients is rare.[14] Some studies suggest that bipolar II patients may experience more frequent episodes and greater risk for rapid cycling,[15] as well as greater burden of depressive symptoms.[16] These differences belie the common misconception that bipolar II is less disabling than bipolar I.

Psychosis

Psychosis is not represented in the diagnostic features for BPD. However, psychotic symptoms are common during both manic/mixed and depressive episodes. A Finnish population-based study found a prevalence of 0.24% for psychotic bipolar I disorder.[17] The lifetime prevalence of psychotic symptoms in a cohort of bipolar patients was approximately 40%.[18] So-called "mood-congruent" psychotic symptoms are often seen—for example, grandiose delusions during mania or delusions of decay and doom during depression. Psychosis typically resolves along with the mood symptoms, though diagnostic criteria acknowledge that psychotic symptoms may linger beyond the end of the mood episode.

Suicide

Suicidal thoughts and attempts are also not required for a diagnosis of BPD, although they are among the criteria for a depressive episode. In one large cohort of bipolar I and II patients, between 25% and 50% reported at least one lifetime suicide attempt.[18] In population-based studies, risk of death from suicide among bipolar patients is estimated at between 10 and 25 times that of the general population,[19,20] similar to that observed in MDD.[20]

Cognitive Symptoms

Increasingly, a subset of patients with BPD has been recognized as experiencing cognitive impairment, both during and outside of mood episodes.[21] Such impairment has been difficult to characterize because it is likely multi-factorial, but clearly contributes to the profound functional impairments experienced by many bipolar patients.[21] Many commonly used pharmacotherapies (including lithium and anticonvulsants) can affect cognition. Likewise, residual mood symptoms, both depressive and manic, may affect cognition—for example, difficulty with concentrating or distractibility may occur. Attention-deficit/hyperactivity disorder (ADHD) has also been suggested to be prevalent among patients with BPD. This finding may represent "true" ADHD, or simply an overlap in the diagnostic criteria of these diagnoses.

Regardless of potential confounding effects, rigorous studies incorporating neuropsychological testing of relatively euthymic patients suggest a plethora of cognitive complaints.[21] Because these studies often use different cognitive batteries among relatively small numbers of patients, it is difficult to arrive at a single cognitive profile that is typical for BPD. Typical findings on neuropsychological testing include impairment in attention and executive function and, in some studies, deficits in working or verbal memory.

FEATURES OF LONGITUDINAL COURSE
Age at Onset and Prodrome

More recent studies suggest that the age of onset of BPD may be somewhat earlier than previously appreciated. In a large cohort study of adults with BPD, nearly one-third of individuals reported the onset of symptoms before age 13, and another one-third became symptomatic between ages 13 and 18 years.[18] In this study, earlier onset was associated with a more chronic and recurrent course, greater functional impairment, and greater Axis I co-morbidity. Unfortunately, most such studies rely on retrospective reporting, and frequently fail to distinguish between the onset of mood symptoms and the onset of a syndromal mood episode. In the NCS-R survey, the mean age at onset for bipolar I disorder was 18.2 years, and for bipolar II disorder it was 20.3 years.[1]

Mood Episodes and Chronicity

Traditional emphasis on the episodic structure of BPD has been complemented with a recognition that, for many patients, symptoms may be chronic and persist beyond discrete episodes (see Figure 5-1). Indeed, such symptoms likely contribute substantially to the disability associated with BPD, estimated to be one of the 10 greatest medical causes of disability world-wide.[22] In general, while hypomania and mania are considered the defining features of BPD, patients spend a far greater amount of time ill—around two-thirds of the time, in one longitudinal study[23]—with depressive symptoms. In general, persistence of sub-syndromal symptoms appears to be common,[24] which may explain in part persistence of functional impairment as well.[25]

Up to 40% of bipolar I patients experience a mixed state at some point in their disease course.[26] Recently, the concept of sub-threshold mixed states has received increasing attention: patients who do not meet the stringent criteria for a mixed state (who do not meet full criteria for both a manic and a depressive episode simultaneously), but nonetheless have some degree of both types of symptoms. Depressive symptoms are common during manic or hypomanic episodes, underscoring the importance of inquiring about both poles. Conversely, during depressive episodes, patients may experience some degree of hypomanic symptoms, such as racing thoughts. The prognostic implications, if any, of these sub-threshold mixed states has not been well studied. However, the change in DSM-5 to incorporate mixed symptoms as modifiers of a manic or depressive episode rather than distinct states is an effort to better capture such symptoms.

Rapid Cycling

DSM-IV-TR criteria described rapid cycling as a course specifier in BPD—that is, an illness feature that may be present at times but not necessarily throughout the course of the illness. Specifically, individuals with at least four syndromal mood episodes within a single year, separated by full recovery or a switch to the opposite pole, are considered to experience rapid cycling. In one cohort of bipolar patients, prevalence of rapid cycling was 20% assessed retrospectively,[27] and rapid cycling was associated with greater illness burden and chronicity.

Antidepressant-induced Mania/Hypomania

A small number of patients experience the onset of mania or hypomania after initiation of antidepressants, which under DSM-5 is considered to represent BPD. The true prevalence and time course of this phenomenon is difficult to estimate, particularly for a switch to hypomania, because in clinical practice, as well as in randomized controlled trials (RCTs), such symptoms of elevated mood may not be aggressively investigated. A patient who sees his or her clinician, 2 weeks after beginning an antidepressant, feeling "great" and congratulating the clinician on the clinician's excellent skills requires careful questioning about manic/hypomanic symptoms, but more often is congratulated in turn on his or her excellent antidepressant response. In one of the largest prospective antidepressant treatment studies to date in MDD,[28] there was little or no evidence of antidepressant-induced mood elevation. Likewise, most randomized trials in MDD report switch-rates of less than 1%. In a cohort study of BPD, ~20% of subjects transitioned directly from depression to mania/hypomania. Importantly, however, this rate was similar regardless of antidepressant treatment exposure, making the point that such transitions are often not associated with antidepressant treatment and may represent part of the natural history of the disorder.

Such switches are typically described as early (often within 2 weeks) and abrupt, though the time course has not been well established and it is possible that patients "switch" after prolonged antidepressant exposure, and perhaps even after antidepressant discontinuation. Some definitions consider any transition within 8 or 12 weeks of antidepressant initiation to represent a switch. Some patients describe colors being more vivid, or having an abrupt urge to undertake new projects. Importantly, the switch must be discriminated from the immense relief many patients experience with resolution of their depressive symptoms. It does not represent simply the absence of depressive symptoms, but the presence of hypomanic/manic symptoms. Again, close longitudinal follow-up may be required to clarify the diagnosis.

Because of its relative rarity, both the short- and long-term prognosis for patients who only experience hypomania or mania after antidepressant initiation is not known. Even among patients with BPD, induction of a switch with one antidepressant does not necessarily imply induction of a switch with another agent. Still, in general, patients with an antidepressant-induced mood elevation require treatment with mood-stabilizing medications for treatment and prevention of future depressive episodes.

Seasonality and Climate

A relationship between season and course of illness in BPD has been reported, but its precise nature remains unclear.

Multiple studies suggest peaks in admissions for mania, generally occurring in late spring/summer.[29-31] One report suggested that most bipolar patients follow one of two patterns: depression in fall or winter, with elevation in spring/summer, or spring-summer depression, with fall-winter mania.[32] Most recently, a large cohort study found depression peaks in February and July, but only in BPD-II.[33] They found depression to be more prevalent among patients with BPD in more northern regions of the US.

Changes in Episode Frequency

A persistent belief about BPD dating back to Kraepelin's descriptions has been that the interval between episodes decreases over time, at least across the first several episodes. This apparent observation contributed in part to earlier hypotheses that posited a "kindling" effect in which episodes beget subsequent episodes. However, it may actually be the result, at least in part, of a statistical artifact first described more than 70 years ago and referred to as "Slater's fallacy."[34] Indeed, more recent analyses suggest that such worsening with time is not the case for many patients.[35]

NEUROBIOLOGY AND PATHOPHYSIOLOGY
Hypotheses

A number of overlapping hypotheses guide current research into the neurobiology of BPD. One set of observations relates to the mechanism of action of lithium, known to be an effective treatment for BPD (see Chapter 8). While its therapeutic mechanism is not known, it does interact with two key pathways in cell signaling: inositol triphosphate (InsP3)-dependent signaling, and the Wnt signaling pathway, the latter because it inhibits glycogen synthesis kinase 3-beta (GSK3B). The Wnt/GSK3 pathway represents a particular area of interest in BPD because it is a convergent site of action of multiple psychotropics, not just lithium, and because some putative schizophrenia and bipolar liability genes influence this pathway.[36] Other clinically-based hypotheses of current interest include the role of circadian rhythm disruption, because of its prevalence in BPD, and models of stress response.

Animal Models

Research into the pathophysiology of BPD has been hindered by the lack of a convincing animal model.[37] Perhaps the best-studied model is the mouse amphetamine-induced hyperactivity model, which is purported to mimic mania (or sometimes psychosis), at least in terms of inducing psychomotor agitation. Another potential mouse model of mania was created by disrupting a gene important in circadian rhythms, CLOCK.[38] Mania-like features in these mice include a marked decrease in sleep and an increase in activity, as well as an increase in the "rewarding" effects of cocaine; most intriguingly, these changes are normalized by the administration of lithium. Circadian rhythm abnormalities have been a focus of investigation because they are so often noted clinically among individuals with BPD.[39] Most recently, additional animal models based on genetic investigation have been reported, with both depressive and manic-like symptoms. In general, results in animal models of BPD highlight the limitations in using rodents to study affective illness.

Post-mortem Studies

Another approach to the study of BPD relies on post-mortem studies of brains from bipolar patients. Neuropathological studies suggest decreased density or morphology of oligodendrocytes.[40] Other studies examine changes in gene expression. Major caveats with this approach include the sensitivity of these studies to post-mortem handling of samples and the mode of death (e.g., duration of agonal period), as well as difficulty in discriminating medication effects from the effects of a primary disease. Still, such studies suggest differences between brains of bipolar patients and normal controls. For example, one small study found down-regulation of genes related to myelination and oligodendrocytes similar to that observed in the brains of patients with schizophrenia.[41] Other recent post-mortem data suggest changes in histone acetylation in some individuals with bipolar disorder.[42]

Neuroimaging Studies

Structural brain imaging has identified regional differences in multiple brain structures among bipolar patients, predominantly cortical and sub-cortical areas implicated in limbic circuitry. While studies of the prefrontal cortex as a whole are inconsistent, a number of reports find decreased volume in individual regions among bipolar patients (reviewed by Strakowski and colleagues[43]). Among sub-cortical structures, perhaps the most consistent findings are of increased volume in the striatum and amygdala. Notably, data from twin and early-onset cohorts suggest that striatal changes may represent "trait" markers of bipolarity, present early in the disease process.

Functional imaging in BPD is complicated by the need to consider variation in mood states, and particularly by practical difficulties in imaging truly manic patients. Region-specific differences by mood state have been noted in regions of prefrontal cortex; for example, one study found decreased perfusion of sub-genual prefrontal cortex during depression and increased perfusion during mania.[44] Similar increases have been noted in basal ganglia perfusion among manic patients.[45] Studying euthymic bipolar patients provides an opportunity to elucidate potential trait markers of bipolarity. In one such study, on a cognitive task, bipolar patients demonstrated greater activation than healthy controls in regions including the ventrolateral prefrontal cortex and amygdala.[46]

Neurochemical studies applied to BPD include positron-emission tomography (PET) and magnetic resonance spectroscopy (MRS). To date, no consistently replicated patterns for binding of serotonergic or dopaminergic ligands have been identified (reviewed by Strakowski and associates[43]). With MRS, multiple studies have reported a decrease in *N*-acetyl aspartate (NAA) concentration, considered a measure of neuronal health, in the prefrontal cortex.[47] Likewise, in the basal ganglia and anterior cingulate, elevations of choline (considered a marker of integrity of cell membrane) have been identified.[48] Finally, regional changes in other metabolites (i.e., lactate, glutamate/gamma-aminobutyric acid [GABA]) have also been described.[49] Taken together, these results describe an emerging pattern of metabolic abnormalities, though one whose precise nature remains to be elucidated.

Genetic Studies

The familiality of BPD was established by numerous studies indicating that, among first-degree family members of individuals with BPD, the risk for BPD is between 7 and 10 times that found in the general population.[50] Notably, the risk for MDD is also increased roughly twofold. Twin studies indicate that up to 80% of the risk for BPD is inherited. Family and twin studies also indicate an overlap in risk with schizophrenia and schizoaffective disorder. Recent studies utilize genome-wide data to estimate the amount of BPD risk explained by common genetic variation (up to 30%), and provide further support for the genetic overlap of BPD with schizophrenia, MDD, and other psychiatric illness.

To date, at least six areas of the genome have been identified as conferring risk for BPD, including a sub-unit of L-type voltage-gated calcium channels. Studies of rarer chromosomal deletions or duplications have not yet consistently identified areas of risk.

A related area of investigation is the role of epigenetic changes in BPD—in particular, modification of chromatin. Early adversity may increase risk for BPD,[51] and both acute and chronic stress may exert epigenetic effects.[52] Intriguingly, some psychotropics, such as clozapine, appear to influence expression of chromatin-modifying enzymes.[53]

EVALUATION, TESTS, AND LABORATORY WORK-UP
Diagnosis of Bipolar Disorder

The diagnosis of BPD relies on a careful clinical assessment to identify current or past manic, hypomanic, mixed, or major depressive episodes. One study suggested that many patients wait 10 years or more for a "correct" diagnosis of BPD, although that figure may be inflated by the inclusion of patients whose initial episode is depressive.[54] A number of tools have been developed to facilitate diagnosis, but none is a substitute for detailed questioning about the mood and associated symptoms for each episode type.

A crucial and often-overlooked aspect of diagnosis in BPD is the importance of longitudinal assessment. Despite careful history-taking, in the setting of an acute episode it may sometimes be difficult to arrive at a definitive diagnosis. For example, a depressed patient may report "always" being depressed and neglect to recall periods of mood elevation consistent with hypomania.

Differential Diagnosis

A number of Axis I and II disorders may mimic BPD; general medical conditions may also yield symptoms of a mood episode. The following sections review specific diagnoses to be considered in the differential diagnosis, but several principles apply broadly. First, diagnosis requires identification of mood episodes, not simply isolated symptoms of mania or depression. Thus, the substance-abusing patient who reports "mood swings" will not necessarily be diagnosed with BPD. Second, longitudinal follow-up is often the key in clarifying the diagnosis. While difficult to implement in practice, a willingness by the clinician to make a provisional diagnosis, and to re-visit it once additional data have been gathered, eliminates some of the misplaced pressure to make an immediate diagnosis with inadequate data.

Schizophrenia and Schizoaffective Disorder

While psychosis is common among bipolar patients, the key feature that distinguishes schizophrenia and BPD is the presence of psychotic symptoms outside of mood episodes, which is not seen in BPD. In acutely psychotic and agitated patients, it may be difficult to distinguish a schizophrenic psychotic episode from a bipolar mixed state. In such cases longitudinal follow-up is required to clarify the diagnosis: in a bipolar patient, psychotic symptoms should resolve along with mood symptoms.

Schizoaffective patients, like bipolar patients, may experience both depressive and manic episodes. However, once again the presence of psychotic symptoms in the absence of a mood episode defines the diagnosis as a primary psychotic rather than affective one—that is, schizoaffective disorder rather than BPD.

Major Depressive Disorder

To distinguish MDD from BPD requires careful questioning to exclude mixed symptoms and past episodes of mood elevation. For cross-sectional evaluation, such as in a patient having a first episode, there is no single feature (other than identifying a prior episode) that distinguishes bipolar depression from MDD. The first-episode problem is particularly acute given that up to two-thirds of those with BPD recall a depressive episode preceding a manic episode. There are, however, features that may help to stratify risk; these features include current symptoms and sociodemographic/longitudinal factors.

Among current symptoms, those of atypical depression—that is, "reverse" neurovegetative signs (such as increased appetite or carbohydrate craving and hypersomnia) have been associated with bipolar depression. However, atypical depressive features are common among individuals with MDD as well, and the cohesiveness of atypical depression itself has been questioned. Likewise, some authors suggest that irritability during a depressive episode is a marker for bipolarity. Certainly irritability should prompt further questioning for mixed/manic symptoms, but the high prevalence of irritability during depressive episodes again mandates that it not be used to make a diagnosis. Psychotic features may be more commonly seen in BPD than MDD, though here too they are not diagnostic. Last, a comparison of individuals with MDD or BPD participating in RCTs found that overall depression severity was greater among the bipolar subjects, with psychic anxiety more common and somatic symptoms less common in this group.

Among other risk factors, perhaps the best characterized is family history (see the section on risk factors, earlier in this chapter). Another well-investigated risk factor is early age of illness onset. In general, the median age of onset for MDD is later than for BPD. Therefore, those with earlier onset of mood symptoms—particularly onset in childhood or adolescence—must be followed closely for BPD. Greater recurrence of depressive episodes has also been associated with BPD.

Anxiety Disorders

Distinguishing anxiety from BPD is complicated by the high rate of co-morbidity: identifying one disorder does not exclude the other. Between 85% and 90% of individuals in one survey reported at least one co-morbid anxiety disorder;[1] a large cohort study of BPD reported co-morbidity in around 60%.[18] Among the most common co-morbid conditions appear to be social phobia, generalized anxiety, post-traumatic stress disorder (PTSD), and panic disorder. One under-recognized consideration is that patients with severe anxiety may report symptoms suggestive of mania or hypomania. In particular, many anxious patients will report that their thoughts race, or that they experience psychomotor restlessness. These symptoms are often intermittent and worse when patients are most anxious, which may help to distinguish them from those with BPD.

Substance Use Disorders

As with anxiety, rates of co-occurrence between substance use disorders and BPD are quite high; determining that a patient has a substance use disorder does not end the need for screening for BPD, and vice versa. Between 40% and 60% of patients with BPD report a lifetime substance use disorder, with alcohol abuse being the most common.[1,18] What complicates the recognition of BPD is that abused substances may cause symptoms that mimic both depression and mania, as well as mixed states. For example, cocaine binges not only represent injudicious/risk-seeking behavior, but are often associated with a decreased need for sleep, pressured speech, or increased social behavior, and increased impulsivity in other domains. Likewise, the impulsivity experienced during a period of mood elevation may increase the likelihood of substance abuse.

Traditional teaching holds that BPD may be recognized among patients with substance use disorder by identifying mood episodes during periods of sobriety. However, this neglects the common phenomenon of depressive symptoms during early sobriety, as well as the fact that many patients fail to achieve a prolonged period of sobriety during which a mood episode might be detected. More useful may be the principle that mood symptoms among non-bipolar individuals are typically confined to, and change in parallel with, periods of substance intoxication or withdrawal. So, for example, a patient might be impulsive, agitated, and euphoric during a cocaine binge, but these symptoms should parallel the course of intoxication and would be unlikely to persist for days after the last cocaine use. In practice, definitively identifying BPD in a patient with frequent and severe substance use can be difficult.

Borderline Personality Disorder

Many symptoms overlap between DSM-5 definitions of BPD and borderline personality disorder.[55] Notable features in common include irritability, lability, impulsivity, and suicidality. These features may be particularly difficult to distinguish in a patient believed to have current rapid cycling,[56] with rapid fluctuation in mood state. However, several aspects of presentation bear consideration. First, symptoms of personality disorders are typically more pervasive and less episodic; while they may wax and wane over time, they would typically not "remit" in the way a mood episode would. Second, while borderline patients likely satisfy multiple manic or depressive criteria, they would not be expected to meet full criteria at a given time—that is, to have a full-blown hypomanic or manic episode.

Secondary Mania

In 1978, a group of clinicians described a small cohort of patients who developed manic symptoms in the context of medical illness, particularly after exposure to certain medications, such as corticosteroids.[57] Typically, in such cases there are other clues that the culprit is not BPD *per se*: late onset in a patient with no prior mood symptoms, close temporal correlation with a previously implicated medication, or presence of other neurological or systemic symptoms. As noted later, further medical work-up is often warranted when such features are present.

Bipolar Spectrum Illness

Symptoms common in BPD, including irritability, mood lability, and impulsivity, are also seen across many psychiatric disorders. This observation has led some authors to speculate about the concept of a bipolar spectrum: that is, bipolar I and II lie along a continuum with other disorders (such as substance abuse and binge-eating).[58]

The concept of a bipolar spectrum is often invoked in individuals with recurrent MDD, particularly those with features of illness suggestive of BPD: those with irritability or highly recurrent illness, for example.[59] In these cases it is sometimes invoked to justify using bipolar pharmacotherapies by analogy, hypothesizing that recurrent MDD that fails to respond to antidepressants might respond to a drug such as lithium. To date, while the bipolar spectrum is an appealing concept, it is not clear that it is a scientifically useful one. In particular, recent investigations suggest that bipolar spectrum illness as traditionally applied has little or no predictive validity.[60]

CONSEQUENCES OF MISDIAGNOSIS

With the increased attention to recognizing BPD, the consequences of mis-diagnosing BPD also bear a note. Some bipolar pharmacotherapies may be effective in the treatment of other disorders, but in general a patient incorrectly diagnosed with BPD is likely to receive sub-optimal treatment. Moreover, these treatments all carry some degree of potential toxicity, to which these patients may be unnecessarily exposed.

ROLE OF DIAGNOSTIC TESTING (INCLUDING NEUROIMAGING AND OTHER BIOMARKERS)

At present, there is no useful diagnostic test for BPD, nor is there a useful predictor of prognosis. A study of radiographic findings among psychiatric patients underscored the lack of utility for brain imaging in unselected populations. However, such tests may in the proper context be useful for diagnosis by excluding general medical conditions that contribute to so-called secondary mania or other mood symptoms. Medical work-up should be considered in presentations of BPD that appear to be atypical (e.g., with a later onset of illness, with an association with neurological signs, or with evidence of other systemic illnesses). For work-up of depressive symptoms. For manic/hypomanic symptoms, structural magnetic resonance imaging (MRI) helps to exclude stroke or tumor; an electroencephalogram (EEG) is rarely useful (because of poor sensitivity) for excluding temporal lobe epilepsy.

TOOLS FOR SCREENING, DIAGNOSIS, AND SYMPTOM MONITORING

Surprisingly, no single screen for BPD has been convincingly validated in clinical populations. One instrument frequently advocated for improving the recognition of BPD is the Mood Disorder Questionnaire (MDQ).[61] This patient-report questionnaire essentially incorporates the DSM criteria for mania and depression. A population-based validation study in which MDQ results were compared to Structured Clinical Interview for Diagnosis (SCID) criteria suggested that its sensitivity is poor (28%) and its specificity is 97%. A similar tool is the Bipolar Spectrum Diagnostic Scale,[62] which also uses self-report for screening. As with any screening measures, their performance depends on the prevalence of the disorder in the population being screened. In general, both measures perform well for excluding BPD when the prior probability is low (approximately 10% prevalence, as might be seen in a cohort of depressed patients), with a negative predictive value of 92% to 97%, but are not useful for confirming a diagnosis, with a positive predictive value as low as 16%—that is, the rate of false positives is extremely high. As such, neither measure can substitute for a clinician's interview, including careful history-taking. They may be most useful in initiating a discussion about BPD, for example, when completed by patients in the office waiting room.

Most research assessment tools for BPD rely on DSM criteria. While cumbersome to use in its entirety in routine practice, the mood and psychosis modules from the SCID require relatively little training to use and are helpful in ensuring comprehensive assessment of mood episodes.

For assessing depressive symptoms, validated self-report measures (the Beck Depression Inventory, the Quick Inventory of Depressive Symptoms) and clinician-rated measures (Hamilton Depression Rating Scale, Montgomery-Asberg Depression Rating Scale) are available. Of note, both the MADRS and the 17-item HAM-D do not capture reverse neurovegetative signs, and the latter weights insomnia relatively strongly, which may limit their application in bipolar depression. Self-report measures are less well-validated in BPD, though there is no reason to imagine they would perform differently in this population. Finally, the 7-point Clinical Global Impression (CGI) scale has been adapted for BPD, with one report suggesting it may capture clinical improvement in randomized trials that is not otherwise measured by other rating scales.[63] Self-report measures of depression can be applied clinically to monitor treatment response or characterize residual symptoms.

Manic symptoms are typically characterized by the Young Mania Rating Scale (YMRS), a clinician-rated scale, or the Mania Rating Scale, derived from the SAD. While a self-report form of the YMRS has been developed, because patient insight into symptoms may be impaired[64] and patients may tend to minimize symptoms during hypomania/mania, its utility could be limited, particularly among more severely ill patients.

In some cases daily mood charting (Figure 5-2) may be applied to quantify the extent of mood elevation or depression. In this approach, patients rate the extent of manic and depressive symptoms each day, along with details, such as medication compliance and sleep schedule. Beyond paper-based charts, a number of electronic mood diaries now make such mood monitoring relatively simple. The value of such charts is primarily in the measurement of changes in symptoms over time in response to different interventions, or in identification of mood cycling.

TREATMENT

Treatment goals in BPD include remission of acute episodes and prevention of recurrence.[65] Less obvious, but also crucial, given the potential chronicity of symptoms and the side-effect burdens with many treatments, treatment is aimed at preventing the consequences of BPD, including functional impairment[21] and suicide.

Determination of Mood State and Symptom Severity

The importance of characterizing mood state before initiation of treatment cannot be over-emphasized. Patients in a mixed state, for example, may complain of depressed mood, and failure to inquire about manic symptoms may result in inappropriate treatment (such as initiation of an antidepressant). More broadly, characterizing symptoms is important in monitoring treatment response, particularly given the prevalence of a partial or an incomplete response to treatment and the consequences (in terms of functional impairment and recurrence risk) of incomplete response.

Treatment strategies are typically divided into two stages: an acute phase (focused on eliminating or managing acute symptoms) and a maintenance phase (focused on prevention of recurrence and maximization of function). To some extent this dichotomy is false: acute treatments are often selected with an eye toward future use in maintenance, while maintenance treatments often require adjustment to manage residual

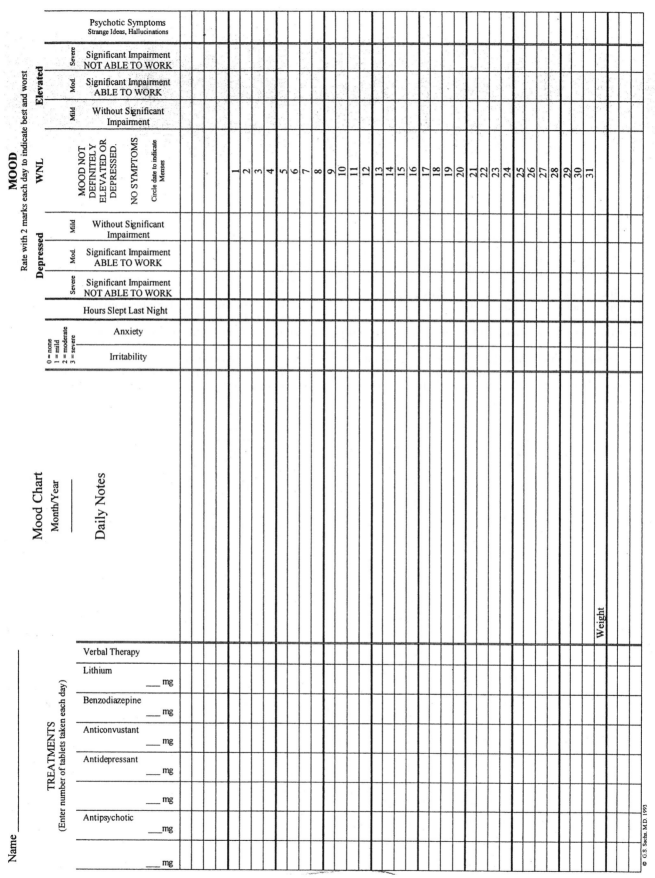

Figure 5-2. Mood chart. *(Source:* www.manicdepressive.org/images/moodchart.pdf. © *G.S. Sachs, MD, 1993.)*

or sub-threshold symptoms. Still, it provides a useful framework for consideration of treatment options.

Treatment Strategies

The number of pharmacological interventions available for the treatment of BPD has grown over the past decade, with increased application of anticonvulsants and antipsychotics. Many of these interventions continue to be actively studied, particularly in the maintenance phase of treatment. Multiple guidelines or algorithms have been developed to aid the clinician in evidence-based treatment of BPD. Internationally, a number of groups have developed their own guidelines, including the Canadian Network for Mood and Anxiety Treatments (CANMAT), the British Association for Psychopharmacology (BAP), and others. In general, these guidelines are remarkably consistent in their approach to treatment. One recent addition is the Clinical Practice Guidelines from the US Department of Veterans Affairs, released in 2010. The following section summarizes evidence-based treatments for each phase of illness. For further details, including information regarding dosing and safety, the interested reader is referred to chapters addressing individual treatment options (see Chapters 3, 7, 9). Traditional discussions of bipolar pharmacotherapy rely on the concept of a mood stabilizer, most often used as short-hand for lithium, valproate, and in some cases carbamazepine. With the broadening of the bipolar pharmacopoeia in the past decade, however, this term is less useful and more difficult to define.[66] In the following

discussion, interventions are discussed instead in terms of their efficacy in achieving specific treatment goals: acute treatment versus prevention of recurrence, and depression versus mania.

General Treatment Strategies

Most guidelines begin by emphasizing the value of psychoeducation and disease management strategies, which are supported by multiple RCTs.[67–69] These approaches focus on educating patients about the illness, and particularly recognizing symptoms, and understanding and adhering to treatment. Recent studies particularly support the utility of group-based cognitive and behavioral interventions.

Approach to Mania

As with any acute episode, the first element of managing mania is to ensure safety for patients and those around them; this may require hospitalization. Medical contributors (including drugs of abuse) to mania should be ruled-out. Antidepressants, which may precipitate or exacerbate mania, should be discontinued.

Multiple first-line agents have been established for mania (Figure 5-3). Those with greatest evidence of efficacy include lithium, valproate, and second-generation antipsychotics (SGAs). Among the SGAs, there appears to be little difference in efficacy.[70] Whether they are used alone or in combination typically depends on the severity of illness—combination therapy may have modestly greater efficacy. If a single

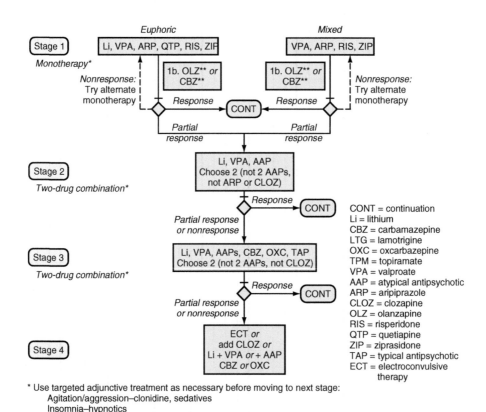

Figure 5-3. Algorithm for treatment of BPD—currently hypomanic/manic. *(Copyright 2005, Texas Department of State Health Services, all rights reserved.)*

pharmacotherapy does not achieve improvement within a short period, a second one may be added, or the patient may be switched to an alternative first-line agent. A number of other pharmacotherapies have been studied in mania; RCTs suggest that gabapentin, topiramate, and lamotrigine are not efficacious in acute treatment (see Chapter 9). Benzodiazepines are sometimes used as adjunctive treatments among manic patients, specifically to reduce agitation and promote sleep; they have shown greater efficacy than placebo in RCTs for agitation.

A question of substantial clinical interest has been whether combining multiple antimanic agents achieves better response than monotherapy. Meta-analyses do suggest modest advantage in efficacy for combination therapy, though this must be weighed against an increase in adverse effects.[70] Generally, monotherapy is preferred for less ill patients, whereas combination therapy is used for those who are more ill (e.g., hospitalized).

Approach to Mixed States

Treatment for mixed states is similar to that for manic states. Most atypical antipsychotics (AAPs) show similar efficacy among mixed and non-mixed manias. While one study suggested that lithium might be less effective in these patients than in euphoric mania, this is by no means a consistent finding. Valproate and the atypical antipsychotics generally appear to have similar efficacy across forms of mania.[70] Similarly, antimanic agents generally show similar efficacy against psychotic mania, but antipsychotics are typically advised either as monotherapy or combination therapy in these patients.

The approach to mixed states generally follows that of mania. One study suggested that lithium was relatively less effective in mixed mania than in euphoric mania.[71]

Approach to Depression

Multiple strategies have shown efficacy in the treatment of bipolar depression in RCTs (Figure 5-4). Efficacy for lithium, valproate, and carbamazepine has been suggested but not definitively established in RCTs (see Chapters 8 and 9). Multiple SGAs, including quetiapine and olanzapine (the latter in combination with fluoxetine), as well as lurasidone, were more effective than placebo.[25,72] A head-to-head study found slightly greater improvement with the olanzapine–fluoxetine combination than with lamotrigine, despite better tolerability in the lamotrigine arm.[73] The anticonvulsant lamotrigine has also been extensively studied in bipolar depression as well, with suggestive but not consistent evidence

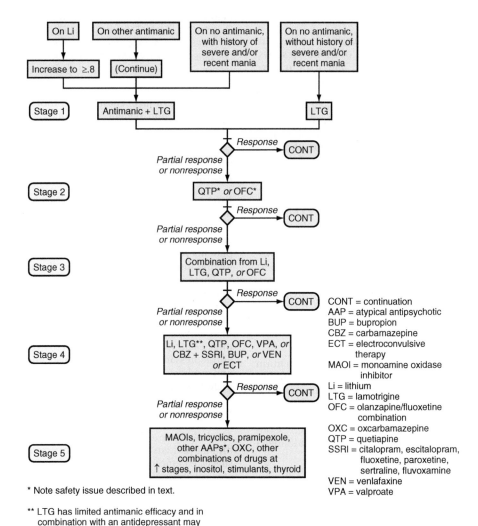

Figure 5-4. Algorithm for treatment of BPD—currently depressed. *(Copyright 2005, Texas Department of State Health Services, all rights reserved.)*

of benefit (see Chapter 9), except in combination with lithium.[74]

The efficacy of antidepressants in patients already treated with an antimanic/prophylactic medication, such as lithium, is not clear. A study of paroxetine or imipramine versus placebo, in addition to lithium, failed to find an advantage for antidepressant treatment, except in a secondary analysis examining individuals with lower (less than 0.8 mEq/L) lithium levels.[75] In the largest study to date, addition of bupropion or paroxetine to a traditional mood stabilizer likewise yielded no benefit compared to placebo.[76]

Furthermore, antidepressants appear to increase the risk of a switch—that is, transitioning directly to manic, hypomanic, or mixed states. While the risk of "switch" into mania is no greater than placebo when these medications are used along with a traditional mood stabilizer,[76,77] in the absence of evidence of efficacy, most guidelines suggest that they are better avoided. However, recent expert consensus statements acknowledge that some individuals with BPD may benefit from antidepressants in conjunction with mood stabilizers.[78] That is, antidepressants may have benefit for some individual patients, even though they fail to benefit bipolar patients as a group; for example, it has not been determined whether they benefit symptoms of co-morbid anxiety in these patients.

Approach to Maintenance Treatment

Most studies of lithium and valproate suggest that they are effective in the prevention of recurrence of mood episodes. The optimum therapeutic dose of each, and their relative benefit for prevention of manic versus depressive recurrence, is debated.[79,80] Two RCTs also found efficacy for lamotrigine in the prevention of depressive recurrence[81] (see Chapter 9). Evidence of benefit in preventing manic recurrence was much more modest. Numerous SGAs have also been shown to prevent recurrence of mood episodes. Despite the efficacy of these interventions, BPD remains highly recurrent for many patients, with residual mood symptoms one of the primary risk factors (Figure 5-5).

As in acute treatment, the role of antidepressants in maintenance is not established. As noted previously, antidepressants may contribute to an increase in mood episode frequency. On the other hand, one study suggested that discontinuing antidepressants among patients who achieved remission was associated with a greater risk of recurrence. In practice, most guidelines suggest avoiding antidepressants in long-term treatment where possible. Long-term benzodiazepine treatment has also been suggested to increase recurrence risk.[82]

Use of Psychosocial Interventions

Psychosocial interventions have received increasing attention in the management of BPD, with some but not all studies showing efficacy. In a large multi-center trial, interventions including cognitive-behavioral therapy (CBT), interpersonal/social rhythm therapy (IPSRT), and family-focused therapy increased rates of recovery from an acute episode.[83] Conversely, IPSRT showed no acute benefit in another randomized trial.[84]

A group psychoeducation approach incorporating elements of CBT also reduced recurrence in one large study.[69] A trial of IPSRT during acute episodes found reduced recurrence regardless of whether IPSRT was continued beyond that episode.[84] On the other hand, a large RCT of CBT found no benefit in preventing recurrence,[85] while another did not reduce recurrence beyond the first year,[86] despite evidence of cost-effectiveness.[87]

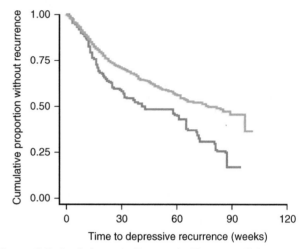

— With residual manic symptoms			
N = 156	46	16	2
— Without residual manic symptoms			
N = 702	309	164	19
Total			
N = 858	355	180	21

Figure 5-5. Survival curve (Systematic Treatment Enhancement Program for Bipolar Disorder [STEP-BD]). *(From Perlis RH, Ostacher MJ, Patel JK, et al. Predictors of recurrence in bipolar disorder: primary outcomes from the Systematic Treatment Enhancement Program for Bipolar Disorder (STEP-BD), Am J Psychiatry 163:217–224, 2006.)*

This pattern has persisted with more recent studies: some, but not all, find benefit, not unlike acute pharmacotherapy trials.

SPECIAL CONSIDERATIONS IN TREATMENT
Features of Course

Psychotic symptoms are common during both manic and depressive episodes.[18] Typical management involves the use of an antipsychotic, although at least one study suggested similar efficacy for valproate in psychotic mania.[88] Whether these patients require ongoing treatment with an antipsychotic following the acute episode is not well studied.

There is limited evidence to support the widespread belief that rapid cycling is associated with differential treatment response. Therefore, most treatment guidelines suggest the use of appropriate interventions for the presenting or predominant mood type (e.g., mania, hypomania, depression, and mixed state), with particular effort to avoid the use of standard antidepressants. Clinicians are also encouraged to consider and address other factors that may contribute to cycling, including substance abuse and thyroid disease.

Psychiatric and Medical Co-Morbidity

Alcohol abuse and dependence is extremely prevalent among bipolar patients, and requires concurrent treatment. One RCT suggested efficacy for divalproex among bipolar patients with alcohol abuse.[89] Behavioral strategies have also been shown to be effective. In general, management of co-morbidity in BPD is under-studied, despite its prevalence.

Bipolar II

With a few exceptions, nearly all RCTs in BPD have focused on bipolar I patients, and evidence among bipolar II patients is extremely limited.[90] Therefore, treatment recommendations typically suggest that bipolar II patients be treated "by analogy"—that is, that interventions shown to be effective in bipolar I disorder be used. The two placebo-controlled trials of quetiapine in bipolar depression did include both bipolar I and II patients, with pooled results suggesting less benefit among individuals with bipolar II.

Pregnancy

Most studies find that, on average, recurrence risk neither increases nor decreases during pregnancy. The post-partum period, however, is a period of dramatically increased risk for recurrence, with bipolar patients at particular risk for post-partum psychosis. Whether this is a result of hormonal changes or other factors (such as sleep disruption) during the post-partum period has not been well studied. Treatment of BPD during pregnancy is beyond the scope of this chapter; the interested reader is referred to Viguera and co-workers.[91] In general, all pharmacological treatment strategies carry some risk to the fetus, although this must be balanced against the substantial consequences of recurrence during or after pregnancy.

Childhood, Adolescence, and Geriatric Patients

Regardless of the accuracy with which BPD can be diagnosed in childhood, retrospective studies in adults make it clear that many individuals with BPD were symptomatic before age 18.[18] As such, there remains a need to understand whether adult bipolar interventions are safe and effective in children. In geriatric populations, similar treatment approaches are generally adopted but with more attention paid to potential toxicities. So, for example, lithium may be used but at lower target levels, recognizing that brain levels may correspond poorly to plasma levels in this group. Notably, pharmacovigilance studies suggest that atypical antipsychotics may increase stroke risk among older patients, particularly those with dementia, so use of SGAs requires more caution in this group.

PROGNOSIS

By comparison with other chronic and recurrent medical illnesses, remarkably few data exist to guide clinicians in the estimation of prognosis. The few diagnostic features associated with differential prognosis are rarely replicated, with some exceptions. A greater number of recent episodes, or more days ill in the prior year, do appear to predict earlier recurrence.[92] Also not surprisingly, residual mood symptoms—both manic and depressive—following an acute episode appear to be predictive of earlier recurrence.

Earlier onset of mood symptoms has been associated with a more severe illness course, with greater chronicity, and with recurrence.[18] One study also suggested that individuals with a first depressive rather than manic episode might also be at greater risk for a chronic and depressive course.[93]

An open question is whether interventions targeting those prognostic factors that may be modifiable might improve outcome. For example, more aggressive treatment of residual mood symptoms to target remission, as has been emphasized in MDD, might reduce recurrence risk, though this has not been formally studied.

MEDICAL CO-MORBIDITY AMONG BIPOLAR PATIENTS

A persistent concern is the observation that bipolar patients are at elevated risk of morbidity and mortality from multiple causes, not only suicide.[20,94] In particular, they show elevated incidences of cardiovascular risk factors (including obesity, hyperlipidemia, and diabetes), with risk compounded by greater rates of tobacco use compared to the general population. Several explanations have been suggested for this co-morbidity: it may be another feature of the disorder itself, or a consequence of poorer health maintenance arising from chronic illness. Moreover, many first-line treatments for BPD can precipitate or exacerbate these risk factors. With the discovery that variations in calcium channel genes are associated with BPD risk, it is also possible that systemic effects of such risk genes have previously been overlooked. Indeed, the increased rate of migraine in individuals with BPD may represent one such co-morbidity.

CONTROVERSIES
Child Bipolar

Perhaps no single area of BPD research and clinical practice has prompted as much controversy as the diagnosis and treatment of BPD in children and adolescents. Two key questions for debate are the reliability of the BPD diagnosis, particularly in younger children, and the validity of this diagnosis—that is, to what extent children diagnosed with BPD grow up to be adults with BPD. These issues are often conflated with broader concerns about exposing children to psychotropic medications that are not yet well studied in this population. Cross-sectional/retrospective studies suggest that many bipolar adults are symptomatic as children, while small prospective studies suggest that children diagnosed with BPD often continue to be symptomatic and have a bipolar-like course of illness. To truly understand the continuity between child and adult BPD, long-term prospective cohort studies will be required. Such studies can definitively establish the validity of childhood-onset BPD by examining the proportion of children diagnosed with BPD whose symptoms persist into adulthood.

Access the complete reference list and multiple choice questions (MCQs) online at https://expertconsult.inkling.com

KEY REFERENCES

1. Merikangas KR, Akiskal HS, Angst J, et al. Lifetime and 12–month prevalence of bipolar spectrum disorder in the National Comorbidity Survey Replication. *Arch Gen Psychiatry* 64(5):543–552, 2007.
2. Hirschfeld RM, Calabrese JR, Weissman MM, et al. Screening for bipolar disorder in the community. *J Clin Psychiatry* 64(1):53–59, 2003.
10. Angst J, Marneros A. Bipolarity from ancient to modern times: conception, birth and rebirth. *J Affect Disord* 67(1–3):3–19, 2001.
11. Salvatore P, Baldessarini RJ, Centorrino F, et al. Weygandt's *On the Mixed States of Manic-Depressive Insanity*: a translation and commentary on its significance in the evolution of the concept of bipolar disorder. *Harv Rev Psychiatry* 10(5):255–275, 2002.
16. Judd LL, Akiskal HS, Schettler PJ, et al. A prospective investigation of the natural history of the long-term weekly symptomatic status of bipolar II disorder. *Arch Gen Psychiatry* 60(3):261–269, 2003.
18. Perlis RH, Miyahara S, Marangell LB, et al. Long-term implications of early onset in bipolar disorder: data from the first 1000 participants in the Systematic Treatment Enhancement Program for Bipolar Disorder (STEP-BD). *Biol Psychiatry* 55(9):875–881, 2004.
20. Osby U, Brandt L, Correia N, et al. Excess mortality in bipolar and unipolar disorder in Sweden. *Arch Gen Psychiatry* 58(9):844–850, 2001.
24. Tohen M, Stoll AL, Strakowski SM, et al. The McLean first-episode psychosis project: six month recovery and recurrence outcome. *Schizophr Bull* 18:172–185, 1992.

25. Tohen M, Vieta E, Calabrese J, et al. Efficacy of olanzapine and olanzapine-fluoxetine combination in the treatment of bipolar I depression. *Arch Gen Psychiatry* 60(11):1079–1088, 2003.

29. Lee HC, Tsai SY, Lin HC. Seasonal variations in bipolar disorder admissions and the association with climate: a population-based study. *J Affect Disord* 97(1–3):61–69, 2007.

34. Oepen G, Baldessarini RJ, Salvatore P, et al. On the periodicity of manic-depressive insanity, by Eliot Slater (1938): translated excerpts and commentary. *J Affect Disord* 78(1):1–9, 2004.

38. Roybal K, Theobold D, Graham A, et al. Mania-like behavior induced by disruption of CLOCK. *Proc Natl Acad Sci U S A* 104(15):6406–6411, 2007.

44. Drevets WC, Price JL, Simpson JR Jr, et al. Subgenual prefrontal cortex abnormalities in mood disorders. *Nature* 386(6627):824–827, 1997.

51. Gilman SE, Dupuy JM, Perlis RH. Risks for the transition from major depressive disorder to bipolar disorder in the National Epidemiologic Survey on Alcohol and Related Conditions. *J Clin Psychiatry* 73(6):829–836, 2012. doi:10.4088/JCP.11m06912.

52. Tsankova NM, Berton O, Renthal W, et al. Sustained hippocampal chromatin regulation in a mouse model of depression and antidepressant action. *Nat Neurosci* 9:519–525, 2006. 10.1038/nn1659.

53. Kurita M, Holloway T, Garcia-Bea A, et al. HDAC2 regulates atypical antipsychotic responses through the modulation of mGlu2 promoter activity. *Nat Neurosci* 15:1245–1254, 2012. doi:10.1038/nn.3181.

57. Krauthammer C, Klerman GL. Secondary mania: manic syndromes associated with antecedent physical illness or drugs. *Arch Gen Psychiatry* 35(11):1333–1339, 1978.

60. Perlis RH, Uher R, Ostacher M, et al. Association between bipolar spectrum features and treatment outcomes in outpatients with major depressive disorder. *Arch Gen Psychiatry* 68(4):351–360, 2011. doi:10.1001/archgenpsychiatry.2010.179.

65. Hirschfeld RA, Bowden CL, Gitlin MJ, et al. Practice guideline for the treatment of patients with bipolar disorder (revision). *Am J Psychiatry* 159(Suppl. 4):1–11, 2002.

68. Simon GE, Ludman EJ, Bauer MS, et al. Long-term effectiveness and cost of a systematic care program for bipolar disorder. *Arch Gen Psychiatry* 63(5):500–508, 2006.

70. Perlis RH, Welge JA, Vornik LA, et al. Atypical antipsychotics in the treatment of mania: a meta-analysis of randomized, placebo-controlled trials. *J Clin Psychiatry* 67(4):509–516, 2006.

72. Calabrese JR, Keck PE Jr, Macfadden W, et al. A randomized, double-blind, placebo-controlled trial of quetiapine in the treatment of bipolar I or II depression. *Am J Psychiatry* 162(7):1351–1360, 2005.

73. Brown EB, McElroy SL, Keck PE Jr, et al. A 7-week, randomized, double-blind trial of olanzapine/fluoxetine combination versus lamotrigine in the treatment of bipolar I depression. *J Clin Psychiatry* 67(7):1025–1033, 2006.

74. van der Loos MLM, Mulder PGH, Hartong EG, et al. Efficacy and safety of lamotrigine as add-on treatment to lithium in bipolar depression: a multicenter, double-blind, placebo-controlled trial. *J Clin Psychiatry* 70(2):223–231, 2009. Published online 2008 December 30.

75. Nemeroff CB, Evans DL, Gyulai L, et al. Double-blind, placebo-controlled comparison of imipramine and paroxetine in the treatment of bipolar depression. *Am J Psychiatry* 158(6):906–912, 2001.

79. Perlis RH, Sachs GS, Lafer B, et al. Effect of abrupt change from standard to low serum levels of lithium: a reanalysis of double-blind lithium maintenance data. *Am J Psychiatry* 159(7):1155–1159, 2002.

81. Goodwin GM, Bowden CL, Calabrese JR, et al. A pooled analysis of 2 placebo-controlled 18-month trials of lamotrigine and lithium maintenance in bipolar I disorder. *J Clin Psychiatry* 65(3):432–441, 2004.

82. Perlis RH, Ostacher MJ, Miklowitz DJ, et al. Benzodiazepine use and risk of recurrence in bipolar disorder: a STEP-BD report. *J Clin Psychiatry* 71(2):194–2010, 2010.

83. Miklowitz DJ, Otto MW, Frank E, et al. Psychosocial treatments for bipolar depression: a 1-year randomized trial from the Systematic Treatment Enhancement Program. *Arch Gen Psychiatry* 64(4):419–426, 2007.

87. Lam DH, McCrone P, Wright K, et al. Cost-effectiveness of relapse-prevention cognitive therapy for bipolar disorder: 30-month study. *Br J Psychiatry* 186:500–506, 2005.

92. Perlis RH, Ostacher MJ, Patel JK, et al. Predictors of recurrence in bipolar disorder: primary outcomes from the Systematic Treatment Enhancement Program for Bipolar Disorder (STEP-BD). *Am J Psychiatry* 163(2):217–224, 2006.

6

The Pharmacotherapy of Anxiety Disorders

Eric Bui, MD, PhD, Mark H. Pollack, MD, Gustavo Kinrys, MD, Hannah Delong, BA, Débora Vasconcelos e Sá, BA, MSc, and Naomi M. Simon, MD, MSc

KEY POINTS

- A variety of pharmacological agents are effective for the treatment of anxiety disorders.

- The SSRIs and SNRIs are first-line pharmacological agents for the treatment of anxiety disorders.

- Benzodiazepines are effective, rapidly acting and well-tolerated, but are associated with the risk of abuse and dependence, and lack efficacy for co-morbid depression.

- Anticonvulsants, atypical antipsychotics, adrenergic antagonists, and other agents also play role in the treatment of anxiety disorders.

- Many patients remain symptomatic despite standard treatments; this necessitates the creative use of available interventions (alone and in combination), and spurs the development of novel therapeutics.

OVERVIEW

Anxiety disorders are associated with both significant distress and dysfunction. In this chapter we will review the pharmacotherapy of panic disorder with or without co-morbid agoraphobia, generalized anxiety disorder (GAD), and social anxiety disorder (SAD); the treatment of posttraumatic stress disorder (PTSD), and obsessive-compulsive disorder (OCD). Table 6-1 includes dosing information and common side effects associated with the pharmacological agents commonly used for the treatment of anxiety, referred to in the following sections.

PANIC DISORDER AND AGORAPHOBIA

Pharmacotherapy of panic disorder is aimed at preventing panic attacks, diminishing anticipatory and generalized anxiety, reversing phobic avoidance, improving overall function and quality of life, and treating co-morbid conditions (such as depression). As for all anxiety disorders, the goal of pharmacotherapy is to reduce the patient's distress and impairment to the point of remission, and/or to facilitate their participation, if necessary, in other forms of treatment (such as cognitive-behavioral therapy [CBT]).

Antidepressants

The selective reuptake inhibitors (SSRIs) and serotonin-norepinephrine serotonin reuptake inhibitors (SNRIs) have become first-line agents for the treatment of panic disorder as well as other anxiety disorders because of their broad spectrum of efficacy (including benefit for disorders commonly co-morbid with panic disorder, such as major depression), favorable side-effect profile, and lack of cardiotoxicity. Currently, paroxetine, both the immediate ([Paxil] and controlled-release formulations [Paxil-CR]), sertraline (Zoloft), fluoxetine

(Prozac) and extended-release venlafaxine Effexor-XR) are Food and Drug Administration (FDA)-approved for the treatment of panic disorder, though other SSRIs including citalopram (Celexa), and escitalopram (Lexapro),[1] and fluvoxamine (Luvox)[2] have also demonstrated anti-panic efficacy in both open and double-blind trials. A recently introduced SNRI, duloxetine (Cymbalta), has also been reported effective for panic disorder in case reports,[3] and in an open-label trial[4] though no randomized controlled trials (RCTs) are currently reported.

A recent meta-analysis on 50 clinical trials (yielding over 5,000 participants) confirmed that citalopram, paroxetine, fluoxetine, and venlafaxine were superior to placebo in the treatment of panic disorder.[5] Finally, while the majority of data supporting the efficacy of pharmacological agents for panic disorder derive from short-term trials, several long-term studies have also demonstrated sustained efficacy over time.[6]

Because the SSRI/SNRIs have the potential to cause initial restlessness, insomnia, and increased anxiety, and because panic patients are commonly sensitive to somatic sensations, the starting doses should be low, typically half (or less) of the usual starting dose (e.g., fluoxetine 5 to 10 mg/d, sertraline 25 mg/d, paroxetine 10 mg/d [or 12.5 mg/d of the controlled-release formulation], controlled-release venlafaxine 37.5 mg/d), to minimize the early anxiogenic effect. Doses can usually begin to be raised, after about a week of acclimation, to achieve typical therapeutic levels, with further gradual titration based on clinical response and side effects, although even more gradual upward titration is sometimes necessary in particularly sensitive or somatically-focused individuals. Although the nature of the dose–response relationship for the SSRIs in panic is still being assessed, available data support doses for this indication in the typical antidepressant range, and sometimes higher, i.e., fluoxetine 20 to 40 mg/d, paroxetine 20 to 60 mg/d (25 to 72.5 mg/d of the controlled-release formulation), sertraline 100 to 200 mg/d, citalopram 20 to 60 mg/d, escitalopram 10 to 20 mg/d, fluvoxamine 150 to 250 mg/d, and controlled-release venlafaxine 75 to 225 mg/d (although some patients may respond at lower doses). In some cases of refractory panic, even higher doses may be clinically useful, although additional data examining such dosing is needed.

SSRI and SNRI administration may be associated with adverse effects that include sexual dysfunction, sleep disturbance, weight gain, headache, dose-dependent increases in blood pressure (with venlafaxine), gastrointestinal disturbance, potential risk of bleeding (with anticoagulants, aspirin or NSAIDs), and provocation of increased anxiety (particularly at initiation of therapy) that may make their administration problematic for some individuals.[7-9] The SSRIs/SNRIs are usually administered in the morning (though for some individuals, agents such as paroxetine and others may be sedating and better tolerated with bedtime dosing); emergent sleep disruption can usually be managed by the addition of hypnotic agents. The typical 2–3 week lag in onset of therapeutic efficacy for the SSRI/SNRIs can be problematic for acutely distressed individuals. There is also an FDA class warning for risk of emergent suicidal thoughts and behaviors based on short-term studies that suggests close monitoring is advised for individuals age 24 or younger, with use balancing risk and

TABLE 6-1A Dosing of selective Serotonin Reuptake Inhibitors

Agent	Initial Dose (mg/day)	Typical Dose Range (mg/day)	Limitations/Primary Side Effects
Selective Serotonin Reuptake Inhibitors (SSRIs)/Serotonin-Norepinephrine Reuptake Inhibitors (SNRIs)			
Citalopram (Celexa)	10	20–40	Initial jitteriness, GI distress, sedation or insomnia, hypertension (venlafaxine), sexual dysfunction, urinary hesitation (duloxetine), discontinuation syndrome
Duloxetine (Cymbalta)	30	60–90	
Escitalopram (Lexapro)	5–10	10–20	
Fluoxetine (Prozac)	10	20–80	
Fluvoxamine (Luvox)	50	150–300	
Paroxetine (Paxil)	10	20–60	
Paroxetine controlled release (Paxil-CR)	12.5	25–75	
Sertraline (Zoloft)	25	50–200	
Venlafaxine extended release (Effexor-XR)	37.5	75–225	

TABLE 6-1B Dosing of Tricyclic Antidepressants (TCAs) and Monoamine Oxidase Inhibitors (MAOIs)

Agent	Initial Dose (mg/day)	Typical Dose Range (mg/day)	Limitations/Primary Side Effects
Tricyclic Antidepressants (TCAs)			
Imipramine (e.g., Tofranil)	10–25	100–300	Jitteriness, sedation, dry mouth, weight gain, cardiac conduction effects, orthostasis, variably anticholinergic
Clomipramine (Anafranil)	25	25–250	
Monoamine Oxidase Inhibitors (MAOIs)			
Phenelzine (e.g., Nardil)	15–30	45–90	Diet restrictions, hypertensive reactions, serotonin syndrome
Tranylcypromine (e.g., Parnate)	10	30–60	
Benzodiazepines			
Alprazolam (Xanax)	0.25 QID	2–8	Sedation, discontinuation difficulties, potential for abuse, psychomotor and memory impairment, interdose rebound anxiety (for shorter-acting agents)
Clonazepam (Klonopin)	0.25 at bedtime	1–5	
Lorazepam (Ativan)	0.5 TID	3–12	
Oxazepam (Serax)	15	30–60	

TABLE 6-1C Dosing of Other Agents

Agent	Initial Dose (mg/day)	Typical Dose Range (mg/day)	Limitations/Primary Side Effects
Anticonvulsants			
Gabapentin (Neurontin)	300	600–6,000	Light-headedness, sedation
Pregabalin (Lyrica)	200	300–600	Light-headedness, sedation
Lamotrigine (Lamictal)	25	50–500	GI distress, rash (rare Stevens-Johnson)
Valproic acid (Valproate)	250	500–2,000	GI distress, sedation, weight gain (rare polycystic ovary disease, hepatotoxicity, pancreatitis)
Antipsychotics			
Aripiprazole (Abilify)	15	15–45	Extrapyramidal symptoms, metabolic syndrome, weight gain, sedation, akathisia, prolonged QTc, blood pressure changes, neuroleptic malignant syndrome
Olanzapine (Zyprexa)	2.5	5–15	
Quetiapine (Seroquel)	25	50–500	
Risperidone (Risperdal)	0.25	0.5–3	
Trifluoperazine (Stelazine)	2.5	2.5–40	
Ziprasidone (Geodon)	20	40–160	
Beta-blockers			
Atenolol	25	50–100	Bradycardia, depression, hypotension, light-headedness, sedation; monotherapy efficacy limited to performance anxiety
Propranolol (Inderal)	10–20	10–160	
Other Agents			
Buspirone (BuSpar)	5 TIB	15–60/day	Dysphoria; limited efficacy

clinical need. In addition, some data suggesting possibly dose-dependent QTc prolongation with citalopram in those aged 60 and up has led to recommendations to limit dose to 20 mg/day and EKG monitoring in some populations.

Although results from a recent meta-analysis of 50 trials suggest the following increasing order of effectiveness among SSRIs/SNRIs, citalopram, sertraline, paroxetine, fluoxetine, and venlafaxine, for panic symptoms, they found a different order for associated overall anxiety symptoms,[5] and there is no clear evidence of a differential efficacy between agents in the SSRI or SNRI classes to guide selection. On the other hand, potentially relevant differences in their side-effect profiles (e.g., potential for weight gain and discontinuation-related symptomatology), differences in their potential for drug interactions, and the availability of generic formulations may be clinically relevant.[10-12]

Tricyclic Antidepressants (TCAs)

Imipramine (Tofranil) was the first pharmacological agent shown to be efficacious in panic disorder, and tricyclic antidepressants (TCAs) were typically the first-line, "gold standard" pharmacological agents for panic disorder until they were supplanted by the SSRIs, SNRIs, and benzodiazepines. Numerous, RCTs demonstrate the efficacy of imipramine and clomipramine for panic disorder, with supportive evidence for other TCAs.[13,14] There is some evidence that clomipramine may have superior anti-panic properties when compared with the other TCAs, possibly related to its greater potency for serotonergic uptake. The efficacy of the TCAs is comparable to that of the newer agents[15-17] for panic disorder, but they are now used less frequently due to their greater side-effect burden,[18] including associated anticholinergic effects, orthostasis, weight gain, cardiac conduction delays, and greater lethality in overdose. The side-effect profile of the TCAs is associated with a high drop-out rate (30%–70%) in most studies. The SSSIs/SNRIs appear to have a broader spectrum of efficacy than the TCAs, which are less efficacious for conditions such as SAD[19] and, with the exception of the more serotonergic TCA, clomipramine, less effective for OCD. This is of particular importance as both SAD and OCD may present with co-morbid panic disorder.

Similar to recommendations for the use of the SSRIs/SNRIs, treatment with the TCAs should be initiated with lower doses (e.g., 10 mg/d for imipramine) to minimize the "activation syndrome" (involving restlessness, jitteriness, palpitations, and increased anxiety) noted upon initiation of treatment. Typical antidepressant doses (e.g., 100–300 mg/d for imipramine) may ultimately be used to control the symptoms of panic disorder. In cases of poor response or intolerability to treatment with standard doses, use of TCA plasma levels, especially for imipramine, nortriptyline (Pamelor), and desipramine (Norpramin), may be informative.

Monoamine Oxidase Inhibitors

Despite their reputation for efficacy, the monoamine oxidase inhibitors (MAOIs) have not been systematically studied in panic disorder as defined by the current nomenclature; there is, however, at least one study pre-dating the use of current diagnostic criteria that likely included panic-disordered patients and reported results consistent with efficacy for the MAOI phenelzine.[20] Although clinical lore suggests that MAOIs may be particularly effective for patients with panic disorder refractory to other agents, there is actually no data to address this issue. Because of the need for careful dietary monitoring (including proscriptions against tyramine-containing foods and ingestion of sympathomimetic and other agents) to reduce the risks of hypertensive reactions and serotonin syndrome,

the MAOIs are typically used after lack of response to safer and better tolerated agents.[21,22] Use of MAOIs is also associated with a side-effect profile that includes insomnia, weight gain, orthostatic hypotension, and sexual disturbance.

Optimal doses for phenelzine range between 60 and 90 mg/d, while doses of tranylcypromine generally range between 30 and 60 mg/d. Though reversible inhibitors of monoamine oxidase_A (RIMAs) have in general a more benign side-effect profile and lower risk of hypertensive reactions than irreversible MAOIs (such as phenelzine), RCTs of brofaromine and of moclobemide in panic disorder report inconsistent efficacy; neither agent has become available in the US.[23-27] A transdermal patch for the MAOI selegiline (that does not require dietary proscriptions at its lowest dose) became available in the US with an indication for treatment of depression; to date, systematic evaluation of its efficacy for panic or other anxiety disorders has not been reported.

Benzodiazepines

Despite guidelines[28] for the use of antidepressants as first-line anti-panic agents, benzodiazepines are still commonly prescribed for the treatment of panic disorder.[29,30] Two high-potency benzodiazepines, alprazolam (immediate and extended-release forms) and clonazepam, are FDA-approved for panic disorder; however, other benzodiazepines of varying potency, such as diazepam,[30,31] adinazolam, and lorazepam,[32-34] at roughly equipotent doses have also demonstrated anti-panic efficacy in RCTs. Benzodiazepines remain widely used for panic and other anxiety disorders, likely due to their effectiveness, tolerability, rapid onset-of-action, and ability to be used on an "as needed" basis for situational anxiety. It should be noted; however, that "as needed" dosing for monotherapy of panic disorder is rarely appropriate, as this strategy generally exposes the patient to the risks associated with benzodiazepine use without the benefit of adequate and sustained dosing to achieve and maintain comprehensive efficacy. Further, from a cognitive-behavioral perspective, "as needed" dosing engenders dependency on the medication as a safety cue and interferes with exposure to and mastery of avoided situations.

Despite their generally favorable tolerability, benzodiazepines may be associated with side effects that include sedation, ataxia, and memory impairment (particularly problematic in the elderly and those with prior cognitive impairment).[35] Despite concerns that ongoing benzodiazepine administration will result in the development of therapeutic tolerance (i.e., loss or therapeutic efficacy or dose escalation), available studies of their long-term use suggest that benzodiazepines remain generally effective for panic disorder over time,[36,37] and do not lead to reports of significant dose escalation.[38] Of interest, a recent randomized, naturalistic, parallel-group study, found that after 3 years of treatment, individuals receiving clonazepam were slightly better, and reported fewer side effects, than those receiving paroxetine.[39,40] However, even after a relatively brief period of regular dosing, rapid discontinuation of benzodiazepines may result in significant withdrawal symptoms (including increased anxiety and agitation)[41]; for instance, in one study, over two-thirds of patients with panic disorder, discontinuing alprazolam, experienced a discontinuation syndrome.[42] Discontinuation of longer-acting agents (such as clonazepam) may result in fewer and less intense withdrawal symptoms with an abrupt taper. Patients with a high level of sensitivity to somatic sensations may find withdrawal-related symptoms particularly distressing, and a slow taper as well as the addition of CBT[43] during discontinuation may be helpful to reduce distress associated with benzodiazepine discontinuation. A gradual taper is recommended for all patients treated with daily benzodiazepines for more than a few weeks, to reduce the likelihood of withdrawal symptoms (including in rare cases, seizures). Though individuals with a predilection for substance abuse[44] are at risk for abuse of benzodiazepines, those without this diathesis do not appear to share this risk.[38] However, benzodiazepines and alcohol may negatively interact in combination,[45] and the concomitant use of benzodiazepines in patients with current co-morbid alcohol abuse or dependence can be problematic (thus further supporting the use of antidepressants as first-line anti-panic agents in this population with co-morbid illness). In addition, given the high rates of co-morbid depression associated with panic disorder, it is worth noting that benzodiazepines are not in general effective for treatment of depression and may in fact induce or intensify depressive symptoms in those with co-morbid depression.[46] A meta-analysis reported that, although benzodiazepines may be as effective as antidepressants on PD symptoms, they might be less so on depressive symptoms. [47]

Although benzodiazepines are commonly prescribed for the treatment of panic disorder, benzodiazepine monotherapy has decreased somewhat.[29] Treatment with a combination of an antidepressant and a benzodiazepine compared to an antidepressant alone results in acceleration of therapeutic effects as early as the first week, although by weeks 4 or 5 of treatment, combined treatment (whether maintained or tapered and discontinued) shows no advantage over monotherapy.[48,49] Thus, the data suggest that co-administration improves the rapidity of response when co-initiated with antidepressants, but that ongoing use may not be necessary after the initial weeks of antidepressant pharmacotherapy. Recent data suggest some benefit of the augmentation with a benzodiazepine for individuals who remain symptomatic on antidepressant monotherapy.[50]

Other Agents

The data addressing the potential efficacy of bupropion (a relatively weak reuptake inhibitor of norepinephrine [noradrenaline] and dopamine) for the treatment of panic disorder is mixed, with a small study of the immediate-release formulation administered at high doses demonstrating no benefit,[51] but a more recent open-label study employing standard doses of the extended-release formulation suggesting potential benefit.[52] Similarly, there is mixed support for the potential efficacy for panic disorder of another noradrenergic agent, reboxetine,[53,54] with a meta-analysis reporting that this agent may be ineffective in treating both panic and anxiety symptoms in panic-disordered patients.[5]

There is suggestive evidence from case reports that buspirone (an azapirone 5-HT$_{1A}$ partial agonist) may be useful as an adjunct to antidepressants and benzodiazepines[55] and acutely, although not over the long term, to CBT[56] for panic disorder, but appears ineffective as monotherapy.[57,58]

Beta-blockers reduce the somatic symptoms of arousal associated with panic and anxiety, but may be more useful as augmentation for incomplete response rather than as initial monotherapy.[59] Pindolol, a beta-blocker with partial antagonist effects at the 5-HT$_{1A}$ receptor, was effective in a small double-blind RCT[60] of patients with panic disorder remaining symptomatic despite initial treatment.

Atypical antipsychotics, including olanzapine,[61] risperidone,[62] and aripiprazole,[63,64] have demonstrated potential efficacy as monotherapy or as augmentation for the treatment of patients with panic disorder refractory to standard interventions in a number of small, open-label trials or case series. More recently, a randomized, single-blind comparison of low-dose risperidone to paroxetine in the treatment of panic attacks failed to show any significant difference.[65] However,

evidence for treatment-emergent weight gain, hyperlipidemia, and diabetes with some of the atypical agents, as well as the lack of large RCTs examining their efficacy and safety in panic disorder to date, do not support the routine first-line use of these agents for panic disorder, but rather consideration for patients whose panic disorder has not sufficiently responded to standard interventions.

On the basis of limited data, some anticonvulsants appear to have a potential role in the treatment of panic disorder, in individuals with co-morbid disorders (such as bipolar disorder and substance abuse), for which the use of antidepressants and benzodiazepines, respectively, are associated with additional risk. Small studies support the potential efficacy of valproic acid,[66,67] but not carbamazepine[68] for the treatment of panic disorder. Gabapentin did not demonstrate significant benefit compared to placebo for the overall sample of patients with panic disorder in a large RCT, but a post-hoc analysis found efficacy for those with at least moderate panic severity.[69] Another related compound, the alpha$_2$ delta calcium channel antagonist pregabalin, has demonstrated utility for GAD,[70] but there are no published reports to date in panic disorder.

GENERALIZED ANXIETY DISORDER

The pharmacotherapy of generalized anxiety disorder (GAD) is aimed at reducing or eliminating excessive and uncontrollable worry, somatic and cognitive symptoms associated with motor tension and autonomic arousal (e.g., muscle tension, restlessness, difficulty concentrating, disturbed sleep, fatigue, and irritability), and common co-morbidities (including depression) that comprise the syndrome. The anxiety characteristic of GAD is typically persistent and pervasive rather than episodic and situational. GAD severity, however, may worsen in response to situational stressors. Thus, while GAD pharmacotherapy is generally chronic, adjustments may be required in response to worsening during prolonged periods of stress.

Antidepressants

Selective serotonin Reuptake Inhibitors and Serotonin Norepinephrine Reuptake Inhibitors

As is true for panic and the other anxiety disorders, the SSRIs and SNRIs are generally considered first-line agents for the treatment of GAD because of their favorable side-effect profile compared to older antidepressants (e.g., TCAs), lack of abuse or dependency liability compared to the benzodiazepines, and a broad spectrum of efficacy for common co-morbidities, such as depression. Similar to considerations for their use in individuals with panic disorder, SSRIs, SNRIs, and other antidepressants should be initiated in patients with GAD at half or less than the usual starting dose in order to minimize jitteriness and anxiety. Currently, the SSRIs paroxetine and escitalopram and the SNRIs (including the extended-release formulation of venlafaxine [Effexor-XR] and duloxetine [Cymbalta]) have received FDA approval for GAD; however, all agents in these classes including sertraline are likely effective for GAD without convincing evidence for significant divergence in efficacy between them, but with some differences in their side-effect profiles.[71] Long-term trials with SSRIs and SNRIs demonstrate that continued treatment for 6 months is associated with significantly decreased rates of relapse relative to those who discontinued the drug following acute treatment; further, ongoing treatment appears associated with continued gains in the quality of improvement as evinced by a greater proportion of individuals reaching remission over time.[72,73]

Tricyclic Antidepressants

A number of studies have demonstrated the efficacy of the prototypic TCA imipramine for the treatment of GAD, with RCTs showing generally comparable efficacy but slower speed-of-onset relative to a benzodiazepine comparator,[74] and a greater side-effect burden relative to an SSRI comparator.[75]

Benzodiazepines

Benzodiazepines have been widely used for the treatment of generalized anxiety for close to half a century. Although recent guidelines[76] have emphasized the use of antidepressants for the treatment of anxiety states including GAD, particularly in the common scenario in which co-morbid depression is present. Benzodiazepines remain broadly prescribed, either as co-therapy or monotherapy for GAD, because of their ease of use, rapid and generally reliable anxiolytic effect, and relatively favorable side-effect profile.

Given their apparent equivalent efficacy, the selection of an appropriate benzodiazepine should be made by matching the pharmacokinetic properties of the agent with the situational parameters and patient's clinical profile. Agents that are slowly metabolized and have multiple metabolites (such as diazepam and chlordiazepoxide) and those with long half-lives (such as clonazepam) may be easier to taper rapidly and are generally associated with fewer intra-dose breakthrough symptoms compared to shorter-acting and more rapidly metabolized agents (such as oxazepam or lorazepam); the latter agents may be better suited for brief intermittent anxiolysis or individuals likely to be slower metabolizers (e.g., the elderly or those with hepatic disease).[77] The regular use of benzodiazepines for more than 2 or 3 weeks may be associated with physiological dependence and the potential for significant withdrawal symptoms with discontinuation. Discontinuation of benzodiazepines is best done with a gradual taper to minimize withdrawal symptoms. For some patients switching from a short-acting to a longer-acting agent (e.g., alprazolam to clonazepam) may facilitate discontinuation, although the available evidence suggests that differences in ease of discontinuation disappear during a slow as opposed to rapid taper. The addition of CBT during the tapering process may facilitate benzodiazepine discontinuation by giving the patient skills for the management of recurrent anxiety and withdrawal, and addressing concerns about their ability to function without benzodiazepines.[43] There are few data supporting the utility of augmentation with agents such as anticonvulsants or antidepressants to facilitate discontinuation, although they may prove useful on a case-by-case basis. Moreover, the abuse liability of benzodiazepines may be problematic in individuals predisposed to substance abuse or dependence, although available evidence does not support concerns about dose escalation or therapeutic tolerance for the majority of individuals taking benzodiazepines.[38] Pharmacodynamic interactions due the co-administration of benzodiazepines with alcohol or other sedating agents, however, may be problematic because of the additive potential for CNS depression. In addition, benzodiazepines are less effective than antidepressants in the treatment of anxiety with significant co-morbid depression[78] and in fact have the potential to worsen extant depression. Thus, benzodiazepines are not recommended as first-line treatment for GAD.

Buspirone

Buspirone is a 5-HT$_{1A}$ partial agonist belonging to the azapirone class that is FDA-approved for use in generalized anxiety, although it has demonstrated somewhat inconsistent effectiveness in clinical practice. However, case reports and small series suggest it may be useful as an adjunct to standard therapies for refractory panic and other anxiety disorders[55,79] as well as depression[80]; it may also have weak antidepressant effects at higher doses.[81] Buspirone has a generally favorable side-effect profile, though a gradual onset of effect; the average therapeutic dose is in the range of 30–60 mg/d, typically administered as twice-a-day dosing. A review of the literature reporting on 36 trials involving azapirones, including buspirone, found no evidence for their superiority over antidepressants, and suggest they may be less effective than benzodiazepines.[82]

Anticonvulsants

The alpha-$_2$ delta calcium channel antagonist pregabalin has received approval for the treatment of GAD in Europe, but not in the US. Pregabalin has demonstrated efficacy in seven large randomized placebo-controlled trials,[83] including a number which showed efficacy of pregabalin for co-morbid depressive symptoms[84-86] as well as studies showing a similar speed of therapeutic onset (as early as 1 week) to a benzodiazepine comparator.[70,87] The typical therapeutic dose range for pregabalin is 300–600 mg/d, with the most common adverse events being somnolence and dizziness. Recent data suggest that while low doses of pregabalin are efficacious, there is additional benefit gained by increasing the dose up to 450 mg per day, but that beyond 450 mg, reduction in anxiety symptoms does not continue to improve. Gabapentin, a related compound, has also been suggested potentially effective for the treatment of GAD, though at the level of case reports rather than RCTs. The selective GABA reuptake inhibitor tiagabine demonstrated efficacy for the treatment of GAD in one randomized, placebo-controlled trial at doses of 4–16 mg/d,[88] though a subsequent series of RCTs failed to confirm this initial observation and do not support the routine use of tiagabine as an anxiolytic.[89,90]

Antipsychotics

Conventional antipsychotics have long been used in clinical practice for the treatment of anxiety; in fact, based on a large placebo-controlled randomized trial of trifluroperazine (2–6 mg/d),[91] the agent received an FDA indication for the short-term treatment of non-psychotic anxiety. However, concerns regarding the potential development of extrapyramidal symptoms (EPS) and tardive dyskinesia (TD) have limited the use of typical antipsychotics for the treatment of anxiety. More recently a number of atypical antipsychotics including olanzapine,[92] risperidone,[62,93] aripiprazole, and ziprasidone[94] have demonstrated efficacy in RCTs, and case series and reports for the treatment of GAD,[92] typically though not exclusively as augmentation in individuals refractory to standard interventions. In addition, five recent RCTs provide strong support for the efficacy of quetiapine (50 mg to 300 mg) monotherapy in the treatment of GAD.[95-99] In particular, one of them showed that by day 4 of treatment, quetiapine was associated with significantly greater reduction in anxiety compared to escitalopram, though the difference was not significant by endpoint (week 8).[98] In addition, the efficacy of the atypicals as mood stabilizers for bipolar disorder,[100] their potential efficacy for refractory depression,[101] and lack of abuse potential suggest they may prove useful for individuals with co-morbid anxiety, mood and substance use disorders, particularly those refractory to more standard interventions, though there is currently relatively little systematic data addressing this issue. Decisions regarding the use of the atypicals should involve consideration of their potential for significant adverse effects as well, including sedation, weight gain, and metabolic syndrome.

Other agents

Riluzole

The efficacy of riluzole, an anti-glutamatergic agent, traditionally used in the treatment of amyotrophic lateral sclerosis (ALS) was examined in individuals with GAD, in an 8-week, open-label, fixed-dose study of 100 mg/d.[102] Riluzole appeared to be effective and generally well-tolerated; although its expense makes it unlikely that its use will be widely adopted, the report does suggest a potential role for anti-glutamatergic agents for the treatment of anxiety.

Chamomile

Chamomile as infusion has been commonly used for sleep for decades. Recently, one of its compounds, apigenin, which may have GABA-ergic actions, has been identified as a potential active agent. A small RCT (chamomile 220–1,100 mg, 1.2% apigenin vs. placebo) suggests that chamomile may be useful in the treatment of GAD.[103]

Kava

Similarly, kava roots have been consumed throughout the Pacific Ocean cultures of Polynesia, as a drink with sedative and anesthetic properties. Although earlier reports were inconclusive,[104,105] a recent RCT provides some support for the efficacy of its active agent kavalactones (120–240 mg) in the treatment of GAD.[106]

SOCIAL ANXIETY DISORDER

The pharmacotherapy of social anxiety disorder (SAD) is aimed at reducing the patient's anticipatory anxiety prior to and distress during social interaction and performance situations, reducing avoidance of social and performance situations, and improving associated impairments in quality of life and function.

Selective serotonin Reuptake Inhibitors and Serotonin Norepinephrine Reuptake Inhibitors

Selective serotonin and SNRIs have become first-line pharmacotherapy for the treatment of SAD because of their greater efficacy for this condition, broad-spectrum effects for other anxiety disorders, efficacy for co-morbid depression in contrast to the benzodiazepines, better tolerability than the TCAs, more favorable safety profile than the monoamine oxidase inhibitors (MAOIs), and lack of abuse potential. Currently, the SSRIs paroxetine and sertraline as well as the SNRI venlafaxine (extended-release) have FDA-approved indications for SAD, though available evidence suggests that other agents from these classes, including fluvoxamine,[107–111] citalopram, and escitalopram.[112–114] Regarding fluoxetine, the reported study results have been mixed.[115–117] Finally, some recent data suggest the efficacy of the SNRI duloxetine for the treatment of SAD as well.[118] A meta-analysis of the efficacy of second-generation antidepressants in SAD[119] suggests that escitalopram, paroxetine, sertraline, and venlafaxine produced significantly more responders than placebo and that there were no differences in terms of efficacy among them.

As noted, individuals with SAD are at increased risk for alcohol and other substance abuse, which may in some cases reflect an attempt to "self medicate" anxiety in social situations. A small, randomized placebo-controlled study,[120] in individuals with SAD and active alcohol use disorders, suggested that treatment with the SSRI paroxetine decreased the anxiety and may have reduced the alcohol use as well.

Treatment with the SSRIs and SNRIs for SAD is typically initiated at low doses (e.g., paroxetine 10 mg/d, sertraline 25 mg/d, venlafaxine-extended release 37.5 mg/d) and titrated up against therapeutic response and tolerability (e.g., paroxetine 20–60 mg/d, sertraline 50–200 mg/d, and venlafaxine 75–225 mg/d). There is usually a therapeutic lag in efficacy of 2–3 weeks following initiation of SSRI/SNRI therapy for SAD, although full response can occur over weeks to months, particularly when social anxiety-related avoidance is present, and a return to avoided situations should be encouraged alongside pharmacotherapy to both assess and optimize outcomes. Typical treatment-emergent adverse effects include nausea, headache, dizziness, sedation, increased anxiety, and sexual dysfunction.

Beta-blockers

Beta-blockers, including propranolol (Inderal) and atenolol (Tenormin) are effective for the treatment of non-generalized social anxiety (i.e., "performance anxiety") about public speaking or other performance situations.[121,122] Beta-blockers blunt the symptoms of physiological arousal associated with anxiety or fear, such as tachycardia and tremor, which are often the focus of an individual's apprehension in performance situations and lead to an escalating cycle of arousal, agitation, and further elevations in social anxiety. Beta-blockers are effective for the treatment of performance anxiety, at least in part by blocking these physiological symptoms of arousal, interrupting the escalating fear cycle, and thus mitigating the individual's escalating concern and focus on their anxiety.

Though effective for physiological symptoms of arousal, beta-blockers are not as effective at reducing the emotional and cognitive aspects of social anxiety and thus are not first-line agents for generalized SAD. Results from a double-blind, placebo-controlled study of the beta-blocker atenolol and the MAOI phenelzine found the beta-blocker ineffective for individuals with generalized social anxiety.[123]

Beta-blockers (e.g., propranolol [10–80 mg/d] or atenolol [50–150 mg/d]) are typically administered "as needed" 1–2 hours before a performance situation. The use of beta-blockers may be associated with orthostatic hypotension, lightheadedness, bradycardia, sedation, and nausea. Atenolol is less lipophilic[124] and thus less centrally active than propranolol, and, therefore, may be less sedating. In practice, it is best to administer a "test dose" of the beta-blocker prior to use in an actual performance-related event in order to establish the tolerability of an effective dose and minimize disruptive side effects during a performance that could further increase anxiety.

Monoamine Oxidase Inhibitors

Before they were supplanted by the SSRIs and SNRIs, the MAOIs were the "gold-standard" pharmacological treatment for SAD. Interest in their use in SAD grew in part from initial observations of their efficacy for the atypical subtype of depression characterized in part by marked sensitivity to rejection,[125] and they were subsequently demonstrated effective in RCTs in SAD.[123]

Though clearly effective, the use of MAOIs is associated with troubling side effects including orthostatic hypotension, paresthesias, weight gain, and sexual dysfunction, as well as the need for careful attention to diet and use of concomitant medication because of the risk of potentially fatal hypertensive reactions and serotonin syndrome if the proscriptions are violated. Concerns about the use of MAOIs may have contributed in part to the under-recognition and treatment of SAD[126] that existed until demonstration of the efficacy of the generally safer and easier-to-use SSRIs and SNRIs for this syndrome.

Among the MAOIs, phenelzine has been the best studied for SAD,[123,127,128] although tranylcypromine also appears effective.[129] In a study comparing cognitive-behavioral group therapy (CBGT), phenelzine, an educational-supportive group, and a placebo for the treatment of SAD (n=133),[130] 77% of patients taking phenelzine, were responders at 12 weeks compared to 41% of those in the placebo group (p < 0.005); phenelzine appeared to be more effect than CBGT on some measures during acute treatment, but the psychosocial intervention resulted in better maintenance of benefit after treatment discontinuation.[131]

Phenelzine is typically initiated at 15 mg PO BID, and is less likely than reuptake inhibitors (such as the TCAs, SSRIs, or SNRIs) to exacerbate anxiety during initiation of treatment. The usual therapeutic dose range of phenelzine is 60 to 90 mg/d, with some refractory patients responding to higher doses. Careful attention to adherence to a diet free of tyramine-containing foods and avoidance of sympathomimetic and other serotonergic drugs is important to avoid the risk of hypertensive or serotonergic crisis, and assessment of the ability of an individual patient to maintain these restrictions is a critical component of the risk–benefit analysis of MAOI usage.

Interest in the reversible inhibitors of MAO$_A$ (RIMAs) was stimulated by the significant safety concerns attendant to the administration of the irreversible MAOIs, such as phenelzine. Because they can be displaced from MAO when a substrate (such as tyramine) is presented, the RIMAs do not carry with them the need for strict dietary prohibitions and the risk of hypertensive crisis and serotonin syndrome associated with the irreversible MAOIs. Unfortunately, while some clinical trials have reported positive results with RIMAs (such as moclobemide and brofaromine) for SAD, others have not.[132] Further, while moclobemide is available in some countries, it is generally not perceived as effective as standard MAOIs and is not available in the US. There are no systematic data available to date regarding the efficacy of the selegiline transdermal patch for the treatment of SAD.

Benzodiazepines

Although benzodiazepines are commonly used for many anxiety disorders (including SAD) there are relatively few systematic data addressing their use for this indication. However, the available data do suggest efficacy for these agents with response noted as soon as early as 2 weeks in non-depressed individuals with SAD.[127,133,134] Benzodiazepines may also help enhance response to an antidepressant; results from a randomized, double-blind placebo-controlled study demonstrated that the addition of clonazepam 1–2 mg/d to flexibly, dosed paroxetine (20–40 mg/d) resulted in greater improvement than paroxetine alone in generalized SAD.[135]

As noted, benzodiazepines have the advantage of a relatively rapid onset of effect, a favorable side-effect profile, and efficacy on an as-needed basis for situational anxiety. The use of benzodiazepines, however, may be associated with treatment-emergent adverse effects (including sedation, ataxia, and cognitive and psychomotor impairment), as well as the development of physiological dependence with regular use. Further, they are generally not effective for depression that commonly presents as co-morbid with SAD, and may worsen it. Their potential for abuse in those with a diathesis or a history of alcohol or substance abuse, and their potential negative interaction with concurrent alcohol use, is relevant given the increased rates of alcohol and substance use amongst social phobics. Benzodiazepines are initiated at low dose (e.g., clonazepam 0.25–0.5 mg qHS) to minimize emergent adverse effects (such as sedation) and then titrated up as tolerated to therapeutic doses (e.g., clonazepam 1–4 mg/d or its equivalent).

For maintenance treatment, in order to optimize a continuous anxiolytic effect, longer-acting benzodiazepines (such as clonazepam) are associated with less inter-dose rebound anxiety than shorter-acting agents and are generally preferred, whereas a shorter-acting agent with a more rapid onset of effect (such as alprazolam or lorazepam) may be more appropriate if used on an as-needed basis for performance situations. Monotherapy with as-needed dosing of benzodiazepines alone is not, however, recommended for non-"performance only" social anxiety disorder, and as-needed benzodiazepine use may interfere with the reduction of social anxiety and related avoidance with cognitive behavioral treatments.[136]

Other medications

Although TCAs are useful for a number of anxiety disorders including panic disorder, PTSD, GAD, and, in the case of clomipramine, OCD, results from open[19] and double-blind placebo-controlled trials[137] suggest they are not effective for the treatment of SAD. Small open trials have suggested the efficacy of bupropion in SAD.[138] Although the noradrenergic and serotonergic antidepressant mirtazapine has been reported to be effective for SAD in open-label studies,[139,140] as well as in a RCT conducted specifically in women,[141] a recent randomized placebo-controlled trial failed to replicate these results in a sample (n = 60) including adults of both genders.[142] Available evidence does not support the use of buspirone as a monotherapy for the treatment of SAD, although one report suggests that it may have a role as an adjunct for patients incompletely responsive to SSRI therapy.[79] Small studies and case series suggest the potential efficacy of atypical antipsychotics, including olanzapine,[143] risperidone,[62] and quetiapine[144,145] for the treatment of SAD, but their use is generally reserved for patients remaining symptomatic despite more standard interventions. A number of anticonvulsants have demonstrated potential efficacy for the treatment of SAD. Gabapentin, a GABA (an alpha-$_2$ delta calcium channel antagonist), demonstrated efficacy for SAD in a double-blind, placebo-controlled, parallel-group trial with doses of ranging from 900 to 3,600 mg daily, with most patients receiving greater than 2,100 mg/d.[146] A related compound, pregabalin, currently indicated for the treatment of neuropathic pain and as adjunctive treatment for partial seizures, also demonstrated efficacy for the treatment of SAD at a dose of 600 mg/d, although the side-effect burden at this higher dose was significant.[147] Valproic acid, an anticonvulsant mood-stabilizer, was reported effective for SAD, in an open trial with flexible dosing of 500–2,500 mg/d.[148] Levetiracetam demonstrated promising potential for the treatment of SAD in open trial,[149] but recent RCT data failed to show any efficacy over placebo.[150,151] An open-label trial suggests the potential efficacy of topiramate[152] and tiagabine[153] for the treatment of SAD; however, to date, no RCTs have confirmed these findings.

Though the adjunctive use of pindolol, a beta-blocker with 5-HT$_{1A}$ autoreceptor antagonist properties, has in some, but not all, studies accelerated or augmented response to antidepressants for depression,[154] it was ineffective in one placebo-controlled randomized augmentation trial in social phobics.[155] Other medications, such as the pre-synaptic adrenergic agonist clonidine[156] and the 5-HT$_3$ receptor ondansetron,[157] have been reported helpful for social anxiety in case reports, but there are few systematic data following up on these observations.

CONCLUSIONS AND FUTURE DIRECTIONS

The increased recognition of the prevalence, early-onset, chronicity, and morbid impact of the anxiety disorders has spurred development efforts to find more effective and better-tolerated pharmacotherapies for this condition. Though the SSRIs/SNRIs and benzodiazepines have demonstrated efficacy and favorable tolerability compared to older classes of agents, many patients remain symptomatic despite standard treatment; only a minority remit. In addition to creative uses of available agents alone and in combination, a variety of other pharmacological agents with novel mechanisms of actions, including corticotropin releasing factor (CRF) antagonists, neurokinin (NK)-substance P antagonists, metabotropic glutamate receptor agonists, GABA-ergic agents and receptor modulators, and compounds with a variety of effects on serotonin, noradrenergic, and dopaminergic receptors and their subtypes are in various stages of development. In addition, specific agents targeting ways to enhance outcomes with cognitive-behavioral therapy for anxiety disorders, such as the NMDA receptor antagonist D-cycloserine, remain an active area of translational research.[158,159] These efforts may provide more effective and better-tolerated agents for the treatment of anxiety in the future.

🅰 Access a list of MCQs for this chapter at https://expertconsult.inkling.com

REFERENCES

1. Stahl SM, Gergel I, Li D. Escitalopram in the treatment of panic disorder: a randomized, double-blind, placebo-controlled trial. *J Clin Psychiatry* 64(11):1322–1327, 2003.
2. Irons J. Fluvoxamine in the treatment of anxiety disorders. *Neuropsychiatr Dis Treat* 1(4):289–299, 2005.
3. Crippa JA, Zuardi AW. Duloxetine in the treatment of panic disorder. *Int J Neuropsychopharmacol* 9(5):633–634, 2006.
4. Simon NM, Kaufman RE, Hoge EA, et al. Open-label support for duloxetine for the treatment of panic disorder. *CNS Neurosci Ther* 15(1):19–23, 2009.
5. Andrisano C, Chiesa A, Serretti A. Newer antidepressants and panic disorder: a meta-analysis. *Int Clin Psychopharmacol* 28(1):33–45, 2013.
6. Pollack MH, Allgulander C, Bandelow B, et al. WCA recommendations for the long-term treatment of panic disorder. *CNS Spectr* 8(8 Suppl. 1):17–30, 2003.
7. Dannon PN, Iancu I, Cohen A, et al. Three year naturalistic outcome study of panic disorder patients treated with paroxetine. *BMC Psychiatry* 4:16, 2004.
8. Modell JG, Katholi CR, Modell JD, et al. Comparative sexual side effects of bupropion, fluoxetine, paroxetine, and sertraline. *Clin Pharmacol Ther* 61(4):476–487, 1997.
9. Ballenger JC, Wheadon DE, Steiner M, et al. Double-blind, fixed-dose, placebo-controlled study of paroxetine in the treatment of panic disorder. *Am J Psychiatry* 155(1):36–42, 1998.
10. Fava M, Judge R, Hoog SL, et al. Fluoxetine versus sertraline and paroxetine in major depressive disorder: changes in weight with long-term treatment. *J Clin Psychiatry* 61(11):863–867, 2000.
11. Fava M. Prospective studies of adverse events related to antidepressant discontinuation. *J Clin Psychiatry* 67(Suppl. 4):14–21, 2006.
12. Pollack MH, Lepola U, Koponen H, et al. A double-blind study of the efficacy of venlafaxine extended-release, paroxetine, and placebo in the treatment of panic disorder. *Depress Anxiety* 24(1):1–14, 2007.
13. Pollack MH. The pharmacotherapy of panic disorder. *J Clin Psychiatry* 66(Suppl. 4):23–27, 2005.
14. Rosenbaum JF, Pollack MH, Fredman SJ. The pharmacotherapy of panic disorder. In Rosenbaum JF, Pollack MH, editors: *Panic disorder and its treatment*, New York, 1998, Marcel Dekker Inc., pp 153–180.
15. Bakker A, van Dyck R, Spinhoven P, et al. Paroxetine, clomipramine, and cognitive therapy in the treatment of panic disorder. *J Clin Psychiatry* 60(12):831–838, 1999.
16. den Boer JA, Westenberg HG, Kamerbeek WD, et al. Effect of serotonin uptake inhibitors in anxiety disorders; a double-blind comparison of clomipramine and fluvoxamine. *Int Clin Psychopharmacol* 2(1):21–32, 1987.
17. Noyes R Jr, Perry P. Maintenance treatment with antidepressants in panic disorder. *J Clin Psychiatry* 51(Suppl. A):24–30, 1990.
18. Bakish D, Hooper CL, Filteau MJ, et al. A double-blind placebo-controlled trial comparing fluvoxamine and imipramine in the treatment of panic disorder with or without agoraphobia. *Psychopharmacol Bull* 32(1):135–141, 1996.
19. Simpson HB, Schneier FR, Campeas RB, et al. Imipramine in the treatment of social phobia. *J Clin Psychopharmacol* 18(2):132–135, 1998.
20. Sheehan DV, Ballenger J, Jacobsen G. Treatment of endogenous anxiety with phobic, hysterical, and hypochondriacal symptoms. *Arch Gen Psychiatry* 37(1):51–59, 1980.
21. Livingston MG, Livingston HM. Monoamine oxidase inhibitors. An update on drug interactions. *Drug Saf* 14(4):219–227, 1996.
22. Lippman SB, Nash K. Monoamine oxidase inhibitor update. Potential adverse food and drug interactions. *Drug Saf* 5(3):195–204, 1990.
23. van Vliet IM, Westenberg HG, Den Boer JA. MAO inhibitors in panic disorder: clinical effects of treatment with brofaromine. A double blind placebo controlled study. *Psychopharmacology (Berl)* 112(4):483–489, 1993.
24. van Vliet IM, den Boer JA, Westenberg HG, Slaap BR. A double-blind comparative study of brofaromine and fluvoxamine in outpatients with panic disorder. *J Clin Psychopharmacol* 16(4):299–306, 1996.
25. Bakish D, Saxena BM, Bowen R, et al. Reversible monoamine oxidase-A inhibitors in panic disorder. *Clin Neuropharmacol* 16(Suppl. 2):S77–S82, 1993.
26. Loerch B, Graf-Morgenstern M, Hautzinger M, et al. Randomised placebo-controlled trial of moclobemide, cognitive-behavioural therapy and their combination in panic disorder with agoraphobia. *Br J Psychiatry* 174:205–212, 1999.
27. Tiller JW, Bouwer C, Behnke K. Moclobemide and fluoxetine for panic disorder. International Panic Disorder Study Group. *Eur Arch Psychiatry Clin Neurosci* 249(Suppl. 1):S7–S10, 1999.
28. Practice guideline for the treatment of patients with panic disorder. Work Group on Panic Disorder. American Psychiatric Association. *Am J Psychiatry* 155(5 Suppl.):1–34, 1998.
29. Bruce SE, Vasile RG, Goisman RM, et al. Are benzodiazepines still the medication of choice for patients with panic disorder with or without agoraphobia? *Am J Psychiatry* 160(8):1432–1438, 2003.
30. Noyes R Jr, Burrows GD, Reich JH, et al. Diazepam versus alprazolam for the treatment of panic disorder. *J Clin Psychiatry* 57(8):349–355, 1996.
31. Dunner DL, Ishiki D, Avery DH, et al. Effect of alprazolam and diazepam on anxiety and panic attacks in panic disorder: a controlled study. *J Clin Psychiatry* 47(9):458–460, 1986.
32. Charney DS, Woods SW. Benzodiazepine treatment of panic disorder: a comparison of alprazolam and lorazepam. *J Clin Psychiatry* 50(11):418–423, 1989.
33. Schweizer E, Fox I, Case G, et al. Lorazepam vs. alprazolam in the treatment of panic disorder. *Psychopharmacol Bull* 24(2):224–227, 1988.
34. Schweizer E, Pohl R, Balon R, et al. Lorazepam vs. alprazolam in the treatment of panic disorder. *Pharmacopsychiatry* 23(2):90–93, 1990.
35. Stewart SA. The effects of benzodiazepines on cognition. *J Clin Psychiatry* 66(Suppl. 2):9–13, 2005.
36. Nagy LM, Krystal JH, Woods SW, et al. Clinical and medication outcome after short-term alprazolam and behavioral group treatment in panic disorder. 2.5 year naturalistic follow-up study. *Arch Gen Psychiatry* 46(11):993–999, 1989.
37. Pollack MH, Otto MW, Tesar GE, et al. Long-term outcome after acute treatment with alprazolam or clonazepam for panic disorder. *J Clin Psychopharmacol* 13(4):257–263, 1993.
38. Soumerai SB, Simoni-Wastila L, Singer C, et al. Lack of relationship between long-term use of benzodiazepines and escalation to high dosages. *Psychiatr Serv* 54(7):1006–1011, 2003.
39. Nardi AE, Freire RC, Mochcovitch MD, et al. A randomized, naturalistic, parallel-group study for the long-term treatment of panic disorder with clonazepam or paroxetine. *J Clin Psychopharmacol* 32(1):120–126, 2012.
40. Nardi AE, Valenca AM, Freire RC, et al. Randomized, open naturalistic, acute treatment of panic disorder with clonazepam or paroxetine. *J Clin Psychopharmacol* 31(2):259–261, 2011.

41. Pecknold JC, Swinson RP, Kuch K, et al. Alprazolam in panic disorder and agoraphobia: results from a multicenter trial. III. Discontinuation effects. *Arch Gen Psychiatry* 45(5):429–436, 1988.

42. Rickels K, Schweizer E, Weiss S, et al. Maintenance drug treatment for panic disorder. II. Short- and long-term outcome after drug taper. *Arch Gen Psychiatry* 50(1):61–68, 1993.

43. Otto MW, Pollack MH, Sachs GS, et al. Discontinuation of benzodiazepine treatment: efficacy of cognitive-behavioral therapy for patients with panic disorder. *Am J Psychiatry* 150(10):1485–1490, 1993.

44. Kan CC, Hilberink SR, Breteler MH. Determination of the main risk factors for benzodiazepine dependence using a multivariate and multidimensional approach. *Compr Psychiatry* 45(2):88–94, 2004.

45. Gaudreault P, Guay J, Thivierge RL, et al. Benzodiazepine poisoning. Clinical and pharmacological considerations and treatment. *Drug Saf* 6(4):247–265, 1991.

46. Greenblatt DJ, Shader RI, Abernethy DR. Drug therapy. Current status of benzodiazepines. *N Engl J Med* 309(6):354–358, 1983.

47. Mitte K. A meta-analysis of the efficacy of psycho- and pharmacotherapy in panic disorder with and without agoraphobia. *J Affect Disord* 88(1):27–45, 2005.

48. Pollack MH, Simon NM, Worthington JJ, et al. Combined paroxetine and clonazepam treatment strategies compared to paroxetine monotherapy for panic disorder. *J Psychopharmacol* 17(3):276–282, 2003.

49. Goddard AW, Brouette T, Almai A, et al. Early coadministration of clonazepam with sertraline for panic disorder. *Arch Gen Psychiatry* 58(7):681–686, 2001.

50. Simon NM, Otto MW, Worthington JJ, et al. Next-step strategies for panic disorder refractory to initial pharmacotherapy: a 3-phase randomized clinical trial. *J Clin Psychiatry* 70(11):1563–1570, 2009.

51. Sheehan DV, Davidson J, Manschreck T, et al. Lack of efficacy of a new antidepressant (bupropion) in the treatment of panic disorder with phobias. *J Clin Psychopharmacol* 3(1):28–31, 1983.

52. Simon NM, Emmanuel N, Ballenger J, et al. Bupropion sustained release for panic disorder. *Psychopharmacol Bull* 37(4):66–72, 2003.

53. Versiani M, Cassano G, Perugi G, et al. Reboxetine, a selective norepinephrine reuptake inhibitor, is an effective and well-tolerated treatment for panic disorder. *J Clin Psychiatry* 63(1):31–37, 2002.

54. Bertani A, Perna G, Migliarese G, et al. Comparison of the treatment with paroxetine and reboxetine in panic disorder: a randomized, single-blind study. *Pharmacopsychiatry* 37(5):206–210, 2004.

55. Gastfriend DR, Rosenbaum JF. Adjunctive buspirone in benzodiazepine treatment of four patients with panic disorder. *Am J Psychiatry* 146(7):914–916, 1989.

56. Bouvard M, Mollard E, Guerin J, et al. Study and course of the psychological profile in 77 patients expressing panic disorder with agoraphobia after cognitive behaviour therapy with or without buspirone. *Psychother Psychosom* 66(1):27–32, 1997.

57. Sheehan DV, Raj AB, Sheehan KH, et al. Is buspirone effective for panic disorder? *J Clin Psychopharmacol* 10(1):3–11, 1990.

58. Sheehan DV, Raj AB, Harnett-Sheehan K, et al. The relative efficacy of high-dose buspirone and alprazolam in the treatment of panic disorder: a double-blind placebo-controlled study. *Acta Psychiatr Scand* 88(1):1–11, 1993.

59. Munjack DJ, Crocker B, Cabe D, et al. Alprazolam, propranolol, and placebo in the treatment of panic disorder and agoraphobia with panic attacks. *J Clin Psychopharmacol* 9(1):22–27, 1989.

60. Hirschmann S, Dannon PN, Iancu I, et al. Pindolol augmentation in patients with treatment-resistant panic disorder: A double-blind, placebo-controlled trial. *J Clin Psychopharmacol* 20(5):556–559, 2000.

61. Hollifield M, Thompson PM, Ruiz JE, et al. Potential effectiveness and safety of olanzapine in refractory panic disorder. *Depress Anxiety* 21(1):33–40, 2005.

62. Simon NM, Hoge EA, Fischmann D, et al. An open-label trial of risperidone augmentation for refractory anxiety disorders. *J Clin Psychiatry* 67(3):381–385, 2006.

63. Worthington JJ 3rd, Kinrys G, Wygant LE, et al. Aripiprazole as an augmentor of selective serotonin reuptake inhibitors in depression and anxiety disorder patients. *Int Clin Psychopharmacol* 20(1):9–11, 2005.

64. Hoge EA, Worthington JJ 3rd, Kaufman RE, et al. Aripiprazole as augmentation treatment of refractory generalized anxiety disorder and panic disorder. *CNS Spectr* 13(6):522–527, 2008.

65. Prosser JM, Yard S, Steele A, et al. A comparison of low-dose risperidone to paroxetine in the treatment of panic attacks: a randomized, single-blind study. *BMC Psychiatry* 9:25, 2009.

66. Woodman CL, Noyes R Jr. Panic disorder: treatment with valproate. *J Clin Psychiatry* 55(4):134–136, 1994.

67. Lum M, Fontaine R, Elie R. Divalproex sodium's antipanic effect in panic disorder: A placebo-controlled study. *Biol Psychiatry* 27(Suppl. 1):164A–165A, 1990.

68. Uhde TW, Stein MB, Post RM. Lack of efficacy of carbamazepine in the treatment of panic disorder. *Am J Psychiatry* 145(9):1104–1109, 1988.

69. Pande AC, Pollack MH, Crockatt J, et al. Placebo-controlled study of gabapentin treatment of panic disorder. *J Clin Psychopharmacol* 20(4):467–471, 2000.

70. Rickels K, Pollack MH, Feltner DE, et al. Pregabalin for treatment of generalized anxiety disorder: a 4-week, multicenter, double-blind, placebo-controlled trial of pregabalin and alprazolam. *Arch Gen Psychiatry* 62(9):1022–1030, 2005.

71. Bielski RJ, Bose A, Chang CC. A double-blind comparison of escitalopram and paroxetine in the long-term treatment of generalized anxiety disorder. *Ann Clin Psychiatry* 17(2):65–69, 2005.

72. Montgomery SA, Sheehan DV, Meoni P, et al. Characterization of the longitudinal course of improvement in generalized anxiety disorder during long-term treatment with venlafaxine XR. *J Psychiatr Res* 36(4):209–217, 2002.

73. Stocchi F, Nordera G, Jokinen RH, et al. Efficacy and tolerability of paroxetine for the long-term treatment of generalized anxiety disorder. *J Clin Psychiatry* 64(3):250–258, 2003.

74. Rickels K, Downing R, Schweizer E, et al. Antidepressants for the treatment of generalized anxiety disorder. A placebo-controlled comparison of imipramine, trazodone, and diazepam. *Arch Gen Psychiatry* 50(11):884–895, 1993.

75. Rocca P, Fonzo V, Scotta M, et al. Paroxetine efficacy in the treatment of generalized anxiety disorder. *Acta Psychiatr Scand* 95(5):444–450, 1997.

76. Allgulander C, Bandelow B, Hollander E, et al. WCA recommendations for the long-term treatment of generalized anxiety disorder. *CNS Spectr* 8(8 Suppl. 1):53–61, 2003.

77. Ballenger JC. Benzodiazepines. In Schatzberg AF, Nemeroff CB, editors: *Textbook of psychopharmacology*, Washington, DC, 1998, American Psychiatric Press, pp 271–286.

78. Rickels K, Schweizer E. The treatment of generalized anxiety disorder in patients with depressive symptomatology. *J Clin Psychiatry* 54(Suppl.):20–23, 1993.

79. Van Ameringen M, Mancini C, Wilson C. Buspirone augmentation of selective serotonin reuptake inhibitors (SSRIs) in social phobia. *J Affect Disord* 39(2):115–121, 1996.

80. Appelberg BG, Syvalahti EK, Koskinen TE, et al. Patients with severe depression may benefit from buspirone augmentation of selective serotonin reuptake inhibitors: results from a placebo-controlled, randomized, double-blind, placebo wash-in study. *J Clin Psychiatry* 62(6):448–452, 2001.

81. Strand M, Hetta J, Rosen A, et al. A double-blind, controlled trial in primary care patients with generalized anxiety: a comparison between buspirone and oxazepam. *J Clin Psychiatry* 51(Suppl.):40–45, 1990.

82. Chessick CA, Allen MH, Thase M, et al. Azapirones for generalized anxiety disorder. *Cochrane Database Syst Rev* (3):CD006115, 2006.

83. Boschen MJ. A meta-analysis of the efficacy of pregabalin in the treatment of generalized anxiety disorder. *Can J Psychiatry* 56(9):558–566, 2011.

84. Stein DJ, Baldwin DS, Baldinetti F, et al. Efficacy of pregabalin in depressive symptoms associated with generalized anxiety disorder: a pooled analysis of 6 studies. *Eur Neuropsychopharmacol* 18(6):422–430, 2008.

85. Kasper S, Herman B, Nivoli G, et al. Efficacy of pregabalin and venlafaxine-XR in generalized anxiety disorder: results of

a double-blind, placebo-controlled 8-week trial. *Int Clin Psychopharmacol* 24(2):87–96, 2009.

86. Montgomery SA, Tobias K, Zornberg GL, et al. Efficacy and safety of pregabalin in the treatment of generalized anxiety disorder: a 6-week, multicenter, randomized, double-blind, placebo-controlled comparison of pregabalin and venlafaxine. *J Clin Psychiatry* 67(5):771–782, 2006.

87. Feltner DE, Crockatt JG, Dubovsky SJ, et al. A randomized, double-blind, placebo-controlled, fixed-dose, multicenter study of pregabalin in patients with generalized anxiety disorder. *J Clin Psychopharmacol* 23(3):240–249, 2003.

88. Pollack MH, Roy-Byrne PP, Van Ameringen M, et al. The selective GABA reuptake inhibitor tiagabine for the treatment of generalized anxiety disorder: results of a placebo-controlled study. *J Clin Psychiatry* 66(11):1401–1408, 2005.

89. Pollack M, Tiller J, Zie F, et al. *Tiagabine in adult patients with generalized anxiety disorder: results from three randomized, double-blind, placebo-controlled, parallel-group studies.* Submitted for Publication.

90. Pollack MH, Tiller J, Xie F, et al. Tiagabine in adult patients with generalized anxiety disorder: results from 3 randomized, double-blind, placebo-controlled, parallel-group studies. *J Clin Psychopharmacol* 28(3):308–316, 2008.

91. Mendels J, Krajewski TF, Huffer V, et al. Effective short-term treatment of generalized anxiety disorder with trifluoperazine. *J Clin Psychiatry* 47(4):170–174, 1986.

92. Pollack MH, Simon NM, Zalta AK, et al. Olanzapine augmentation of fluoxetine for refractory generalized anxiety disorder: a placebo controlled study. *Biol Psychiatry* 59(3):211–215, 2006.

93. Brawman-Mintzer O, Knapp RG, Nietert PJ. Adjunctive risperidone in generalized anxiety disorder: a double-blind, placebo-controlled study. *J Clin Psychiatry* 66(10):1321–1325, 2005.

94. Snyderman SH, Rynn MA, Rickels K. Open-label pilot study of ziprasidone for refractory generalized anxiety disorder. *J Clin Psychopharmacol* 25(5):497–499, 2005.

95. Bandelow B, Chouinard G, Bobes J, et al. Extended-release quetiapine fumarate (quetiapine XR): a once-daily monotherapy effective in generalized anxiety disorder. Data from a randomized, double-blind, placebo- and active-controlled study. *Int J Neuropsychopharmacol* 13(3):305–320, 2010.

96. Katzman MA, Brawman-Mintzer O, Reyes EB, et al. Extended release quetiapine fumarate (quetiapine XR) monotherapy as maintenance treatment for generalized anxiety disorder: a long-term, randomized, placebo-controlled trial. *Int Clin Psychopharmacol* 26(1):11–24, 2011.

97. Khan A, Joyce M, Atkinson S, et al. A randomized, double-blind study of once-daily extended release quetiapine fumarate (quetiapine XR) monotherapy in patients with generalized anxiety disorder. *J Clin Psychopharmacol* 31(4):418–428, 2011.

98. Merideth C, Cutler AJ, She F, et al. Efficacy and tolerability of extended release quetiapine fumarate monotherapy in the acute treatment of generalized anxiety disorder: a randomized, placebo controlled and active-controlled study. *Int Clin Psychopharmacol* 27(1):40–54, 2012.

99. Mezhebovsky I, Magi K, She F, et al. Double-blind, randomized study of extended release quetiapine fumarate (quetiapine XR) monotherapy in older patients with generalized anxiety disorder. *Int J Geriatr Psychiatry* 28(6):615–625, 2013.

100. Ketter TA, Nasrallah HA, Fagiolini A. Mood stabilizers and atypical antipsychotics: bimodal treatments for bipolar disorder. *Psychopharmacol Bull* 39(1):120–146, 2006.

101. Rapaport MH, Gharabawi GM, Canuso CM, et al. Effects of risperidone augmentation in patients with treatment-resistant depression: Results of open-label treatment followed by double-blind continuation. *Neuropsychopharmacology* 31(11):2505–2513, 2006.

102. Mathew SJ, Amiel JM, Coplan JD, et al. Open-label trial of riluzole in generalized anxiety disorder. *Am J Psychiatry* 162(12):2379–2381, 2005.

103. Amsterdam JD, Li Y, Soeller I, et al. A randomized, double-blind, placebo-controlled trial of oral Matricaria recutita (chamomile) extract therapy for generalized anxiety disorder. *J Clin Psychopharmacol* 29(4):378–382, 2009.

104. Connor KM, Payne V, Davidson JR. Kava in generalized anxiety disorder: three placebo-controlled trials. *Int Clin Psychopharmacol* 21(5):249–253, 2006.

105. Connor KM, Davidson JR. A placebo-controlled study of Kava kava in generalized anxiety disorder. *Int Clin Psychopharmacol* 17(4):185–188, 2002.

106. Sarris J, Stough C, Bousman CA, et al. Kava in the treatment of generalized anxiety disorder: a double-blind, randomized, placebo-controlled study. *J Clin Psychopharmacol* Apr 30 2013.

107. Asakura S, Tajima O, Koyama T. Fluvoxamine treatment of generalized social anxiety disorder in Japan: a randomized double-blind, placebo-controlled study. *Int J Neuropsychopharmacol* 10(2):263–274, 2007.

108. Davidson J, Yaryura-Tobias J, DuPont R, et al. Fluvoxamine-controlled release formulation for the treatment of generalized social anxiety disorder. *J Clin Psychopharmacol* 24(2):118–125, 2004.

109. Owen RT. Controlled-release fluvoxamine in obsessive-compulsive disorder and social phobia. *Drugs Today (Barc)* 44(12):887–893, 2008.

110. Stein MB, Fyer AJ, Davidson JR, et al. Fluvoxamine treatment of social phobia (social anxiety disorder): a double-blind, placebo-controlled study. *Am J Psychiatry* 156(5):756–760, 1999.

111. van Vliet IM, den Boer JA, Westenberg HG. Psychopharmacological treatment of social phobia; a double blind placebo controlled study with fluvoxamine. *Psychopharmacology (Berl)* 115(1–2):128–134, 1994.

112. Furmark T, Appel L, Michelgard A, et al. Cerebral blood flow changes after treatment of social phobia with the neurokinin-1 antagonist GR205171, citalopram, or placebo. *Biol Psychiatry* 58(2):132–142, 2005.

113. Kasper S, Stein DJ, Loft H, et al. Escitalopram in the treatment of social anxiety disorder: randomised, placebo-controlled, flexible-dosage study. *Br J Psychiatry* 186:222–226, 2005.

114. Lader M, Stender K, Burger V, et al. Efficacy and tolerability of escitalopram in 12- and 24-week treatment of social anxiety disorder: randomised, double-blind, placebo-controlled, fixed-dose study. *Depress Anxiety* 19(4):241–248, 2004.

115. Davidson JR, Foa EB, Huppert JD, et al. Fluoxetine, comprehensive cognitive behavioral therapy, and placebo in generalized social phobia. *Arch Gen Psychiatry* 61(10):1005–1013, 2004.

116. Kobak KA, Greist JH, Jefferson JW, et al. Fluoxetine in social phobia: a double-blind, placebo-controlled pilot study. *J Clin Psychopharmacol* 22(3):257–262, 2002.

117. Clark DM, Ehlers A, McManus F, et al. Cognitive therapy versus fluoxetine in generalized social phobia: a randomized placebo-controlled trial. *J Consult Clin Psychol* 71(6):1058–1067, 2003.

118. Simon NM, Worthington JJ, Moshier SJ, et al. Duloxetine for the treatment of generalized social anxiety disorder: a preliminary randomized trial of increased dose to optimize response. *CNS Spectr* 15(7):367–373, 2010.

119. Hansen RA, Gaynes BN, Gartlehner G, et al. Efficacy and tolerability of second-generation antidepressants in social anxiety disorder. *Int Clin Psychopharmacol* 23(3):170–179, 2008.

120. Randall CL, Johnson MR, Thevos AK, et al. Paroxetine for social anxiety and alcohol use in dual-diagnosed patients. *Depress Anxiety* 14(4):255–262, 2001.

121. Brantigan CO, Brantigan TA, Joseph N. Effect of beta blockade and beta stimulation on stage fright. *Am J Med* 72(1):88–94, 1982.

122. Gossard D, Dennis C, DeBusk RF. Use of beta-blocking agents to reduce the stress of presentation at an international cardiology meeting: results of a survey. *Am J Cardiol* 54(1):240–241, 1984.

123. Liebowitz MR, Schneier F, Campeas R, et al. Phenelzine vs atenolol in social phobia. A placebo-controlled comparison. *Arch Gen Psychiatry* 49(4):290–300, 1992.

124. Conant J, Engler R, Janowsky D, et al. Central nervous system side effects of beta-adrenergic blocking agents with high and low lipid solubility. *J Cardiovasc Pharmacol* 13(4):656–661, 1989.

125. Welkowitz LA, Liebowitz MR. Pharmacologic treatment of social phobia and performance anxiety. In Noyes R, Roth M, Burrows GD, editors: *Handbook of anxiety*, vol. 4, London, 1990, Elsevier Science Publishers, pp 233–250.

126. Liebowitz MR, Gorman JM, Fyer AJ, et al. Social phobia. Review of a neglected anxiety disorder. *Arch Gen Psychiatry* 42(7):729–736, 1985.

127. Gelernter CS, Uhde TW, Cimbolic P, et al. Cognitive-behavioral and pharmacological treatments of social phobia. A controlled study. *Arch Gen Psychiatry* 48(10):938–945, 1991.
128. Versiani M, Nardi AE, Mundim FD, et al. Pharmacotherapy of social phobia. A controlled study with moclobemide and phenelzine. *Br J Psychiatry* 161:353–360, 1992.
129. Versiani M, Mundim FD, Nardi AE, et al. Tranylcypromine in social phobia. *J Clin Psychopharmacol* 8(4):279–283, 1988.
130. Heimberg RG, Liebowitz MR, Hope DA, et al. Cognitive behavioral group therapy vs phenelzine therapy for social phobia: 12-week outcome. *Arch Gen Psychiatry* 55(12):1133–1141, 1998.
131. Hart TA, Turk CL, Heimberg RG, et al. Relation of marital status to social phobia severity. *Depress Anxiety* 10(1):28–32, 1999.
132. Noyes R Jr, Moroz G, Davidson JR, et al. Moclobemide in social phobia: a controlled dose-response trial. *J Clin Psychopharmacol* 17(4):247–254, 1997.
133. Davidson JR, Potts N, Richichi E, et al. Treatment of social phobia with clonazepam and placebo. *J Clin Psychopharmacol* 13(6):423–428, 1993.
134. Otto MW, Pollack MH, Gould RA, et al. A comparison of the efficacy of clonazepam and cognitive-behavioral group therapy for the treatment of social phobia. *J Anxiety Disord* 14(4):345–358, 2000.
135. Seedat S, Stein MB. Double-blind, placebo-controlled assessment of combined clonazepam with paroxetine compared with paroxetine monotherapy for generalized social anxiety disorder. *J Clin Psychiatry* 65(2):244–248, 2004.
136. Hoge E, Pollack MH. Pharmacotherapy of social anxiety disorder: current practice and future promise. In Pollack M, Simon NM, Otto MW, editors: *Social anxiety disorder: research and practice*, New York, 2003, Professional Publishing Group, Ltd., pp 157–186.
137. Emmanuel N, Johnson M, Villareal G. *Imipramine in the treatment of social phobia: a double-blind study.* Presented at American College of Neuropsychopharmacology 36 meeting, 1997, Waikoloa, Hawaii.
138. Emmanuel NP, Brawman-Mintzer O, Morton WA, et al. Bupropion-SR in treatment of social phobia. *Depress Anxiety* 12(2):111–113, 2000.
139. Van Veen JF, Van Vliet IM, Westenberg HG. Mirtazapine in social anxiety disorder: a pilot study. *Int Clin Psychopharmacol* 17(6):315–317, 2002.
140. Mrakotsky C, Masek B, Biederman J, et al. Prospective open-label pilot trial of mirtazapine in children and adolescents with social phobia. *J Anxiety Disord* 22(1):88–97, 2008.
141. Muehlbacher M, Nickel MK, Nickel C, et al. Mirtazapine treatment of social phobia in women: a randomized, double-blind, placebo-controlled study. *J Clin Psychopharmacol* 25(6):580–583, 2005.
142. Schutters SI, Van Megen HJ, Van Veen JF, et al. Mirtazapine in generalized social anxiety disorder: a randomized, double-blind, placebo-controlled study. *Int Clin Psychopharmacol* 25(5):302–304, 2010.
143. Barnett SD, Kramer ML, Casat CD, et al. Efficacy of olanzapine in social anxiety disorder: a pilot study. *J Psychopharmacol* 16(4):365–368, 2002.
144. Schutters SI, van Megen HJ, Westenberg HG. Efficacy of quetiapine in generalized social anxiety disorder: results from an open-label study. *J Clin Psychiatry* 66(4):540–542, 2005.
145. Vaishnavi S, Alamy S, Zhang W, et al. Quetiapine as monotherapy for social anxiety disorder: a placebo-controlled study. *Prog Neuropsychopharmacol Biol Psychiatry* 31(7):1464–1469, 2007.
146. Pande AC, Davidson JR, Jefferson JW, et al. Treatment of social phobia with gabapentin: a placebo-controlled study. *J Clin Psychopharmacol* 19(4):341–348, 1999.
147. Pande AC, Feltner DE, Jefferson JW, et al. Efficacy of the novel anxiolytic pregabalin in social anxiety disorder: a placebo-controlled, multicenter study. *J Clin Psychopharmacol* 24(2):141–149, 2004.
148. Kinrys G, Pollack MH, Simon NM, et al. Valproic acid for the treatment of social anxiety disorder. *Int Clin Psychopharmacol* 18:169–172, 2003.
149. Simon NM, Worthington JJ, Doyle AC, et al. An open-label study of levetiracetam for the treatment of social anxiety disorder. *J Clin Psychiatry* 65(9):1219–1222, 2004.
150. Stein MB, Ravindran LN, Simon NM, et al. Levetiracetam in generalized social anxiety disorder: a double-blind, randomized controlled trial. *J Clin Psychiatry* 71(5):627–631, 2010.
151. Zhang W, Connor KM, Davidson JR. Levetiracetam in social phobia: a placebo controlled pilot study. *J Psychopharmacol* 19(5):551–553, 2005.
152. Van Ameringen M, Mancini C, Pipe B, et al. An open trial of topiramate in the treatment of generalized social phobia. *J Clin Psychiatry* 65(12):1674–1678, 2004.
153. Dunlop BW, Papp L, Garlow SJ, et al. Tiagabine for social anxiety disorder. *Hum Psychopharmacol* 22(4):241–244, 2007.
154. Martinez D, Broft A, Laruelle M. Pindolol augmentation of antidepressant treatment: recent contributions from brain imaging studies. *Biol Psychiatry* 48(8):844–853, 2000.
155. Stein MB, Sareen J, Hami S, et al. Pindolol potentiation of paroxetine for generalized social phobia: a double-blind, placebo-controlled, crossover study. *Am J Psychiatry* 158(10):1725–1727, 2001.
156. Goldstein S. Treatment of social phobia with clonidine. *Biol Psychiatry* 22(3):369–372, 1987.
157. Bell J, De Vaugh-Geiss J. *Multi-center trail of a 5-HT3 antagonist, ondansetron, in social phobia.* Presented at 33rd Annual Meeting of the American College of Neuropsychopharmacology, 1994, San Juan, Puerto Rico.
158. Hofmann SG, Smits JA, Rosenfield D, et al. D-Cycloserine as an augmentation strategy with cognitive-behavioral therapy for social anxiety disorder. *Am J Psychiatry* 170(7):751–758, 2013.
159. Davis M. NMDA receptors and fear extinction: implications for cognitive behavioral therapy. *Dialogues Clin Neurosci* 13(4):463–474, 2011.

7   Antipsychotic Drugs

Oliver Freudenreich, MD, Donald C. Goff, MD, and David C. Henderson, MD

KEY POINTS

- All antipsychotics share dopamine$_2$ blockade as the presumed main mechanism of action.
- Primary symptom targets of antipsychotics are positive symptoms (disorganization, delusions, and hallucinations) and agitation; their efficacy for negative symptoms and cognitive deficits of schizophrenia is questionable. Increasingly, antipsychotics are used for treatment of mood disorders.
- Historically, antipsychotics have been grouped into first-generation antipsychotics (typical or conventional antipsychotics, which are all characterized by their risk of extrapyramidal symptoms [EPS]) and second-generation antipsychotics (with a reduced risk of EPS; hence they are called "atypical" antipsychotics). However, antipsychotics within each class are not necessarily interchangeable.
- The main risks of first-generation antipsychotics are neurological side effects (e.g., dystonias, akathisia, parkinsonism, tardive dyskinesia [TD]); for most second-generation antipsychotics, metabolic problems (e.g., weight gain, dyslipidemia, hyperglycemia) have emerged as major problems.
- First- and second-generation antipsychotics are equally effective for non-refractory patients with schizophrenia. For refractory patients, olanzapine, and in particular clozapine, have been the most efficacious.
- Clozapine has minimal or no risk of inducing EPS and is the most effective antipsychotic. However, its clinical use is limited to refractory patients because of serious side effects (including metabolic problems and agranulocytosis that requires white blood cell count monitoring).
- Currently available antipsychotics have variable efficacy and tolerability and need to be selected on the basis of individualized risk–benefit assessments (i.e., balancing the degree of symptomatic response with day-to-day tolerability and long-term medical morbidity, particularly cardiovascular risk).

INTRODUCTION

In this chapter, we will review the basic pharmacology of antipsychotics, emphasizing the differential efficacy and side-effect profiles between first- and second-generation antipsychotics, including clozapine, based on the schizophrenia literature. While antipsychotics are used more broadly than for the treatment of schizophrenia, antipsychotic agents have received FDA approval for additional indications, particularly for the treatment of mood disorders for which they are used routinely. A recent meta-analysis found that antipsychotics were significantly more effective for mania than were mood stabilizers.[1]

HISTORY
Chlorpromazine and the Early Agents

In 1952, Henri Laborit, a French naval surgeon, was experimenting with combinations of preoperative medications to reduce the autonomic stress of surgical procedures. He tried a newly-synthesized antihistamine, chlorpromazine, and was impressed by its calming effect. He noted that patients seemed indifferent about their impending surgery, yet they were not overly sedated. Convinced that the medication had potential for the care of psychiatric patients, Laborit urged colleagues to test his hypothesis. Eventually a surgical colleague told his brother-in-law, the psychiatrist Pierre Deniker, about Laborit's discovery.

Deniker and Jean Delay, who was the chairman of his department at the Hôpital Sainte-Anne in Paris, experimented with chlorpromazine and found remarkable tranquilizing effects in their most agitated and psychotic patients.[2,3] By 1954, Delay and Deniker had published six papers on their clinical experience with chlorpromazine. They noted in 1955 that both chlorpromazine and the dopamine-depleting agent reserpine shared antipsychotic efficacy and neurological side effects that resembled Parkinson's disease. They coined the term *neuroleptic* to describe these effects. In 1956 Frank Ayd[4,5] described acute dystonia and fatal hyperthermia with chlorpromazine. The first reports of tardive dyskinesia (TD) were published by Sigwald and colleagues in 1959.[6]

Smith Kline purchased chlorpromazine from the French pharmaceutical company Rhône-Poulenc, and in 1954 chlorpromazine received approval from the Food and Drug Administration (FDA) for the treatment of psychosis. Almost immediately the care of psychotic patients was transformed. In the US the traditional practice of life-long "warehousing" of individuals with schizophrenia in large state psychiatric hospitals gave way to the new outpatient community psychiatry movement. An additional 10 antipsychotic compounds were rapidly synthesized and approved for clinical use. This included a series of phenothiazines, the thioxanthenes (that were derived from phenothiazines), and haloperidol, which was synthesized from meperidine by Paul Janssen in 1958. In 1967 haloperidol, the last "neuroleptic," was approved by the FDA and, because of its relative selectivity for dopamine$_2$ (D$_2$) receptors and paucity of non-neurological side effects, became the market leader.

By 1964, several multi-center trials sponsored by the Veterans Administration and the National Institutes of Mental Health (NIMH) were completed, comparing the rapidly growing list of antipsychotic agents. These landmark studies each enrolled several hundred patients and were the first large clinical trials to be conducted in the new field of psychopharmacology. The phenothiazines were found to be highly effective and superior to placebo, barbiturates, and reserpine. With the exception of promazine and mepazine, the phenothiazines were found to be of equivalent efficacy, although they differed in their side-effect profiles. In the NIMH collaborative study of over 400 acutely ill patients, 75% of patients were at least moderately improved with chlorpromazine, thioridazine, or fluphenazine, compared to only 23% with placebo.[7] While reports of efficacy were impressive, the goal of identifying differences in efficacy between drugs that might allow matching of specific drugs with subgroups of patients was not realized.

The discovery by Carlsson and Lindqvist[8] in 1963 that chlorpromazine increased turnover of dopamine in the brain led to the hypothesis that dopamine receptor-blockade was responsible for antipsychotic effects. This was confirmed in 1976 by Creese and colleagues,[9] who demonstrated that the antipsychotic potency of a wide range of agents correlated closely with affinity for the D_2 receptor, which explained the equivalency of efficacy between agents since all were acting via the same mechanism. The dopamine hypothesis led to a reliance on animal models sensitive to D_2 blockade as a screen for discovering potential antipsychotic drugs, with the result that new mechanisms were not intentionally explored.

Clozapine, the First Atypical Antipsychotic

The discovery of the first antidepressant, imipramine, led to the synthesis of related heterotricyclic compounds, among which clozapine, a dibenzodiazepine derivative, was synthesized in 1958 by the Swiss company Wander. Clozapine was initially a disappointment, because it did not produce in animal models the behavioral effects associated with an antidepressant or the neurological side effects associated with an antipsychotic. Clinical trials proceeded in Europe but were halted in 1975 after reports of 17 cases of agranulocytosis in Finland, 8 of which were fatal.[10] However, the impression among researchers that clozapine possessed unique clinical characteristics led the manufacturer, Sandoz, to sponsor a pivotal multicenter trial comparing clozapine with chlorpromazine in neuroleptic-resistant patients prospectively shown to be refractory to haloperidol. The dramatic results reported by Kane and colleagues in 1988[11] demonstrated the superiority of clozapine for essentially all domains of symptoms and a relative absence of neurological side effects, prompting a second revolution in the pharmacotherapy of schizophrenia. To this date, clozapine remains the most effective antipsychotic for treatment-refractory schizophrenia.

Other Atypical Agents

Starting in the mid-1980s, Paul Janssen and colleagues began experimenting with serotonin 5-HT$_2$ antagonism added to D_2 blockade after demonstrating that this combination reduced neurological side effects of haloperidol in rats.[12] When the 5-HT$_2$ antagonist ritanserin was added to haloperidol in patients with schizophrenia, EPS were diminished and negative symptoms improved.[13] This led to development of risperidone, a D_2 and 5-HT$_{2A}$ antagonist, the first agent designed to follow clozapine's example as an "atypical antipsychotic" with the goal of reduced EPS and enhanced efficacy. Multicenter trials comparing multiple fixed doses of risperidone with haloperidol at a single, relatively high dose of 20 mg/day demonstrated reduced EPS, improved negative symptoms, and, in a subset of relatively resistant patients, greater antipsychotic efficacy.[14,15] Olanzapine, a chemical derivative of clozapine, similarly demonstrated reduced EPS and superior efficacy compared to haloperidol. Risperidone and olanzapine

TABLE 7-1 Timeline of Antipsychotics in the United States

First-Generation Antipsychotics (11 Agents)*	
Chlorpromazine (Thorazine)	1954
Haloperidol (Haldol)	1967

Second-Generation Antipsychotics (10 Agents)	
Clozapine (Clozaril)	1989
Risperidone (Risperdal)	1993
Olanzapine (Zyprexa)	1997
Quetiapine (Seroquel)	1997
Ziprasidone (Geodon)	2001
Aripiprazole (Abilify)	2002
Paliperidone (Invega)	2006
Iloperidone (Fanapt)	2009
Asenapine (Saphris)	2009
Lurasidone (Latuda)	2010

Note: The year given for each agent denotes the year of FDA approval.
*Only the first and last agents are listed for first-generation antipsychotics.

rapidly replaced the first generation of neuroleptics, particularly after clinicians became convinced that the risk of TD was substantially lower. However, it soon became apparent that risperidone markedly elevated serum prolactin levels and that olanzapine produced weight gain in some patients to a degree previously seen only with clozapine. Quetiapine, ziprasidone, and aripiprazole were subsequently approved in the US, based largely on reduced EPS; these agents did not convincingly demonstrate superior efficacy compared to older neuroleptics. Like risperidone and olanzapine, these last three agents acted via D_2 and 5-HT$_{2A}$ receptors; aripiprazole differed from the other second-generation antipsychotics by possessing partial agonist activity at the D_2 receptor rather than full antagonism. Risperidone became the first atypical agent available as a long-acting injection in the form of "risperidone microspheres". Recently, several additional atypical agents have become available, including a metabolite of risperidone (i.e., paliperidone) and asenapine, iloperidone, and lurasidone (Tables 7-1 and 7-2).

A series of case reports, pharmacoepidemiological studies, and, eventually, direct physiological investigations linked atypical antipsychotics with insulin resistance, a heightened risk for diabetes mellitus (DM), and dyslipidemia (primarily elevation of triglycerides). In response, the FDA issued a class warning for DM, although over time, the evidence most strongly implicated clozapine and olanzapine.

The CATIE Study

In 1999, the NIMH, recognizing that almost all information regarding the new antipsychotics had come from industry-supported efficacy trials of uncertain generalizability, awarded a competitive contract to Dr. Jeffrey Lieberman to conduct a large, multi-center trial to assess the effectiveness and tolerability of these agents under more representative treatment conditions. Results of this seminal Clinical Antipsychotic Trials of Intervention Effectiveness (CATIE) study were first published in 2005 (Figure 7-1).[16] The study was conducted at 57 sites across the US and included 1,493 representative patients with schizophrenia who were randomly assigned to risperidone, olanzapine, quetiapine, ziprasidone, or the conventional comparator, perphenazine, for an 18-month double-blind trial. Dosing was flexible; the range of doses for each

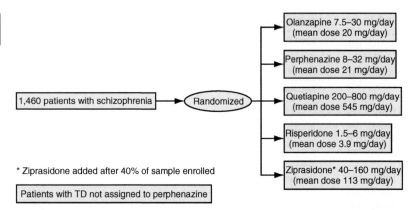

Results
Limitations of CATIE:
- Not powered to detect differences in rates of tardive dyskinesia
- Did not study medication-naïve patients
- Aripiprazole was not available for study
- Optimal dosing of all drugs may not have been achieved

Conclusions of CATIE:
- Olanzapine most effective agent in phase I, but associated with greater metabolic side effects
- Perphenazine comparable to the other atypical agents in effectiveness and tolerability and the most "cost effective"
- Risperidone associated with greater hyperprolactinemia, but well-tolerated
- Clozapine extremely effective in phase II (open label) for nonresponders
- No single antipsychotic is consistently effective or tolerable for all patients—several trials may be necessary to identify the optimal agent for an individual patient

Figure 7-1. CATIE phase 1: double-blind, randomized 18-month trial.

TABLE 7-2 Affinity of Antipsychotic Drugs for Human Neurotransmitter Receptors (Ki, nM)

Receptor	Clozapine	Risperidone	Olanzapine	Quetiapine	Ziprasidone	Aripiprazole	Iloperidone	Haloperidol	Lurasidone
D_1	290	580	52	1,300	130	410	320	120	
D_2	130	2.2	20	180	3.1	0.52	6.3	1.4	1.68
D_3	240	9.6	50	940	7.2	9.1	7.1	2.5	
D_4	47	8.5	50	2,200	32	260	25	3.3	
$5\text{-}HT_{1A}$	140	210	2,100	230	2.5		93	3,600	6.75
$5\text{-}HT_{1D}$	1,700	170	530	>5,100	2			>5,000	
$5\text{-}HT_{2A}$	8.9	0.29	3.3	220	0.39	20	5.6	120	2.03
$5\text{-}HT_{2C}$	17	10	10	1,400	0.72		43	4,700	
$5\text{-}HT_6$	11	2,000	10	4,100	76	160	63	6,000	
$5\text{-}HT_7$	66	3	250	1,800	9.3	15	110	1,100	0.495
α_1	4	1.4	54	15	13	57	1.4	4.7	47.9
α_2	33	5.1	170	1,000	310		160	1,200	40.7
H_1	1.8	19	2.8	8.7	47		470	440	1000
m_1	1.8	2,800	4.7	100	5,100			1,600	1000

(Adapted from Miyamoto S, Duncan GE, Goff DC, et al. Therapeutics in schizophrenia. In Meltzer H, Nemeroff C, editors: Neuropsychopharmacology: the fifth generation of progress, Philadelphia, 2002, Lippincott Williams & Wilkins. The binding affinities for lurasidone were adapted from Ishibashi T, Horisawa T, Tokuda K, et al. Pharmacological profile of lurasidone, a novel antipsychotic agent with potent 5-hydroxytryptamine 7 (5-HT7) and 5-HT1A receptor activity. J Pharmacol Exp Ther 334(1):171–181, 2010.)

drug was selected based on patterns of clinical use (in consultation with the manufacturers). Ziprasidone became available and was added after the study was roughly 40% completed. Patients with TD at study entry were not randomized to perphenazine, and their data were excluded from analyses comparing the atypical agents with perphenazine. Patients who failed treatment with their first assigned agent could be randomized again in subsequent phases; one re-randomization pathway featured open-label clozapine for treatment-resistant patients and one pathway featured ziprasidone for treatment-intolerant patients. The secondary randomization pathway did not include perphenazine.

One striking finding of the CATIE study was that only 26% of subjects completed the 18-month trial still taking their originally-assigned antipsychotic. The primary measure of effectiveness, "all cause discontinuation," significantly favored olanzapine over the other agents. The superior effectiveness of olanzapine was also reflected in significantly fewer hospitalizations and fewer discontinuations due to lack of efficacy. While risperidone-treated patients were numerically less likely to discontinue due to intolerance, this difference was not statistically significant. In addition to greater effectiveness, olanzapine was associated with greater cardiovascular risk; patients treated with olanzapine had more weight gain and elevation

TABLE 7-3 First-Generation Antipsychotic Doses

	Equivalent Dose	Typical Dose Acute/maintenance
	(mg)*	*(mg/day)*
LOW POTENCY		
Chlorpromazine	100	300–1,000/300–600
Thioridazine	100	300–800/300–600
MEDIUM POTENCY		
Loxapine	10	30–100/30–60
Perphenazine	10	12–64/8–32**
HIGH POTENCY		
Trifluoperazine	5	15–50/15–30
Thiothixene	5	15–50/15–30
Fluphenazine	2	6–20/6–12
Haloperidol	2	6–20/6–12

*Equivalent dose (or "chlorpromazine equivalents") reflects the potency of antipsychotics compared to 100 mg of chlorpromazine as the reference.
**CATIE dose range 8 mg to 32 mg/day.
(Adapted from Buchanan RW, Kreyenbuhl J, Kelly DL, et al. The 2009 schizophrenia PORT psychopharmacological treatment recommendations and summary statements. Schizophrenia Bulletin 36(1):71–93, 2010.)

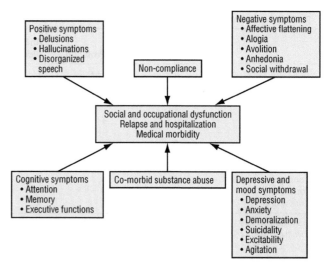

Figure 7-2. Targets for the treatment of schizophrenia.

of hemoglobin A_{1c}, total cholesterol, and triglycerides. The other atypical agents did not significantly differ from perphenazine in either efficacy or tolerability. Overall, the results suggested that no single antipsychotic is likely to be optimal for all, or for most, patients. The duration of the CATIE trial was not long enough to detect differences between agents in the incidence of TD.

CURRENTLY AVAILABLE ANTIPSYCHOTIC AGENTS

All marketed antipsychotic agents share the common property of dopamine (D_2) receptor blockade. The 11 agents approved in the US between 1953 (chlorpromazine) and 1967 (haloperidol) are commonly referred to as *conventional neuroleptics* or *first-generation antipsychotics* (Table 7-3). As a group they possess equivalent efficacy, but differ in their potency and side effects. Reflecting their common property of D_2 blockade, these agents all can produce EPS, TD, and hyperprolactinemia. Clozapine was the first of the *second-generation antipsychotics*, also known as *atypical antipsychotics*. Currently there are 10 atypical antipsychotics approved in the US; these agents generally produce fewer EPS, less elevation of prolactin, and less risk of TD than first-generation antipsychotics. Clozapine has clearly demonstrated greater efficacy than the first-generation agents. Of the other second-generation antipsychotics, only olanzapine was found to be more effective than the first-generation comparator in the CATIE study. Risperidone and its metabolite, paliperidone are unique among the atypical agents in producing marked prolactin elevation. Aripiprazole is the only antipsychotic with partial agonist rather than antagonist activity at the D_2 receptor; this property is believed to limit neurological side effects. Because aripiprazole was not included in the CATIE study, it is unclear if D_2 partial agonism has implications for effectiveness. The most comprehensive meta-analysis, published by Leucht and colleagues in 2013,[17] found substantial differences in side effects and small but statistically significant differences in efficacy between currently available antipsychotics, arguing against a simple categoriza-

tion as first- or second-generation even though this terminology continues to be used (for lack of a better one).

GENERAL CLINICAL CONSIDERATIONS

For schizophrenia, the primary target symptoms for antipsychotic agents fall into three categories: psychotic symptoms (e.g., hallucinations, delusions, disorganization); agitation (e.g., distractibility, affective lability, tension, increased motor activity); and negative symptoms (e.g., apathy, diminished affect, social withdrawal, poverty of speech). Although cognitive deficits are an important contributor to disability in schizophrenia, cognitive deficits usually are not considered a target for antipsychotic agents because they are not very responsive to current agents. Agitation responds to most antipsychotics rapidly and often fully, whereas response of psychotic symptoms is quite variable and negative symptoms rarely exhibit more than modest improvement[18] (Figure 7-2).

The time course of antipsychotic response also can be quite variable. In the 1970s, the treatment of psychosis with relatively large doses of intramuscular (IM) haloperidol, known as "rapid neuroleptization," was advocated, based on the clinical impression that agitation and psychosis responded quickly to this aggressive treatment approach.[19] For the next two decades, the consensus shifted to the view that psychotic symptoms require weeks of antipsychotic treatment before responding. More recently, Kapur and colleagues[20] analyzed data from studies of IM administration of atypical antipsychotics and documented antipsychotic effects within hours of administration, independent of tranquilization. Most likely, tranquilization, or the improvement of agitation and irritability, occurs rapidly with most agents whereas psychotic symptoms may begin to improve quickly in some patients and only after a delay of several weeks in others. Maximal response to antipsychotic treatment can require months. The pharmacological treatment of psychotic symptoms is similar to the treatment of infection with antibiotics—the clinician needs to choose a proper dose and then await therapeutic results while monitoring side effects.

The degree of antipsychotic efficacy ranges from complete resolution of psychosis in a substantial number of patients to minimal or no benefit in others. In between, some patients experience diminished delusional conviction, or may persist in their delusional conviction but no longer interpret new

TABLE 7-4 Antipsychotic Side Effects

	EPS	Tardive Dyskinesia	Prolactin	Anticholinergic Side Effects	Sedation	Weight Gain	Diabetes	Dyslipidemia
Chlorpromazine	++	+++	+++	++++	++++	+++	+++	++
Perphenazine	+++	+++	+++	++	++	++	–	+
Haloperidol	++++	+++	+++	–	+	+– –		
Clozapine	–	–	–	++++	++++	++++	++++	++++
Risperidone	++	+	++++	–	++	++	++	+
Olanzapine	+	+	+	+	+++	++++	++++	++++
Quetiapine	–	?	–	++*	+++	++	+++†	+++†
Ziprasidone	+	?	+	–	+	+	–	–
Aripiprazole	+	?	–	–	+	+	–	–
Asenapine	++	?	+	–	++	+	–?	–?
Iloperidone	–	?	–	–	+	++	++?	?
Lurasidone	+/++	?	+	–	+	+/–	–	–?

*Elevated urinary hesitancy, dry mouth, constipation in CATIE study, probably not mediated via muscarinic acetylcholine receptors.
†Possibly dose related.(Henderson DC, Copeland PM, Borba CP, et al. Glucose metabolism in patients with schizophrenia treated with olanzapine or quetiapine: a frequently sampled intravenous glucose tolerance test and minimal model analysis. J Clin Psychiatry 67(5):789–797, 2006.)

experiences within the delusional framework. Other patients continue to hear voices, but muted, or less frequently, or with greater insight. Some patients are surprisingly stable and functional despite chronic, attenuated psychotic symptoms. A major benefit from antipsychotics is prevention of relapse by maintenance treatment.[21]

Negative symptoms have been found to respond to both conventional and atypical antipsychotics, although a full resolution of negative symptoms is rare.[18] It remains controversial whether "primary" negative symptoms improve with pharmacotherapy. Examples of "secondary" negative symptoms include social withdrawal resulting from paranoia, and apathy resulting from depression. The most common etiology of secondary negative symptoms is neuroleptic-induced parkinsonism; the improvement of negative symptoms following a switch to an atypical agent sometimes represents resolution of iatrogenic parkinsonian side effects caused by the previous conventional neuroleptic.

DRUG SELECTION

Selection of an antipsychotic agent usually is guided by the side-effect profile and by available formulations (e.g., tablet, rapidly-dissolving or sublingual preparation, liquid, IM immediate-release, or long-acting injectable preparations). The "atypical" antipsychotics have largely supplanted conventional agents because of their reduced burden of neurological side effects, although the good efficacy and tolerability of perphenazine in CATIE has led to a reappraisal of the use of low-dose mid-potency first-generation antipsychotics. TD remains a concern for first-generation antipsychotics (but not limited to them), even if used at low doses. Increasingly, a drug's metabolic side-effect profile is taken into account when selecting an agent. Because of the considerable heterogeneity in response and susceptibility to side effects, it is not possible to predict the optimal agent for an individual patient; sequential trials may be needed. As listed in Table 7-4, side effects likely to influence tolerability and compliance include sedation or activation, weight gain, neurological side effects, and sexual dysfunction. With an increased emphasis on reducing iatrogenic cardiovascular risk factors (i.e., metabolic syndrome), it is becoming more common to switch patients from a high-risk to a low-risk antipsychotic.[22] A switch strategy is often more effective than behavioral interventions.

BOX 7-1 Side Effects Associated with Low-Potency First-Generation Antipsychotics

- Sedation
- Hypotension
- Weight gain
- Anticholinergic symptoms (dry mouth, urinary retention, constipation, blurred vision)
- Impaired heat regulation (hyperthermia or hypothermia)
- Pigmentary retinopathy (thioridazine > 800 mg/day)
- Cardiac conduction effects (chlorpromazine, thioridazine)

The potential therapeutic benefits of clozapine (including greater efficacy for psychosis, negative symptoms, agitation or tension, suicidal ideation, and relapse) are quite broad.[11,23,24] Because of the risk of agranulocytosis, clozapine is reserved for patients who fail to respond to other antipsychotics.

Based on epidemiological studies, all antipsychotics carry a black box warning with regard to an increased risk of death when used for behavioral problems in elderly patients with dementia.[25,26]

FIRST-GENERATION ("TYPICAL") ANTIPSYCHOTICS

Examining representative first-generation antipsychotics, it has been shown that roughly a 65% occupancy of striatal D_2 receptors is necessary for antipsychotic efficacy, whereas neurological side effects emerge when D_2 occupancy levels exceed approximately 80%.[27] Among the conventional antipsychotics, low-potency agents (such as chlorpromazine) have relatively low affinity for the D_2 receptor and hence require higher doses (roughly 50-fold greater than haloperidol). In addition, they are less selective for D_2 receptors and so are associated with a wider range of side effects, including orthostatic hypotension, anticholinergic side effects, sedation, and weight gain (Box 7-1). Perphenazine, which was the conventional antipsychotic selected to represent this class in the CATIE study, is a mid-potency agent that requires doses roughly three-fold greater than are necessary with haloperidol. High-potency conventional agents (such as haloperidol and fluphenazine) are more selective for D_2 receptors and more likely to produce

EPS, such as acute dystonias, parkinsonism, and akathisia. Because affinity for the D_2 receptor is readily measured and is inversely correlated with the typical therapeutic dose for each compound, conversion ratios to calculate equivalent dosing between conventional agents, typically expressed in "chlorpromazine equivalents," can be calculated (see Table 7-3).

Haloperidol is available for parenteral (including intravenous [IV]) administration, and both haloperidol and fluphenazine are available in long-acting injectable depot preparations. Although considerable inter-individual variability exists, daily oral doses of haloperidol between 5 and 15 mg are adequate for the large majority of chronic patients; increasing the dose further may only aggravate side effects without improving antipsychotic efficacy. IM and IV administration require roughly half the dose of oral doses. Great care should be taken with the elderly, in whom 0.5 to 2 mg of haloperidol at bedtime may often be sufficient. If a patient has not previously received antipsychotic medication, it is best to start at a low dose before arriving at a standard therapeutic dose which is between 1 and 4 mg orally. A large number of studies have indicated that an optimal response with haloperidol generally corresponds with trough serum concentrations between 5 and 15 ng/ml,[28] although clinical titration remains the most reliable approach in most situations. In the setting of serious medical illness and delirium, particularly if other medications with anticholinergic or hypotensive side effects are administered, haloperidol is often used. Patients need to be monitored for torsades de pointes if haloperidol is given IV.[29]

The mid-potency antipsychotic loxapine is available as a rapidly-acting aerosolized preparation for inhalation to manage agitation in the setting of psychosis or mania.[30] It shows efficacy within 10 minutes after inhalation and might obviate the need for IM administration of an antipsychotic to patients who need rapid tranquilization.

In the US, fluphenazine and haloperidol are available as long-acting depot preparations (decanoates) that are administered IM. Since 2011, shortages of depot haloperidol and fluphenazine supplies have created disruptions in treatment for some patients and led to uncertainty about the future availability of these medications.

EXTRAPYRAMIDAL SYMPTOMS AND TARDIVE DYSKINESIA

Akathisia is an extremely unpleasant sensation of motor restlessness that is primarily experienced in the lower extremities in patients receiving antipsychotics.[31] Akathisia usually manifests as pacing, although some patients experience akathisia as leg discomfort rather than restlessness, and it can develop after a single dose. Akathisia increases non-adherence and has been associated with self-injurious behaviors, as well as a worsening of psychosis. Untrained staff can mistake akathisia for psychotic agitation, resulting in an unfortunate escalation of the antipsychotic dose. A switch to a different antipsychotic with a low liability for akathisia usually resolves the problem. Because akathisia is dose dependent, lowering the dose may provide relief. Alternatively, propranolol 10 to 20 mg two to four times daily is often helpful.[32] The antidepressant mirtazepine which has antagonism at serotonin$_{2A}$ receptors that are implicated in the pathophysiology of akathisia has been shown in double-blind trials to reduce akathisia.[33]

Dystonias are sustained spasms that can affect any muscle group. Neuroleptic-induced dystonias usually occur within the first 4 days of initiating neuroleptic treatment, or after a dose increase, and often affect the neck, tongue, or back. Dystonia may also manifest as lateral deviation of the eyes (opisthotonus) or stridor (laryngeal spasm). Younger patients started on high-potency first-generation antipsychotic

medication are at high risk for developing acute dystonic reactions during the first week of exposure to antipsychotic medication.[34] The incidence of dystonia decreases by about 4% per year of age until it is almost negligible after age 40. Dystonia is a frightening and uncomfortable experience. The occurrence of dystonia early in treatment seriously jeopardizes future compliance with antipsychotic medication, so it is important to anticipate and treat this side effect aggressively. The best method of prevention comes from use of a second-generation atypical antipsychotic. When high-potency neuroleptics are started, prophylaxis with anticholinergic agents (such as benztropine 1 to 2 mg twice daily) substantially reduces the likelihood of dystonic reactions in high-risk patients.[35] Prophylaxis with anticholinergics is risky in the elderly because of their sensitivity to adverse effects, but is usually unnecessary since the elderly are at very low risk for dystonia. Dystonia is uncommon with atypical agents and occurs very rarely with quetiapine and clozapine.

Antipsychotic-induced parkinsonism mimics the tremor, stiffness, gait disturbance, and diminished facial expression characteristic of idiopathic Parkinson's disease. It easily can be mistaken for depression or for negative symptoms of schizophrenia,[36] although the presence of tremor and rigidity usually distinguishes this side effect. Parkinsonian side effects are most common with high-potency first-generation antipsychotics and occur in a bi-modal age distribution with maximal risk in the young and in the elderly. Symptoms frequently improve with a reduction in the dose of the antipsychotic or with addition of an antiparkinsonian agent (such as benztropine 1 to 2 mg twice daily or amantadine 100 mg twice or three times daily).[37] Because anticholinergic agents can produce an array of troublesome side effects (including constipation, dry mouth, dental caries, blurred vision, urinary retention, and memory impairment), particularly in the elderly, long-term use of these agents should be avoided. In addition, anticholinergics might impede cognitive gains hoped for when using cognitive-behavioral therapy or cognitive remediation.[38,39] The atypical agents as a class produce substantially fewer parkinsonian side effects, and both clozapine and quetiapine are essentially free of EPS, making them the drugs of choice for patients with idiopathic Parkinson's disease complicated by psychosis.[40] Box 7-2 describes EPS.

TD rarely appears after less than 6 months of treatment with an antipsychotic agent, but once present it may be

---

BOX 7-2 Extrapyramidal Symptoms

AKATHISIA

Restlessness in lower extremities; often results in pacing
Can occur after the first dose
Risk factors: use of high-potency first-generation agents in high doses

DYSTONIA

Acute muscle spasm: can be very distressing
Usually occurs within the first 4 days after starting the drug
Risk factors: youth and use of high-potency first-generation antipsychotics

PARKINSONISM

Tremor, bradykinesia, rigidity—often confused with negative symptoms
Usually does not become evident until after several weeks of treatment
Risk factors: use of high-potency first-generation antipsychotics, high doses, youth, and old age

irreversible.[39] TD usually takes the form of involuntary, choreiform (quick, non-rhythmic) movements of the mouth, tongue, or upper extremities, although a dystonic form has also been described.[41] The risk for developing TD with first-generation agents is about 5% per year of exposure, with a life-time risk possibly as high as 50% to 60%.[42] The incidence of TD is much higher in the elderly, although a substantial proportion of these cases may represent spontaneously occurring dyskinesias.[43] Patients who develop parkinsonian side effects early in the course of treatment also appear to be at heightened risk for TD. The best treatment of TD is prevention since options are limited once TD is established. Clozapine has not been linked to TD, and switching a patient who develops TD to clozapine increases the likelihood of spontaneous improvement of TD.[44] Lowering the dose of a first-generation antipsychotic or switching to a second-generation agent can occasionally produce "withdrawal dyskinesias," which typically resolve within 6 weeks, or may unmask an underlying dyskinesia that was previously suppressed by the antipsychotic medication.[45] In severe cases, tetrabenazine or deep brain stimulation can been tried.[46,47] Box 7-3 describes TD.

NEUROLEPTIC MALIGNANT SYNDROME

Neuroleptic malignant syndrome (NMS) is a rare, potentially lethal complication of neuroleptic treatment characterized by hyperthermia, rigidity, confusion, diaphoresis, autonomic instability, elevated creatine phosphokinase (CPK), and leukocytosis (Box 7-4).[48] The symptoms of NMS may evolve gradually over time, usually starting with mental status changes and culminating in fever and elevated CPK. NMS probably occurs in fewer than 1% of patients receiving conventional

antipsychotic agents, although subsyndromal cases may be much more common.[49,50] Parallels have been drawn between NMS and malignant hyperthermia (resulting from general anesthesia), largely on the basis of common clinical characteristics. Patients with a history of either NMS or malignant hyperthermia, however, appear to be at no increased risk for developing the other syndrome, and analysis of muscle biopsy specimens has not consistently demonstrated a physiological link between the two conditions.[49] Lethal catatonia is a spontaneously occurring syndrome that may be indistinguishable from NMS and has been described in the absence of neuroleptic treatment.[51] In addition, antipsychotic agents may impair temperature regulation and so may produce low-grade fever in the absence of other symptoms of NMS.[52] The clinician's immediate response to NMS should be to discontinue medication and hospitalize the patient to provide IV fluids and cooling. Whether bromocriptine or dantrolene facilitates recovery remains the subject of debate.[53] It is important that re-institution of antipsychotic medication be delayed at least 2 weeks until after the episode of NMS has resolved.[54] NMS has been described with all antipsychotics including clozapine.[55] It has been suggested that a variant of NMS without rigidity may result from use of second-generation antipsychotics, although if such a syndrome occurs, it is probably quite rare: perhaps with the exception of clozapine where NMS can display few EPS, second-generation antipsychotics produce the typical clinical picture of NMS with rigidity.[56]

SECOND-GENERATION ("ATYPICAL") ANTIPSYCHOTICS

The second-generation agents (Table 7-5) are generally better tolerated with regards to EPS, producing fewer neurological side effects (dystonia, akathisia, and parkinsonism) than the first-generation agents and possibly less TD (see Table 7-4). While relatively free of EPS in most patients at doses of less than 6 mg daily, risperidone (and its metabolite paliperidone) requires careful titration to avoid EPS at higher doses and is unique among the atypical agents in producing sustained hyperprolactinemia.[57] However, attention over the past decade has focused on effects of second-generation antipsychotics on glucose metabolism and lipids[58] and the associated metabolic syndrome (Table 7-6). A large number of cases of treatment-emergent DM have been reported, which in some cases resolved after discontinuation of the antipsychotic.[59,60] In the CATIE study, olanzapine produced significantly greater weight gain, impairment of glucose metabolism, and dyslipidemia than the other agents[16]; this has since been confirmed in a meta-analysis that found clozapine and olanzapine to be the drugs with the highest metabolic liability.[61] Nonetheless, intermediate risk drugs, such as quetiapine, may carry similar risks when used in doses necessary to treat psychotic symptoms.[62] Possible differences between second-generation antipsychotics in risk for causing DM may be obscured in part by the considerable variability between individual patients for weight gain, the potential delay between initiation of treatment and elevation of glucose levels, and a possible propensity for abnormal glucose metabolism associated with schizophrenia independent of drug treatment.[63] All patients treated with an antipsychotic should therefore be monitored regularly for weight gain, DM, and hyperlipidemia, with particular attention paid to more frequent monitoring for patients who receive high-risk drugs (i.e., olanzapine and clozapine) (Table 7-7). Olanzapine and aripiprazole have few or no cardiac effects and can be initiated at a full therapeutic dose. Clozapine, risperidone, quetiapine, ziprasidone, and iloperidone have α-adrenergic effects that necessitate dose titration to avoid orthostatic hypotension. Clozapine produces more

---

BOX 7-3 Tardive Dyskinesia

Late-developing, chronic choreiform (non-rhythmic, quick) movements, most commonly oral-buccal muscles and tongue

RISK FACTORS

Old age
More than 6 months of first-generation neuroleptic exposure
History of parkinsonian side effects
Diabetes
Risk is reduced with second-generation agents

BOX 7-4 Neuroleptic Malignant Syndrome

TRIAD

1. Rigidity
2. Fever
3. Altered mental status

PRESENTATION (MAY GRADUALLY EVOLVE, USUALLY IN THE FOLLOWING ORDER):

- Confusion and fluctuating levels of consciousness
- Rigidity (can be less pronounced with clozapine)
- Diaphoresis
- Mutism
- Autonomic instability
- Hyperthermia
- Elevated creatine phosphokinase

(Based on Gurrera RJ, Caroff SN, Cohen A, et al. An international consensus study of neuroleptic malignant syndrome diagnostic criteria using the Delphi method. J Clin Psychiatry 72(9):1222–1228, 2011.)

TABLE 7-5 Second-Generation Antipsychotic Doses

	Typical Dose (mg/day)	High Dose* (mg/day)	Potential Dose-Limiting Side Effects
Risperidone	3–6	6–12	EPS
Olanzapine	10–20	30–40	Sedation
Quetiapine	300–600	600–1,200**	Sedation
Ziprasidone	80–160	160–320***	Akathisia
Aripiprazole	10–20	20–40	
Clozapine	100–400	400–900****	Sedation, orthostatic hypotension, seizures
Iloperidone	12–24	24	Orthostatic hypotension
Asenapine	10–20	20	Sedation; EPS
Lurasidone	40–80	160	EPS

*Evidence for benefit of higher dose available for olanzapine only.
**Two controlled trials have <u>not</u> found benefit from high-dose quetiapine.[111,112]
***One controlled trial has not found benefit from high-dose ziprasidone.[114]
****Dose should be guided by clozapine serum levels. An optimal highest dose has not been established. (Remmington G, Agid O, Foussias G, et al. Clozapine and therapeutic drug monitoring: is there sufficient evidence for an upper threshold? *Psychopharmacology* 225(3):505–518, 2013.)
EPS, Extrapyramidal symptom.

TABLE 7-6 Identification of the Metabolic Syndrome

Risk Factor (three or more required for diagnosis)	Defining Level
Abdominal obesity	Waist circumference
Men	>40 in (> 102 cm)
Women	>35 in (> 88 cm)
Triglycerides	≥150 mg/dl
HDL cholesterol	
Men	<40 mg/dl
Women	<50 mg/dl
Blood pressure	≥130/85 mmHg
Fasting blood glucose	≥100 mg/dl

HDL, High-density lipoprotein.
(Adapted from Expert panel on detection, evaluation, and treatment of high blood cholesterol in adults. JAMA 285:2486–2497, 2001.)

BOX 7-5 Clozapine

CLINICAL EFFICACY

Effective in 30% of treatment-resistant patients at 6 weeks
Prevents relapse
Stabilizes mood
Improves polydipsia and hyponatremia
Reduces hostility and aggression
Reduces suicidality
Possibly reduces cigarette smoking and substance abuse

ADVERSE EFFECTS

Common Side Effects

Sedation
Tachycardia
Sialorrhea (impairs esophageal motility)
Dizziness
Constipation (can lead to bowel impaction)
Hypotension
Fever (usually within first 3 weeks, lasting a few days)
Weight gain

Serious Side Effects

Agranulocytosis*
Seizures*
Myocarditis*
Orthostatic hypotension with syncope or cardiorespiratory arrest*
Pulmonary embolus
Diabetes mellitus

*Clozapine-specific black box warnings

hypotension and tachycardia than other atypical agents; both are generally easily managed. Ziprasidone's approval was delayed when it became clear that it prolongs the QT interval more than other second-generation antipsychotics (but less than thioridazine).[64]

Clozapine

Clozapine (Box 7-5) is a tricyclic dibenzodiazepine derivative approved for the treatment of treatment-resistant schizophrenia and for the reduction of suicidal behavior in patients with schizophrenia or schizoaffective disorder. Clozapine binds to a wide array of central nervous system (CNS) receptors (including dopaminergic [all five subtypes], muscarinic cholinergic receptors, histaminergic, noradrenergic, and serotonergic). In addition, it appears to modulate glutamatergic NMDA-receptor sensitivity and the release of brain-derived neurotropic factor (BDNF). The absence of neurological side effects has been attributed to serotonin 5-HT$_{2A}$ antagonism, a high D$_2$ dissociation constant (loose binding) that results in relatively low levels of D$_2$ receptor occupancy at therapeutic doses, strong anticholinergic activity, and preferential binding to limbic over striatal dopamine receptors. However, the exact mechanism by which clozapine achieves greater efficacy than other agents remains a mystery, despite almost 20 years of research.

Peak plasma levels of clozapine are attained approximately 2 hours after oral administration. It is metabolized primarily by hepatic microsomal enzymes CYP 1A2 and, to a lesser extent, 3A4 and 2D6, with a mean half-life of 8 hours following a single dose and 12 hours after repeated dosing. Only the desmethyl metabolite is active. Clozapine blood levels are significantly lowered by cigarette smoking and by other hepatic enzyme-inducers (including phenytoin and rifampin) and elevated by CYP 1A2 and 3A4 inhibitors (such as fluvoxamine and erythromycin). Fluvoxamine has been shown to increase clozapine plasma concentrations by as much as four-fold.[65] Some patients may experience a doubling of clozapine blood levels after smoking cessation, with attendant sedation and worsening of other side effects. Several studies have indicated that clozapine is most likely to be effective at trough serum concentrations of 350 ng/ml or greater.[66] In a prospective, double-blind trial, patients randomly assigned to treatment with a clozapine dose adjusted to produce a serum concentration between 200 and 300 ng/ml responded more fully than

TABLE 7-7 Recommendations for Monitoring Patients Starting Antipsychotics*

	Baseline	4 Weeks	8 Weeks	12 Weeks	Quarterly	Annually
Personal/family history	X					X
Weight (body mass index [BMI])	X	X	X	X	X	
Waist circumference	X			X	X	
Blood pressure	X			X	X	
Fasting plasma glucose†	X			X		X**
Fasting lipid profile	X			X		X**

Consider an intervention (weight reduction program or switch antipsychotic) if:
- 5% or greater increase in weight
- 1 point increase in BMI
- 1 inch or greater increase in waist circumference
- Criteria met for metabolic syndrome

*The monitoring recommendations are derived from the literature about second-generation antipsychotics. However, first-generation antipsychotics (particularly low-potency antipsychotics) are not devoid of metabolic problems.
**More frequent monitoring (e.g., every 3 months until stable, then every 6 months) is indicated for patients on high-risk drugs (clozapine, olanzapine)
†Hemoglobin A1c can be used insteadHemoglobin A1c can be used instead.
(Adapted in part from American Diabetes Association, American Psychiatric Association, American Association of Clinical Endocrinologists, North American Association for the Study of Obesity. Consensus development conference on antipsychotic drugs and diabetes and obesity. Diabetes Care 27:596–601, 2004 and Goff DC, Cather C, Evins AE, et al. Medical morbidity and mortality in schizophrenia: guidelines for psychiatrists. J Clin Psychiatry 66(2):183–194; quiz 147, 273–184, 2005.)

did patients assigned to lower concentrations; moreover, their response was comparable to patients assigned to higher concentrations.[67]

In the pivotal study comparing clozapine to chlorpromazine in patients prospectively defined as treatment resistant, clozapine produced significantly greater improvement in measures of psychosis, negative symptoms, depression, and anxiety.[11] Thirty percent of the clozapine-treatment group responded compared to 4% treated with chlorpromazine; a subsequent study indicated that the response rate may increase to as high as 60% with trials lasting 6 months or longer.[68] Clozapine has also been found to improve aggression and hostility,[69] reduce relapse,[70] and decrease suicidality.[24,70] Open-label studies have found impressive mood-stabilizing effects of clozapine in patients with refractory bipolar or schizoaffective disorder.[71] Clozapine may also improve polydipsia with hyponatremia,[72] reduce arrest rates,[73] and facilitate a decrease in cigarette smoking.[74]

Potentially serious side effects (such as agranulocytosis, seizures, DM, and myocarditis) have limited clozapine treatment to the most refractory patients; the more common side effects of weight gain, sialorrhea, orthostatic hypotension, constipation, and sedation further complicate its use (see Box 7-5).[75] Because of the risk of agranulocytosis, patients must meet a minimum threshold for their neutrophil count before starting the drug and must continue to meet safety criteria with weekly blood tests during the first 6 months of treatment, biweekly tests for the second 6 months, and then monthly bloods tests for as long as the patient takes the drug (Box 7-6 and Box 7-7). Results of all white blood cell (WBC) counts are monitored and stored in national databases; an analysis of these records from the period 1990 to 1991 indicated that 0.8% of patients who were started on clozapine developed agranulocytosis, and 0.01% of patients died of agranulocytosis.[76] The risk of developing agranulocytosis peaked in the 3rd month. While most cases of agranulocytosis occur during the first 6 to 12 months of treatment, 10% of patients developed agranulocytosis after 2 years of treatment, even after a decade.[77] Patients usually recover from clozapine-induced agranulocytosis within 14 to 24 days of stopping the drug, but re-challenge with clozapine is not allowed because of the very high rate of recurrence.[78,79]

Some patients with habitually low WBC counts due to ethnicity (benign ethnic neutropenia [BEN]) can safely be treated with clozapine if they are pre-treated with lithium,

BOX 7-6 Clozapine-Induced Agranulocytosis

- Granulocytes < 500/mm^3
- Risk factors: Ashkenazi Jews (HLA-B38, DR4, DQw3) and Finns
- Preservation of other cell lines (platelets and RBCs)
- Maximum risk: 4–18 weeks (77% of cases)
- Recovery usually within 14 days if drug stopped
- No cross-reactivity with other drugs, but avoid carbamazepine, captopril, sulfonamides, propylthiouracil, and other drugs that might affect bone marrow or WBCs
- Because of sensitization: Do not rechallenge!

RBCs, Red blood cells; WBCs, white blood cells.

BOX 7-7 Monitoring for Agranulocytosis

WBC count must be ≥ 3,500 and ANC ≥ 2,000 to initiate clozapine
Weekly CBC for 6 months, if all WBC counts ≥ 3,500 and ANCs ≥ 2,000; then biweekly for 6 months, then monthly
Repeat CBC if:
- ANC = 1,500–2,000 or WBC count = 3,000–3,500, or
- WBC count drops by 3,000 or ANC drops by 1,500 from previous test, or
- Three consecutive weekly drops

If ANC = 1,500–2,000 or WBC count = 3,000–3,500, proceed with twice-weekly CBCs
Hold drug if ANC < 1,500 or WBC count < 3,000
Discontinue if ANC < 1,000 or WBC count < 2,000: do not re-challenge

ANC, Absolute neutrophil count; CBC, complete blood count; WBC, white blood cell.

which stimulates the bone marrow to boost WBC counts to levels acceptable for prescribing clozapine.[80]

Of additional concern are the recent findings of myocarditis and cardiomyopathy occurring in 0.01% to 0.2% of patients treated with clozapine, of which approximately 20% were fatal.[81] These cases commonly manifested within the first month of treatment with fever, dyspnea, a "flu-like illness," and chest pain; abnormal laboratory findings included a reduced ventricular ejection fraction on echocardiogram, T-wave changes on the electrocardiogram (ECG), eosinophilia, and an elevated CPK.[82,83]

Seizures have been reported in 5% to 10% of patients treated with clozapine.[84] Seizure risk appears to be related to both rapid dose escalation and to high plasma concentrations. High rates of obesity, DM, and dyslipidemia have also been associated with clozapine. In one 5-year naturalistic study, weight gain with clozapine reached a mean plateau of 31 lb after approximately 4 years and almost 37% of patients developed DM.[58] Whereas the striking abdominal adiposity associated with clozapine treatment might explain the elevated rate of DM, markedly decreased insulin sensitivity has been documented in non-obese patients treated with clozapine compared to risperidone-treated patients matched for age and weight.[85]

Given the rare but serious risks of agranulocytosis and myocarditis and the more common risks of seizures and metabolic complications, clozapine should be reserved for patients who fail at least two other trials of antipsychotics. However, the potential therapeutic benefits of clozapine often outweigh the risks of medical morbidity. One study using the Clozapine National Registry found a higher mortality rate in patients after they stopped clozapine than while they were taking it, due to an almost 90% reduction in suicide associated with clozapine treatment.[86] A second epidemiological study (FIN11 study) found a lower all-cause mortality rate and no increased deaths from cardiovascular causes over an 11-year period for clozapine-treated patients compared to other antipsychotics.[87]

Risperidone and Paliperidone

Risperidone is a benzisoxazole derivative that received FDA approval for the treatment of schizophrenia in 1994 and later for bipolar mania. It is characterized by a very high affinity for the 5-HT$_{2A}$ receptor and by moderate affinity for D$_2$, H$_1$, and α_1- and α_2-adrenergic receptors. Risperidone has essentially no activity at muscarinic acetylcholine receptors. Risperidone has a high affinity and low dissociation constant for the D$_2$ receptor, making it "tightly bound" and thereby more likely to produce EPS at high doses than some more "loosely bound" agents. At typical clinical doses, risperidone was found to occupy 65% to 69% of D$_2$ receptors 12 to 14 hours after the last dose; a mean occupancy of 79% was found in patients treated with a risperidone dose of 6 mg/day.[88]

Risperidone is rapidly absorbed after oral administration with peak plasma levels achieved within 1 hour. It is metabolized by hepatic microsomal enzyme CYP 2D6 to form the active metabolite 9-hydroxyrisperidone, which exhibits a pattern of receptor binding similar to that of the parent compound. 9-Hydroxyrisperidone is in turn metabolized by N-dealkylation. The half-life of the "active moiety" (risperidone plus 9-hydroxyrisperidone) is approximately 20 hours. CYP 2D6 activity, which varies dramatically between "rapid" and "poor" metabolizers, determines the ratio of risperidone to 9-hydroxyrisperidone serum concentrations and influences the half-life of the active moiety. Drugs that inhibit CYP 2D6, such as paroxetine and fluoxetine, may increase risperidone levels with the risk of neurological side effects.[89]

In the North American registration trials, risperidone doses of 6, 10, and 16 mg/day (but not 2 mg/day) produced significantly greater reductions compared to high-dose haloperidol (20 mg/day) in all five domains of the Positive and Negative Syndromes Scale (PANSS),[90] whereas risperidone was similar in efficacy to the first-generation antipsychotic perphenazine in the CATIE trial and in an earlier study.[16] In a flexibly-dosed, double-blind, randomized study, Csernansky and colleagues[91]

found almost twice the relapse rate with haloperidol compared to risperidone. Increasing the risperidone dose above 8 mg/day has not improved response in patients who did not fully respond to a treatment with a typical dose.[92]

Risperidone is well tolerated at doses low enough to avoid EPS (generally below 6 mg/day). In the CATIE trial, risperidone at a mean dose of 3.9 mg/day was the best-tolerated agent, although differences between agents were not statistically significant. Weight gain with risperidone is intermediate compared to other atypical agents and is quite variable. Woerner and colleagues[93] found a cumulative TD rate of 7.2% over 2 years of treatment in elderly, antipsychotic-naive patients who were prospectively followed. Risperidone causes a small increase in the QTc interval (a mean prolongation of 10 ms at a dose of 16 mg/day).[94]

Risperidone differs from other second-generation antipsychotics in causing persistent hyperprolactinemia. In one large study, galactorrhea or amenorrhea occurred in 8% to 12% of women treated with risperidone (4 to 6 mg/day), and sexual dysfunction or gynecomastia was reported in 15% of men.[95] Side effects tend not to correlate with serum prolactin concentrations. Hyperprolactinemia in patients with pituitary tumors has been shown to lower estrogen and testosterone levels, which may secondarily result in osteopenia. Similarly, risperidone-induced hyperprolactinemia might increase the risk for osteoporosis.[96]

The active metabolite of risperidone, 9-hydroxyrisperidone, was re-named paliperidone and approved for the treatment of schizophrenia in 2006. It is equipotent to risperidone with which it shares its receptor and side-effect profile including significant prolactin elevation. Its typical dose range is 3 to 6 mg/day but doses up to 12 mg/day can be given. As the end-product of oxidative metabolism, paliperidone is primarily renally excreted and does not rely on P450 metabolism (59% excreted unchanged in urine).

Both risperidone and paliperidone are available as long-acting injectable formulations. The long-acting risperidone formulation (Consta) consists of polymer microspheres containing risperidone, which, immediately before injection, are suspended in a water-based diluent. Following injection, the microspheres begin to release risperidone after a delay of 3 to 4 weeks, after which levels persist for about 4 weeks. Microspheres are administered by gluteal injection every 2 weeks (dose range 12.5 and 50 mg); oral dosing of risperidone should continue until the third injection (4 weeks after the first). If an increase in the dose is necessary, oral supplementation should be provided for 3 to 4 weeks after increasing the dose of risperidone microspheres. Paliperidone is also available as a long-acting injectable formulation (paliperidone palmitate) for monthly IM injections at a dose between 39 and 234 mg. A loading strategy (i.e., 234 mg once, followed by 117 mg 1 week later) produces therapeutic steady-state drug levels rapidly and can be started in inpatient settings. After treatment initiation it is given as a monthly IM injection at a dose between 39 mg and 234 mg. Before administering a long-acting injectable antipsychotic, tolerability of the oral preparation should first be established.

Olanzapine

Olanzapine, a thienobenzodiazepine derivative chemically related to clozapine, was approved by the FDA in 1997 for the treatment of schizophrenia and subsequently approved for bipolar mania. Olanzapine binds to dopamine D$_1$, D$_2$, D$_4$, and D$_5$; serotonin 5-HT$_{2A}$ and 5-HT$_{2C}$; muscarinic M$_{1-5}$; histaminergic H$_1$; and α_1-adrenergic receptors.

Following oral administration, olanzapine is well absorbed, producing peak concentrations in 4 to 6 hours. Olanzapine is metabolized via glucuronidation and oxidation by CYP 450 1A2 with a mean half-life of 24 to 36 hours. Like clozapine, olanzapine's metabolism is induced by cigarette smoking and slowed by CYP 1A2 inhibitors, although to a lesser degree because of alternative metabolic pathways.

In an early fixed-dose registration trial, olanzapine (at doses ranging from 5 to 15 mg/day) displayed a near-linear dose–response relationship; antipsychotic effects were comparable to haloperidol at 15 mg/day, but olanzapine (15 mg/day) demonstrated significantly greater improvement of negative symptoms, fewer EPS, and less prolactin elevation compared to haloperidol at 15 mg/day.[97] A larger flexible-dose trial found higher completion rates, response rates, and greater improvement over a broad range of symptom domains with a mean olanzapine dose of 13 mg/day compared to a mean haloperidol dose of 12 mg/day.[98] Additional analyses of data from these studies found a significant reduction in rates of TD with olanzapine,[99] and a path analysis suggested that olanzapine's superior efficacy for negative symptoms was a primary effect and not due to effects on EPS or depression.[100] In contrast, Rosenheck and colleagues[101] found in a study conducted at Veterans Affairs Medical Centers that outcomes were quite similar between patients randomized to olanzapine and to haloperidol plus prophylactic benztropine except for reduced rates of akathisia and TD. In the CATIE study, olanzapine at a mean dose of 20 mg/day was the antipsychotic with the best efficacy.[16] Since the original designation of 10 mg/day as the recommended dose at the time of olanzapine's introduction, typical clinical doses have steadily climbed to the 15 to 20 mg/day range. One study indicated that escalation of the mean dose to 30 mg/day may improve efficacy in some treatment-resistant patients.[92]

Olanzapine may cause sedation, which some patients experience as a welcome treatment for insomnia whereas others are distressed by difficulty awakening in the morning. Even at high doses, olanzapine is relatively free of EPS[92] and prolactin elevation. However, weight gain and dyslipidemia and metabolic dysregulation are common and a major long-term concern. In the CATIE study, patients randomized to olanzapine gained an average of 2 lb per month and 30% gained more than 7% of their body weight.[16] Olanzapine was also associated with significant elevation of glycosylated hemoglobin, triglycerides, and total cholesterol. Weight gain or metabolic side effects caused 9% of olanzapine-treated patients to discontinue their medication. Both olanzapine and clozapine have been linked to insulin resistance and to DM—an effect that may occur in the absence of obesity.[85] Patients should be carefully screened for metabolic risk factors before initiating olanzapine and should be monitored according to established guidelines (see Table 7-7).[102,103]

A long-acting injectable olanzapine formulation (olanzapine pamoate) can be given every 2 to 4 weeks. Very rarely (approximately 1 event per 1,700 injections), the injection can cause confusion, severe drowsiness or coma due to excessive olanzapine plasma concentrations, resembling alcohol intoxication.[104,105] Termed post-injection delirium/sedation syndrome (PDSS), it requires patients to be observed for 3 hours after receiving the injection which can only be given by certified prescribers and facilities who are able to manage PDSS.

Quetiapine

Quetiapine was approved in 1997 for the treatment of schizophrenia and later for the treatment of acute bipolar mania. Quetiapine has a high affinity for serotonin 5-HT_{2A}, α_1- and α_2-adrenergic, and histaminergic H_1 receptors and a relatively low affinity for D_2 receptors. Whereas maximal D_2 occupancy levels of approximately 60% are achieved 2 to 3 hours after a single dose, because of quetiapine's high dissociation constant and short half-life, D_2 occupancy drops to less than 30% after 12 hours.[106]

Quetiapine is rapidly absorbed following oral administration, with peak plasma concentrations achieved in 1 to 2 hours. It is primarily metabolized via CYP P450 3A4, producing two active metabolites. Quetiapine metabolism is significantly influenced by drugs that inhibit 3A4 (such as ketoconazole) or induce 3A4 (such as carbamazepine). The half-life of quetiapine is approximately 6 hours; despite this short half-life, quetiapine is frequently prescribed as a once-daily dose, at bedtime, with good results.[107] No significant association has been identified between quetiapine blood levels and clinical response.[108]

In controlled clinical trials, quetiapine demonstrated efficacy for global psychopathology, psychotic symptoms, and negative symptoms greater than placebo and it was comparable to haloperidol or chlorpromazine. Whereas one large multiple fixed-dose trial found no dose–response relationship within a range of doses from 150 to 750 mg/day,[109] another study found superior efficacy when patients were randomly assigned to a higher range of doses (approximately 750 mg/day) compared to low (approximately 250 mg/day).[110] In the CATIE study, quetiapine at a mean dose of 543 mg/day was less effective than olanzapine but it did not differ statistically from the other antipsychotics in tolerability or effectiveness.[16] Doses above 800 mg/day have not been found to have added therapeutic benefit.[111,112]

Common side effects reported with quetiapine include somnolence and dizziness. Quetiapine is very sedating; however, because of its short half-life, bedtime dosing may minimize daytime sedation. Mild orthostatic hypotension was observed in trials that followed a conservative schedule of dose titration, starting with quetiapine 25 mg twice daily. Initiation at higher doses may cause significant orthostatic hypotension, particularly in the elderly, due to quetiapine's adrenergic effects. Reports of dry mouth are probably attributable to its adrenergic mechanisms, since quetiapine is essentially free of muscarinic activity. Quetiapine has consistently demonstrated extremely low levels of EPS and prolactin elevation, comparable to placebo. Quetiapine is intermediate among the second-generation antipsychotics in producing weight gain and in estimates for risk for producing dyslipidemia and DM. In the CATIE study, quetiapine was similar to risperidone in producing a mean 0.5 lb weight gain per month, compared to a 2 lb per month weight gain with olanzapine and weight loss with perphenazine and ziprasidone.[18] Early concerns about a possible link with cataracts have not been supported in post-marketing surveillance, nor was a link detected in the CATIE study. While QTc prolongation is not clinically significant at typical doses, quetiapine overdoses have been associated with cardiac arrhythmias.[113]

Ziprasidone

Ziprasidone was approved in 2001 for the treatment of schizophrenia. Like other second-generation agents, it has a favorable ratio of serotonin 5-HT_2 to dopamine D_2 affinities. In addition, it is an antagonist with high affinity for serotonin 5-HT_{1D} and 5-HT_{2C} receptors and an agonist at the 5-HT_{1A} receptor. Ziprasidone differs from other agents in its moderate reuptake blockade of serotonin and norepinephrine (noradrenaline).

After oral administration, absorption of ziprasidone is significantly more rapid when administered within 1 hour of a meal compared to fasting. In one study, a fatty meal increased total absorption compared to fasting by 68% and decreased the serum half-life from 6.6 hours to 4.7 hours.[104] Ziprasidone is metabolized by several pathways. Approximately two-thirds of ziprasidone's metabolism is via aldehyde oxidase and the remainder is by CYP450 3A4 and 1A2 hepatic microsomal enzymes. Clinically significant drug–drug interactions have not been reported.

In early trials, ziprasidone exhibited efficacy comparable to haloperidol at doses above 120 mg/day,[105] but with fewer EPS and without sustained elevation of prolactin. Ziprasidone did not become available for inclusion in the CATIE trial until after approximately 40% of subjects had entered and been randomized. At a mean dose of 113 mg/day ziprasidone was less effective than olanzapine and did not differ from the other antipsychotics. Notably, ziprasidone was associated with a mean weight loss of 0.3 lb per month, normalization of lipids, and a lowering of prolactin levels. In a recent study of patients with schizophrenia who remained symptomatic after at least 3 weeks of treatment with ziprasidone at a dose of 160 mg/day, increasing the dose to a maximum of 320 mg/day did not improve outcomes.[114]

Side effects commonly associated with ziprasidone include insomnia or somnolence, nausea, anxiety, and headache. The finding of a mean QTc prolongation of 15.9 ms raised concerns about the risk of torsades de pointes, particularly when administered to patients with underlying cardiac conduction defects or other cardiac risk factors. However, QTc intervals greater than 500 ms have been extremely rare, and a large post-marketing surveillance study of over 18,000 patients (Ziprasidone Observational Study of Cardiac Outcomes [ZODIAC]) did not find an increased rate of non-suicide deaths compared to olanzapine-treated patients.[115] Despite the reassuring safety data, cardiac risk factors should be assessed before initiating this agent.

Aripiprazole

Aripiprazole is a dihydroquinolinone, structurally unrelated to the other antipsychotics. It was approved for the treatment of schizophrenia in 2002 and subsequently for bipolar or mixed mania. It exhibits a novel mechanism of action as a partial agonist at the D_2 receptor with approximately 30% activity compared to dopamine. In addition, aripiprazole has high affinity as a partial agonist at serotonin 5-HT$_{1A}$ and as a full antagonist at 5-HT$_{2A}$. Aripiprazole has moderate affinity for α_1-adrenergic and histamine H$_1$ receptors, as well as the serotonin reuptake site. At typical clinical doses of 15 to 30 mg/day, aripiprazole exhibited D_2 receptor occupancy greater than 80%[116] and was not associated with EPS at occupancy levels greater than 90%, presumably the result of partial agonism.

Aripiprazole is well absorbed and reaches peak plasma levels within 3 to 5 hours of an oral dose. It is metabolized primarily by CYP 450 2D6 and 3A4 to dehydroaripiprazole, an active metabolite with a pharmacological profile similar to aripiprazole. The half-lives of aripiprazole and dehydroaripiprazole are 75 and 94 hours, respectively. Because of this unusually long half-life, a period of approximately 2 weeks is required to achieve steady-state drug levels following a change in dosing. Aripiprazole's metabolism may be altered by inhibitors and inducers of CYP 450 3A4 and 2D6.

In registration studies, aripiprazole at doses ranging from 15 to 30 mg/day exhibited efficacy comparable to haloperidol (10 mg/day) and risperidone (6 mg/day). Compared to haloperidol, patients treated with aripiprazole had significantly less prolactin elevation, had less akathisia, and required less anticholinergic treatment for EPS. No differences in efficacy or tolerability were identified between aripiprazole doses of 15, 20, and 30 mg/day. In a 26-week placebo-controlled

trial, aripiprazole was found to prevent relapse.[117] Because aripiprazole was not included in the CATIE trial, its relative effectiveness compared to other agents remains unclear.

Aripiprazole has generally been found to be well tolerated, with side effects largely restricted to insomnia, somnolence, headache, agitation, nausea, and anxiety. It has not differed from placebo in prolactin elevation, EPS, or QTc prolongation. Aripiprazole can lower prolactin (to below the lower normal of prolactin levels in some cases), and it can be used adjunctively to reverse antipsychotic-induced hyperprolactinemia.[118] In a prospective study of first-time users of antipsychotics, aripiprazole caused weight gain, but does not seem to have major effects on glucose or lipid metabolism.[119]

A long-acting injectable aripiprazole formulation (extended-release suspension for monthly IM injections) was approved in 2013 for the maintenance treatment of schizophrenia. This preparation has been shown to reduce relapse rate in a 1-year trial.[120]

Iloperidone

Iloperidone was approved for the treatment of schizophrenia in 2009. Like risperidone, it belongs to the class of benzisoxazole antipsychotics. It has high affinity for D_2/5-HT$_{2A}$ receptors, consistent with other atypicals, and the D_3 and norepinephrine α_1-receptor. In addition, it has moderate affinities for D_4, 5-HT$_6$ and 5-HT$_7$ receptors. It is not anticholinergic.

Iloperidone is well absorbed in 2 to 4 hours. While food slows its absorption, it does not alter overall bioavailability and can be given without regards to meals. It is extensively metabolized by 3A4 and 2D6, leading to two active metabolites, P88 and P95.

The effective dose range for iloperidone is 12 to 24 mg/day, given as twice daily dosing (half-life 18 hours). Iloperidone needs to be titrated slowly over the course of at least 1 week or more (e.g., starting with 1 mg twice daily, and daily increases by a maximum of 2 mg twice daily [4 mg/day]; to 2 mg, 4 mg, 6 mg, 8 mg, 10 mg, and 12 mg twice daily) to minimize orthostatic hypotension.[121] In registration trials, orthostatic hypotension was observed in 5% of patients given 20 to 24 mg/day of drug versus 1% given placebo. Consistent with iloperidone's prominent α-blocking properties, retrograde ejaculation and priapism have been observed. Other side effects reported in clinical trials include tachycardia, dizziness, dry mouth, nasal congestion, somnolence, and dyspepsia. Headache, insomnia, and anxiety were reported as well. Iloperidone can cause modest prolactin elevation but little EPS, which might be a relative advantage. It has been associated with dose-dependent weight gain but its overall propensity for metabolic problems remains to be defined. Iloperidone can increase the QTc interval in a dose-dependent fashion.[122] Its use needs thus to be preceded by an assessment of cardiac safety, including possible drug interactions that could alter iloperidone drug levels. In known poor metabolizers of 2D6, half the dose should be used.

Asenapine

Asenapine was approved in 2009 for the treatment of schizophrenia and the acute treatment of manic or mixed mood episodes of bipolar disorder, either as monotherapy or in conjunction with lithium or valproate. Its chemical structure is unique among antipsychotics (a dibenzo-oxepino pyrrole). It has high affinity for a host of receptors, including dopamine$_{1-4}$, 5-HT$_{1A}$ (partial agonist)/$_B$, 5-HT$_{2A,B,C}$, 5-HT$_{5/6/7}$ and $\alpha_{1/2}$-receptors; it has negligible muscarinic receptor affinity but moderate H$_{1/2}$ receptor affinity.

Due to poor gastrointestinal absorption, asenapine is formulated as a sublingual tablet that gets rapidly absorbed. For 10 minutes after the dose, there should be no eating or drinking; if asenapine is swallowed as an oral tablet, the bioavailability is less than 2%.[123] For schizophrenia and adjunctive treatment of mood episodes, the starting dose is 5 mg twice daily that can be adjusted to 10 mg twice daily; for mania monotherapy, the recommended starting dose is 10 mg twice daily. Asenapine is cleared via glucuronidation by UGT1A4 and oxidative metabolism, mostly via CYP1A2.

The most prominent side effects in asenapine registration trials were somnolence and EPS, dose-related akathisia and oral hypoesthesia as well as dizziness and dysgeusia. Asenapine is not weight-neutral but its propensity for weight gain and metabolic disturbances remains to be elucidated. In a 52-week extension trial, 15% of patients gained 7% of body weight or more.[124] Allergic reactions and syncope have been reported as rare but dangerous side effects. Prolactin levels can be increased with asenapine. The registration trials found modest QTc prolongation ranging from 2 to 5 ms for doses up to 40 mg/day, which should be taken into account before prescribing asenapine.

Lurasidone

In 2010, the benzisothiazole antipsychotic lurasidone was approved by the FDA for schizophrenia. It has high affinity binding for dopamine$_2$ receptors, 5-HT$_{2A}$ receptors, and 5-HT$_7$ receptors.[125] Moderate binding exists for α_{2C}; partial antagonism 5-HT$_{1A}$; antagonism for α_{2A}. It does not appreciably bind histamine$_1$ and muscarinic M$_1$ receptors. Lurasidone has a half-life of 18 hours. Its total absorption is increased by two-fold with food, and it should be taken with a meal of at least 350 calories (no effect of fat composition). It is mostly metabolized via 3A4 and blood levels of lurasidone may be significantly affected by CYP3A4 inducers or inhibitors. The recommended starting dose, which is also an effective dose, is 40 mg/day given once daily but doses up to 160 mg/day have been studied.[126] Lurasidone can increase prolactin levels, and it can cause insomnia and EPS including akathisia, particularly at higher doses.[127] In contrast, its propensity for weight gain and metabolic disturbances seems to be low.[128] It effects on the QTc interval are minimal.

DRUG INTERACTIONS WITH ANTIPSYCHOTIC AGENTS

Antipsychotic drugs are most likely to interact with other medications as a result of alterations of hepatic metabolism or when combined with drugs that produce additive side effects (such as anticholinergic effects) or when combined with drugs that impair cardiac conduction. Most conventional antipsychotic agents are extensively metabolized by the 2D6 isoenzyme of the hepatic P450 enzyme system, whereas atypical agents generally have more variable hepatic metabolism, typically involving isoenzymes 3A4, 1A2, and 2D6.[129] Fortunately, because the therapeutic index (risk ratio) of antipsychotic drugs is quite large, interactions with agents that inhibit hepatic metabolism are unlikely to be life-threatening but may increase side effects. Among the atypical antipsychotics, clozapine can produce the most serious adverse effects when blood levels are dramatically elevated; obtundation and cardiovascular effects have been associated with inhibition of clozapine metabolism by fluvoxamine or erythromycin.[65,130] Addition of 2D6 inhibitors (e.g., some SSRIs) to conventional antipsychotics would be expected to increase EPS, but in one placebo-controlled trial this was not clinically significant despite

substantial increases in blood levels of haloperidol and fluphenazine.[131] Drugs that induce hepatic metabolism (such as certain anticonvulsants [e.g., carbamazepine, phenobarbital, phenytoin]) may lower antipsychotic blood concentrations substantially and cause loss of therapeutic efficacy.[132]

Great care must be taken if low-potency agents (such as chlorpromazine, thioridazine, and clozapine) are combined with other highly anticholinergic drugs because the additive anticholinergic activity may produce confusion, urinary retention, or constipation. In addition, low-potency antipsychotic agents can depress cardiac function and can significantly impair cardiac conduction when added to class I antiarrhythmic agents (such as quinidine or procainamide). Ziprasidone and iloperidone also significantly affect cardiac conduction and should not be combined with low-potency phenothiazines or the antiarrhythmic agents.[64]

ONGOING CHALLENGES

Two major challenges remain: antipsychotics are not effective for all patients with psychosis, and they pose significant long-term medical risks to patients who need maintenance treatment. Very little guidance is available from controlled trials for additional interventions if a schizophrenia patient remains symptomatic despite treatment with an adequate dose of clozapine. Early reports described improvement of positive and negative symptoms with the addition of risperidone to clozapine, consistent with the hypothesis that achieving a higher degree of D$_2$ blockade might enhance clozapine's effectiveness for some patients.[133] Subsequent placebo-controlled trials produced inconsistent results, and therefore the role of clozapine augmentation in refractory cases remains controversial and poorly substantiated.[134] As a result, polypharmacy for refractory disease remains a widely used, expensive practice with little support from clinical trials, particularly for patients with serious mental illness. Some forms of secondary psychosis (e.g., psychosis in setting of dementia) show little if any benefit from a treatment which in addition might increase mortality.

For those patients who benefit sufficiently from treatment, prevention of antipsychotic-induced metabolic problems has become a major clinical focus, and creating integrated treatment settings that allow for appropriate medical management of psychiatric patients who receive antipsychotics is a major health care systems goal. Currently, even simple preventive measures (i.e., guideline-concordant metabolic monitoring) remain a major hurdle in many settings,[135] hindering progress in preventing premature death from iatrogenic contributions.[136] The use of metformin to blunt antipsychotic-induced weight gain and metabolic problems has been shown to be an effective prevention strategy in both early course[137] and chronic schizophrenia patients.[138] Patients can benefit from a switch to antipsychotics with less metabolic liability,[22] and some patients can safely reduce polypharmacy.[139] Such proactive management strategies are necessary to reduce the multimorbidity that characterizes many patients who are treated with antipsychotics.[140] In addition to metabolic problems, there remain concerns about neurotoxicity from antipsychotics over and above disease-related changes as suggested by brain volume loss in treatment studies of patients with schizophrenia.[141,142] Recently, a long-term follow-up of a randomized first episode clinical trial comparing early antipsychotic drug discontinuation with maintenance treatment in symptomatically remitted first-episode patients found that the less aggressive approach with early drug discontinuation led to better long-term functional outcomes compared to those patients assigned to maintenance treatment.[143]

Despite the short-comings of antipsychotics, not treating patients with schizophrenia with an antipsychotic has been shown to have an increased overall mortality rate that needs to be taken into account when considering the risk–benefit equation.[87,144-147]

Access the complete reference list and multiple choice questions (MCQs) online at https://expertconsult.inkling.com

KEY REFERENCES

9. Creese I, Burt DR, Snyder SH. Dopamine receptor binding predicts clinical and pharmacological potencies of antischizophrenic drugs. *Science* 192(4238):481–483, 1976.
11. Kane J, Honigfeld G, Singer J, et al. Clozapine for the treatment-resistant schizophrenic. A double-blind comparison with chlorpromazine. *Arch Gen Psychiatry* 45(9):789–796, 1988.
16. Lieberman JA, Stroup TS, McEvoy JP, et al. Effectiveness of antipsychotic drugs in patients with chronic schizophrenia. *N Engl J Med* 353(12):1209–1223, 2005.
17. Leucht S, Cipriani A, Spinelli L, et al. Comparative efficacy and tolerability of 15 antipsychotic drugs in schizophrenia: a multiple-treatments meta-analysis. *Lancet* 328(9896):951–962, 2013.
20. Kapur S, Arenovich T, Agid O, et al. Evidence for onset of antipsychotic effects within the first 24 hours of treatment. *Am J Psychiatry* 162(5):939–946, 2005.
21. Leucht S, Tardy M, Komossa K, et al. Antipsychotic drugs versus placebo for relapse prevention in schizophrenia: a systematic review and meta-analysis. *Lancet* 379(9831):2063–2071, 2012.
22. Stroup TS, Byerly MJ, Nasrallah HA, et al. Effects of switching from olanzapine, quetiapine, and risperidone to aripiprazole on 10-year coronary heart disease risk and metabolic syndrome status: results from a randomized controlled trial. *Schizophr Research* 146(1–3):190–195, 2013.
24. Meltzer HY, Alphs L, Green AI, et al. Clozapine treatment for suicidality in schizophrenia: International Suicide Prevention Trial (InterSePT). *Arch Gen Psychiatry* 60(1):82–91, 2003.
27. Farde L, Wiesel FA, Halldin C, et al. Central D2-dopamine receptor occupancy in schizophrenic patients treated with antipsychotic drugs. *Arch Gen Psychiatry* 45(1):71–76, 1988.
42. Kane JM, Woerner M, Weinhold P, et al. Incidence of tardive dyskinesia: five-year data from a prospective study. *Psychopharmacol Bull* 20(3):387–389, 1984.
48. Gurrera RJ, Caroff SN, Cohen A, et al. An international consensus study of neuroleptic malignant syndrome diagnostic criteria using the Delphi method. *J Clin Psychiatry* 72(9):1222–1228, 2011.
58. Henderson DC, Cagliero E, Gray C, et al. Clozapine, diabetes mellitus, weight gain, and lipid abnormalities: A five-year naturalistic study. *Am J Psychiatry* 157(6):975–981, 2000.
76. Alvir JM, Lieberman JA, Safferman AZ, et al. Clozapine-induced agranulocytosis. Incidence and risk factors in the United States. *N Engl J Med* 329(3):162–167, 1993.
83. Ronaldson KJ, Fitzgerald PB, Taylor AJ, et al. A new monitoring protocol for clozapine-induced myocarditis based on an analysis of 75 cases and 94 controls. *Aust N Z J Psychiatry* 45(6):458–465, 2011.
85. Henderson DC, Cagliero E, Copeland PM, et al. Glucose metabolism in patients with schizophrenia treated with atypical antipsychotic agents: a frequently sampled intravenous glucose tolerance test and minimal model analysis. *Arch Gen Psychiatry* 62(1):19–28, 2005.
87. Tiihonen J, Lonnqvist J, Wahlbeck K, et al. 11-year follow-up of mortality in patients with schizophrenia: a population-based cohort study (FIN11 study). *Lancet* 374(9690):620–627, 2009.
93. Woerner MG, Correll CU, Alvir JM, et al. Incidence of tardive dyskinesia with risperidone or olanzapine in the elderly: results from a 2-year, prospective study in antipsychotic-naive patients. *Neuropsychopharmacology* 36(8):1738–1746, 2011.
102. Goff DC, Cather C, Evins AE, et al. Medical morbidity and mortality in schizophrenia: guidelines for psychiatrists. *J Clin Psychiatry* 66(2):183–194, 2005.
115. Strom BL, Eng SM, Faich G, et al. Comparative mortality associated with ziprasidone and olanzapine in real-world use among 18,154 patients with schizophrenia: The Ziprasidone Observational Study of Cardiac Outcomes (ZODIAC). *Am J Psychiatry* 168(2):193–201, 2011.
134. Sommer IE, Begemann MJ, Temmerman A, et al. Pharmacological augmentation strategies for schizophrenia patients with insufficient response to clozapine: a quantitative literature review. *Schizophr Bull* 38(5):1003–1011, 2012.
137. Wu RR, Zhao JP, Jin H, et al. Lifestyle intervention and metformin for treatment of antipsychotic-induced weight gain: a randomized controlled trial. *JAMA* 299(2):185–193, 2008.
138. Jarskog LF, Hamer RM, Catellier DJ, et al. Metformin for weight loss and metabolic control in overweight outpatients with schizophrenia and schizoaffective disorder. *Am J Psychiatry* 170(9):1032–1040, 2013.
139. Essock SM, Schooler NR, Stroup TS, et al. Effectiveness of switching from antipsychotic polypharmacy to monotherapy. *Am J Psychiatry* 168(7):702–708, 2011.
141. Andreasen NC, Liu D, Ziebell S, et al. Relapse duration, treatment intensity, and brain tissue loss in schizophrenia: a prospective longitudinal MRI study. *Am J Psychiatry* 170(6):609–615, 2013.
143. Wunderink L, Nieboer RM, Wiersma D, et al. Recovery in remitted first-episode psychosis at 7 years of follow-up of an early dose reduction/discontinuation or maintenance treatment strategy: Long-term follow-up of a 2-year randomized clinical trial. *JAMA Psychiatry* 70(9):913–920, 2013.
144. Buchanan RW, Kreyenbuhl J, Kelly DL, et al. The 2009 schizophrenia PORT psychopharmacological treatment recommendations and summary statements. *Schizophr Bull* 36(1):71–93, 2010.

8 Lithium and Its Role in Psychiatry

Roy H. Perlis, MD, MSc, and Michael J. Ostacher, MD, MPH, MMSc

KEY POINTS

- Lithium remains a first-line treatment for all phases of bipolar disorder, including mania, depression, and prevention of recurrence.
- While not examined in a controlled trial, abundant evidence supports a role for lithium in decreasing the risk of suicide.
- Lithium has a narrow therapeutic window, necessitating careful titration and close monitoring of plasma levels.
- Lithium toxicity may cause confusion and ataxia.
- Drugs that affect lithium levels include non-steroidal anti-inflammatory drugs (NSAIDs) and diuretics.

HISTORICAL CONTEXT

The history of lithium's use in psychiatry parallels the development of modern psychopharmacology. The first specific description of the application of lithium to treat mania occurred in 1949, by an Australian named John Cade, who observed that lithium had calming effects on animals and then treated a series of 10 agitated manic patients. In fact, however, descriptions of lithium treatment date back to at least the United States Civil War. An 1883 textbook by Union Army Surgeon General William Hammond recommended the use of lithium bromide to treat manic or agitated patients, though he later downplayed the importance of lithium. In the early 1900s, a Danish physician, Lange, published a case series reporting the treatment of manic patients with lithium carbonate. There is little evidence that lithium was studied further, however, until Garrod proposed that lithium urate could be used to treat gout, opening the door to its broader therapeutic application.

Unfortunately, despite early studies by Mogen Schou and others, lithium's wider adoption in the US was hindered by concerns about lithium toxicity. Lithium chloride had been used as a sodium substitute in the 1940s, until several deaths were reported from lithium toxicity among hyponatremic patients. Thus, lithium was initially perceived as too dangerous for clinical application, and it was only in 1970 that lithium was approved by the United States Food and Drug Administration (FDA) for the treatment of mania.[1]

LITHIUM'S MECHANISM OF ACTION

The mechanisms by which lithium exerts its therapeutic effects are not entirely clear, but the signaling pathways with which it interacts are becoming better understood. Two major pathways are influenced by lithium. In the first, re-cycling of inositol is inhibited by lithium, which influences inositol 1,4,5-triphosphate ($InsP_3$)-dependent signaling.[2-4] $InsP_3$ signaling acts in part by regulating intra-cellular calcium release and protein kinase activation, with broad effects. At a neuronal level, lithium, like valproate, has been shown to increase the spread of growth cones, which are necessary for synapse formation. This effect is reversed by addition of myoinositol, providing some support for the importance of $InsP_3$ in lithium's effect.

In the second, lithium inhibits glycogen synthesis kinase 3-beta (GSK3B),[4-7] an important enzyme in pathways including the Wnt signaling cascade.[8] Notably, mice expressing lower levels of GSK3B exhibit behaviors similar to mice treated chronically with lithium.[9] Signaling through the GSK3B pathway may also be central to the observed neuroprotective effects of lithium.[10] Of course, both $InsP_3$ and GSK3B pathways have convergent effects—both influence the serine/threonine kinase Akt-1,4 for example. Expression of other genes (typically in lymphocytes) has been shown in single studies to be influenced by lithium administration, though the relevance of these effects to lithium's effects on mood or other phenotypes is unknown.

PHARMACOKINETICS AND PHARMACODYNAMICS

Lithium is absorbed through the gut and distributes rapidly through body water, achieving peak plasma concentrations 1 to 2 hours after a single dose. (Slower-release forms may require 4 to 5 hours to reach peak concentration, because of transit time through the gut.) As a monovalent cation like sodium, lithium's clearance relies entirely on renal function. It is not metabolized by the liver, nor is it significantly protein bound while circulating. In general, the half-life for renal excretion is approximately 24 hours, so steady-state serum levels are typically reached after 5 days. For this reason, lithium levels are typically checked about 5 days after initiation or dose change. Because lithium distributes throughout the body, it is influenced by lean body mass—for example, among geriatric patients, lithium levels for a given dose tend to be greater than among younger patients with greater lean body (including muscle) mass. Magnetic resonance spectroscopy studies suggest that brain lithium levels are highly correlated with plasma levels, though less so in patients at the extremes of age—that is, it is possible to have supra-therapeutic levels in the central nervous system (CNS) while maintaining a normal plasma lithium level.

Drugs that affect renal function, particularly re-absorption, can have profound effects on lithium clearance. Perhaps most notably from a clinical perspective, non-steroidal anti-inflammatory drugs (NSAIDs) or other COX-2 inhibitors may decrease renal blood flow and thereby increase lithium levels by up to 25%. Diuretics likewise affect lithium levels, though the nature of their effect depends on their site of action. In the kidney, lithium is primarily re-absorbed in the proximal renal tubules, with some subsequent absorption in the loop of Henle. Importantly, in contrast to sodium, no significant absorption occurs in the distal tubules. Therefore, thiazide diuretics, which act distally, will tend to increase lithium levels by up to 50%, while those that act more proximally generally have less of an effect on lithium levels.

More broadly, hydration status can affect lithium levels: individuals who become salt-avid (e.g., because of hypovolemia or hyponatremia, perhaps in the context of vomiting and diarrhea or self-induced injury, such as long-distance-running) will cause their lithium levels to increase.

EVIDENCE FOR LITHIUM'S EFFICACY
Lithium in Acute Mania

Beginning with Schou's study of lithium versus placebo for acute mania, lithium has repeatedly shown efficacy for the treatment of mania,[11] with the first large randomized study of lithium treatment of acute mania finding lithium comparably effective to the antipsychotic chlorpromazine.[12] Since then, multiple studies have found lithium to be superior to placebo and comparable or superior to other agents in the acute management of bipolar mania; few studies have found superiority for other drugs over lithium. A systematic review found 12 acute mania trials comparing lithium to placebo or another agent that met their criteria for data-pooling. This review of studies of lithium for acute mania found superiority for lithium over placebo and chlorpromazine, with equivalence to valproate and carbamazepine.[13]

As pointed out by Grunze,[14] however, few studies of lithium in acute mania were undertaken with the methodological rigor required today for regulatory approval of a drug's use. By coincidence, the first rigorously designed study to demonstrate the efficacy of lithium for acute mania was Bowden's seminal study of divalproex sodium for the treatment of acute mania in 1994, which was designed to study that drug for FDA approval; by including lithium as an active comparator, the study also demonstrated lithium's efficacy.[15] This study was adequately powered (i.e., it included a large enough sample of patients to find a high probability of finding a statistically significant difference between treatments with a low probability of error), compared a drug to an agent known to be effective (lithium), and it included a placebo arm. Additionally, it was not biased by inclusion based on prior response to lithium. In this 3-week study, lithium was superior to placebo and equivalent in efficacy to divalproex sodium with a 50% response rate (defined as a 50% drop in mania scale scores) for lithium compared to 26% for placebo.[15] Since that study, pooled data from trials of topiramate for mania failed to demonstrate a benefit for that drug, but it did re-confirm the efficacy of lithium for acutely manic patients.[16] The percentage of patients with a 50% or greater reduction in the Young Mania Rating Scale (YMRS) at day 21 was 28% with placebo (n = 427), 27% with topiramate (n = 433), and 46% with lithium (n = 227). Lithium was statistically better than placebo and topiramate on all psychometric measures other than the Montgomery-Asberg Depression Rating Scale (MADRS).

Monotherapy treatment in any phase of bipolar disorder, however, is increasingly rare, and is especially so in the treatment of acute mania.[17] It appears that mania outcomes, in terms of time to response and proportion of patients who remit, may be improved with the addition of antipsychotics to lithium.[18] The adjunctive use of typical (including haloperidol) and atypical (e.g., aripiprazole, asenapine, olanzapine, quetiapine, and risperidone) antipsychotics with lithium carbonate has been found to improve outcomes compared to lithium alone. The atypical antipsychotic ziprasidone, however, did not improve outcomes significantly compared to placebo when added to lithium.

Lithium in Acute Bipolar Depression

The options for the pharmacological treatment of major depressive episodes in bipolar disorder, unlike those for mania, remain few. In spite of being recommended as first-line treatment in recent bipolar treatment guidelines, there are few data to support the use of lithium as an acute antidepressant in bipolar disorder. A comprehensive review by Bauer and Mitchner[19] identified only three placebo-controlled trials of lithium for bipolar depression (with a total of 62 subjects).

While these trials showed a positive benefit for lithium, none was a randomized, parallel-group study; instead, they used a within-subject design in which each subject was started on lithium or placebo and then switched to the other. It is unlikely, unfortunately, that there will be any large, well-designed trials of lithium to answer this question, most prominently because there is no pharmaceutical manufacturer producing lithium that has any financial incentive to undertake such a study.

Lithium, used as monotherapy, appears to be as effective for the treatment of bipolar depression as the combination of lithium and an antidepressant. In a study comparing imipramine, paroxetine, and placebo added to lithium carbonate for the treatment of a major depressive episode in bipolar disorder, neither antidepressant added benefit beyond lithium alone.[20] Response rates (defined as a Hamilton Depression Rating Scale [HAM-D] score of 7 or lower) were 35% for lithium alone, compared to 39% for imipramine, and 46% for paroxetine. In a secondary analysis, subjects with lower lithium levels (less than 0.8 mEq/L) had a lower response rate compared to the adjunctive antidepressant group, suggesting, perhaps, that higher lithium levels are as effective as lithium plus an antidepressant in the treatment of bipolar depression.

Lithium for Maintenance Treatment and Relapse Prevention of Bipolar Disorder

Lithium is the archetypal maintenance treatment for bipolar disorder. From Prien's first maintenance study of lithium (comparing it to chlorpromazine), to more recent studies using lithium as a comparator for maintenance studies of other drugs, lithium has clear benefit for maintaining response and preventing relapse in bipolar disorder.[12,21] Lithium's clearest benefit in long-term use is in the prevention of relapse to mania, although relapse to depression is more common in patients with bipolar disorder. As is the case with lithium in acute mania, lithium's efficacy compared to placebo was only confirmed in later studies designed to establish regulatory approval for newer drugs, including divalproex sodium and lamotrigine. Earlier studies were beset with methodological problems, including on–off rather than parallel group designs, lack of diagnostic clarity (e.g., the inclusion of unipolar patients), and rapid or abrupt lithium discontinuation in stable patients. Concerns about sudden discontinuation of lithium are genuine, as there is a high rate of manic relapse in these patients; inclusion of patients from these studies might artificially inflate the difference between lithium and placebo in maintenance treatment.[22,23]

Geddes and colleagues[24] have completed the definitive systematic review of lithium for maintenance treatment in bipolar disorder. Having reviewed 300 studies, they included only five in their meta-analysis, limiting inclusion to randomized, double-blind, placebo-controlled trials. They found that lithium was more effective than placebo in preventing relapses to any mood episode (random effects relative risk = 0.65, 95% confidence interval [CI] = 0.50 to 0.84) and to mania (relative risk = 0.62, 95% CI = 0.40 to 0.95), with a non-significant effect on relapse to depression (relative risk = 0.72, 95% CI = 0.49 to 1.07).[24] The average risk of relapse of any kind in 1 to 2 years of follow-up was 60% for placebo, compared to 40% for lithium; this can be understood as lithium preventing one relapse for every five patients treated compared to placebo. Relapse rates to mania were 14% for lithium compared to 24% for placebo, while relapse rates to depression were 25% for placebo compared to 32% for lithium. There are some limitations and criticisms of this study, however. The outcomes were not defined uniformly across the included studies; one study included in the analysis had exclusively bipolar II subjects, and the follow-up period of 1 to 2 years is too short to adequately evaluate the benefit of lithium (as some have argued that the maintenance benefit of lithium is only apparent after 2 years of treatment).[23,25]

Lithium was compared to olanzapine for the prevention of relapse of bipolar I disorder in a randomized, controlled, double-blind trial.[26] Bipolar I patients were stabilized on a combination of lithium and olanzapine, randomized to one or the other drug, and followed for 12 months. There was no difference between drugs on the primary outcome measure or time to symptomatic relapse (YMRS or HAM-D scores of 15 or greater), although there were fewer relapses to mania/mixed (but not depressive) episodes in the olanzapine-treated group.

A number of studies have examined outcomes for subjects stabilized on an antipsychotic added to lithium or valproate and then randomized to remain on lithium or valproate and the antipsychotic or lithium or valproate plus placebo. Notably, these studies include aripiprazole, quetiapine, and ziprasidone; they are enriched designs intended to study the impact of the antipsychotic primarily, but do suggest that those patients who are stabilized on lithium or valproate plus one of those antipsychotics remain on both drugs.

A study was completed specifically to examine whether combination treatment with lithium and valproate together is more effective than either of those two drugs as monotherapy to prevent recurrence in bipolar I disorder. BALANCE is a randomized, open-label trial of lithium, divalproex sodium, or the combination for maintenance treatment in bipolar disorder. Participants were stabilized on both drugs during a 4 to 8-week open-label run-in phase (to screen for tolerability), then randomized to continue on lithium (titrated to at 0.4–1.0 mmol/L), divalproex sodium (750 mg, 1,250 mg, or valproic acid serum concentration at least 50 μg/ml), or the combination, with the primary outcome measure being time to intervention for a mood episode. While combination treatment was superior to divalproex sodium (hazard ratio 0.59, 95% CI 0.42–0.83) and lithium was also superior to divalproex (HR 0.71, 95% CI 0.71–1.00), combination therapy was not superior to lithium (HR 0.82, 95% CI 0.58–1.17). This suggests that the role for valproate monotherapy (i.e., not in combination with lithium) is limited, and that lithium alone or in combination with valproate is the preferred treatment.

There remains some controversy about what adequate maintenance lithium levels should be. In order to minimize adverse effects and to increase patient acceptance of lithium treatment, lowest effective doses should be the goal. A randomized, double-blind study by Gelenberg and co-workers[27] stabilized patients on a standard serum level of lithium (0.8 to 1 mmol/L), then assigned them to either remain at that level or to be maintained with a lower serum lithium level (0.4 to 0.6 mmol/L). Patients in the higher lithium level group had fewer relapses than those randomly assigned to lower lithium levels.[27] A re-analysis of the data, however, controlling for the rate at which the lithium dose was lowered, found no difference between groups, suggesting that lower maintenance lithium levels may be adequate for some patients.[28]

Lithium in Rapid-cycling Bipolar Disorder

Rapid cycling is no longer included as a course specifier in DSM-5, but continues to be used conceptually by clinicians. Rapid-cycling is defined in DSM-IV-TR as four or more distinct mood episodes (either of opposite poles, or of the same pole after at least 8 weeks of partial or full recovery) within a 12-month period; patients with this course are notoriously difficult to treat and to stabilize. Some have concluded that lithium is less effective than other drugs (e.g., divalproex

sodium) for this specific course of bipolar disorder, but an ambitious clinical trial and a large body of naturalistic data suggest that lithium is no less ineffective than other compounds for rapid-cycling.[29-32] Calabrese and colleagues[31] compared lithium to divalproex sodium in rapid-cycling patients stabilized on both drugs and found no difference between drugs on time-to-episode-recurrence. As testament to the difficulty of treating rapid-cycling, only 60 of the original 254 subjects, who were randomized to the two study conditions, achieved stabilization. In a cohort of 360 patients treated for bipolar disorder in Sardinia, time to recurrence was no different for the patients with or without a rapid-cycling course.[32]

Lithium in Suicide Prevention

Lithium may have anti-suicide effects in patients with mood disorders. While there are no prospective, randomized studies designed to examine lithium's potential to reduce suicide and suicide attempts, a number of meta-analyses, smaller independent studies, and a study from two large health insurance databases generally substantiate lithium's value as a prophylactic agent against suicidal behavior in bipolar disorder.

The strongest evidence for decreased suicide in patients treated with lithium comes from a meta-analysis by Cipriani and co-workers[33] of all randomized studies of lithium (either versus placebo or another drug) in mood disorders (including bipolar disorder and major depressive disorder [MDD]).[33]

They found that lithium-treated patients had significantly fewer suicides and deaths from all causes. In an examination of 32 trials, 1,389 patients were randomly assigned to lithium treatment and 2,069 to other compounds. Seven trials reported any deaths by suicide; subjects treated with lithium were less likely to commit suicide (2 versus 11 suicides; odds ratio = 0.26; 95% CI = 0.09 to 0.77). When suicides plus suicidal behavior (i.e., deliberate self-harm) were examined, the results also favored the lithium-treated group (odds ratio = 0.21; 95% CI = 0.08 to 0.50). In the 11 trials reporting any deaths, all-cause mortality was lower in the lithium group (data from 11 trials; 9 versus 22 deaths; odds ratio = 0.42, 95% CI = 0.21 to 0.87).

In an analysis of databases from two large health maintenance organizations in the US, Goodwin and Goldstein[34] found a strong effect favoring lithium compared to divalproex sodium or other anticonvulsants. The incidence of emergency department admissions for suicide attempts (31.3 versus 10.8 per 1,000 person-years; P < 0.001), suicide attempts resulting in hospitalization (10.5 versus 4.2 per 1,000 person-years; P < 0.001), and death by suicide (1.7 versus 0.7 per 1,000 person-years; P = 0.04) was lower in the group receiving at least one prescription for lithium. When adjusted for a number of demographic factors (including age and psychiatric and medical co-morbidity), they found that the risk of death by suicide was 2.7 times that for patients prescribed divalproex for a diagnosis of bipolar disorder compared to those prescribed lithium (95% CI = 1.1 to 6.3; P = 0.04).[34] The non-randomized nature of the sample, however, leaves open the concern that the groups were clinically different, and the results confounded by indication.[35] For instance, it is not known how many of the patients in the divalproex group had previously failed to respond to lithium and were thus a treatment-resistant group, and whether there were co-morbidities (such as anxiety disorders, personality disorders, or substance use disorders) that were present to a greater degree in the non–lithium-treated subjects. In any case, the results are strongly in favor of lithium and are consistent with other examinations of the effect of lithium on suicide.

Another meta-analysis of 33 studies investigating long-term lithium treatment between the years 1970 and 2000 yields a result that favors lithium as a potential means of suicide prevention.[36] Of the 19 studies comparing groups with and without lithium treatment, 18 found a lower risk of suicide in the treatment group and one had no suicides in either group.[36] Overall, the meta-analysis demonstrated a 13-fold reduction in suicidality for patients with an affective illness, leading to a largely reduced suicide risk (which nevertheless remained larger than that estimated for the general population). The rates of suicide associated with lithium treatment (0.109% to 0.224% annually) are 10 times greater than the international base rate (0.017%).[36]

Lithium discontinuation itself may increase suicide risk. Rapid or accelerated lithium discontinuation (as may be practiced by non-compliant individuals who decide to simply stop taking their medications) may increase risk for suicidal behavior. In a sample of 165 patients who decided to discontinue lithium for a variety of reasons (whether electively or for some medical reason), there was a 14-fold increase in all suicidal acts following discontinuation of lithium.[37] It is unclear whether the risk of suicide following lithium discontinuation exceeds that found in untreated affective illness. Lithium discontinuation may increase suicidal behavior due to higher relapse rates, higher than would be expected even if subjects had been treated with placebo or had been on no medication at all.[23] Ultimately, although the effects of lithium are promising in the realm of suicide prevention, they have not yet been definitively determined (and are likely never to be).

Lithium in Children and Adolescents
Pediatric Bipolar Disorder

There are no randomized, controlled, parallel group trials of lithium treatment of acute mania in children or adolescents. This is unfortunate, as the use of lithium in children without clear benefit may be inappropriate due to its known side effects. Open-label data are suggestive of an anti-manic effect, but without randomization or a control group, these data are difficult to interpret.[38] Kafantaris and co-workers[39] published a discontinuation study of adolescents with acute mania who were stabilized for 4 weeks on lithium, then randomly assigned to double-blind discontinuation over 2 weeks. They found no differences in rate of symptom-worsening between the group continued on lithium (10 of 19, 52.6%) versus the group switched to placebo (13 of 21, 61.9%), but their follow-up period may have been too short to detect a meaningful difference.[39]

A small, randomized, placebo-controlled, 6-week study of lithium in adolescents (n = 25, average age 16.3 years) with bipolar disorder and substance dependence disorder (including alcohol, cannabis, stimulants, and sedative/hypnotics) showed that lithium (average serum level 0.9 mEq/L) appears to improve both disorders.[40] Urine screens and measures of psychopathology improved in this group, although the results were preliminary and have yet to be replicated in a larger sample using more rigorous methodology.

Conduct Disorder

Lithium has been of some interest for use in treating symptoms of aggression associated with conduct disorder in children. In the largest study of this, 40 children (33 boys, 7 girls, with an average age of 12.5 years) were randomly assigned to lithium or placebo for 4 weeks.[41] Sixteen of 20 subjects in the lithium-treated group were considered responders on consensus ratings compared to 6 of 20 in the placebo group (P = 0.04), while Overt Aggression Scale scores decreased significantly for the lithium group compared to the placebo group (P = 0.04). There were significant side effects, however,

potentially limiting the utility of the treatment, and the follow-up period was short.

Other Uses of Lithium

While well validated for use in the treatment of bipolar disorder, lithium has been studied with greater or lesser success through randomized trials in the treatment of other psychiatric illnesses, including unipolar MDD, schizophrenia, and alcohol dependence.

Augmentation of Antidepressants in Treatment-refractory Major Depressive Disorder

The use of lithium as an agent to prevent relapse in MDD has been somewhat controversial, although the accumulation of evidence suggests that it may be effective in a small number of difficult-to-treat, refractory patients. While some of the earlier placebo-controlled trials found lithium augmentation to be of no benefit, a few larger studies with improved methodology suggested a benefit for lithium over placebo; a meta-analysis that included nine double-blind, placebo-controlled trials found a statistically significant difference in response rates to lithium augmentation compared to placebo in trials that used a minimum lithium carbonate dose of 800 mg/day or a serum level of 0.5 mEq/L or greater.[42] More recently, however, a small, double-blind, placebo-controlled trial of lithium augmentation found no benefit for lithium, and a recent large head-to-head comparison between lithium carbonate and triiodothyronine (T_3) found that only a small proportion of patients improved with lithium.[43,44]

Nierenberg and associates[43] found no benefit for lithium in a placebo-controlled trial. Thirty-five non-responders to 6 weeks of treatment with nortriptyline were treated with lithium carbonate or placebo; only 12.5% of the lithium-treated subjects improved, compared to 20% on placebo. As part of the Sequential Treatment Alternatives to Relieve Depression (STAR*D) study, lithium carbonate was compared to T_3 as an augmentation strategy in a 14-week randomized, open-label trial for 142 patients who had failed to improve on citalopram followed by a second treatment (either a switch to another antidepressant or augmentation with another agent), and found similarly low response rates for lithium.[44]

Remission rates were 15.9% with lithium augmentation (mean dose = 859.8 mg, SD = 373.1) and 24.7% with T_3 augmentation (mean dose = 45.2 µg, SD = 11.4) after a mean of 9.6 weeks of treatment, although the difference between treatments was not statistically significant. Lithium, however, was more frequently associated with side effects than was T_3 (P = 0.045), and more participants in the lithium group left treatment because of side effects (23.2% versus 9.6%; P = 0.027).

Relapse Prevention in Major Depressive Disorder

Several efforts have been made to examine the potential benefit of lithium in preventing relapse in MDD. In an early study, Prien and colleagues[45] found no additional benefit of the combination of lithium and imipramine over imipramine monotherapy. Lithium monotherapy was less successful than imipramine or combination treatment in this study.

In a small cohort (n = 29) of patients who responded to lithium augmentation in a 6-week open-label treatment phase and remained well over a 2- to 4-week stabilization period, those randomized to continue lithium had lower relapse rates in 4 months of follow-up (0 of 14) compared to those on placebo (7 of 15, including one suicide).[42] Serum lithium levels were moderate, averaging between 0.65 and

0.72 mmol/L. One methodological limitation of the study is that lithium was discontinued over a 1-week washout period, raising the possibility that rapid lithium discontinuation may have contributed to the high relapse rate (and perhaps to the suicide in the placebo arm).

Lithium in Psychotic Disorders

Lithium is ineffective in the treatment of psychosis, but it has been studied as an adjunct to antipsychotics in the treatment of patients with schizophrenia and schizoaffective disorders. In the last published randomized trial of lithium in schizophrenia, a double-blind, placebo-controlled, crossover design study of 21 patients with schizophrenia, little benefit was found for lithium compared to placebo on most measures of illness severity.[46] The benefit for lithium in patients with schizophrenia or schizoaffective disorder has only been studied in samples of a similar size, and results are not definitively in favor of its use.[47-50]

Lithium in Alcohol Dependence

A Veterans Administration study of lithium in depressed and non-depressed alcoholics failed to find a benefit for the drug.[51]

In a year-long study of 286 alcoholics without depression and 171 alcoholics with depression, no significant differences between alcoholics who took lithium and those who took placebo were found on any study measure (including number of alcoholics who became abstinent, number of days of drinking, number of alcohol-related hospitalizations, changes in rating of severity of alcoholism, and change in severity of depression). No significant differences were found when the data from medication-compliant subjects were reviewed.

PRINCIPLES OF LITHIUM TREATMENT
Predictors of Lithium Response

Few if any reliable predictors of lithium response have been identified. Indeed, on closer look many of the purported predictors have proven to be untrue. Thus, the bulk of evidence suggests that patients with rapid-cycling bipolar disorder respond well to lithium. Likewise, there is little convincing evidence that discontinuation of lithium decreases the likelihood of subsequent response to lithium. There is no evidence that males or females respond differentially to lithium.

Individuals with a positive family history of bipolar disorder (rather than schizophrenia) do appear to respond better to lithium. This is often interpreted, incorrectly, to mean that lithium response itself is familial, which has not been established.

Laboratory Monitoring

The standard evaluation (i.e., with evaluation of renal function, thyroid function, and cardiac rhythm) for a patient beginning lithium flows from its major potential toxicities. Specifically, standard guidelines advise checking electrolytes, blood urea nitrogen (BUN) and creatinine, thyroid-stimulating hormone (TSH), and an electrocardiogram (ECG) in individuals 40 years or older.

Lithium levels should be checked at least 5 days after each dose change, or any time a patient reports the new onset of symptoms potentially suggestive of lithium toxicity.

Guidelines also recommend following electrolytes, BUN, and creatinine up to every 2 months for the first 6 months, with a lithium level, BUN, creatinine, and thyroid function tests every 6 months to 1 year thereafter.

TABLE 8-1 Medications That Commonly Interact with Lithium

Medication	Effect
COMMON	
Diuretics: thiazide, loop (e.g., furosemide)	↑
ACE inhibitors	↑
NSAIDs	↑
Metronidazole	↑
Tetracycline	↑
Diuretics: osmotic, potassium-sparing, acetazolamide	↓
Theophylline/aminophylline	↓
Drugs that alkalinize urine	↓
Caffeine	↓
RARE BUT NOTABLE	
Antipsychotics	Risk of neurotoxicity
Bupropion	Increased seizure risk
SSRIs	Serotonin syndrome
Iodide salts	Hypothyroidism

ACE, Angiotensin-converting enzyme; NSAIDs, non-steroidal anti-inflammatory drugs; SSRIs, selective serotonin reuptake inhibitors.

Lithium Dosing

Lithium carbonate is available in 300 mg capsules or tablets, as well as 300 and 450 mg slow-release forms. A liquid, lithium citrate, is also available, in 300 mg/5 ml form. For most patients, the immediate-release lithium carbonate is initiated first, with a switch to another form only to maximize tolerability if necessary.

The narrow therapeutic window for lithium treatment (see Pharmacokinetics and Pharmacodynamics, earlier in this chapter) complicates lithium dosing. Indeed, in its early application lithium levels of 0.8 to 1.2mEq/L were advised, while more recently levels of 0.6 to 0.8—and perhaps even lower in some cases—have been advocated. The optimal dose is driven, not merely by considerations of efficacy, but by tolerability as well: that is, the "best" dose for prevention of recurrence may be too high for some patients to tolerate. Drug–drug interactions must be considered, and a list of selected interactions is provided in Table 8-1.

Typically, the clinician will begin with 600 mg once daily at bedtime and then increase it to 900 mg at bedtime. After 5 days, a lithium level is checked and the dose is increased or decreased as required to attain a level in the 0.6 to 0.8 mEq/L range. While nomograms exist for predicting the necessary lithium dose based on an initial test dose, because of concerns about lithium toxicity, the authors generally prefer to observe the level that results from 900 mg before titrating further.

Some data suggest that lithium may be better tolerated by patients, and possibly less likely to cause renal complications, when dosed once daily. If tolerability of a single dose becomes a problem—for example, in terms of sedation or gastrointestinal distress—divided dosing may be used. This need not be morning and night; some patients prefer dinnertime and bedtime.

Adverse Effects and Their Management

Hypothyroidism has been reported to be common in patients treated with lithium, with some studies describing a prevalance of up to 35%. However, more recent studies suggest that it is substantially less common, and is seen more often among women than men. When hypothyroidism occurs, it is typically managed with the addition of thyroid (T$_4$) treatment.

Lithium has a number of renal effects, which range from bothersome to potentially life-threatening. Perhaps the most common, polyuria (including nocturia) and consequent polydipsia, arise when lithium prevents distal tubule re-absorption of free water, antagonizing the actions of anti-diuretic hormone. When necessary, they may be addressed with careful addition of a diuretic. Amiloride is often used first, as it has little effect on lithium levels. Thiazide diuretics may also be used if required, though they will increase lithium levels and often require a dose decrease of 50% and close monitoring of lithium levels. When edema (particularly common in the lower extremities) is seen in a patient with normal renal function, the diuretic spironolactone may be used, though again lithium levels and renal function will require close monitoring.

Of greater concern, long-term treatment with lithium is associated with reduction in creatinine clearance in about 10% of patients, indicating a decrease in glomerular filtration rate (GFR). Small studies suggest that glomerulosclerosis and interstitial fibrosis are seen among some patients receiving long-term lithium treatment. Beyond a certain point, this deterioration may accelerate and dramatically increase the risk of lithium toxicity, as small perturbations in GFR can have large effects on lithium levels. When creatinine rises above baseline by 25% or more, consultation with a nephrologist may be helpful to rule out other contributors to reduction in GFR (e.g., renal complications of diabetes mellitus [DM]), and discontinuation of lithium often becomes necessary once GFR decreases beyond a certain point.

While rare, lithium can cause a depression of firing at the sino-atrial node, contributing to sinus arrhythmias. Lithium may also cause benign ECG abnormalities, most typically an appearance resembling hypokalemia, including widening of the QRS complex and increased PR interval.

Weight gain is common among lithium-treated patients, and while the mechanism is not known, it is not merely a result of lithium-induced edema. Some studies suggest that up to half of lithium-treated patients will experience a 5% to 10% increase in weight. As with any medication-induced weight gain, early and aggressive intervention is warranted, focusing on both diet and exercise. A specific concern among lithium-treated patients with polydipsia is the consumption of sodas or juices high in sugar.

Cognitive complaints are common among lithium-treated patients, sometimes characterized as feeling "foggy" or "cloudy." Adjunctive thyroid hormone is sometimes used in an attempt to ameliorate these symptoms; however, there is no well-established means of treating such complaints, other than decreasing lithium dose.

Other Bothersome Adverse Effects

Gastrointestinal adverse effects are common among lithium-treated patients, and may include upper (nausea, vomiting, and dyspepsia) and lower (diarrhea and cramping) gastrointestinal symptoms. Because slow-release formulations are absorbed lower in the gut, they are more often associated with the latter symptoms, while immediate-release formulations are more often associated with the former symptoms. In many cases, dividing dosages or dosing with food can minimize or eliminate these symptoms. If this is not the case, a switch to lithium citrate (in liquid form) may be helpful, though some patients object to the taste of this preparation.

Tremor is common with lithium treatment, even at therapeutic levels and particularly following each dose when peak levels are achieved. This tremor, which resembles a benign physiological tremor, may be exacerbated by caffeine and by anxiety. It is typically managed by changing the timing of the lithium dose (to ensure that peak levels occur during sleep)

BOX 8-1 Signs of Lithium Toxicity

LEVELS ABOVE 1.5 mEq/L*
Lethargy/fatigue
Coarse tremor
Nausea/vomiting
Diarrhea
Visual changes (blurring)
Vertigo
Hyperreflexia
Dysarthria
Ataxia
Confusion

LEVELS ABOVE 2.5–3 mEq/L
Seizure
Coma
Arrhythmia

*Absence of significant symptoms does not rule out toxicity; likewise, some symptoms may be apparent at levels as low as 1 mEq/L.

BOX 8-2 Management of Lithium Toxicity

If patient is comatose/obtunded, protect airway.
In cases of suspected overdose, consider gastric lavage. For lithium levels above 4 mEq/L,* or above 3 mEq/L and severely symptomatic, or in other cases where volume load will not be tolerated, initiate dialysis.
Hold further lithium doses.
Begin IV normal saline, 150–200 ml/h (as long as able to tolerate volume load).
Address other electrolyte abnormalities.
Follow lithium levels approximately every 2–3 h. Initiate work-up to determine cause of toxicity.

*Recommendations vary about when to initiate dialysis, though most sources agree that levels above 4 mEq/L merit immediate dialysis.

and when necessary by adding a beta-adrenergic blocker. This may be used on either an as-needed or a standing basis, depending on patient preference. Propranolol is often initiated first to establish an effective dose, then changed to atenolol for the convenience of once-daily dosing.

Both psoriasis and acne exacerbations have been associated with lithium treatment. Typically these do not require treatment discontinuation as they can be controlled with dermatological treatments.

Presentation of lithium toxicity develops as lithium levels rise above 1, and particularly beyond 1.2 mEq/L; initial symptoms may include slurring of speech, ataxia/unsteady gait, confusion, and agitation. Box 8-1 shows signs and symptoms of lithium toxicity, and Box 8-2 shows management of acute toxicity.

Lithium in Pregnancy and Breast-feeding

Lithium use during the first trimester of pregnancy has been associated with a potentially life-threatening cardiac abnormality, known as Ebstein's anomaly, a spectrum of changes that typically includes insufficiency of the tricuspid valve and hypoplasia of the right ventricle. The risk appears to be about 10-fold greater among children of lithium-treated patients compared to those in the general population, though the absolute risk is still quite low (on the order of 1 in 2,000).

This risk must be balanced against the substantial dangers to the fetus of a mother with uncontrolled bipolar disorder during pregnancy.

The changes in maternal fluid status during pregnancy typically cause a larger volume of distribution for lithium, which can lead to a decrease in lithium levels, entailing closer monitoring of lithium during pregnancy and in some cases a dose increase. At the time of delivery, fluid shifts may likewise lead to an increase in lithium levels. However, discontinuing lithium in the peripartum period is no longer routinely advised, as it has become clear that the risk of bipolar recurrence is extremely high in this period.

Levels of lithium in breast milk are substantial, approaching 50% of maternal plasma levels. For this reason, lithium-treated mothers should not breast-feed, as the effects of lithium on newborn development are not well studied and the risk for toxicity is high.

Lithium Adherence

Recent studies document very low rates of lithium adherence in bipolar disorder, particularly in a cohort of patients participating in a health maintenance organization.[52] These studies highlight the importance of careful lithium dosing and aggressive management of adverse effects.

CURRENT CONTROVERSIES AND FUTURE DIRECTIONS

Several recent reviews have raised concern that lithium is being under-used relative to other, potentially less effective treatments. This has been attributed to lithium receiving less attention in medical education, and more generally because of the marketing efforts for newer, on-patent alternatives for the treatment of bipolar disorder.

If lithium's mechanism of action can be better understood, it might facilitate the identification of targets for drug therapy in bipolar disorder—that is, proteins that might be targeted by drugs that could exert similar effects to lithium, without its toxicity. Alternatively, it may be possible to explain why some patients fail to respond to lithium, and "sensitize" them by combining lithium with other agents. Further mechanistic and pharmacogenetic studies of lithium will be crucial in this regard.

Access the complete reference list and multiple choice questions (MCQs) online at https://expertconsult.inkling.com

KEY REFERENCES

4. Chalecka-Franaszek E, Chuang DM. Lithium activates the serine/threonine kinaseAkt-1 and suppresses glutamate-induced inhibition of Akt-1 activity in neurons. *Proc Natl Acad Sci USA* 96(15):8745–8750, 1999.
9. O'Brien WT, Harper AD, Jove F, et al. Glycogen synthase kinase-3 beta haploinsufficiency mimics the behavioral and molecular effects of lithium. *J Neurosci* 24(30):6791–6798, 2004.
12. Prien RF, Caey EM Jr, Klett CJ. Comparison of lithium carbonate and chlorpromazine in the treatment of mania. Report of the Veterans Administration and National Institute of Mental Health Collaborative Study Group. *Arch Gen Psychiatry* 26:146–153, 1972.
15. Bowden CL, Brugger AM, Swann AC, et al. Efficacy of divalproex vs lithium and placebo in the treatment of mania. The Depakote Mania Study Group. *JAMA* 271(12):918–924, 1994.
18. Perlis RH, Welge JA, Vornik LA, et al. Atypical antipsychotics in the treatment of mania: a meta-analysis of randomized, placebo-controlled trials. *J Clin Psychiatry* 67(4):509–516, 2006.
20. Nemeroff CB, Evans DL, Gyulai L, et al. Double-blind, placebo-controlled comparison of imipramine and paroxetine in the treatment of bipolar depression. *Am J Psychiatry* 158(6):906–912, 2001.
21. Prien RF, Caffey EM, Klett CJ. Prophylactic efficacy of lithium carbonate in manic-depressive illness: report of the Veterans Administration and National Institute of Mental Health Collaborative Study Group. *Arch Gen Psychiatry* 28:337–341, 1973.
22. Suppes T, Baldessarini RJ, Faedda GL, et al. Risk of recurrence following discontinuation of lithium treatment in bipolar disorder. *Arch Gen Psychiatry* 48:1082–1088, 1991.
23. Goodwin GM. Recurrence of mania after lithium withdrawal: implications for the use of lithium in the treatment of bipolar affective disorder. *Br J Psychiatry* 164:149–152, 1994.
24. Geddes JR, Burgess S, Hawton K, et al. Long-term lithium therapy for bipolar disorder: systematic review and meta-analysis of randomized controlled trials. *Am J Psychiatry* 161:217–222, 2004.
25. Young AH, Newham JI. Lithium for maintenance therapy in bipolar disorder. *J Psychopharmacol* 20:17–22, 2006.
26. Tohen M, Greil W, Calabrese JR, et al. Olanzapine versus lithium in the maintenance treatment of bipolar disorder: a 12-month, randomized, double-blind, controlled clinical trial. *Am J Psychiatry* 162(7):1281–1290, 2005.
27. Gelenberg AJ, Kane JM, Keller MB, et al. Comparison of standard and low serum levels of lithium for maintenance treatment of bipolar disorder. *N Engl J Med* 321:1489–1493, 1989.
28. Perlis RH, Sachs GS, Lafer B, et al. Effect of abrupt change from standard to low serum levels of lithium: a reanalysis of double-blind lithium maintenance data. *Am J Psychiatry* 159:1155–1159, 2002.
30. Bowden CL, Calabrese JR, McElroy SL, et al. A randomized, placebo-controlled 12-month trial of divalproex and lithium in treatment of outpatients with bipolar I disorder. Divalproex Maintenance Study Group. *Arch Gen Psychiatry* 57:481–489, 2000.
31. Calabrese JR, Bowden CL, Sachs G, et al. A placebo-controlled 18-month trial of lamotrigine and lithium maintenance treatment in recently depressed patients with bipolar I disorder. *J Clin Psychiatry* 64:1013–1024, 2003.
32. Baldessarini RJ, Tondo L, Floris G, et al. Effects of rapid cycling on response to lithium maintenance treatment in 360 bipolar I and II disorder patients. *J Affect Disord* 61:13–22, 2006.
33. Cipriani A, Wilder H, Hawton K, et al. Lithium in the prevention of suicidal behaviour and all-cause mortality in patients with mood disorders: a systematic review of randomized trials. *Am J Psychiatry* 162:1805–1819, 2005.
37. Tondo L, Baldessarini RJ. Reduced suicide risk during lithium maintenance treatment. *J Clin Psychiatry* 61(Suppl. 9):97–104, 2000.
41. Malone RP, Delaney MA, Luebbert JF, et al. A double-blind placebo-controlled study of lithium in hospitalized aggressive children and adolescents with conduct disorder. *Arch Gen Psychiatry* 57(7):649–654, 2000.
42. Bauer M, Döpfmer S. Lithium augmentation in treatment-resistant depression: meta-analysis of placebo-controlled studies. *J Clin Psychopharmacol* 19:427–434, 1999.
45. Prien RF, Kupfer DJ, Mansky PA, et al. Drug therapy in the prevention of recurrences in unipolar and bipolar affective disorders. Report of the NIMH Collaborative Study Group comparing lithium carbonate, imipramine, and a lithium carbonate-imipramine combination. *Arch Gen Psychiatry* 41(11):1096–1104, 1984.
48. Calabrese JR, Shelton MD, Rapport DJ, et al. Lithium combined with neuroleptics in chronic schizophrenic and schizoaffective patients. *J Clin Psychiatry* 42(3):124–128, 1981.
52. Johnson RE, McFarland BH. Lithium use and discontinuation in a health maintenance organization. *Am J Psychiatry* 153(8):993–1000, 1996.

9 The Use of Antiepileptic Drugs in Psychiatry

Michael J. Ostacher, MD, MPH, MMSc, and Honor Hsin, MD, PhD

KEY POINTS

- A "kindling hypothesis" of mood instability led to the search for anticonvulsant medications that might improve the course of illness in bipolar disorder (BPD).
- Divalproex sodium (valproate) and carbamazepine (in extended-release form) are effective in the treatment of acute mania.
- Lamotrigine is effective in the prevention of relapse to a new mood state in BPD, especially to major depression.
- The risk of the development of polycystic ovarian syndrome is elevated in women of childbearing age with BPD treated with divalproex sodium.
- Other anticonvulsants (such as gabapentin, topiramate, zonisamide, pregabalin, tiagabine, and oxcarbazepine) have been ineffective in the treatment of BPD, worsen the course of illness, or lack data from randomized trials to support their use; none can be recommended for the treatment of any phase of BPD.

OVERVIEW: HISTORICAL CONTEXT

There has been great hope for the utility of anticonvulsants in the treatment of bipolar disorder (BPD), but in this hope lies a cautionary tale. In the 1980s, work on BPD (especially that of Robert Post, MD, at the NIMH) suggested that the mood instability that characterized the illness bore a resemblance to characteristics of epilepsy, and hypotheses about the pathophysiologic origins of bipolar disorder evolved.[1,2] Post and others have suggested that a stress model of kindling may be responsible for the onset of mood episodes, and that worsening of the course of illness over time may be due to either kindling or sensitization phenomena.[1,2] These hypotheses led directly to the use of carbamazepine (effective as a treatment for partial seizures) for the treatment of mania, and, later, to the use of valproate in BPD. Many anticonvulsants (with different mechanisms for seizure reduction in epilepsy) have been used in BPD, but only three—valproate, lamotrigine, and carbamazepine—have proved effective in any phase of the illness.

Although anticonvulsant therapy in BPD remains attractive, its historical use has often exceeded the limit of the evidence base. The use of gabapentin as a treatment for BPD became popular in the late 1990s, propelled in part by the drug's favorable qualities: no need for blood monitoring, few interactions with other drugs, simple metabolism, and the perception of good tolerability. Even as studies demonstrated its ineffectiveness for mania (gabapentin was significantly worse than placebo as an adjunctive treatment for mania), its use persisted. Ultimately, Pfizer Incorporated (which had acquired Warner-Lambert, gabapentin's original marketing company) settled a $430 million civil and criminal lawsuit with the United States Justice Department for the inappropriate marketing of the drug.[3] Although the kindling hypothesis has not been abandoned with regard to an understanding of the pathophysiology of BPD, there remains limited evidence in support of the phenomenon.[4] In the NIMH Collaborative Study of Depression, no evidence was found for cycle length shortening in a cohort of patients (followed prospectively) with BPD.[5]

It is likely that the efficacy of anticonvulsant drugs in BPD is independent of their efficacy in epilepsy, in that the mechanisms of mood improvement and relapse prevention may not be the same as those that underlie seizure prevention. Sodium channel inhibition is unlikely to be the primary mechanism underlying efficacy of these compounds in BPD, for example, as newer-generation carbamazepine family drugs and many other anticonvulsants have failed to demonstrate efficacy in BPD.[6] Of the three anticonvulsants currently in use, possible common mechanisms of action include inhibition of phosphatidylinositol recycling, inhibition of glycogen synthase kinase 3-beta signaling, and/or inhibition of histone deacetylases, culminating in the modulation of synaptic plasticity and/or neuronal survival mechanisms.[7] At this point, however, these hypotheses are speculative and the biological mechanisms of anticonvulsant therapy in BPD remain unclear.

Valproic Acid

The acute anti-manic efficacy of valproic acid has been established by several controlled studies, as these randomized and placebo-controlled studies have found divalproex sodium to be an effective and safe treatment for a manic episode, even in cases where lithium treatment previously failed.[8,9] In comparison with lithium, a randomized, open-label trial of 300 patients with acute mania showed no difference between the two medications in mania remission or tolerability at 12 weeks.[10] A meta-analysis of multiple different anti-manic treatments showed that valproate was slightly (but not significantly) less efficacious than lithium, and slightly better tolerated (although as a class, antipsychotics were overall more effective than anticonvulsants and lithium in treating acute mania).[11] The Food and Drug Administration (FDA) has approved divalproex sodium as a treatment for acute mania. There also appears to be a linear relationship between valproate serum concentration and symptom response, and the target dosage with optimal response in acute mania is above 94 μg/ml.[12]

Valproate is not approved by the FDA for maintenance treatment of BPD; in fact, there is growing evidence in disfavor of such a role. The largest trial of valproate for BPD maintenance to date (n = 372) failed to find a difference between valproate, lithium, and placebo for the primary outcome measure (time to any mood episode) for up to 1 year.[13] More recently, a large randomized, open-label trial (the BALANCE study; n = 330) compared valproate and lithium monotherapies in BPD maintenance with combination lithium and valproate, for up to 2 years.[14] This innovative study examined physician intervention for a mood episode as the primary outcome, and utilized an initial run-in period where patients were stabilized on both medications before randomization to different maintenance arms, which ensured patient tolerance to either medication. The study found that patients on combination lithium and valproate were significantly less likely to relapse compared to patients on valproate alone, and were as equally likely to relapse as patients on lithium alone. The study was not designed to compare valproate and lithium monotherapies directly, although it appeared that lithium monotherapy was more effective than valproate alone. Thus valproate monotherapy is not recommended for maintenance therapy of BPD. For patients on valproate alone, the study indicates there is a potential benefit of adding lithium for maintenance, although the question remains whether patients should simply be on lithium alone in the first place. It is intriguing that the same investigators who demonstrated a role for divalproex sodium in acute mania treatment conducted a second, randomized double-blind study of the same drug in the same setting, but subsequently found no difference between divalproex sodium and placebo in acute mania.[15] The investigators attributed this discrepancy to methodological differences in study design (lower drug dose, allowance of early study termination, more liberal use of adjunctive medications, and 2:1 randomization in favor of study drug); however, in the context of other well-established options for acute mania treatment and BPD maintenance therapy, one wonders whether overall use of valproate for any phase of BPD should be limited.

Anticonvulsants, including valproate, are often viewed as more effective in rapid cycling than is lithium. However, it appears that this may not be the case. In a rigorous and ambitious double-blind study, rapid-cycling patients were stabilized on open-label lithium and divalproex sodium and then randomized in a double-blind fashion to either lithium or divalproex and followed prospectively.[16] There were no significant differences between the lithium-treated or the valproate-treated groups in time to drop-out or time to additional psychopharmacology.

Lastly, there is inadequate data to support a role for valproate in acute bipolar depression. Two independent meta-analyses of four randomized placebo-controlled trials suggested possible efficacy in acute depressive symptoms of BPD; however, the study sizes were very small (n = 9–28).[17,18] These findings will need to be replicated before valproate can be recommended for this indication.

Lamotrigine

Lamotrigine represents a significant advance in the long-term management of bipolar depression, especially given the prominent burden of depression and depressive relapses in BPD.[19-23] Lamotrigine is approved for the maintenance treatment of BPD, and is efficacious when compared to placebo in maintenance studies.[24] Long-term studies found an overall reduction in bipolar depressive relapse compared with placebo. In a key study in which patients who were most recently depressed were first stabilized on lamotrigine and randomly assigned to maintenance treatment with lamotrigine, lithium, or placebo, the overall sustained response rate was 57% with lamotrigine, compared with 46% for lithium, and 45% for placebo; this indicates that lamotrigine is effective in the prevention of relapse to depression when compared with placebo.[21] It is important to note, however, that a substantial proportion (43%) of bipolar patients remained unprotected against a depression relapse by continuation lamotrigine.

The evidence for efficacy of lamotrigine in the treatment of acute bipolar depression, on the other hand, remains limited. No single trial of the drug for acute bipolar depression found the drug better than placebo on the primary outcome measure of the study.[25] One widely referenced study found that while lamotrigine was not statistically different from placebo for total Hamilton Depression Rating Scale (HDRS) scores, it was superior on several other measures, including the Montgomery-Asberg Depression Rating Scale (MADRS) and the Clinical Global Impression Improvement (CGI-I) scale.[19]

This effect has never been replicated in individual trials, but a meta-analysis and meta-regression of pooled individual data from all five lamotrigine trials in acute bipolar depression (both bipolar I and II disorders) found that response (defined as a ≥ 50% decrease in scores) on both the HDRS and the MADRS was significantly greater than for placebo.[26] The effect size was small, however, and the number-needed-to-treat was about 11; a finding the authors note is at the "margins" of clinical utility. Remission was greater than placebo on the MADRS, but not the HDRS. The antidepressant effect of lamotrigine was greatest in the most severely depressed subjects in a subgroup analysis. These data suggest that any potential benefit of lamotrigine in acute depression is likely to be small, except perhaps in severely depressed patients. It is notable that the study of lamotrigine in maintenance of bipolar depression was designed to follow patients after they were first stabilized on lamotrigine for an acute depressive episode[21]; taken together, these studies suggest that lamotrigine should be continued for maintenance therapy in patients who responded to lamotrigine during acute bipolar depression, and that the patients most likely to respond are those who are most severely depressed.

A small randomized, double-blind study was performed comparing lamotrigine versus placebo as add-on medications to lithium in acutely depressed bipolar patients, and showed that lamotrigine plus lithium significantly improved MADRS scores at the end of week 8 versus lithium alone.[27] In order to be eligible for the study, however, patients had to be depressed despite taking a therapeutic dose of lithium for at least 2 weeks (most had been taking for at least 3 months), suggesting that this study population was likely enriched for non-responders to lithium monotherapy. The study also consisted of only 124 patients, and needs to be replicated. Subsequent follow-up of these patients showed that lamotrigine plus lithium was approximately as effective as lithium alone for preventing mood relapse or recurrence up to 68 weeks; however, the small sample size and the study design precluded formal statistical analyses.[28] At this point, evidence for any additional benefit of lamotrigine–lithium combination therapy in treating BPD, versus either of these medications alone, remains limited.

Lamotrigine has not demonstrated efficacy for the acute treatment of mania. Multiple treatments meta-analysis of antimanic drugs also indicated that lamotrigine is not more effective than placebo in treating acute mania.[11] No single trial found benefit for lamotrigine in the prevention of manic episodes; however, pooled analysis revealed a small but significant effect size for the prevention of mania.[21,24,29] While lamotrigine is more effective than lithium in the prevention of depressive episodes, lithium appears to be more effective than lamotrigine in preventing manic episodes.

No validated treatments for treatment-refractory bipolar depression exist, but a small, randomized, open-label trial of adjunctive lamotrigine, risperidone, or inositol in subjects who had depression in spite of trials of two consecutive standard antidepressants of adequate dose and duration was conducted as part of the Systematic Treatment Enhancement Program for Bipolar Disorder (STEP-BD).[30] An equipoise randomization process allowed subjects to choose to be randomized to any pair of the study treatments. While no differences were found in primary pair-wise comparisons in randomized patients (n = 66), a secondary, post-hoc analysis found that 8 weeks of sustained recovery were seen in 23.8% of the lamotrigine-treated patients, 17.4% of inositol-treated patients, and 4.6% of risperidone-treated patients. These data must be viewed cautiously, as they are from a secondary analysis, but they represent one of few studies for the treatment of refractory bipolar depression.

Carbamazepine

Carbamazepine was the first anticonvulsant studied as a treatment of mania. More than 19 studies (most of which were small case series or open trials) evaluated carbamazepine for the treatment of mania, and until recently it was used in BPD despite little scientific support for its use. More recently, carbamazepine (in extended-release form) was found to be effective for acute mania in two large placebo-controlled trials.[31,32] Multiple treatments meta-analysis of anti-manic drugs showed that carbamazepine was similar to valproate in terms of efficacy and acceptability in treating acute mania; however, all anticonvulsants as a class were outperformed by atypical antipsychotics.[11] There are no data directly establishing carbamazepine as an effective maintenance treatment in BPD. A meta-analysis of four small studies comparing efficacy of carbamazepine versus lithium in BPD maintenance suggested a possible similarity in relapse rates; however, this was tempered by the finding that carbamazepine use was associated with significantly more study withdrawals due to adverse effects.[33] At present, there are insufficient data to suggest that carbamazepine is more effective in these patients than any other treatment.

PHARMACOKINETICS, PHARMACODYNAMICS, ADVERSE EFFECTS, AND MONITORING
Valproic Acid

Valproic acid (di-n-propylacetic acid) is an anticonvulsant drug chemically unrelated to other psychiatric medications. One of the more commonly used preparations is divalproex sodium (Depakote), a compound of sodium valproate and valproic acid in a 1:1 molar ratio. Valproate is available as tablets (both delayed- and extended-release), capsules, enteric-coated capsules, sprinkles, and syrup. Absorption is different across the different preparations and it is delayed by ingestion of food. This may be of some importance when one switches from one preparation to another. Peak plasma levels are achieved between 2 and 4 hours after ingestion of the direct-release preparation, and the half-life ranges from 6 to 16 hours. More than 90% of plasma valproic acid is protein-bound. The time of dosing is determined by possible side effects, and, if tolerated, a once-a-day dosing could be employed. The therapeutic plasma levels generally used for the treatment of mania are the same as those used for anticonvulsant therapy (50–100 µg/ml), and the total daily dosage required to achieve these levels ranges from 500 mg to greater than 1,500 mg, although one study suggests a direct relationship between plasma valproate levels and response in acute mania, suggesting optimal levels in acute treatment of greater than 90 µg/ml.[12]

Valproic acid is metabolized by the hepatic CYP 2D6 system but, unlike carbamazepine, does not auto-induce its own metabolism. Concomitant administration of carbamazepine will decrease plasma levels of valproic acid, and drugs that inhibit the CYP system (e.g., selective serotonin reuptake inhibitors [SSRIs]) can cause an increase in valproic acid levels. Valproate is known to increase the plasma levels of lamotrigine, so it is recommended that the lamotrigine dose be lowered in patients taking valproate. Dose-related and common initial side effects include nausea, tremor, and lethargy. Gastric irritation and nausea can be reduced by dividing the dose or by using enteric-coated preparations. Valproic acid has been associated with potentially fatal hepatic failure, usually occurring within the first 6 months of treatment and most frequently occurring in children under age 2 years and in persons with pre-existing liver disease. Transient, dose-related elevations in liver enzymes can occur in up to 44% of patients. Any change in hepatic function should be followed closely, and patients should be warned to report symptoms of hepatic failure (such as malaise, weakness, lethargy, edema, anorexia, or vomiting). Multiple cases of valproate-associated pancreatitis have also been reported, as has multi-organ failure. These can occur at any point during treatment.

Valproic acid may produce teratogenic effects, including spina bifida (1%) and other neural tube defects. Other potential side effects include weight gain, inhibition of platelet aggregation, hair loss, and severe dermatological reactions (such as Stevens-Johnson syndrome).

There is additional worry that valproate may cause endocrine abnormalities in women. Two hundred and thirty women were evaluated for polycystic ovarian syndrome (PCOS) as part of an ancillary study during the Systematic Treatment Enhancement Program for Bipolar Disorder (STEP-BD). Criteria for PCOS are met when oligomenorrhea (defined as ≤ 9 cycles in the past year) coincides with at least one feature of hyperandrogenism (including hirsutism, acne, male-pattern alopecia, or elevated serum androgen levels); it can ultimately result in an increased risk of type 2 diabetes mellitus, cardiovascular disease, and some types of cancer.[34] Joffe and associates[34] compared the rate of new-onset PCOS in women with BPD taking valproate compared to the rate in those taking other anticonvulsants and lithium. Nine (10.5%) of the 86 valproate users developed treatment-emergent oligomenorrhea with hyperandrogenism, compared to 2 (1.4%) of the 144 valproate non-users. The relative risk for developing PCOS on valproate versus on non-valproate mood stabilizers was 7.5 (95% confidence interval, 1.7 to 34.1, p = 0.02).[34] The onset of oligomenorrhea usually began within 12 months of the beginning of valproate treatment.[34] A later analysis found that discontinuation of valproate in women with valproate-associated PCOS may result in an improvement of the PCOS reproductive features, as these symptoms resolved in three of the four women who discontinued valproate, but persisted in all three women who continued on valproate.[35]

Because of the risk of PCOS in women of child-bearing age who are exposed to valproate-containing products, the use of valproate as a first-line treatment for BPD is not recommended in these patients.

Lamotrigine

Lamotrigine was originally developed and approved for use as an anticonvulsant. The mechanism of action of lamotrigine in BPD is not precisely known, although lamotrigine appears to block voltage-gated sodium channels in vitro, and decrease pre-synaptic release of glutamate.[36] Lamotrigine is a weak dihydrofolate reductase inhibitor in vitro and in animal studies, but no effect on folate concentrations has been noted in human studies.[36] It is absorbed within 1–3 hours and has a half-life of 25 hours. Non-serious rash can arise in approximately 8% of adults, but serious rash that requires hospitalization is seen in up to 0.5% of lamotrigine-treated individuals.[36] Because of the possibility of Stevens-Johnson syndrome, toxic epidermal necrolysis, or angioedema, all rashes should be regarded as potentially serious and monitored closely, and to minimize serious rashes the dose should be increased at the rate suggested in the package insert. One randomized, open-label trial of rash precautions during the use of lamotrigine found no benefit from taking additional dermatological precautions (e.g., avoiding use of any other new drugs during dosage titration), but found an overall rash rate of approximately 8% while also finding that only 5.3% of subjects discontinued lamotrigine due to this adverse effect.[37] Dosing is adjusted upward for patients who are simultaneously taking antiepileptics, such as carbamazepine, that induce the metabolism of lamotrigine, and downward for those patients who are simultaneously taking antiepileptics, such as valproate, that may inhibit the clearance of the drug. There is no known relationship between lamotrigine drug levels and response in BPD.

Post-marketing surveillance has revealed an increased risk of fetal anomalies in children born to women exposed to lamotrigine during early pregnancy, specifically oral cleft deformities.[36] One study in the US found five cases of oral clefts in infants in a study of 684 pregnancies (i.e., 7.3 in 1,000 cases) where the mother was taking lamotrigine and no other antiepileptic drugs.[38] This is 10.4-times higher (95% confidence interval 4.3 to 24.9) than a comparison group of unexposed infants (where the prevalance was 0.7 in 1,000).[38] Other large-scale studies have not found such an elevated rate, however, and it remains controversial whether the rate elevation is due to reporting bias.[39]

Carbamazepine

Carbamazepine, an anticonvulsant drug structurally related to the tricyclic antidepressants (TCAs), has variable absorption and metabolism. Carbamazepine is rapidly absorbed (peak plasma levels within 4–6 hours). Eighty percent of plasma carbamazepine is protein-bound. Half-life ranges from 13 to 17 hours. Carbamazepine is metabolized by the hepatic CYP 2D6 system.

Carbamazepine induces the CYP enzymes, causing an increase in the rate of its own metabolism over time (as well as that of other drugs metabolized by the CYP system). Because of this, the dose of the drug should be monitored by serum levels every 2 to 3 months and raised if necessary. Concomitant administration of carbamazepine with oral contraceptives, warfarin, theophylline, doxycycline, haloperidol, TCAs, or valproic acid leads to decreased plasma levels of these other drugs. Concomitant administration of drugs that inhibit the CYP system will increase plasma levels of carbamazepine. These drugs include fluoxetine, cimetidine, erythromycin, isoniazid, calcium channel blockers, and propoxyphene. Concomitant administration of phenobarbital, phenytoin, and primidone causes a decrease in carbamazepine levels through induction of the CYP enzymes.

Based on its use as an anticonvulsant, dosages of carbamazepine typically range from 400 mg to 1,200 mg/day, and therapeutic plasma levels range from 4 to 12 µg/ml. The relationship between blood levels and response in mania is unknown.

Carbamazepine frequently causes lethargy, sedation, nausea, tremor, ataxia, and visual disturbances during the acute-treatment phase. Some patients can develop mild leukopenia or thrombocytopenia during this phase, although it typically does not progress. Carbamazepine causes a rare but severe form of aplastic anemia or agranulocytosis—estimated to occur with an incidence of about 2 to 5 per 100,000, which is 11 times the incidence in the general population. Although the vast majority of these reactions occur during the first 3 months of therapy, some cases have been reported as late as 5 years after the start of therapy treatment. If the white blood cell count drops below 3,000 cells/mm³, the medication should be discontinued.

Carbamazepine has also been associated with fetal anomalies, including a risk of spina bifida (1%), low birth weight, and small head circumference. It has also been shown to have effects on cardiac conduction, slowing atrioventricular conduction. Other reported side effects include inappropriate secretion of antidiuretic hormone with concomitant hyponatremia, decreased thyroid hormone levels without changes in levels of thyroid-stimulating hormone, severe dermatological reactions (such as Stevens-Johnson syndrome), and hepatitis.

Because of the cardiac, hematological, endocrine, and renal side effects associated with carbamazepine, patients should have the drug initiated with care. A recent physical examination, complete blood count (CBC) with platelet count, liver function tests, thyroid function tests, and renal function tests are necessary before the start of the drug. The CBC (with platelets) and liver function tests should be monitored every 2–3 weeks during the initial 3–4 months of treatment, and yearly after stabilization of the dose. Any abnormalities in the tests listed above should be evaluated, especially decreases in neutrophils and sodium. As with TCAs, carbamazepine shares the risk of hypertensive crisis when co-administered with monoamine oxidase inhibitors, and so this combination should be avoided.

OTHER ANTICONVULSANTS
Oxcarbazepine

Oxcarbazepine, a keto-analog of carbamazepine, is purported to have fewer side effects and drug–drug interactions than carbamazepine, but evidence of its efficacy in mania is absent. There are no published placebo-controlled studies of oxcarbazepine in adults with BPD, and the single published double-blind, placebo-controlled trial of oxcarbazepine in children and adolescents with BPD found no difference between drug and placebo.[40] There are a few small studies comparing oxcarbazepine with other anti-manic agents that have not found any difference in efficacy.[41] Because it is now available as a generic drug, it is unlikely that any definitive trials of this drug for BPD will ever be completed.

Gabapentin

Gabapentin was for a time a popular treatment for mania, likely because of perceptions of good tolerability and ease of use and because of aggressive marketing by the drug's manufacturer, Warner-Lambert. Two double-blind studies failed to detect anti-manic or antidepressant effect of gabapentin (one found an antidepressant effect for lamotrigine, however).[42] One double-blind, placebo-controlled study of adjunctive gabapentin in acute mania actually found that the anti-manic response to placebo was statistically significantly greater than for the drug.[43] Current evidence does not support the use of gabapentin in any phase of BPD.

Levetiracetam

Levetiracetam is an adjunctive treatment for complex partial seizures, and its mechanism of antiepileptic action remains unknown. It has had mixed results in several open-label trials as monotherapy or adjunctive therapy in bipolar mania. In one open-label trial, a proportion of the subjects had marked mood worsening.[44] Recently, a randomized, double-blind trial of adjunctive levetiracetam versus placebo in the treatment of acute bipolar depression showed no difference between the two groups in mean change of HDRS ratings at week 6.[45] At this time, more evidence is needed to determine the safety and efficacy of the compound before it can be used in BPD.

Pregabalin

Pregabalin binds voltage-gated calcium channels, and is used in the treatment of fibromyalgia and neuropathic pain. It has also been approved in Europe, but not the US, for the treatment of anxiety. A recent meta-analysis of randomized controlled trials in generalized anxiety disorder showed a small, but statistically significant, effect of pregabalin on the Hamilton Anxiety Rating Scale (HARS), compared to placebo.[46] For BPD, one open-label trial found that the use of adjunctive pregabalin in treatment-refractory bipolar patients improved mood in 41% of patients, as measured by CGI-BP; however, these data are preliminary.[47] The authors of the study also cited an unpublished double-blind, placebo-controlled trial by Pfizer, Inc., that showed no difference between pregabalin and placebo in the treatment of acute mania. Thus, further data are needed to support the use of pregabalin in the treatment of BPD, although there is substantial evidence supporting its use in generalized anxiety disorder.

Tiagabine

Tiagabine is a potent selective inhibitor of the principal neuronal gamma-aminobutyric acid (GABA) transporter (GAT-1) in the cortex and hippocampus, and it is marketed as an antiepileptic compound. There are no published parallel-group trials of tiagabine in BPD. While there has been hope for this drug as a monotherapy or adjunctive treatment for mania, there have been serious concerns about adverse effects in patients treated with it, including syncope and seizures. A recent Cochrane review found little rigorous data for tiagabine in BPD to recommend its use.[48]

Topiramate

Topiramate is an anticonvulsant that inhibits voltage-gated sodium channels, antagonizes kainate and alpha-amino-3-hydroxy-5-methyl-4-isoxazole propionic acid (AMPA) glutamate receptors, and potentiates the $GABA_A$ receptor, although its mechanism of action in the treatment of seizures remains unknown. Although case reports and uncontrolled trials suggested efficacy for topiramate in the treatment of acute bipolar mania, controlled trials have not demonstrated this effect.[49] These do not appear to be failed trials (i.e., ones in which the study was not able to demonstrate an effect that was actually there), as the active comparator in some of the trials, lithium, was effective in reducing manic symptoms in those studies.

Zonisamide

The antiepileptic mechanism of zonisamide is unknown. Recently, a randomized, double-blind trial of adjunctive zonisamide in the treatment of acute bipolar mania/hypomania showed no difference in efficacy between zonisamide and placebo adjunctive groups.[50] In a large, open-label, 56-week trial of zonisamide for acute and continuation treatment in BPD, McElroy and associates[51] found that while some patients may have had improvements in mood, a high proportion of subjects dropped out of the study due to adverse effects or worsening of mood. Any beneficial effects of zonisamide on weight loss may be mitigated by concerns about the safety of the drug in BPD.

CONCLUSION

In spite of great promise, anticonvulsants, as a class of medications, have limited usefulness in the treatment of BPD (Table 9-1). Three anticonvulsants have proven effective in different phases of BPD (valproate, lamotrigine, and carbamazepine), but each has specific (and not broad) efficacy in the disorder. Other anticonvulsants have proved ineffective in rigorous trials or have not been adequately studied.

It is difficult to argue that unproven anticonvulsants have a place in the treatment of any phase of BPD—even if they have

TABLE 9-1 Anticonvulsants for Bipolar Disorder

	Acute Mania	Acute Depression	Maintenance
Valproate	+	–	–
Carbamazepine	+	–	–
Lamotrigine	–	+/–	+

a theoretically favorable side-effect profile—as there are now multiple evidence-based treatments for acute mania, acute depression, and relapse prevention in BPD. There is ongoing concern in the epilepsy literature that anticonvulsants, such as zonisamide and topiramate, may induce mood syndromes in patients with seizure disorders.[52] While BPD is often a life-threatening and disabling illness, anticonvulsants without proven efficacy in BPD must be used with caution in this illness, and it is prudent to wait until firm evidence allows clinicians and patients to make informed decisions regarding defined benefits and known harm before initiating these agents.

Access a list of MCQs for this chapter at https://expertconsult .inkling.com

REFERENCES

1. Post RM, Uhde TW, Putnam F, et al. Kindling and carbamazepine in affective illness. *J Nerv Ment Dis* 170(12):717–731, 1982.
2. Post RM. Cocaine psychoses: a continuum model. *Am J Psychiatry* 132(3):225–231, 1975.
3. Lenzer J. Pfizer pleads guilty, but drug sales continue to soar. *BMJ* 328(7450):1217, 2004.
4. Bender RE, Alloy LB. Life stress and kindling in bipolar disorders: review of the evidence and integration with emerging biopsychosocial theories. *Clin Psychol Rev* 31(3):383–398, 2011.
5. Turvey CL, Coryell WH, Solomon DA, et al. Long-term prognosis of bipolar I disorder. *Acta Psychiatr Scand* 99(2):110–119, 1999.
6. Bialer M. Why are antiepileptic drugs used for nonepileptic conditions? *Epilepsia* 53(Suppl. 7):26–33, 2012.
7. Rogawski MA, Loscher W. The neurobiology of antiepileptic drugs for the treatment of nonepileptic conditions. *Nature Med* 10(7):685–692, 2004.
8. Bowden CL, Swann AC, Calabrese JR, et al. A randomized, placebo-controlled, multicenter study of divalproex sodium extended release in the treamtent of acute mania. *J Clin Psychiatry* 67(10):1501–1510, 2006.
9. Pope HG, McElroy SL, Keck PE, et al. Valproate in the treamtent of acute mania. A placebo-controlled study. *Arch Gen Psychiatry* 48(1):62–68, 1991.
10. Bowden C, Gogus A, Grunze H, et al. A 12-week, open, randomized trial comparing sodium valproate to lithium in patients with bipolar I disorder suffering from a manic episode. *Int Clin Psychopharm* 23(5):254–262, 2008.
11. Cipriani A, Barbui C, Salanti G, et al. Comparative efficacy and acceptability of antimanic drugs in acute mania: a multiple-treatments meta-analysis. *Lancet* 378(9799):1306–1315, 2011.
12. Allen MH, Hirschfeld RM, Wozniak PJ, et al. Linear relationship of valproate serum concentration to response and optimal serum levels for acute mania. *Am J Psychiatry* 163(2):272–275, 2006.
13. Bowden CL, Calabrese JR, McElroy SL, et al. A randomized, placebo-controlled 12-month trial of divalproex and lithium in treatment of outpatients with bipolar I disorder. Divalproex Maintenance Study Group. *Arch Gen Psychiatry* 57:481–489, 2000.
14. BALANCE investigators and collaborators, Geddes J, Goodwin GM, et al. Lithium plus valproate combination therapy versus monotherapy for relapse prevention in bipolar I disorder (BALANCE): a randomised open-label trial. *Lancet* 375(9712):385–395, 2010.
15. Hirschfeld RMA, Bowden CL, Vigna NV, et al. A randomized, placebo-controlled, multicenter study of divalproex sodium extended-release in the acute treatment of mania. *J Clin Psychiatry* 71(4):426–432, 2010.

16. Calabrese JR, Shelton MD, Rapport DJ, et al. A 20-month, double-blind, maintenance trial of lithium versus divalproex in rapid cycling bipolar disorder. *Am J Psychiatry* 162:2152–2161, 2005.

17. Bond DJ, Lam RW, Yatham LN. Divalproex sodium versus placebo in the treatment of acute bipolar depression: a systematic review and meta-analysis. *J Affect Disord* 124(3):228–234, 2010.

18. Smith LA, Cornelius VR, Azorin JM, et al. Valproate for the treatment of acute bipolar depression: systematic review and meta-analysis. *J Affect Disord* 124(3):228–234, 2010.

19. Calabrese JR, Bowden CL, Sachs GS, et al. A double-blind placebo-controlled study of lamotrigine monotherapy in outpatients with bipolar I depression. Lamictal 602 Study Group. *J Clin Psychiatry* 60:79–88, 1999.

20. Calabrese JR, Suppes T, Bowden CL, et al. A double-blind, placebo-controlled, prophylaxis study of lamotrigine in rapid-cycling bipolar disorder. Lamictal 614 Study Group. *J Clin Psychiatry* 61:841–850, 2000.

21. Calabrese JR, Bowden CL, Sachs G, et al. A placebo-controlled 18-month trial of lamotrigine and lithium maintenance treatment in recently depressed patients with bipolar I disorder. *J Clin Psychiatry* 64:1013–1024, 2003.

22. Judd LL, Akiskal HS, Schettler PJ, et al. The long-term natural history of the weekly symptomatic status of bipolar I disorder. *Arch Gen Psychiatry* 59:530–537, 2002.

23. Judd LL, Akiskal HS, Schettler PJ, et al. A prospective investigation of the natural history of the long-term weekly symptomatic status of bipolar II disorder. *Arch Gen Psychiatry* 60:261–269, 2003.

24. Goodwin GM, Bowden CL, Calabrese JR, et al. A pooled analysis of 2 placebo-controlled 18-month trials of lamotrigine and lithium maintenance in bipolar I disorder. *J Clin Psychiatry* 65:432–441, 2004.

25. Calabrese JR, Huffman RF, White RL, et al. Lamotrigine in the acute treatment of bipolar depression: results of five double-blind, placebo-controlled clinical trials. *Bipolar Disord* 10(2):323–333, 2008.

26. Geddes JR, Calabrese JR, Goodwin GM. Lamotrigine for treatment of bipolar depression: independent meta-analysis and meta-regression of individual patient data from five randomised trials. *Br J Psychiatry* 194(1):4–9, 2009.

27. van der Loos MDM, Mulder PGH, Hartong EGThM, LamLit Study Group. Efficacy and safety of lamotrigine as add-on treatment to lithium in bipolar depression: a multicenter, double-blind, placebo-controlled trial. *J Clin Psychiatry* 70(2):223–231, 2009.

28. van der Loos MDM, Mulder P, Hartong EGThM, LamLit Study Group. Long-term outcome of bipolar depressed patients receiving lamotrigine as add-on to lithium with the possibility of the addition of paroxetine in nonresponders: a randomized, placebo-controlled trial with a novel design. *Bipolar Disord* 13(1):111–117, 2011.

29. Bowden CL, Calabrese JR, Sachs G, et al. A placebo-controlled 18-month trial of lamotrigine and lithium maintenance treatment in recently manic or hypomanic patients with bipolar I disorder. *Arch Gen Psychiatry* 60:392–400, 2003.

30. Nierenberg AA, Ostacher MJ, Calabrese JR, et al. Treatment-resistant bipolar depression: a STEP-BD equipoise randomized effectiveness trial of antidepressant augmentation with lamotrigine, inositol, or risperidone. *Am J Psychiatry* 163:210–216, 2006.

31. Weisler RH, Kalali AH, Ketter TA, SPD417 Study Group. A multicenter, randomized, double-blind, placebo-controlled trial of extended-release carbamazepine capsules as monotherapy for bipolar disorder patients with manic or mixed episodes. *J Clin Psychiatry* 65(4):478–484, 2004.

32. Weisler RH, Keck PE Jr, Swann AC, SPD417 Study Group. Extended-release carbamazepine capsules as monotherapy for acute mania in bipolar disorder: a multicenter, randomized, double-blind, placebo-controlled trial. *J Clin Psychiatry* 66(3):323–330, 2005.

33. Ceron-Litvoc D, Soares BG, Geddes J, et al. Comparison of carbamazepine and lithium in treatment of bipolar disorder: a systematic review of randomized controlled trials. *Hum Psychopharmacol Clin Exp* 24:19–28, 2009.

34. Joffe H, Cohen LS, Suppes T, et al. Valproate is associated with new-onset oligoamenorrhea with hyperandrogenism in women with bipolar disorder. *Biol Psychiatry* 59(11):1078–1086, 2006.

35. Joffe H, Cohen LS, Suppes T, et al. Longitudinal follow-up of reproductive and metabolic features of valproate-associated polycystic ovarian syndrome features: a preliminary report. *Biol Psychiatry* 60(12):1378–1381, 2006.

36. Lamictal (lamotrigine) package insert, 2006, GlaxoSmithKline.

37. Ketter TA, Greist JH, Graham JA, et al. The effect of dermatologic precautions on the incidence of rash with addition of lamotrigine in the treatment of bipolar I disorder: a randomized trial. *J Clin Psychiatry* 67(3):400–406, 2006.

38. Holmes LB, Baldwin EJ, Smith CR, et al. Increased frequency of isolated cleft palate in infants exposed to lamotrigine during pregnancy. *Neurology* 70(22):2152–2158, 2008.

39. Hunt SJ, Craig JJ, Morrow JI. Comment on: Increased frequency of isolated cleft palate in infants exposed to lamotrigine during pregnancy. *Neurology* 72(12):1108, 2009.

40. Wagner KD, Kowatch RA, Emslie GJ, et al. A double-blind, randomized, placebo-controlled trial of oxcarbazepine in the treatment of bipolar disorder in children and adolescents. *Am J Psychiatry* 163(7):1179–1186, 2006.

41. Vasudev A, Macritchie K, Vasudev K, et al. Oxcarbazepine for acute affective episodes in bipolar disorder. *Cochrane Database Syst Rev* 7(12):CD004857, 2011.

42. Frye MA, Ketter TA, Kimbrell TA, et al. A placebo-controlled study of lamotrigine and gabapentin in refractory mood disorders. *J Clin Psychopharmacol* 20:607–614, 2000.

43. Pande AC, Crockatt JG, Janney CA, et al. Gabapentin in bipolar disorder: a placebo-controlled trial of adjunctive therapy. Gabapentin Bipolar Disorder Study Group. *Bipolar Disord* 2:249–255, 2000.

44. Post RM, Altshuler LL, Frye MA, et al. Preliminary observations on the effectiveness of levetiracetam in the open adjunctive treatment of refractory bipolar disorder. *J Clin Psychiatry* 66(3):370–374, 2005.

45. Saricicek A, Maloney K, Muralidharan A, et al. Levetiracetam in the management of bipolar depression: a randomized, double-blind, placebo-controlled trial. *J Clin Psychiatry* 72(6):744–750, 2011.

46. Boschen MJ. A meta-analysis of the efficacy of pregabalin in the treatment of generalized anxiety disorder. *Can J Psychiatry* 56(9):558–566, 2011.

47. Schaffer LC, Schaffer CB, Miller AR, et al. An open trial of pregabalin as an acute and maintenance adjunctive treatment for outpatients with treatment resistant bipolar disorder. *J Affect Disord* 147(1–3):407–410, 2013.

48. Vasudev A, Macritchie K, Rao SNK, et al. Tiagabine in the maintenance treatment of bipolar disorder. *Cochrane Database Syst Rev* 7(12):CD005173, 2012.

49. Kushner SF, Khan A, Lane R, et al. Topiramate monotherapy in the management of acute mania: results of four double-blind placebo-controlled trials. *Bipolar Disord* 8(1):15–27, 2006.

50. Dauphinais D, Knable M, Rosenthal J, et al. Zonisamide for bipolar disorder, mania, or mixed states: a randomized, double blind, placebo-controlled adjunctive trial. *Psychopharmacol Bull* 44(1):5–17, 2011.

51. McElroy SL, Suppes T, Keck PE Jr, et al. Open-label adjunctive zonisamide in the treatment of bipolar disorders: a prospective trial. *J Clin Psychiatry* 66(5):617–624, 2005.

52. Mula M, Sander JW. Negative effects of antiepileptic drugs on mood in patients with epilepsy. *Drug Saf* 30(7):555–567, 2007.

10 Stimulants and Other Medications for ADHD

Jefferson B. Prince, MD, Timothy E. Wilens, MD, Thomas J. Spencer, MD, and Joseph Biederman, MD

KEY POINTS

- Attention-deficit/hyperactivity disorder (ADHD) is a common disorder in children, adolescents, and adults.
- While the phenotype of ADHD changes across the life span, ADHD persists in many children, adolescents, and adults.
- Formulations of stimulant and non-stimulant medications are Food and Drug Administration-approved as pharmacological treatments for ADHD in children, adolescents, and adults.
- Co-morbid psychiatric and learning disorders are common in patients with ADHD across the life span.
- When treating ADHD and co-morbid disorders, clinicians must prioritize and treat the most severe condition first, and regularly re-assess the symptoms of ADHD and the co-morbid disorder.

OVERVIEW

Attention-deficit/hyperactivity disorder (ADHD) is a common psychiatric condition shown to occur in 3% to 10% of school-age children worldwide, up to 8% of adolescents and up to 4% of adults.[1-5] The classic triad of impaired attention, impulsivity, and excessive motor activity characterizes ADHD, although many patients may manifest only inattentive symptoms.[6,7] ADHD usually persists, to a significant degree, from childhood through adolescence and into adulthood.[8,9] Most children, adolescents, and adults with ADHD suffer significant functional impairment(s) in multiple domains,[10] as well as co-morbid psychiatric or learning disorders.[5,11-18]

Studies demonstrate that ADHD is frequently co-morbid with oppositional defiant disorder (ODD), conduct disorder (CD), multiple anxiety disorders (panic disorder, obsessive-compulsive disorder [OCD], tic disorders), mood disorders (e.g., depression, dysthymia, and bipolar disorder [BPD]), learning disorders (e.g., auditory processing problems and dyslexia), and substance use disorders (SUDs) and often complicates the development of patients with autism spectrum disorders (ASDs). Co-morbid psychiatric, learning, and developmental disorders need to be assessed in all patients with ADHD and the relationship of these symptoms with ADHD delineated.[1,19,20]

Before using medications, clinicians should complete a through clinical evaluation that includes a complete history of symptoms, a differential diagnosis, a review of prior assessments/treatments, a medical history, and a description of current physical symptoms (including questions about the physical history, including either a personal or family history of cardiovascular symptoms or problems). Before treatment with medications, it is usually important to measure baseline levels of height, weight, blood pressure, and pulse and to monitor them over the course of treatment (see http://

www.fda.gov/Drugs/DrugSafety/PostmarketDrugSafety InformationforPatientsandProviders/DrugSafetyInformation forHeathcareProfessionals/ucm165858.htm for the most recent recommendations by the Food and Drug Administration [FDA] about monitoring for children and http://www.fda.gov/drugs/drugsafety/ucm279858.htm for the most recent recommendations about monitoring for adults). Clinicians and patients/families should select an initial treatment, either a stimulant or a non-stimulant; decide on a target dose (either absolute or weight-based) titration schedule; and decide how to monitor tolerability and response to treatment (using rating scales, anchor points, or both). Patients should be educated about the importance of adherence, safely maintaining medications (e.g., as in college students), and additional types of treatment (e.g., coaching and organizational help) that may be helpful.

STIMULANTS

For over 60 years stimulants have been used safely and effectively in the treatment of ADHD[21] and they are among the most well-established treatments in psychiatry.[22,23] The stimulants most commonly used include methylphenidate (MPH), a mixture of amphetamine salts (MAS) and dextroamphetamine (DEX). The recent development of various novel delivery systems has significantly advanced the pharmacotherapy of ADHD (see Table 10-1 for a list of these medications).

Pharmacodynamic Properties of Stimulants

Stimulants increase intra-synaptic concentrations of dopamine (DA) and norepinephrine (NE).[24-27] MPH primarily binds to the DA transporter protein (DAT), blocking the re-uptake of DA, increasing intra-synaptic DA.[25,27] While amphetamines diminish pre-synaptic re-uptake of DA by binding to DAT, these compounds also travel into the DA neuron, promoting release of DA from reserpine-sensitive vesicles in the pre-synaptic neuron.[25,26] In addition, stimulants (amphetamine > MPH) increase levels of NE and serotonin (5-HT) in the inter-neuronal space.[24] Although group studies comparing MPH and amphetamines generally demonstrate similar efficacy,[19,20] their pharmacodynamic differences may explain why a particular patient may respond to, or tolerate, one stimulant preferentially over another. It is necessary to appreciate that while the efficacy of amphetamine and MPH is similar, their potency differs, such that 5 mg of amphetamine is approximately equally potent to 10 mg of MPH.

Methylphenidate

As originally formulated, MPH was produced as an equal mixture of d,l-threo-MPH and d,l-erythro-MPH. The erythro isomers of MPH appear to produce side effects, and thus MPH is now manufactured as an equal racemic mixture of d,l-threo-MPH.[28] Behavioral effects of immediate-release MPH peak 1 to 2 hours after administration, and tend to dissipate within 3 to 5 hours. After oral administration immediate-release MPH is readily absorbed, reaching peak plasma concentration in 1.5 to 2.5 hours, and has an elimination half-life of

TABLE 10-1 Available FDA-approved Treatments for Attention-Deficit/Hyperactivity Disorder

Generic Name (Brand Name)	Formulation and Mechanism	Duration of Activity	How Supplied	Usual Absolute and (Weight-based) Dosing Range	FDA-approved Maximum Dose for ADHD
MPH (Ritalin)*	Tablet of 50:50 racemic mixture d,l-threo-MPH	3–4 hours	5, 10, and 20 mg tablets	(0.3–2 mg/kg/day)	60 mg/day
Dex-MPH (Focalin)*	Tablet of d-threo-MPH	3–5 hours	2.5, 5, and 10 mg tablets (2.5 mg Focalin equivalent to 5 mg Ritalin)	(0.15–1 mg/kg/day)	20 mg/day
MPH (Methylin)*	Tablet of 50:50 racemic mixture d,l-threo-MPH	3–4 hours	5, 10, and 20 mg tablets	(0.3–2 mg/kg/day)	60 mg/day
MPH-SR (Ritalin-SR)*	Wax-based matrix tablet of 50:50 racemic mixture d,l-threo-MPH	3–8 hours Variable	20 mg tablets (amount absorbed appears to vary)	(0.3–2 mg/kg/day)	60 mg/day
MPH (Metadate ER)*	Wax-based matrix tablet of 50:50 racemic mixture d,l-threo-MPH	3–8 hours Variable	10 and 20 mg tablets (amount absorbed appears to vary)	(0.3–2 mg/kg/day)	60 mg/day
MPH (Methylin ER)*	Hydroxypropyl methylcellulose base tablet of 50:50 racemic mixture d,l-threo-MPH; no preservatives	8 hours	10 and 20 mg tablets 2.5, 5, and 10 mg chewable tablets 5 mg/5 ml and 10 mg/5 ml oral solution	(0.3–2 mg/kg/day)	60 mg/day
MPH (Ritalin LA)*	Two types of beads give bimodal delivery (50% immediate-release and 50% delayed-release) of 50:50 racemic mixture d,l-threo-MPH	8 hours	20, 30, and 40 mg capsules; can be sprinkled	(0.3–2 mg/kg/day)	60 mg/day
D-MPH (Focalin XR)	Two types of beads give bimodal delivery (50% immediate-release and 50% delayed-release) of d-threo-MPH	12 hours	5, 10, 15, 20, 25, 30, 35, and 40 mg capsules	0.15–1 mg/kg/day	30 mg/day in youth; 40 mg/day in adults
MPH (Metadate CD)*	Two types of beads give bimodal delivery (30% immediate-release and 70% delayed-release) of 50:50 racemic mixture d,l-threo-MPH	8 hours	20 mg capsule; can be sprinkled	(0.3–2 mg/kg/day)	60 mg/day
MPH (Daytrana)*	MPH transdermal system	12 hours (patch worn for 9 hours)	10, 15, 20, and 30 mg patches	0.3–2 mg/kg/day	30 mg/day
MPH (Concerta)*	Osmotic pressure system delivers 50:50 racemic mixture d,l-threo-MPH	12 hours	18, 27, 36, and 54 mg caplets	(0.3–2 mg/kg/day)	72 mg/day
MPH (Quillivant XR)	Extended-release liquid	12 hours	25 mg/5 ml	(0.3–2 mg/kg/day)	60 mg/day
AMPH† (Dexedrine Tablets)	d-AMPH tablet	4–5 hours	5 mg tablets	(0.15–1 mg/kg/day)	40 mg/day
AMPH† (Dextrostat)	d-AMPH tablet	4–5 hours	5 and 10 mg tablets	(0.15–1 mg/kg/day)	40 mg/day
AMPH† (Dexedrine Spansules)	Two types of beads in a 50:50 mixture short and delayed-absorption of d-AMPH	8 hours	5, 10, and 15 mg capsules	(0.15–1 mg/kg/day)	40 mg/day
Mixed salts of AMPH† (Adderall)	Tablet of d,l-AMPH isomers (75% d-AMPH and 25% l-AMPH)	4–6 hours	5, 7.5, 10, 12.5, 15, 20, and 30 mg tablets	(0.15–1 mg/kg/day)	40 mg/day
Mixed salts of AMPH*‡ (Adderall-XR)	Two types of beads give bimodal delivery (50% immediate-release and 50% delayed-release) of 75:25 racemic mixture d,l-AMPH	At least 8 hours (but appears to last much longer in certain patients)	5, 10, 15, 20, 25, and 30 mg capsules; can be sprinkled	(0.15–1 mg/kg/day)	30 mg/day in children Recommended dose is 20 mg/day in adults

TABLE 10-1 Available FDA-approved Treatments for Attention-Deficit/Hyperactivity Disorder *(Continued)*

Generic Name (Brand Name)	Formulation and Mechanism	Duration of Activity	How Supplied	Usual Absolute and (Weight-based) Dosing Range	FDA-approved Maximum Dose for ADHD
Lisdexamfetamine (Vyvanase)*	Tablets of dextroamphetamine and L-lysine	12 hours	30, 50, and 70 mg tablets		70 mg/day
Atomoxetine*‡ (Strattera)	Capsule of atomoxetine	5 hour plasma half-life but CNS effects appear to last much longer	10, 18, 25, 40, 60, and 80 mg capsules	1.2 mg/kg/day	1.4 mg/kg/day or 100 mg
Guanfacine ER** (Intuniv)	Extended-release tablet of guanfacine	Labeled for once-daily dosing	1,2,3 & 4 mg tablets	Up to 4 mg per day	Up to 4 mg per day
Clonidine ER**(Kapvay)	Extended-release tablet of clonidine	Labeled for twice-daily dosing	0.1 mg tablet	0.1–0.2 mg twice daily	Up to 0.4 mg daily

*Approved to treat ADHD age 6 years and older.
†Approved to treat ADHD age 3 years and older.
‡Specifically approved for treatment of ADHD in adults.
**Approved to treat ADHD in youth 6–17 years old as monotherapy or as adjunctive treatment with stimulant.

2.5–3.5 hours. After oral administration, but prior to reaching the plasma, the enzyme carboxylesterase (CES-1), which is located in the walls of the stomach and liver, extensively metabolizes MPH via hydrolysis and de-esterification, with little oxidation.[29,30] Individual differences in CES-1's hydrolyzing activity may result in variable metabolism and serum MPH levels.[31] While generic MPH has a similar pharmacokinetic profile to Ritalin, it is more rapidly absorbed and peaks sooner.[32] Due to its wax-matrix preparation, the absorption of the sustained-release MPH preparation (Ritalin-SR) is variable,[33] with peak MPH plasma levels in 1 to 4 hours, a half-life of 2 to 6 hours, and behavioral effects that may last up to 8 hours.[34] The availability of the various new extended-delivery stimulant formulations has greatly curtailed use of MPH-SR.

Concerta (OROS-MPH) uses the Osmotic Releasing Oral System (OROS) technology to deliver a 50:50 racemic mixture of d,l-threo-MPH.[35] OROS-MPH, indicated for the treatment of ADHD in children and adolescents, is available in 18, 27, 36, and 54 mg doses and is indicated in doses up to 72 mg daily. The 18 mg caplet of OROS-MPH provides an initial bolus of 4 mg of MPH, delivering the remaining MPH in an ascending pattern, such that peak concentrations are generally reached around 8 hours after dosing; it is labeled for 12 hours of coverage.[28,36] A single morning dose of 18, 27, 36, 54,or 72 mg of OROS-MPH is approximately bioequivalent to 5, 7.5, 10,15,or 20 mg of immediate-release MPH administered three times daily, respectively. The effectiveness and tolerability of OROS-MPH have been demonstrated in children,[37–39] adolescents,[40] and adults[41] with ADHD. Data support OROS-MPH's continued efficacy in many of those with ADHD over the course of 24 months of treatment.[42]

Metadate CD (MPH MR), the first available extended-delivery stimulant preparation to employ beaded technology, is available in capsules of 10, 20, 30, 40, 50, and 60 mg, which may be sprinkled. Using Eurand's Diffucaps technology, MPH MR contains two types of coated beads, IR-MPH and extended-release-MPH (ER-MPH). Metadate delivers 30% of d,l-threo-MPH initially, and 70% of d,l-threo-MPH several hours later. MPH MR is designed to simulate twice-daily (BID) dosing of IR MPH providing approximately 8 hours of coverage. The efficacy of MPH MR capsules has been demonstrated,[43] and it is approved for treatment in youth with ADHD in doses of up to 60 mg/day.[28] An extended-delivery tablet form of Metadate (Metadate ER) is also available in doses of 10 and 20 mg.

Ritalin-LA (MPH-ERC), another beaded-stimulant preparation, which may be sprinkled,[28] is available in capsules of 10, 20, 30, and 40 mg, essentially equivalent to 5, 10, 15 and 20 mg of IR-MPH delivered BID. MPH-ERC uses the beaded Spheroidal Oral Drug Absorption System (SODAS) technology to achieve a bi-modal release profile that delivers 50% of its d,l-threo-MPH initially and another bolus approximately 3 to 4 hours later, providing around 8 hours of coverage. The efficacy of MPH-ERC has been demonstrated in youth with ADHD.[44]

The primarily active form of MPH appears to be the d-threo isomer,[45–47] which is available in both immediate-release tablets (Focalin 2.5, 5, and 10 mg) and, employing the SODAS technology, extended-delivery capsules (Focalin XR 5, 10, 15, and 20 mg). The efficacy of D-MPH is well established in children, adolescents, and adults under open- and double-blind conditions.[48–51] D-MPH is approved to treat ADHD in children, adolescents, and adults in doses of up to 20 mg per day and has been labeled to provide a 12-hour duration of coverage.[28] Although not definitive, 10 mg of MPH appears to be approximately equivalent to 5 mg of d-MPH, and clinicians can reasonably use this estimate in clinical practice.[52]

The MPH transdermal system (MTS; Daytrana) delivers MPH through the skin via the DOT Matrix transdermal system. The patches are applied once daily and intended to be worn for 9 hours, although in clinical practice they can be worn for shorter and longer periods of time. The MTS usually takes effect within 2 hours and provides coverage for 3 hours after removal. MTS is available in 10, 15, 20, and 30 mg patches.[53–55] Since the MPH is absorbed through the skin, it does not undergo first-pass metabolism by CES-1 in the liver, resulting in higher plasma MPH levels.[56] Therefore, patients may require lower doses with MTS compared to oral preparations (10 mg of MTS = 15 mg of extended-release oral MPH). MTS may be a particularly useful treatment option for patients who have difficulty swallowing or tolerating oral stimulant formulations or for patients who need flexibility in the duration of medication effect.

Recently an extended-delivery MPH oral suspension formulation became available (MEROS or Quillivant XR 25 mg/5 ml). Although head-to-head trials haven't been published and clinical experience to date is limited, this formulation appears to provide similar efficacy and duration of effect as other extended-delivery MPH preparations.[57,58] This preparation may be particularly helpful for youth who prefer a liquid preparation or who experience skin reactions to the transdermal patch. Prior to dosing, the manufacturer recommends shaking the contents in the bottle to ensure an even distribution of medication.

Amphetamines

Amphetamine is available in three forms, dextroamphetamine (DEX; Dexedrine), mixed amphetamine salts (MAS; Adderall), and lisdexamfetaminedimesylate (LDX, Vyvanase). DEX tablets achieve peak plasma levels 2 to 3 hours after oral administration, and have a half-life of 4 to 6 hours. Behavioral effects of DEX tablets peak 1 to 2 hours after administration, and last 4 to 5 hours. For DEX spansules, these values are somewhat longer. MAS consist of equal portions of d-amphetamine saccharate, d,l-amphetamine asparate, d-amphetamine sulfate, and d,l-amphetamine sulfate, and a single dose results in a ratio of approximately 3:1 d- to l-amphetamine.[28] The two isomers have different pharmacodynamic properties, and some patients with ADHD preferentially respond to one isomer over another. The efficacy of MAS tablets is well established in ADHD youth[59] and adults.[60] An extended-delivery preparation of MAS is available as a capsule containing two types of Micotrol beads (MAS XR; Adderall XR). The beads are present in a 50:50 ratio, with immediate-release beads designed to release MAS in a fashion similar to MAS tablets, and delayed-release beads designed to release MAS 4 hours after dosing. The efficacy of MAS XR is well established in children,[61,62] adolescents,[63] and adults.[64,65] Furthermore, open treatment with MAS XR appears to be effective in the treatment of many ADHD youths over a 24-month period.[66]

LDX is FDA-approved for treatment of ADHD in children, adolescents, and adults. LDX[28] is an amphetamine pro-drug in which L-lysine, a naturally occurring amino acid, is covalently linked to d-amphetamine. After oral administration, the pro-drug is metabolically hydrolyzed in the body to release d-amphetamine. LDX appears to reduce abuse liability (e.g., misuse, abuse, and overdose) as intravenously and intranasally administered LDX results in similar effects as oral administration.[67,68] It is available in capsules of 20, 30, 40, 50, 60, and 70 mg that appear to be comparable to MAS XR doses of 10, 15, 20, 25, 30, and 35 mg, respectively.

Clinical Use of Stimulants

Guidelines and recent excellent clinical reviews regarding the use of stimulant medications in children, adolescents, and adults in clinical practice have been published.[1,7,19,20,69–72] Treatment with immediate-release preparations generally starts at 5 mg of MPH or amphetamine once daily and is titrated upward every 3 to 5 days until an effect is noted or adverse effects emerge. Typically, the half-life of the short-acting stimulants necessitates at least twice-daily dosing, with the addition of similar or reduced afternoon doses dependent on breakthrough symptoms. In a typical adult, dosing of immediate-release MPH is generally up to 30 mg three to four times daily or amphetamine 15 to 20 mg three to four times a day. Currently, most adults with ADHD will be treated with a stimulant that has an extended delivery. Since there is no way to determine which stimulant will be best tolerated and most effective, it is wise to consider including trials with extended-delivery preparations of both MPH and amphetamine.[73]

Side Effects of Stimulants

Although generally well tolerated, stimulants can cause clinically significant side effects (including anorexia, nausea,

difficulty falling asleep, obsessiveness, headaches, dry mouth, rebound phenomena, anxiety, nightmares, dizziness, irritability, dysphoria, and weight loss).[1,20,74–77] Rates and types of stimulant side effects appear to be similar in ADHD patients, regardless of age. In patients with a current co-morbid mood/anxiety disorder, clinicians should consider whether an adverse effect reflects the co-morbid disorder, a side effect of the treatment, or an exacerbation of the co-morbidity. Moreover, while stimulants can cause these side effects, many ADHD patients experience these problems before treatment; therefore, it is important for clinicians to document these symptoms at baseline.[76] Recommendations about management of some common side effects are listed in Table 10-2.

Growth

The impact of stimulant treatment on growth remains a concern, and the data are conflicting. For instance, in the MTA study, ADHD youth, treated with a stimulant medication continuously over a 24-month period, experienced a deceleration of about 1 cm per year. Despite this slowing, except for those subjects in the lowest percentile for height, these children remained within the normal curves.[78] Recently, Biederman and colleagues reported on growth trajectories in two case-control samples of boys and girls with ADHD compared to controls.[79] Over 10–11 years of follow-up these authors found no significant impact of ADHD or its treatment on growth parameters except in subjects with ADHD and depression, where girls were larger and boys smaller. Despite reassuring data clinicians, parents and patients healthy physical development and these difficulties do not usually pose significant clinical problems for most patients. To effectively address these concerns the AACAP practice parameters for ADHD recommend routine monitoring of height and weight, including serial plotting of growth parameters.[1,20] Crossing two percentile lines of height and/or weight may indicate a clinically significant change in growth that should be addressed clinically. A variety of options may be considered, including a medication holiday, dose adjustment, a change in medication, and/or consultation. Ultimately impact on growth should be balanced with the overall benefits of treatment.

Sleep

Parents often report sleep disturbances in their children with ADHD before[80–83] and during treatment.[84–87] Various strategies (including improving sleep hygiene, making behavioral modifications, adjusting timing or type of stimulant, and switching to an alternative ADHD treatment) have been suggested to help make it easier for patients with ADHD to fall asleep.[88,89] Complementary pharmacological treatments to consider include the following: melatonin (1 to 3 mg), clonidine (0.1 to 0.3 mg),[90] diphenhydramine (25 to 50 mg), trazodone (25 to 50 mg), and mirtazapine (3.75 to 15 mg). Recently, interest in the use of melatonin, a hormone secreted by the pineal gland that helps regulate circadian rhythms,[91] to address sleep problems in children has been growing.[92] Melatonin used alone[93] and in conjunction with sleep hygiene techniques[94] appears to improve sleep in youths with ADHD. In these two well-designed but small studies, the most concerning adverse events included migraine (n = 1), nightmares (n = 1), and aggression (n = 1). Although not yet studied, another consideration is ramelteon, a synthetic melatonin receptor agonist.[95]

Appetite Suppression

Patients treated with stimulants often experience a dose-related reduction in appetite, and in some cases weight loss.[74] Although appetite suppression often decreases over time,[42] clinicians

TABLE 10-2 Pharmacological Strategies in Challenging Cases of Attention-Deficit/Hyperactivity Disorder

Symptoms	Interventions
Worsening or unchanged ADHD symptoms (inattention, impulsivity, hyperactivity)	Change medication dose (increase or decrease) Change timing of dose Change preparation, substitute stimulant Evaluate for possible tolerance Consider adjunctive treatment (antidepressant, alpha-adrenergic agent, cognitive enhancer) Consider adjusting non-pharmacological treatment (cognitive-behavioral therapies or coaching or re-evaluating neuropsychological profile for executive function capacities)
Intolerable side effects	Evaluate if side effect is drug-induced Assess medication response versus tolerability of side effect Aggressive management of side effect (change timing of dose; change preparation of stimulant; adjunctive or alternative treatment)
Symptoms of rebound	Change timing of dose Supplement with small dose of short-acting stimulant or alpha-adrenergic agent 1 hour before symptom onset Change preparation Increase frequency of dosage
Development of tics or Tourette's syndrome (TS) or use with co-morbid tics or TS	Assess persistence of tics or TS If tics abate, re-challenge If tics are clearly worsened with stimulant treatment, discontinue Consider stimulant use with adjunctive anti-tic treatment (haloperidol, pimozide) or use of alternative treatment (antidepressants, alpha-adrenergic agents)
Emergence of dysphoria, irritability, acceleration, agitation	Assess for toxicity or rebound Evaluate development or exacerbation of co-morbidity (mood, anxiety, and substance use [including nicotine and caffeine]) Reduce dose Change stimulant preparation Assess sleep and mood Consider alternative treatment
Emergence of major depression, mood lability, or marked anxiety symptoms	Assess for toxicity or rebound Evaluate development or exacerbation of co-morbidity Reduce or discontinue stimulant Consider use of antidepressant or anti-manic agent Assess substance use Consider non-pharmacological interventions
Emergence of psychosis or mania	Discontinue stimulant Assess co-morbidity Assess substance use Treat psychosis or mania

should give guidance on improving the patient's nutritional options with higher caloric intake to balance the consequences of decreased food intake.[19] While appetite suppression is a common side effect of stimulants, little research has been done studying remedies. Cyproheptadine, in doses of 4 to 8 mg, has recently been reported to improve appetite in ADHD patients with stimulant-associated appetite suppression.[96]

Medication Interactions with Stimulants

The interactions of stimulants with other prescription and non-prescription medications are generally mild and not a major source of concern.[97,98] Concomitant use of sympathomimetic agents (e.g., pseudoephedrine) may potentiate the effects of both medications. Likewise, excessive intake of caffeine may potentially compromise the effectiveness of the stimulants and exacerbate sleep difficulties. Although data on the co-administration of stimulants with tricyclic antidepressants (TCAs) suggest little interaction between these compounds,[99] careful monitoring is warranted when prescribing stimulants with either TCAs or anticonvulsants. Although administering stimulants with ATMX is common in clinical practice, and appears to be safe, well tolerated, and effective based on clinical experience, to date only small samples have been studied; therefore, patients taking this combination

should be monitored closely.[100] In fact, co-administration of stimulants with MAOIs is the only true contraindication.

Despite the increasing use of stimulants for patients with ADHD, many of them may not respond, experience untoward side effects, or manifest co-morbidity, which stimulants may exacerbate or be ineffective in treating.[17,101] Over the last 10 years ATMX has been systematically evaluated and is FDA-approved for the treatment of ADHD in children, adolescents, and adults.[28]

ATOMOXETINE

Unlike the stimulants, atomoxetine (ATMX; Strattera) is unscheduled; therefore, clinicians can prescribe refills. ATMX acts by blocking the NE re-uptake pump on the pre-synaptic membrane, thus increasing the availability of intra-synaptic NE, with little affinity for other monoamine transporters or neurotransmitter receptors.[102] In addition to prominent effects of ATMX on NE re-uptake inhibition, pre-clinical data also show that the noradrenergic pre-synaptic re-uptake protein regulates DA in the frontal lobes and that by blocking this protein ATMX increases DA in the frontal lobes.[103] ATMX is rapidly absorbed following oral administration; food does not appear to affect absorption, and C_{max} occurs 1 to 2 hours after dosing.[104] While the plasma half-life appears to be around 5 hours, the central nervous system (CNS) effects appear to last over 24 hours.[105] ATMX is metabolized primarily in the liver to 4-hydroxyatomoxetine by the cytochrome (CYP) P450 2D6 enzyme.[106,107] Although patients identified as "poor metabolizers" (i.e., with low 2D6 activity) appear to generally tolerate ATMX, these patients seem to have more side effects, and a reduction in dose may be necessary.[108,109] Therefore, in patients who are taking medications that are strong 2D6 inhibitors (e.g., fluoxetine, paroxetine, quinidine), it may be necessary to reduce the dose of ATMX. Clinically, ATMX is often prescribed in conjunction with stimulants. Although the safety, tolerability, and efficacy of this combination have not been fully studied, reports suggest that this combination is well tolerated and effective.[100,110,111] Therefore, although the full safety of administering stimulants and ATMX together has not been fully established, there are good data from which to extrapolate, and clinicians must balance the risks and benefits in each patient.

Clinical Use of Atomoxetine

ATMX should be initiated at 0.5 mg/kg/day and after a few days increased to a target dose of 1.2 mg/kg/day. Although ATMX has been studied in doses of up to 2 mg/kg/day, current dosing guidelines recommend a maximum dosage of 1.4 mg/kg/day. Although some patients have an early response, it may take up to 10 weeks to see the full benefits of ATMX treatment.[112-114] In the initial trials, ATMX was dosed BID (typically after breakfast and after dinner); however, recent studies have demonstrated its efficacy and tolerability in many patients dosed once a day.[115-117] Although the effects of ATMX dosed once daily in the morning or at bedtime appear to be similar (with a mean dose of 1.25 mg/kg/morning or 1.26 mg/kg/night), once-daily ATMX appears to be best tolerated when dosed in the evening. To date, plasma levels of ATMX have not been used to guide dosing. However, Dunn and colleagues[118] found that patients with a plasma level of ATMX greater than 800 ng/ml had more robust responses, although patients treated with higher doses also experienced more side effects.

ATMX may be particularly useful when anxiety, mood symptoms, or tics co-occur with ADHD. For example, a large, 14-week multi-site study of ATMX in adults with ADHD and social anxiety disorder reported clinically significant effects on both ADHD and on anxiety.[119] Although untested, because of its lack of abuse liability,[120] ATMX may be particularly of use in adults with current substance use issues. For instance, Wilens and associates[121] demonstrated in a 12-week controlled trial that treatment with ATMX in recently abstinent alcoholics was associated with improved ADHD and reduced drinking, although absolute abstinent rates were unaffected. Moreover, ATMX has not been reported to have significant or serious drug interactions with alcohol or marijuana.[122]

Side Effects of Atomoxetine

Although generally well tolerated, the most common side effects in children and adolescents taking ATMX include reduced appetite, dyspepsia, and dizziness,[28] although height and weight in long-term use appear to be on target.[113] In adults, ATMX treatment may be associated with dry mouth, insomnia, nausea, decreased appetite, constipation, decreased libido, dizziness, and sweating.[123] Furthermore, some men taking ATMX may have difficulty attaining or maintaining erections. Several easy strategies can be used to manage ATMX's side effects. When patients experience nausea, the dose of ATMX should be divided and administered with food. Sedation is often transient, but may be helped by either administering the dose at night or by dividing the dose. If mood swings occur, patients should be evaluated and their diagnosis reassessed.

Although ATMX treatment is associated with mean increases in heart rate of 6 beats per minute, and increases in systolic and diastolic blood pressure of 1.5 mm Hg, the impact of ATMX on the cardiovascular system appears to be minimal.[124-126] Extensive electrocardiogram (ECG) monitoring indicates that ATMX has no apparent effect on QTc intervals, and ECG monitoring outside of routine medical care does not appear to be necessary. Adults should have their vital signs checked prior to initiating treatment with ATMX and periodically thereafter.

Concerns have been raised that treatment with ATMX may increase the risk of hepatitis. During post-marketing surveillance, two patients (out of 3 million exposures) developed hepatitis during treatment with ATMX.[127] Patients and families should contact their doctors if they develop pruritus, jaundice, dark urine, right upper quadrant tenderness, or unexplained "flu-like" symptoms.[28]

The FDA issued a public health advisory, and the manufacturer later added a black box warning regarding the development of suicidal ideation in patients treated with ATMX.[28] Similar to the selective serotonin re-uptake inhibitors (SSRIs), there was a slight increase in suicidal thinking in controlled trials. Parents and caregivers should be made aware of any such occurrences and should monitor unexpected changes in mood or behavior.

Alpha-adrenergic Agonists

Clonidine, an imidazoline derivative with alpha-adrenergic agonist properties, has been primarily used in the treatment of hypertension.[128] At low doses, it appears to stimulate inhibitory, pre-synaptic autoreceptors in the CNS.[129] In 2010 the FDA approved an extended delivery oral formulation of clonidine, clonidine ER (Kapvay) as a treatment for ADHD in youth aged 6–17 years.[28] This formulation is approved both as monotherapy and as adjunctive treatment with stimulants. Although clonidine reduces symptoms of ADHD,[130] its overall effect is less than the stimulants,[131] and likely smaller than ATMX, TCAs, and bupropion. Clonidine appears to be particularly helpful in patients with ADHD and co-morbid CD or ODD,[132-134] tic disorders,[135,136] ADHD-associated sleep disturbances,[90,137] and may reduce anxiety and hypervigilance in traumatized children.[138]

Clonidine is a relatively short-acting compound with a plasma half-life ranging from approximately 5.5 hours (in children) to 8.5 hours (in adults). Clonidine ER is usually initiated a dose of 0.1 mg HS for several days and titrated up to a maximum recommended dose of 0.2 mg BID. Immediate release clonidine usually initiated at the lowest manufactured dose of a half or quarter tablet of 0.1 mg. Usual daily doses ranges from 3 to 10 μg/kg given generally in divided doses, BID, three times daily (TID), or four times daily (QID), and there is a transdermal preparation. The most common short-term adverse effect of clonidine is sedation, which tends to subside with continued treatment. It can also produce, in some cases, hypotension, dry mouth, vivid dreams, depression, and confusion. A recent summary of the safety of Kapvay is available at http://www.fda.gov/downloads/Advisory Committees/CommitteesMeetingMaterials/PediatricAdvisory Committee/UCM319363.pdf. Overdoses of clonidine in children under 5 years of age may have life-threatening consequences.[139] Since abrupt withdrawal of clonidine has been associated with rebound hypertension, slow tapering is advised.[140,141] In addition, extreme caution should be exercised with the co-administration of clonidine with beta-blockers or calcium channel blockers.[142] Although concerns about the safety of co-administration of clonidine with stimulants have been debated,[143] recent data supports the tolerability, safety, and efficacy of this combination.[144] Current guidelines are to monitor blood pressure when initiating and tapering cloni-dine, but ECG monitoring is not usually necessary.[145]

Guanfacine, the most selective alpha$_{2A}$-adrenergic agonist currently available, appears to act by mimicking NE binding in the pre-frontal cortex.[146] In 2009, an extended delivery formulation guanfacine ER (Intuniv) was FDA-approved for the treatment of ADHD as monotherapy or as adjunctive treatment with stimulants.[28] Guanfacine ER is usually started at 1 mg daily at bedtime and titrated to a maximum dose of 4 mg. Possible advantages of guanfacine over clonidine include less sedation, a longer duration of action, and since it has little affinity for the brainstem imidazoline I1 receptors, may have a milder cardiovascular profile.[146] Recent information from the FDA about post-marketing experience with Intuniv is available at http://www.fda.gov/downloads/AdvisoryCommittees/CommitteesMeetingMaterials/PediatricAdvisoryCommittee/UCM255105.pdf. Anecdotal information suggests that guanfacine may be more useful in improving the cognitive deficits of ADHD. School-aged children with ADHD and co-morbid tic disorder, treated with immediate release guanfacine in doses ranging from 0.5 mg BID to 1 mg TID, showed reduction in both tics and ADHD.[147,148] Guanfacine treatment is associated with minor, clinically insignificant decreases in blood pressure and pulse rate. The adverse effects of guanfacine include sedation, irritability, and depression. Several cases of apparent guanfacine-induced mania have been described, but the impact of guanfacine on mood disorders remains unclear.[149] Alpha-adrenergic medications may be particularly useful in youth with primarily a hyperactive/impulsive and/or aggressive component.[150] However, there is a dearth of data on using the alpha agonists in adults with ADHD.

SUGGESTED MANAGEMENT STRATEGIES ACROSS THE LIFE SPAN

Having made the diagnosis of ADHD, the adult needs to be familiarized with the risks and benefits of pharmacotherapy, the availability of alternative treatments, and the likely adverse effects. Patient expectations need to be explored and realistic goals of treatment need to be clearly delineated.[151] Likewise, the clinician should review with the patient the various pharmacological options available and that each will require systematic trials of the anti-ADHD medications for reasonable durations of time and at clinically meaningful doses. Patients with ADHD who have psychiatric co-morbidity, residual symptomatology despite treatment, or report psychological distress related to their ADHD (e.g., self-esteem issues, self-sabotaging patterns, interpersonal disturbances) should be directed to appropriate psychotherapeutic intervention with clinicians knowledgeable in ADHD treatment.

Recognizing the morbidity associated with ADHD, its effect on psychological, social, and emotional development, as well as co-morbid/residual psychiatric and ADHD symptoms, it is necessary to tailor a comprehensive treatment plan. The foundations of such planning involve education, pharmacotherapy, and psychosocial treatments. Support with educational planning, social interactions, and the work environment is often helpful and complimentary to pharmacotherapy.

The stimulant medications, ATMX, guanfacine ER, and clonidine ER are FDA-approved and are considered the first-line therapy for ADHD across the life span. Although there are no evidence-based guidelines in selecting a first choice of medication for patients with ADHD, it is important to consider issues of co-morbidity, tolerability, efficacy, and duration of action.[1,19,20,70,72] The European Network Adult ADHD published a consensus outlining guidelines regarding ADHD treatment with stimulants. The guidelines recommended that the severity of ADHD and co-morbid disorders should be the first guide to select treatments, with stimulants being the medication of choice. Long-lasting, extended-release formulations are preferred for reasons of adherence to treatment, for protection against abuse, to avoid rebound symptoms, and to provide symptomatic relief throughout the day without the need for multiple doses. Every few days the dose may be increased to optimize response. Frequently, patients benefit from adding immediate-release amphetamine or MPH in combination with longer-acting preparations in order to sculpt the dose to the patient's individual needs,[152] although the efficacy of this practice is not well studied. Additionally, psychotherapy is recommended in combination with stimulant treatment in order to relieve additional impairments.[70]

Consideration of another stimulant or ATMX is recommended when symptoms aren't unresponsive or the patient experiences clinically significant side effects to the initial medication. Given their pharmacodynamic differences,[26] if a MPH product was initially selected, then moving to an amphetamine-based medication is appropriate. Although some patients are able to take ATMX once daily, many benefit from BID dosing.[123] Patients must also be made aware that the full benefits of ATMX may not occur for several weeks and they may not "feel" anything like they may have with the stimulants. Monitoring routine side effects, vital signs, and the misuse of the medication is warranted.

SAFETY OF MEDICATIONS USED TO TREAT ATTENTION-DEFICIT/HYPERACTIVITY DISORDER

The FDA's Pediatric Drugs Advisory Committee (PDAC) reviewed data concerning the cardiovascular (CV) effects of medications used to treat ADHD, as well as concerns regarding psychosis, mania, and suicidal thinking.

Cardiovascular Safety of Attention-Deficit/Hyperactivity Disorder Treatments

Treatment with stimulants is associated with small increases in heart rate and blood pressure that are weakly correlated with dose. There has been concern about CV safety/risk in patients receiving stimulants.[153] However, recent work has shed light on the CV risk of stimulants in adults. Habel and colleagues retrospectively investigated serious CV events in a large group of medication users and non-users (n = 443,198 adults aged 25–64). The authors reported on 806,182 person-years of follow-up (median, 1.3 years per person), and found no relationship between past or current ADHD medication use and serious CV or stroke outcomes. As highlighted by these authors[125] among young and middle-aged adults, current or new use of ADHD medications, compared with non-use or remote use, was not associated with an increased risk of serious cardiovascular events. These results mirror the findings of a similarly-designed study in youth with ADHD[126] and a recent review of the cardiovascular literature related to stimulant exposure in ADHD[154] and seems to suggest that the vital sign changes seen acutely and chronically are usually not clinically significant. Please see Table 10-3 for one way to screen for CV symptoms prior to the initiation of pharmacotherapy and while monitoring treatment.

The PDAC cited the baseline rate of sudden unexplained death in the pediatric population to range from 0.6 to 6 occurrences per 100,000 patient-years.[155] From the FDA's research, the PDAC presented data indicating that the rates of sudden unexplained death in the pediatric population between 1992 and February 2005, treated with MPH, amphetamine, or ATMX, were 0.2, 0.3, and 0.5 cases per 100,000 patient-years,

TABLE 10-3 A Strategy to Screen for Cardiovascular Symptoms

Cardiovascular History	Yes	No	Comment
PERSONAL HISTORY			
Congenital or acquired cardiac disease?			
Coronary artery disease?			
Chest pain?			
Palpitations?			
Shortness of breath?			
Dizziness?			
Syncope?			
Change in exercise tolerance or tolerance to usual physical activities?			
FAMILY HISTORY (<30 YEARS OF AGE)			
Early myocardial infarction?			
Cardiac death?			
Significant arrhythmia(s)?			
Long QT syndrome?			
OBJECTIVE			
Baseline (off medication) blood pressure and heart rate within normal limits			

This tool may be useful for screening at initial assessment and prior to initiation of medication(s) used to treat ADHD. As a part of follow-up visits this tool may be used as one way to monitor ongoing treatment as well as prior to changing medication dose(s). During ongoing treatment we encourage clinicians to inquire about current cardiovascular symptoms, measure pulse and blood pressure as well as changes to family history
[a]Copyright Timothy E. Wilens, MD Published with permission.
[b]If positive on an item, recommend referral to primary care physician or cardiology for further assessment prior to initiating medications
(Adapted from Massachusetts General Hospital Cardiovascular Screen[a,b])

respectively. Based on these data, the PDAC *rejected* adding a black box warning, but recommended that current labeling language for amphetamine drugs on CV risks in patients with structural cardiac abnormalities should be extended to all medications approved for the treatment of ADHD. Details regarding these issues are provided in two recent reviews.[156,157]

The American Heart Association has previously commented on CV monitoring of youths taking psychotropic medications.[145] Despite the generally benign CV effects of these medications, caution is warranted in the presence of a compromised CV system (e.g., untreated hypertension, arrhythmias, and known structural heart defects). It remains prudent to monitor symptoms referable to the CV system (e.g., syncope, palpitations, and chest pain) and vital signs at baseline and with treatment in all patients with ADHD. For most pediatric patients it is not necessary to check an ECG at baseline or with treatment. In patients at risk for CV symptoms, it is important to collaborate with the patient's primary care physician and to ensure that hypertension is not an issue. Recent data from an open-label study of ADHD treatment in adults suggest that if hypertension is well controlled, stimulants may be safely used in the short term.[158] Safety remains the paramount concern; thus, in each case the physician and patient must weigh the risks and benefits of treatment.

Aggression during Treatment with Attention-Deficit/Hyperactivity Disorder Medications

From the FDA's research, the PDAC presented data reporting episodes of aggression with all ADHD medications during clinical trials and in post-marketing surveillance. However, aggression in patients with ADHD usually responds to stimulant treatment.[159] During clinical trials, rates of aggression were observed to be similar with active and placebo treatment. The PDAC recommended that the decision about whether to continue therapy following an aggression event is complex and that the physician and parent should evaluate whether the

risks outweigh the benefits that the child obtains from the treatment.

Psychotic or Manic Symptoms during Treatment with Attention-Deficit/Hyperactivity Disorder Medications

The FDA has received hundreds of reports of psychotic or manic symptoms, particularly hallucinations, associated with ADHD medication use in children and adolescents. FDA drug-safety analysts recommended adding warnings to ADHD medication-labeling advising that ADHD medications should be stopped if a patient experiences signs and symptoms of psychosis or mania. A recent review of stimulant trials revealed that psychotic-like or manic-like symptoms might occur in approximately 0.25% of children (or 1 in 400) treated with stimulant medications.[160]

In conclusion, the PDAC recommended that a medication guide be issued for all ADHD medications describing the potential psychiatric, aggression, and CV risks and that these risks be clearly elucidated in the product labeling of all ADHD medications. However, the PDAC concluded that potential episodes of psychosis, aggression, suicidality, and cardiac events during treatment with ADHD medications in children do not warrant a black box warning.

Currently the only black box warning for stimulants warns about the potential for substance abuse.

ALTERNATIVE (NOT FDA-APPROVED) TREATMENTS FOR ATTENTION-DEFICIT/HYPERACTIVITY DISORDER
Bupropion

Bupropion hydrochloride (Wellbutrin), a unicyclic aminoketone, approved for treatment of depression and as an aid for smoking cessation in adults,[28] has been reported to be moderately helpful in reducing ADHD symptoms in children, adolescents,[161-163] and adults.[164-167] Although helpful, the magnitude of effect of bupropion is less than that seen with either stimulants or ATMX. Bupropion is often used in patients with ADHD and co-morbidities and has been studied in small groups of adolescents with ADHD and nicotine dependence,[168] substance use and mood disorders,[169] substance abuse and conduct disorder,[170] and depression.[171] In light of the high rates of marijuana use in patients with ADHD,[172] it is important for clinicians to note that adolescents treated with bupropion may experience increased irritability during marijuana withdrawal.[173] In addition, bupropion has been helpful in ADHD adults with BPD,[174] substance use[175,176] or with co-existing cardiac abnormalities.[177]

Bupropion modulates both NE and DA. It appears to be more stimulating than other antidepressants, may cause irritability, has been reported to exacerbate tics,[178] and is associated with higher rates of drug-induced seizures than other antidepressants.[28] These seizures appear to be dose-related (>450 mg/day) and more likely to occur in patients with bulimia or a seizure disorder, and thus should be avoided in patients with these problems. In ADHD adults, bupropion IR and SR should be given in divided doses, with no single dose of the IR exceeding 150 mg, or SR 200 mg. Dosing for ADHD appears to be similar to that for depression. The once-daily preparation of bupropion is usually initiated at 150 mg XL once in AM and titrated every 7–14 days to maximum dose of 450 mg XL daily. Common side effects include insomnia, edginess, tremor, and a risk for seizures, primarily with immediate-release preparations.

Tricyclic Antidepressants

Although controlled trials in ADHD youths[179] and adults[180] demonstrate TCAs' efficacy, the effects are less robust than with stimulants. Compared to the stimulants, TCAs have negligible abuse liability, have once-daily dosing, and may be useful in patients with co-morbid anxiety, ODD,[181] tics,[182] and, theoretically, depression (adults). However, given concerns about potential cardiotoxicity and the available of ATMX, guanfacine ER and clonidine ER, use of the TCAs has been significantly curtailed.

Before treatment with a TCA, a baseline ECG should be obtained (as well as inquiry into any family history of early-onset or sudden cardiac arrhythmias).[183] Dosing for ADHD appears to be similar to that for depression. ECGs should be obtained as the dose is increased. Monitoring serum levels of TCAs is more helpful in avoiding toxicity than it is in determining optimal levels for response.

Common short-term adverse consequences of the TCAs include dry mouth, blurred vision, orthostasis, and constipation. Since the anticholinergic effects of TCAs limit salivary flow, they may cause dental problems. Following the sudden death of a number of children receiving desipramine (DMI), concerns were raised regarding the possible cardiac toxicity of TCAs in children.[184] However, epidemiological evaluation of the association between DMI and sudden death in children has not supported a causal relationship.[185] TCAs predictably increase heart rate and are associated with conduction delays, usually affecting the right bundle, thus requiring ECG monitoring.[186] However, these effects, when small, rarely seem to be pathophysiologically significant in non-cardiac patients with normal baseline ECGs. In patients with documented congenital or acquired cardiac disease, pathological rhythm disturbances (e.g., atrioventricular block, supraventricular tachycardia, ventricular tachycardia, and Wolff-Parkinson-White syndrome), family history of sudden cardiac death or cardiomyopathy, diastolic hypertension (>90 mm Hg), or when in doubt about the CV state of the patient, a complete (non-invasive) cardiac evaluation is indicated before initiation

of treatment with a TCA to help determine the risk–benefit ratio of such an intervention. A serious adverse event associated with use of TCAs is overdose. Hence, close supervision of the administration and storage of TCAs is necessary.

Modafinil

Modafinil, a novel stimulant that is distinct from amphetamine, is approved for the treatment of narcolepsy.[28] Unlike the broad activation observed with amphetamine, modafinil appears to activate specific hypothalamic regions.[187,188] Although one controlled trial in ADHD adults was positive,[189] a recent large (n = 330) multi-center (18 locations) randomized, double-blind treatment study in adults with ADHD did not find significant reductions in subjects treated with modafinil compared to those treated with placebo.[190] However, these investigators noted that certain subjects experienced significant benefit and suggest that this agent may warrant further investigation. Although controlled trials of modafinil in children with ADHD demonstrated efficacy,[191–193] the FDA PDAC voted that modafinil is "not approvable" for pediatric ADHD due to possible Stevens-Johnson syndrome (SJS) and toxic epidermal necrolysis (TEN). Clinically, it may be reasonable to consider combining modafinil with stimulants,[194,195] and clinicians should be aware of the potential to exacerbate mania.[196]

NOVEL TREATMENTS FOR ATTENTION-DEFICIT/HYPERACTIVITY DISORDER
Nicotinic Agents

Given the cognitive enhancing properties of nicotine,[197] nicotinic agents have been studied in the treatment of ADHD. Whereas smaller cross-over studies of nicotinic analogs with either full or partial agonistic properties demonstrated efficacy in adults with ADHD,[198–200] follow-up larger multi-site parallel design studies failed to show a significant effect of this compound on reducing ADHD symptomatology[201] and the role of nicotinic agents remains investigational.

Medications Used in the Treatment of Alzheimer's Disease

Although compelling based on efficacy in Alzheimer's disease and some positive initial experience in ADHD patients[202] trials in ADHD adults with donepezil[203] and galantamine[204] were negative. At this time there are no data to support the use of these cholinergic agents in the treatment of ADHD. Recently, Surman and colleagues[205] openly treated 34 ADHD adults with the N-methyl-D-aspartate (NMDA) receptor antagonist memantine. In this pilot study, memantine, titrated to a maximum dose of 10 mg BID, was generally well tolerated and resulted in improvements in measures of ADHD symptoms and neuropsychological measures. These encouraging but preliminary results warrant controlled study.

Metadoxine

Recently, MG01CI, an extended-release formulation of metadoxine has been studied in adults with ADHD. Metadoxine is an ion-pair salt of pyridoxine (vitamin B_6) and 2-pyrrolidone-5-carboxylate used in Europe for over 30 years in the treatment of acute alcohol intoxication and withdrawal. In a short-term controlled trial with MG01CI, subjects experienced improvements in ADHD symptoms as well as neuropsychological measures and overall functioning.[206]

Selegiline

Selegiline (l-deprenyl), an irreversible type B monoamine oxidase inhibitor (MAOI) that is metabolized into amphetamine and methamphetamine, has been compared to MPH in two trials of ADHD youths[207,208] and alone in adults.[209] Previous work with selegiline in children with ADHD and Tourette's syndrome suggests that it may reduce symptoms of ADHD.[210,211] Although to date its role in the treatment of ADHD has been limited by both the availability of alternative treatments and potential for the "cheese reaction," its formulation as a patch,[212] which may diminish this reaction, may increase interest in its use.

PHARMACOTHERAPY OF ATTENTION-DEFICIT/ HYPERACTIVITY DISORDER AND COMMON CO-MORBID PSYCHIATRIC DISORDERS

Attention-Deficit/Hyperactivity Disorder and Aggression

The importance of aggression should not be underestimated, as these patients often suffer severe psychopathology, adversely affect their families/communities, and have high rates of service utilization.[213] Although medications are usually effective in reducing symptoms of ADHD and impulsive aggression,[22,23] these patients usually benefit from multi-modal treatment.[214-216] Medications should initially treat the most severe underlying disorder, after which targeting specific symptoms (e.g., irritability, hostility, hypervigilance, impulsivity, fear, or emotional dysregulation) is appropriate.[217,218] These patients often display aggression before, and during, the course of treatment, making it imperative to document their aggressive behaviors before the introduction of medications and to make these behaviors an explicit target of treatment. The PDAC of the FDA suggests that if and when a patient displays worsening of aggressive behaviors during medication treatment for ADHD, the clinician should make a judgment regarding the tolerability and efficacy of the treatment (see www.fda.gov for the most recent recommendations).

In patients with co-morbid ADHD and ODD/CD, the clinician should first attempt to optimize the pharmacotherapy of ADHD[219] followed by augmentation with behavioral treatments. Supporting this strategy, a meta-analysis of studies from 1975 to 2001 found that stimulants significantly reduced both overt and covert aggression as rated by parents, teachers, and clinicians.[159] During the MTA trial, ADHD youths with and without ODD or CD responded robustly and equally well to stimulant medication.[220] Furthermore, in the MTA study, behavioral therapy without concomitant medication was less effective in subjects with ADHD and ODD/CD. Similarly, in ADHD youth treatment with ATMX, MAS XR, and OROS-MPH reduced ODD symptoms.[42,221-223] While these interventions are often sufficient, a significant number of these patients have severe symptoms that necessitate treatment with additional or alternative medications. Neuroleptic use should be limited to those ADHD patients with severe aggression or disruptive or mood disorders.[224,225]

In recent years the use of atypical antipsychotics in pediatric populations has increased considerably.[226] The American Academy of Child and Adolescent Psychiatry has published treatment recommendations for the use of antipsychotic medications in aggressive youth.[215,216] Clinicians are encouraged to optimize psychosocial/educational interventions, followed by appropriate pharmacotherapy of the primary psychiatric disorder, followed by use of an atypical antipsychotic medication. Treatment with atypical antipsychotics warrants careful monitoring as various side effects may be anticipated. These include sedation or extrapyramidal symptoms (EPS), which usually occur during initiation of therapy, while others, such as akathisia or dyskinesia/dystonias, may develop after several months of therapy. Clinicians are encouraged to monitor these side effects and to document abnormal movements using the Abnormal Involuntary Movement Scale (AIMS) on a periodic basis. Patients treated with atypical antipsychotics should also be monitored for sedation, hyperprolactinemia, CV symptoms, weight gain, and development of a metabolic syndrome. Although not specifically written for children, the American Diabetes Association recommends that while treating patients with atypical antipsychotics clinicians should inquire about a family history of diabetes, as well as regularly monitor patients' body mass index, waist circumference, blood pressure, fasting blood glucose, and fasting lipid profile.[227,228] Safety remains the paramount consideration, and after a period of remission of the aggressive symptoms, consideration should be given to tapering off of the atypical antipsychotic. Tapering atypical antipsychotics should proceed slowly in order to prevent withdrawal dyskinesias and to allow adequate time to adjust to the reduced dose. If there is evidence of severe mood instability, other mood stabilizers should be considered (see below).

Attention-Deficit/Hyperactivity Disorder Plus Anxiety Disorders

Anxiety disorders, including agoraphobia, panic, over-anxious disorder, simple phobia, separation anxiety disorder, and OCD, frequently occur in children, adolescents, and adults with ADHD.[5,11,23,229] The effect of stimulant treatment in youths with ADHD and anxiety has been variable. Earlier studies found increased placebo response, increased side effects, and a reduced response to stimulants in patients with both conditions,[230-232] whereas others observed stimulant treatment to be well tolerated and effective.[23,220,233] Many youths with ADHD and anxiety experience robust improvements with stimulant treatment and may not experience exacerbations of anxiety.[234,235] Of interest, ATMX is reported to reduce anxiety in ADHD youths[236] and adults.[119] The Texas Medication Algorithm Project (TMAP) Consensus Panel recommends beginning pharmacotherapy for patients with ADHD and a co-morbid anxiety disorder with either ATMX aimed at both the ADHD and anxiety or prescribing a stimulant first to address the ADHD, then adding an SSRI to address the anxiety if necessary.[219]

Attention-Deficit/Hyperactivity Disorder Plus Obsessive-compulsive Disorder

Considerable overlap exists between pediatric ADHD and OCD,[237] including rates of ADHD in up to 51% of children and 36% of adolescents with OCD.[238,239] In general, patients with OCD and ADHD require treatment for both conditions. The SSRIs, especially in combination with cognitive-behavioral therapy (CBT), are well-established treatments for pediatric and adult OCD.[240] Although stimulants may exacerbate tics, obsessions, or compulsions, they are frequently used in patients with these conditions, often in combination with SSRIs.[19,241,242] Therefore, clinicians should identify and prioritize treatment of the most severe condition first, then address secondary concerns, while monitoring for signs of worsening symptoms while recognizing that patients successfully treated have much residual morbidity and that CBT is an essential component of long-term management.

Attention-Deficit/Hyperactivity Disorder Plus Tic Disorders

Tics and tic disorders commonly occur in patients with ADHD,[241] as well as in students receiving special education services.[243] A community-based study of 3,006 children (6 to 12 years of age) found that 27% with ADHD also had tics, and 56% with tics had ADHD.[244] Tics occurred more commonly in males (2:1 to 6:1) and in youths with combined-type ADHD. Children, adolescents, and adults may suffer the triad of tics, ADHD, and OCD.[245] Pharmacotherapy of youths with ADHD and tic disorders is challenging. First-line treatment about tics is education. In most patients, tics are mild to moderate in severity, have a fluctuating course, even when taking a tic-suppressing medication and generally decline by early adulthood. Although stimulants may exacerbate tics and are listed as a contraindication to the use of MPH,[28] stimulants have been well tolerated and effective in these patients.[241,242,246,247] Randomized treatment with MPH (26.1 mg/day), clonidine (0.25 mg/day), or MPH plus clonidine (26.1 mg/day plus 0.28 mg/day) was studied in 136 children with ADHD and chronic tic disorders.[241] While MPH treatment improved ADHD and clonidine reduced tics, the greatest effect was observed with the combination treatment. Tic severity reduced with all active treatments and in the following order: clonidine plus MPH, clonidine alone, and MPH alone. No clinically significant CV adverse events were noted. The frequency of tic worsening was similar, and not significantly different, in subjects treated with MPH (20%), clonidine (26%), and placebo (22%). Follow-up of children with ADHD and tics treated with MPH over a 2-year period observed improvements in ADHD symptoms without worsening of tics.[242] Given the data on clonidine, interest in guanfacine treatment has grown, and it appears to be effective in reducing symptoms of both ADHD and tics.[147,148]

Palumbo and colleagues[248] observed similar rates of tics during short-term blinded treatment with placebo (3.7%), IR-MPH (2.3%), or OROS-MPH (4.0%). During 24-month open-label treatment with OROS-MPH, the rate of tics remained steady. However, clinicians must still discuss these issues and obtain informed consent from patients and families before using stimulants in patients with tic disorders. Investigations have demonstrated utility of noradrenergic agents, including DMI[182] and ATMX.[249] Although treatment with ATMX was not associated with significant reductions in tics compared to placebo (with reductions of Yale Global Tic Severity Scale −5.5 ± 6.9 versus −3.3 ± 8.9; P = 0.063), tic severity did not worsen and symptoms of ADHD were significantly improved. In patients who do not tolerate or respond to treatment with stimulants, noradrenergic agents, or alpha-adrenergic agents, or their combination, consideration should be given to treatment with a neuroleptic.[219]

Attention-Deficit/Hyperactivity Disorder Plus Depression

Depression and dysthymia are commonly co-morbid with ADHD.[5,11,17,250,251] In ADHD patients, depression is not an artifact,[252] and it must be distinguished from demoralization.[253] Although there are no formal evidence-based guidelines, clinicians should, in general, assess the severity of ADHD and depression and direct their initial treatment toward the most impairing condition. In treating pediatric depression, clinicians must keep in mind recent black box warnings about antidepressants and the risk of suicide. Excellent information for professionals, parents, and patients can be found at www.parentsmedguide.org. Clinicians are also directed to a review of the treatment of pediatric depression.[254] In adults

with ADHD and depression, TCAs remain a reasonable choice and may be helpful for both conditions. As discussed previously, the use of TCAs requires close monitoring.

Attention-Deficit/Hyperactivity Disorder Plus Bipolar Disorder

Although BPD is recognized in ADHD patients, ADHD may complicate the presentation, diagnosis, and treatment of BPD.[255-257] Differentiating BPD from ADHD can be challenging as these disorders share many features (including symptoms of distractibility, hyperactivity, impulsivity, talkativeness, and sleep disturbance).[258-263] Clinicians are faced with the challenging and important task of differentiating BPD, ADHD, ADHD with emotional dysregulation and the new DSM-5 diagnosis of Disruptive Mood Dysregulation Disorder.[264] Data to guide clinicians in this area are emerging, but often conflicting and may be confusing.[265-268] Previous data show that BPD appears to occur at increased rates in ADHD children and adolescents of both genders at baseline (11%) and during longitudinal 4-year follow-up (23%) compared to matched non-ADHD controls (P < 0.01).[269] A large study of BPD in adults funded by the National Institute of Mental Health (NIMH), the Systematic Treatment Enhancement Program for Bipolar Disorder (STEP-BD), observed that 9.5% of adults who present for treatment of BPD had lifetime co-morbid ADHD, with 6% meeting current criteria.[270,271] An array of information about and rating scales to evaluate BPD can be found at www.manicdepressive.org, www.bpkids.org, and www.schoolpsychiatry.org.

Given the severe morbidity of pediatric BPD, families and patients usually benefit from an integrated and coordinated treatment plan that includes medications (often more than one is necessary and appropriate), psychotherapies (individual, group, and family), educational/occupational interventions (accommodations or modifications in school or work), and psychoeducation and parent/family support (available through national organizations such as the National Alliance for the Mentally Ill and the Child and Adolescent Bipolar Foundation).

Medications are usually a fundamental part of the treatment plan of all patients with BPD. The reader is referred to practice guidelines for both pediatric patients[272] and adults.[273] The adult guidelines do not specifically address pharmacotherapy of BPD in the context of co-morbid ADHD; clinicians should first ensure mood stability before the initiation of treatment for ADHD. Patients with BPD type I without symptoms of psychosis should receive monotherapy with either a mood stabilizer (e.g., lithium, valproic acid, or carbamazepine) or an atypical antipsychotic (e.g., risperidone, olanzapine, or quetiapine).[272,274] In patients with only a partial response, the initial medication should be augmented with either an additional mood stabilizer or an atypical antipsychotic. The combination of lithium and valproic acid has been shown to substantially reduce symptoms of mania and depression in children, and in patients with BPD type I with psychosis, both a mood stabilizer and an atypical antipsychotic should be started concurrently (following the same augmentation strategy).

In patients with ADHD plus BPD, for example, the risk of mania or hypomania needs to be addressed and monitored during treatment of ADHD. Once the mood is euthymic, conservative introduction of anti-ADHD medications along with mood-stabilizing agents should be considered.[275] Scheffer and colleagues[276] recently demonstrated the tolerability and efficacy of MAS XR in reducing ADHD symptoms over the short-term in pediatric bipolar patients after successful mood stabilization with VPA. Similarly, in a small short-term trial in bipolar adults, bupropion successfully reduced symptoms of

ADHD without exacerbating mania.[174] McIntyre and colleagues treated 40 mood-stabilized bipolar I/II adults with LDX for their co-morbid ADHD.[277] Short-term (9-week) treatment with a mean dose of 60 ± 10 mg daily subjects reported significant improvements in self-ratings of ADHD and clinicians observed significant improvements in ADHD symptoms and functioning without exacerbations on mania. Case reports also describe successful treatment of ADHD symptoms in bipolar patients with ATMX[278] alone and in combination with OROS-MPH.[279] However, clinicians should advise patients (and perhaps their families) to monitor any induction or exacerbation/worsening of mania or cycling during treatment with ADHD medications.[280-286] In such situations it is necessary to prioritize the mood stabilization, which may also necessitate the discontinuation of the ADHD treatment until euthymia has been achieved.[272,287]

Attention-Deficit/Hyperactivity Disorder Plus Substance Use Disorders

Many adolescents and young adults with ADHD have either a past or current alcohol or drug use disorder, and co-morbidity within ADHD increases the risk.[17,172,288,289] Patients with ADHD frequently misuse a variety of substances (including alcohol, marijuana, cocaine, stimulants, opiates, and nicotine). In fact, children with ADHD start smoking nicotine an average of 2 years earlier than their non-ADHD peers[290] and have increased rates of smoking as adults, more difficulty quitting smoking,[291,292] and nicotine dependence (achieved more rapidly and lasting longer compared to controls).[293,294] Since the rates of substance abuse in patients with ADHD are increased,[295] concerns persist that stimulant treatment contributes to subsequent substance abuse. Wilens and colleagues[296] performed a pooled analysis of six studies that examined the relationship between stimulant treatment and substance abuse. Their meta-analysis revealed that stimulant treatment resulted in a 1.9-fold reduction in risk for later substance abuse among youths treated with a stimulant for ADHD, as compared to those youths receiving no pharmacotherapy for their ADHD.[296] The protective effect was greater through adolescence and less into adulthood. Longitudinal follow-ups also suggest that stimulant pharmacotherapy of ADHD does not increase risk of developing SUD.[297-299]

A careful history of substance use/misuse/abuse should be completed as part of the ADHD evaluation in adolescents and adults.[300] When substance misuse/abuse/dependence is a clinical concern, the clinician should assess the relative severity of the ADHD and the SUD. Furthermore, addictions often affect cognition, behavior, sleep, and mood/anxiety, which make it challenging to assess ADHD symptoms. Stabilizing the addiction and addressing co-morbid disorder(s) are generally the priority when treating ADHD patients with SUD. Treatment for patients with ADHD and SUD usually includes a combination of addiction treatment/psychotherapy and pharmacotherapy.[301] Patients with ongoing substance abuse or dependence should generally not be treated for their ADHD until appropriate addiction treatments have been undertaken and the patient has maintained a drug- and alcohol-free period. The clinician should begin pharmacotherapy with medications that have little likelihood of diversion or low liability, such as bupropion[175] and ATMX,[121] and, if necessary, progress to the stimulants. When using stimulants in this patient population, it is wise to prescribe an extended-delivery formulation with minimal risk of misuse (e.g., MTS or LDX), as well as to agree on a method for monitoring the SUD and adherence to the treatment plan. Moreover, since stimulants are Schedule II medications, concerns remain regarding their addictive potential. Concerns about possible diversion and misuse of stimulant medications remain, making careful monitoring necessary.[302-304] In these populations use of extended-delivery stimulant preparations, which are more difficult to misuse, or non-stimulants should be considered.[301] When administered orally in their intended dosages, stimulants do not appear to cause euphoria, nor do they appear to be addictive.[305,306]

Attention-Deficit/Hyperactivity Disorder Plus Autism Spectrum Disorders

Children, adolescents and adults with ASD may display a persistent and impairing pattern of hyperactivity, impulsivity, and inattention[307-311]; and when these symptoms can be distinguished from core features of ASD, DSM-5 allows clinicians to diagnose ADHD.[264] In treating this group of patients, clinicians, in collaboration with parents, balance the risks and benefits of treatments. In general, the philosophy is to identify target symptoms and to prioritize impairments.

Interest in the pharmacotherapy of ADHD and ASDs is growing. Although earlier work in small samples supported the use of MPH in doses of 0.3 to 0.6 mg/kg/day, these patients often experienced side effects (such as irritability) that limited stimulant use.[312,313] One of the Research Units in Pediatric Psychopharmacology (RUPP) compared placebo to low, medium, and high doses of MPH in 72 children with pervasive developmental disorder and ADHD.[314] In these subjects, although MPH treatment significantly improved attention and reduced distractibility, hyperactivity, and impulsivity, the effect sizes, according to parent and teacher ratings, were smaller than those usually observed in ADHD children. Furthermore, adverse effects, primarily irritability, led to MPH discontinuation in 18%, and occurred most often during treatment with either the medium or high MPH doses. A recent trial in 24 youth with ASD and ADHD found that MPH was generally well tolerated and efficacious in reducing symptoms of hyperactivity and impulsivity.[315] Similarly, data suggest that ATMX may be useful in ASD patients with ADHD symptoms.[316,317] For a full review of pharmacological treatments in ASDs, the interested reader is referred to excellent recent reviews.[318-320]

Attention-Deficit/Hyperactivity Disorder Plus Epilepsy

Children with epilepsy often display difficulties with behavior and cognition, and anticonvulsants may have cognitive side effects. On the other hand, treatment with anticonvulsants may lead to improved seizure control and result in improved cognition and behavior. Although there is ongoing concern that treatment with stimulants may lower the seizure threshold,[28] recent reviews and data challenge the traditional warning and provide evidence for the safe and effective use of stimulants in patients with epilepsy when appropriate antiepileptic treatment is used.[321-324] Current recommendations for evaluation, diagnosis, and treatment of ADHD acknowledge inconsistent findings in the literature on the overlap of ADHD and epilepsy, but do not recommend the use of routine electroencephalograms (EEGs) in the assessment of ADHD.[1,20,70]

MANAGING SUB-OPTIMAL RESPONSES

Despite the availability of various agents for adults with ADHD, there appear to be a number of individuals who either do not respond to, or are intolerant of adverse effects of, medications used to treat their ADHD. In managing difficult cases, several therapeutic strategies are available (see Table 10-2). If psychiatric adverse effects develop concurrent with a poor medication response, alternative treatments should be pursued. Severe psychiatric symptoms that emerge during the acute phase can be problematic, irrespective of the efficacy of the medications for ADHD. These symptoms may require re-consideration of the diagnosis of ADHD and careful re-assessment of the presence of co-morbid disorders. For example, it is common to observe depressive symptoms in an adult with ADHD when symptoms are independent of the ADHD or treatment. If reduction of dose or change in preparation (i.e., regular versus slow-release stimulants) does not resolve the problem, consideration should be given to alternative treatments. Neuroleptic medications should be considered as part of the overall treatment plan in the face of co-morbid BPD or extreme agitation. Concurrent non-pharmacological interventions (such as behavioral or cognitive therapy) may assist with symptom reduction and functional improvements.

CONCLUSION

In conclusion, the aggregate literature supports that pharmacotherapy provides an effective treatment for children, adolescents, and adults with ADHD and co-morbid disorders. Effective pharmacological treatments for ADHD include stimulants and non-stimulants. Structured psychotherapy may be effective when used adjunctly with medications. Groups focused on coping skills, support, and interpersonal psychotherapy may also be very useful for these patients. For adults who are considering advanced schooling, educational planning and alterations in the school environment may be necessary. Further controlled investigations assessing the efficacy of single and combination agents for patients with ADHD are necessary, with careful attention paid to diagnostics, symptom and neuropsychological outcome, long-term tolerability, and efficacy, as well as their use in specific ADHD sub-groups.

Access the complete reference list and multiple choice questions (MCQs) online at https://expertconsult.inkling.com

KEY REFERENCES

1. Wolraich M, Brown L, Brown RT, et al. ADHD: Clinical practice guideline for the diagnosis, evaluation, and treatment of attention-deficit/hyperactivity disorder in children and adolescents. *Pediatrics* 128(5):1007–1022, 2011.
4. Merikangas KR, He JP, Burstein M, et al. Service utilization for lifetime mental disorders in U.S. adolescents: results of the National Comorbidity Survey-Adolescent Supplement (NCS-A). *J Am Acad Child Adolesc Psychiatry* 50(1):32–45, 2011.
5. Kessler RC, Adler L, Barkley R, et al. The prevalence and correlates of adult ADHD in the United States: results from the National Comorbidity Survey Replication. *Am J Psychiatry* 163(4):716–723, 2006.
7. Volkow ND, Swanson JM. Clinical practice: Adult attention deficit-hyperactivity disorder. *N Engl J Med* 369(20):1935–1944, 2013.
11. Biederman J, Monuteaux MC, Mick E, et al. Young adult outcome of attention deficit hyperactivity disorder: a controlled 10-year follow-up study. *Psychol Med* 36(2):167–179, 2006.
17. Biederman J, Faraone SV, Spencer T, et al. Patterns of psychiatric comorbidity, cognition, and psychosocial functioning in adults with attention deficit hyperactivity disorder. *Am J Psychiatry* 150:1792–1798, 1993.
18. Biederman J, Newcorn J, Sprich S. Comorbidity of attention deficit hyperactivity disorder with conduct, depressive, anxiety, and other disorders. *Am J Psychiatry* 148:564–577, 1991.
19. Greenhill LL, Pliszka S, Dulcan MK, et al. Practice parameter for the use of stimulant medications in the treatment of children, adolescents, and adults. *J Am Acad Child Adolesc Psychiatry* 41(2 Suppl.):26S–49S, 2002.
20. Pliszka S. Practice parameter for the assessment and treatment of children and adolescents with attention-deficit/hyperactivity disorder. *J Am Acad Child Adolesc Psychiatry* 46(7):894–921, 2007. [Epub 2007/06/22].
21. Bradley C. The behavior of children receiving benzedrine. *Am J Psychiatry* 94:577–585, 1937.
23. Moderators and mediators of treatment response for children with attention-deficit/hyperactivity disorder: the Multimodal Treatment Study of children with attention-deficit/hyperactivity disorder. *Arch Gen Psychiatry* 56(12):1088–1096, 1999.
36. Spencer TJ, Biederman J, Ciccone PE, et al. PET study examining pharmacokinetics, detection and likeability, and dopamine transporter receptor occupancy of short- and long-acting oral methylphenidate. *Am J Psychiatry* 163(3):387–395, 2006.
70. Kooij SJ, Bejerot S, Blackwell A, et al. European consensus statement on diagnosis and treatment of adult ADHD: The European Network Adult ADHD. *BMC Psychiatry* 10:67, 2010.
71. Wilens TE, Morrison NR, Prince J. An update on the pharmacotherapy of attention-deficit/hyperactivity disorder in adults. *Expert Rev Neurother* 11(10):1443–1465, 2011.
72. Weiss MD, Weiss JR. A guide to the treatment of adults with ADHD. *J Clin Psychiatry* 65(Suppl. 3):27–37, 2004.
73. Ramtvedt BE, Roinas E, Aabech HS, et al. Clinical gains from including both dextroamphetamine and methylphenidate in stimulant trials. *J Child Adolesc Psychopharmacol* 23(9):597–604, 2013.
75. Graham J, Banaschewski T, Buitelaar J, et al. European guidelines on managing adverse effects of medication for ADHD. *Eur Child Adolesc Psychiatry* 20(1):17–37, 2011.
79. Biederman J, Spencer TJ, Monuteaux MC, et al. A naturalistic 10-year prospective study of height and weight in children with attention-deficit hyperactivity disorder grown up: sex and treatment effects. *J Pediatr* 157(4):635–640, 40 e1, 2010.
86. Barrett JR, Tracy DK, Giaroli G. To sleep or not to sleep: a systematic review of the literature of pharmacological treatments of insomnia in children and adolescents with attention-deficit/hyperactivity disorder. *J Child Adolesc Psychopharmacol* 23(10):640–647, 2013.
89. Cortese S, Brown TE, Corkum P, et al. Assessment and management of sleep problems in youths with attention-deficit/hyperactivity disorder. *J Am Acad Child Adolesc Psychiatry* 52(8):784–796, 2013.
102. Arnsten AF, Pliszka SR. Catecholamine influences on prefrontal cortical function: relevance to treatment of attention deficit/hyperactivity disorder and related disorders. *Pharmacol Biochem Behav* 99(2):211–216, 2011.
125. Habel LA, Cooper WO, Sox CM, et al. ADHD medications and risk of serious cardiovascular events in young and middle-aged adults. *JAMA* 306(24):2673–2683, 2011.
126. Cooper WO, Habel LA, Sox CM, et al. ADHD drugs and serious cardiovascular events in children and young adults. *N Engl J Med* 365(20):1896–1904, 2011.
145. Gutgesell H, Atkins D, Barst R, et al. *Cardiovascular monitoring of children and adolescents receiving psychotropic drugs*, Dallas, 1999, American Heart Association, pp 979–982.
146. Arnsten AF. The use of alpha-2A adrenergic agonists for the treatment of attention-deficit/hyperactivity disorder. *Expert Rev Neurother* 10(10):1595–1605, 2010.
151. Haavik J, Halmoy A, Lundervold AJ, et al. Clinical assessment and diagnosis of adults with attention-deficit/hyperactivity disorder. *Expert Rev Neurother* 10(10):1569–1580, 2010.
154. Hammerness PG, Perrin JM, Shelley-Abrahamson R, et al. Cardiovascular risk of stimulant treatment in pediatric attention-deficit/hyperactivity disorder: update and clinical recommendations. *J Am Acad Child Adolesc Psychiatry* 50(10):978–990, 2011.
157. Wilens TE, Prince JB, Spencer TJ, et al. Stimulants and sudden death: what is a physician to do? *Pediatrics* 118(3):1215–1219, 2006.
160. Ross RG. Psychotic and manic-like symptoms during stimulant treatment of attention deficit hyperactivity disorder. *Am J Psychiatry* 163(7):1149–1152, 2006.
183. Gutgesell H, Atkins D, Barst R, et al. AHA scientific statement: Cardiovascular monitoring of children and adolescents receiving psychotropic drugs. *J Am Acad Child Adolesc Psychiatry* 38(8):979–982, 1999.

219. Pliszka SR, Crismon ML, Hughes CW, et al. The Texas Children's Medication Algorithm Project: revision of the algorithm for pharmacotherapy of attention-deficit/hyperactivity disorder. *J Am Acad Child Adolesc Psychiatry* 45(6):642–657, 2006.

220. Jensen PS, Hinshaw SP, Kraemer HC, et al. ADHD comorbidity findings from the MTA study: comparing comorbid subgroups. *J Am Acad Child Adolesc Psychiatry* 40(2):147–158, 2001.

224. Loy JH, Merry SN, Hetrick SE, et al. Atypical antipsychotics for disruptive behaviour disorders in children and youths. *Cochrane Database Syst Rev* (9):CD008559, 2012.

225. Linton D, Barr AM, Honer WG, et al. Antipsychotic and psychostimulant drug combination therapy in attention deficit/hyperactivity and disruptive behavior disorders: a systematic review of efficacy and tolerability. *Curr Psychiatry Rep* 15(5):355, 2013.

235. Abikoff H, McGough J, Vitiello B, et al. Sequential pharmacotherapy for children with comorbid attention-deficit/hyperactivity and anxiety disorders. *J Am Acad Child Adolesc Psychiatry* 44(5):418–427, 2005.

241. Group TTsSS. Treatment of ADHD in children with tics: A randomized controlled trial. *Neurology* 58(4):527–536, 2002.

251. McIntyre RS, Kennedy SH, Soczynska JK, et al. Attention-deficit/hyperactivity disorder in adults with bipolar disorder or major depressive disorder: results from the international mood disorders collaborative project. *Prim Care Companion J Clin Psychiatry* 12(3):2010.

252. Milberger S, Biederman J, Faraone S, et al. Attention deficit hyperactivity disorder and comorbid disorders: Issues of overlapping symptoms. *Am J Psychiatry* 152(12):1793–1799, 1995.

258. Biederman J, Faraone SV, Wozniak J, et al. Clinical correlates of bipolar disorder in a large, referred sample of children and adolescents. *J Psychiatr Res* 39(6):611–622, 2005.

262. Birmaher B, Axelson D, Goldstein B, et al. Four-year longitudinal course of children and adolescents with bipolar spectrum disorders: the Course and Outcome of Bipolar Youth (COBY) study. *Am J Psychiatry* 166(7):795–804, 2009.

263. Mick E, Spencer T, Wozniak J, et al. Heterogeneity of irritability in attention-deficit/hyperactivity disorder subjects with and without mood disorders. *Biol Psychiatry* 58(7):576–582, 2005.

266. Axelson D, Findling RL, Fristad MA, et al. Examining the proposed disruptive mood dysregulation disorder diagnosis in children in the Longitudinal Assessment of Manic Symptoms study. *J Clin Psychiatry* 73(10):1342–1350, 2012.

268. Barkley RA. Differential diagnosis of adults with ADHD: the role of executive function and self-regulation. *J Clin Psychiatry* 71(7):e17, 2010.

274. Kowatch RA, Youngstrom EA, Horwitz S, et al. Prescription of psychiatric medications and polypharmacy in the LAMS cohort. *Psychiatr Serv* 64(10):1026–1034, 2013.

289. Wilens TE, Martelon M, Joshi G, et al. Does ADHD predict substance-use disorders? A 10-year follow-up study of young adults with ADHD. *J Am Acad Child Adolesc Psychiatry* 50(6):543–553, 2011.

296. Wilens T, Faraone S, Biederman J, et al. Does stimulant therapy of attention-deficit/hyperactivity disorder beget later substance abuse? A meta-analytic review of the literature. *Pediatrics* 111(1):179–185, 2003.

297. Biederman J, Monuteaux MC, Spencer T, et al. Stimulant therapy and risk for subsequent substance use disorders in male adults with ADHD: a naturalistic controlled 10-year follow-up study. *Am J Psychiatry* 165(5):597–603, 2008.

302. McCabe SE, Knight JR, Teter CJ, et al. Non-medical use of prescription stimulants among US college students: prevalence and correlates from a national survey. *Addiction* 100(1):96–106, 2005.

306. Swanson JM, Volkow ND. Serum and brain concentrations of methylphenidate: implications for use and abuse. *Neurosci Biobehav Rev* 27(7):615–621, 2003.

310. Johnston K, Dittner A, Bramham J, et al. Attention deficit hyperactivity disorder symptoms in adults with autism spectrum disorders. *Autism* 6(4):225–236, 2013.

315. Pearson DA, Santos CW, Aman MG, et al. Effects of extended release methylphenidate treatment on ratings of attention-deficit/hyperactivity disorder (ADHD) and associated behavior in children with autism spectrum disorders and ADHD symptoms. *J Child Adolesc Psychopharmacol* 23(5):337–351, 2013.

324. Santos K, Palmini A, Radziuk AL, et al. The impact of methylphenidate on seizure frequency and severity in children with attention-deficit-hyperactivity disorder and difficult-to-treat epilepsies. *Dev Med Child Neurol* 655(7):654–660, 2013.

11 Drug–Drug Interactions in Psychopharmacology

Jonathan E. Alpert, MD, PhD

KEY POINTS

- Drug–drug interactions refer to alterations in drug levels or drug effects (or both) related to the administration of two or more prescribed, recreational, or over-the-counter agents in close temporal proximity.

- Although some drug–drug interactions involving psychotropic medications are life-threatening, most interactions manifest in more subtle ways through increased side-effect burden, aberrant drug levels, or diminished efficacy.

- Pharmacokinetic drug–drug interactions involve a change in the plasma level or tissue concentration of one drug following co-administration of one or more other drugs due to an action of the co-administered agents on one of four key pharmacokinetic processes: absorption, distribution, metabolism, or excretion.

- Pharmacodynamic drug–drug interactions involve an effect of one or more drugs on another drug at biological receptor sites of action and do not involve a change in plasma level or tissue concentration.

- The potential for drug–drug interactions should be carefully considered whenever prescribing medications associated with interactions that are uncommon but catastrophic (e.g., hypertensive crises, Stevens-Johnson syndrome, or cardiac arrhythmias) and medications with low therapeutic indices (e.g., warfarin) or narrow therapeutic windows (e.g., cyclosporine), and when prescribing for frail or clinically brittle patients for whom small variations in side effects or efficacy may be particularly troublesome.

OVERVIEW

An understanding of drug–drug interactions is essential to the practice of psychopharmacology.[1,2] As in other areas of medicine, polypharmacy has become an increasingly accepted approach in psychiatry for addressing difficult-to-treat disorders.[3] Moreover, general medical co-morbidity is common among patients with psychiatric disorders, elevating the likelihood of complex medication regimens.[4,5] Similarly, the widespread use of over-the-counter (OTC) supplements by patients receiving treatment for psychiatric disorders may invite additional risk of drug–drug interactions.[6] When they occur, drug–drug interactions may manifest in myriad ways, from perplexing laboratory tests to symptoms that are difficult to distinguish from the underlying psychiatric and physical conditions under treatment. The comprehensive evaluation of patients with psychiatric disorders therefore requires a careful assessment of potential drug–drug interactions.

Drug–drug interactions refer to alterations in drug levels or drug effects (or both) attributed to the administration of two or more prescribed, illicit, or OTC agents in close temporal proximity. Although many drug–drug interactions involve drugs administered within minutes to hours of each other,

some drugs may participate in interactions days or even weeks after their discontinuation because of prolonged elimination half-lives (e.g., fluoxetine) or due to their long-term impact on metabolic enzymes (e.g., carbamazepine). Some drug–drug interactions involving psychotropic medications are life-threatening, such as those involving the co-administration of monoamine oxidase inhibitors (MAOIs) and drugs with potent serotonergic (e.g., meperidine) or sympathomimetic (e.g., phenylpropanolamine) effects.[7-9] These combinations are therefore absolutely contraindicated. However, most drug–drug interactions in psychopharmacology manifest in somewhat more subtle ways, often leading to poor medication tolerability and compliance due to adverse events (e.g., orthostatic hypotension, sedation, or irritability), diminished medication efficacy, or puzzling manifestations (such as altered mental status or unexpectedly high or low drug levels). Drug combinations that can produce these often less than catastrophic drug–drug interactions are usually not absolutely contraindicated. Some of these combinations may, indeed, be valuable in the treatment of some patients while wreaking havoc for other patients. The capacity to anticipate and to recognize both the major, but rare, and the more subtle, but common, potential drug–drug interactions allows the practitioner to minimize the impact of these interactions as an obstacle to patient safety and to therapeutic success. This is both an important goal and a considerable challenge in psychopharmacology.

While drug–drug interactions are ubiquitous, few studies have systematically assessed *in vivo* drug–drug interactions of most interest to psychiatrists. Fortunately, well-designed studies of drug–drug interactions are an increasingly integral part of drug development. Beyond these studies, however, the literature on drug–drug interactions remains a patchwork of case reports, post-marketing analyses, extrapolation from animal and *in vitro* studies, and extrapolation from what is known about other drugs with similar properties. While these studies often shed some light on the simplest case of a single drug (drug B) exerting an effect on another (drug A), they rarely consider the common clinical scenario in which multiple drugs with numerous potential interactions among them are co-administered. Under these circumstances, the range of possible, if not well-delineated, drug–drug interactions often seems overwhelming.

Fortunately, an increasing range of resources are available (including prescribing software packages and regularly updated websites, such as www.drug-interactions.com) that allow for the prevention and detection of potential interactions. In addition, it is important to recall that numerous factors contribute to inter-individual variability in drug response.[10,11] These factors include treatment adherence, age, gender, nutritional status, disease states, and genetic polymorphisms that may influence risk of adverse events and treatment resistance (Figure 11-1). Drug–drug interactions are an additional factor that influence how patients react to drugs. The importance of these interactions depends heavily on the clinical context. In many cases, the practical impact of drug–drug interactions is likely to be very small compared with other factors that affect treatment response, drug levels, and toxicity. It is reasonable, therefore, to focus special attention on the contexts in which drug–drug interactions are most likely to be clinically problematic.

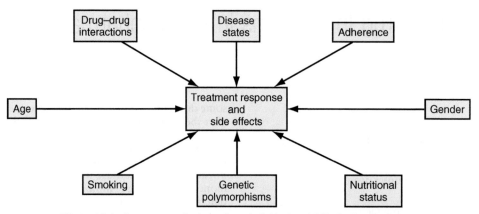

Figure 11-1. Factors contributing to inter-individual variability in drug response.

First, it is crucial to be familiar with the small number of drug–drug interactions in psychopharmacology that, though uncommon, are associated with potentially catastrophic consequences. These include drugs associated with ventricular arrhythmias, hypertensive crisis, serotonin syndrome, Stevens-Johnson syndrome, seizures, and severe bone marrow suppression. In addition, drug–drug interactions are important to consider when a patient's drugs include those with a low therapeutic index (e.g., lithium, digoxin, or warfarin) or a narrow therapeutic window (e.g., indinavir, nortriptyline, or cyclosporine) such that relatively small alterations in pharmacokinetic or pharmacodynamic behavior may jeopardize a patient's well-being. In addition, it is worthwhile to consider potential drug–drug interactions whenever evaluating a patient whose drug levels are unexpectedly variable or extreme, or a patient with a confusing clinical picture (such as clinical deterioration), or with unexpected side effects. Finally, drug–drug interactions are likely to be clinically salient for a patient who is medically frail or elderly, owing to altered pharmacokinetics and vulnerability to side effects, as well as for a patient heavily using alcohol, cigarettes, or illicit drugs, or being treated for a drug overdose.

CLASSIFICATION

Drug–drug interactions may be described as pharmacokinetic, pharmacodynamic, idiosyncratic, or mixed, depending on the presumed mechanism underlying the interaction (Box 11-1). Pharmacokinetic interactions are those that involve a change in the plasma level or tissue distribution (or both) of one drug by virtue of co-administration of another drug. These interactions occur due to effects at one or more of the four pharmacokinetic processes by which drugs are acted on by the body: absorption, distribution, metabolism, and excretion. Because of the importance of these factors, particularly metabolism, in drug–drug interactions, a more detailed description of pharmacokinetic processes follows. An example of a pharmacokinetic drug–drug interaction is the inhibition of the metabolism of lamotrigine by valproic acid,[12] thereby raising lamotrigine levels and increasing the risk of potentially serious adverse events, including hypersensitivity reactions (such as Stevens-Johnson syndrome). In contrast, pharmacodynamic interactions are those that involve a known pharmacological effect at biologically-active (receptor) sites. These interactions occur due to effects on the mechanisms through which the body is acted on by drugs and do not involve a change in drug levels. An example of a pharmacodynamic drug–drug interaction is the interference of the antiparkinsonian effects of a dopamine receptor agonist (such as pramipexole) by a dopamine receptor antagonist (such as risperidone). Mixed interactions are

---

BOX 11-1 Classification of Drug–Drug Interactions

PHARMACOKINETIC

Alteration in blood level or tissue concentration (or both) resulting from interactions involving drug absorption, distribution, metabolism, or excretion

PHARMACODYNAMIC

Alteration in pharmacological effect resulting from interactions at the same or inter-related biologically-active (receptor) sites

MIXED

Alterations in blood levels and pharmacological effects due to pharmacokinetic and pharmacodynamic interactions

IDIOSYNCRACTIC

Sporadic interactions among drugs not accounted for by their currently known pharmacokinetic or pharmacodynamic properties

---

those that are believed to involve both pharmacological and pharmacodynamic effects. Symptoms of serotonin toxicity, such as agitation and confusion that have been observed in some individuals on the combination of paroxetine and dextromethorphan, for example, may reflect the shared pharmacodynamic effect of the two agents at serotonin receptor sites as well as the elevation of dextromethorphan levels due to inhibition of its cytochrome P450 metabolism by paroxetine. Finally, idiosyncratic interactions are those that occur sporadically in a small number of patients in ways that are not yet predicted by the known pharmacokinetic and pharmacodynamic properties of the drugs involved.

PHARMACOKINETICS

As described earlier, pharmacokinetic processes refer to absorption, distribution, metabolism, and excretion, factors that determine plasma levels and tissue concentrations of a drug.[2,11,13] Pharmacokinetics refers to the mathematical analysis of these processes. Advances in analytic chemistry and computer methods of pharmacokinetic modeling and a growing understanding of the molecular pharmacology of the liver enzymes responsible for metabolism of most psychotropic medications have furnished increasingly sophisticated insights into the disposition and interaction of administered drugs. Although pharmacokinetics refers to only one of the two broad mechanisms by which drugs interact, pharmacokinetic interactions involve all classes of psychotropic and non-psychotropic medications. An overview of pharmacokinetic processes is a helpful prelude to a discussion of drug–drug interactions by psychotropic drug class.

Absorption

Factors that influence drug absorption are generally of less importance to drug–drug interactions involving psychiatric medications than are factors that influence subsequent drug disposition, particularly drug metabolism. Factors relevant to absorption generally pertain to orally rather than parenterally administered drugs, for which alterations in gastrointestinal drug absorption may affect the rate (time to reach maximum concentration) or the extent of absorption or both. The extent or completeness of absorption, also known as the fractional absorption, is measured as the area under the curve (AUC) when plasma concentration is plotted against time. The bioavailability of an oral dose of drug refers, in turn, to the fractional absorption for orally compared with intravenously (IV) administered drug. If an agent is reported to have a 90% bioavailability (e.g., lorazepam), this would indicate that the extent of absorption of an orally administered dose is nearly that of an IV-administered dose, although the rate of absorption may well be slower for the oral dose.

Because the upper part of the small intestine is the primary site of drug absorption through passive membrane diffusion and filtration and both passive and active transport processes, factors that speed gastric emptying (e.g., metoclopramide) or diminish intestinal motility (e.g., opiates or marijuana) may facilitate greater contact with, and absorption from, the mucosal surface into the systemic circulation, potentially increasing plasma drug concentrations. Conversely, antacids, charcoal, kaolin-pectin, and cholestyramine may bind to drugs, forming complexes that pass unabsorbed through the gastrointestinal lumen. Changes in gastric pH associated with food or other drugs alter the non-polar, un-ionized fraction of drug available for absorption. In the case of drugs that are very weak acids or bases, however, the extent of ionization is relatively invariant under physiological conditions. Properties of the preparation administered (e.g., tablet, capsule, or liquid) may also influence the rate or extent of absorption, and, for an increasing number of medications (e.g., lithium, bupropion, valproate, and methylphenidate), preparations intended for slow release are available. Finally, the local action of enzymes in the gastrointestinal tract (e.g., monoamine oxidase [MAO] and cytochrome P450 3A4) may be responsible for metabolism of drug before absorption. As described later, this is of critical relevance to the emergence of hypertensive crises that occur when excessive quantities of the dietary pressor tyramine are systemically absorbed in the setting of irreversible inhibition of the MAO isoenzymes for which tyramine is a substrate.

Distribution

Drugs distribute to tissues through the systemic circulation. The amount of drug ultimately reaching receptor sites in tissues is determined by a variety of factors, including the concentration of free (unbound) drug in plasma, regional blood flow, and physiochemical properties of drug (e.g., lipophilicity or structural characteristics). For entrance into the central nervous system (CNS), penetration across the blood–brain barrier is required. Fat-soluble drugs (such as benzodiazepines, neuroleptics, and cyclic antidepressants) distribute more widely in the body than water-soluble drugs (such as lithium), which distribute through a smaller volume of distribution. Changes with age, typically including an increase in the ratio of body fat to lean body mass, therefore result in a net greater volume of lipophilic drug distribution

and potentially greater accumulation of drug in adipose tissue in older than in younger patients.

In general, psychotropic drugs have relatively high affinities for plasma proteins (some to albumin but others, such as antidepressants, to α_1-acid glycoproteins and lipoproteins). Most psychotropic drugs are more than 80% protein-bound. A drug is considered highly protein-bound if more than 90% exists in bound form in plasma. Fluoxetine, aripiprazole, and diazepam are examples of the many psychotropic drugs that are highly protein-bound. In contrast, venlafaxine, lithium, topiramate, zonisamide, gabapentin, pregabalin, milnacipran, and memantine are examples of drugs with minimal protein-binding and therefore minimal risk of participating in drug–drug interactions related to protein-binding. A reversible equilibrium exists between bound and unbound drug. Only the unbound fraction exerts pharmacological effects. Competition by two or more drugs for protein-binding sites often results in displacement of a previously bound drug, which in the free state becomes pharmacologically active. Similarly, reduced concentrations of plasma proteins in a severely malnourished patient or a patient with a disease that is associated with severely lowered serum proteins (such as liver disease or nephrotic syndrome) may be associated with an increase in the fraction of unbound drug potentially available for activity at relevant receptor sites. Under most circumstances, the net changes in plasma concentration of active drug are, in fact, quite small because the unbound drug is available for redistribution to other tissues and for metabolism and excretion, thereby off-setting the initial rise in plasma levels. Nevertheless, clinically significant consequences can develop when protein-binding-interactions alter the unbound fraction of previously highly protein-bound drugs that have a low therapeutic index (e.g., warfarin). For these drugs, relatively small variations in plasma level may be associated with serious untoward effects.

An emerging understanding of the drug transport proteins, of which P-glycoproteins are the best characterized, indicates a crucial role in regulating permeability of intestinal epithelia, lymphocytes, renal tubules, the biliary tract, and the blood–brain barrier. These transport proteins are thought to account for the development of certain forms of drug resistance and tolerance, but are increasingly seen as likely also to mediate clinically-important drug interactions.[2] Little is known yet about their relevance to drug interactions involving psychiatric medications; the capacity of St. John's wort to lower blood levels of several critical medications (including cyclosporine and indinavir) is hypothesized to be related, at least in part, to an effect of the botanical agent on this transport system.[14]

Metabolism

Metabolism is the best-characterized mechanism of all of the pharmacokinetic processes implicated in known drug–drug interactions. Metabolism refers to the biotransformation of a drug to another form, a process that is usually enzyme-mediated and that results in a metabolite that may or may not be pharmacologically active and may or may not be subject to further biotransformations before eventual excretion. Most drugs undergo several types of biotransformation, and many psychotropic drug interactions of clinical significance are based on interference with this process. A growing understanding of hepatic enzymes, and especially the rapidly emerging characterization of the cytochrome P450 isoenzymes and other enzyme systems including the uridine-diphosphate glucuronosyltransferases (UGTs), flavin-containing monooxygenases (FMOs), methyltransferases, and sulfotransferases, has significantly advanced a rational understanding and prediction of drug interactions and individual variation in drug responses.[2,15]

Phase I reactions include oxidation, reduction, and hydrolysis, metabolic reactions that typically result in intermediate metabolites, which are then subject to phase II reactions (including conjugation [e.g., glucuronidation and sulfation] and acetylation). Phase II reactions typically yield highly polar, water-soluble metabolites suitable for renal excretion. Most psychotropic drugs undergo both phase I and phase II metabolic reactions. Notable exceptions include valproic acid and a subset of benzodiazepines (i.e., lorazepam, oxazepam, and temazepam), which skip phase I metabolism and undergo phase II reactions only. In addition, certain medications, including lithium and gabapentin, do not undergo any hepatic biotransformation before excretion by the kidneys.

The synthesis or activity of hepatic microsomal enzymes is affected by metabolic inhibitors and inducers, as well as by distinct genetic polymorphisms (stably inherited traits). Table 11-1 lists enzyme inducers and inhibitors common in clinical settings. These should serve as red flags that beckon further scrutiny for potential drug–drug interactions when they are found on a patient's medication list. Imagine two drugs, drug A and drug B, which are both associated with a metabolic enzyme. Drug B may be an inhibitor or an inducer of that enzyme. Drug A may be normally metabolized by that enzyme and would therefore be called a substrate. If drug B is an inhibitor with respect to the metabolic enzyme, it will impede the metabolism of a concurrently administered substrate (drug A), thereby producing a rise in the plasma levels of that substrate. If drug B is an inducer of that enzyme, it will enhance the metabolism of the substrate (drug A), resulting in a decline in the plasma levels of that substrate (Figure 11-2). In some circumstances an inhibitor (such as grapefruit juice) or inducer (e.g., a cruciferous vegetable, such as brussels sprouts) may not be a drug but rather another ingested substance. Moreover, in some circumstances a drug is not only a substrate of an enzyme but it can also inhibit the metabolism of other substrates relying on that enzyme, in which case it is considered an inhibitor as well as a substrate. Although inhibition is usually immediate, occurring by one or more of a variety of mechanisms (including competitive inhibition or inactivation of the enzyme), induction, which requires enhanced synthesis of the metabolic enzyme, is typically a more gradual process. A fall in plasma levels of a substrate may not be apparent for days to weeks following introduction of the inducer. This is particularly important when a patient's care is being transferred to another setting where clinical deterioration may be the first sign that drug levels have declined. Reciprocally, an elevation in plasma drug concentrations could reflect the previous discontinuation of an inducing factor (e.g., cigarette smoking or carbamazepine) just as it could reflect the more recent introduction of an inhibitor (e.g., fluoxetine or valproic acid).

Although the cytochrome P450 isoenzymes represent only one of the numerous enzyme systems responsible for drug

TABLE 11-1 Commonly Used Drugs and Substances That Inhibit or Induce Hepatic Metabolism of Other Medications

Inhibitors	Inducers
Antifungals (ketoconazole, miconazole, itraconazole)	Barbiturates (e.g., phenobarbital, secobarbital)
Macrolide antibiotics (erythromycin, clarithromycin, triacetyloleandomycin)	Carbamazepine
Fluoroquinolones (e.g., ciprofloxacin)	Oxcarbazepine
Isoniazid	Phenytoin
Antiretrovirals	Rifampin
Antimalarials (chloroquine)	Primidone
Selective serotonin reuptake inhibitors (fluoxetine, fluvoxamine, paroxetine, sertraline)	Cigarettes
Duloxetine	Ethanol (chronic)
Bupropion	Cruciferous vegetables
Nefazodone	Charbroiled meats
β-Blockers (lipophilic) (e.g., propranolol, metoprolol, pindolol)	St. John's wort
Quinidine	Oral contraceptives
Valproate	Prednisone
Cimetidine	
Calcium channel blockers (e.g., diltiazem)	
Grapefruit juice	
Ethanol (acute)	

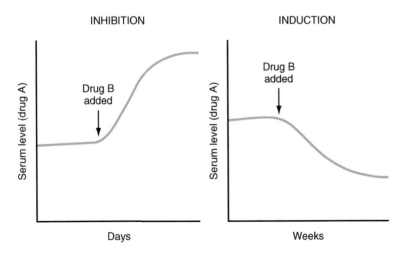

INHIBITION   INDUCTION

Serum level (drug A)   Drug B added

Serum level (drug A)   Drug B added

Days   Weeks

Figure 11-2. Metabolic inhibition and induction. Serum concentrations of drug A rise abruptly if co-administered drug B is an inhibitor of its metabolism, but serum concentrations fall gradually if co-administered drug B is an inducer of its metabolism.

metabolism, they are responsible for metabolizing, at least in part, over 80% of all prescribed drugs. In addition, growing awareness in the 1990s about the capacity of many of the newer antidepressants to inhibit cytochrome P450 isoenzymes fueled great interest in the pattern of interaction of psychotropic and other drugs with these enzymes in the understanding and prediction of drug–drug interactions. The cytochrome P450 isoenzymes represent a family of more than 30 related heme-containing enzymes, largely located in the endoplasmic reticulum of hepatocytes (but also present elsewhere, including the gut and brain), which mediate oxidative metabolism of a wide variety of drugs, as well as endogenous substances (including prostaglandins, fatty acids, and steroids). The majority of antidepressant and antipsychotic drugs are metabolized by, or inhibit, one or more of these isoenzymes. Table 11-2 summarizes the interactions of psychiatric and non-psychiatric drugs with a subset of isoenzymes that have been increasingly well characterized (1A2, 2C subfamily, 2D6, and 3A4). Further information about the relevance of these and other interactions is highlighted in a later section of this chapter in which clinically important drug–drug interactions are reviewed.

In addition to being influenced by pharmacological inducers or inhibitors, a patient's metabolic status is also under genetic control. Knowledge continues to evolve concerning genetic polymorphisms that affect drug metabolism. Within the group of cytochrome P450 isoenzymes, there appears to be a polymodal distribution of metabolic activity in the population with respect to certain isoenzymes (including 2C19 and 2D6). Most individuals are normal ("extensive") metabolizers with respect to the activity of these isoenzymes. A smaller number are "poor metabolizers" with deficient activity of the isoenzyme. Probably very much smaller numbers are ultra-rapid metabolizers (who have more than normal activity of the enzyme) and intermediate metabolizers (who fall between extensive and poor metabolizers). Individuals who are poor metabolizers with respect to a particular cytochrome P450 isoenzyme are expected to have higher plasma concentrations of a drug that is metabolized by that isoenzyme, thereby potentially being more sensitive to, or requiring lower doses of that drug than, a patient with normal activity of that enzyme. They may also have higher-than-usual plasma levels of metabolites of the drug that are produced through other metabolic pathways that are not altered by the polymorphism, thereby potentially incurring pharmacological activity or adverse effects related to these alternative metabolites. Poor metabolizers are relatively impervious to drug interactions involving inhibition of the particular isoenzyme system for which they are already deficient. When the polymorphism is related to an isoenzyme required for conversion of a pro-drug (e.g., tamoxifen, codeine, or tramadol) to its active form, poor metabolizers are also likely to demonstrate a diminished response to those treatments. Studies on genetic polymorphisms affecting the cytochrome P450 system suggest ethnic differences.[16] Approximately 15% to 20% of Asian Americans and African Americans appear to be poor metabolizers with respect to P450 2C19 compared with 3% to 5% of Caucasians. Conversely, the proportion of frankly poor metabolizers with respect to P450 2D6 appears to be higher among Caucasians (approximately 5% to 10%) than among Asian Americans and African Americans (approximately 1% to 3%). Current understanding of the clinical relevance of genetic polymorphisms in drug therapy in psychiatry remains rudimentary. Commercial genotyping tests for polymorphisms of potential relevance to drug–drug metabolism are increasingly available. Further systematic study of their relevance to the understanding and prediction of drug response is needed before such testing can be meaningfully incorporated into routine psychopharmacological practice.

TABLE 11-2 Selected Cytochrome P450 Isoenzyme Substrates, Inhibitors, and Inducers

1A2	Substrates	Acetaminophen, aminophylline, asenapine, caffeine, clozapine, cyclobenzaprine, estradiol, fluvoxamine, haloperidol, mirtazapine, ondansetron, olanzapine, phenacetin, procarcinogens, propranolol, ramelteon, riluzole, ropinirole, tacrine, tertiary amine tricyclic antidepressants (TCAs), theophylline, verapamil, warfarin, zileuton, zolmitriptan
	Inhibitors	Amiodarone, cimetidine, fluoroquinolones, fluvoxamine, grapefruit juice, methoxsalen, ticlopidine
	Inducers	Charbroiled meats, tobacco (cigarette smoking), cruciferous vegetables, modafinil, omeprazole
2C	Substrates	Barbiturates, diazepam, fluvastatin, glipizide, glyburide, irbesartan, losartan, mephenytoin, NSAIDs, nelfinavir, phenytoin, primidone, propranolol, proguanil, proton pump inhibitors, rosiglitazone, tamoxifen, tertiary TCAs, THC, tolbutamide, R-warfarin, S-warfarin
	Inhibitors	Armodafinil, fluoxetine, fluvoxamine, ketoconazole, modafinil, omeprazole, oxcarbazepine, sertraline
	Inducers	Carbamazepine, norethindrone, prednisone, rifampin, secobarbital
2D6	Substrates	Amphetamines, aripiprazole, atomoxetine, β-blockers (lipophilic), codeine, debrisoquine, dextromethorphan, diltiazem, donepezil, duloxetine, encainide, flecainide, galantamine, haloperidol, hydrocodone, iloperidone, lidocaine, mCPP, metoclopramide, mexiletine, nifedipine, ondansetron, phenothiazines (e.g., thioridazine, perphenazine), promethazine, propafenone, risperidone, SSRIs, tamoxifen, TCAs, tramadol, trazodone, venlafaxine
	Inhibitors	Amiodarone, antimalarials, bupropion, cimetidine, citalopram, duloxetine, escitalopram, fluoxetine, methadone, metoclopramide, moclobemide, paroxetine, phenothiazines, protease inhibitors (ritonavir), quinidine, sertraline, terbinafine, TCAs, yohimbine
	Inducers	Dexamethasone, rifampin
3A3/4	Substrates	Alfentanil, alprazolam, amiodarone, amprenavir, aripiprazole, armodafinil, bromocriptine, buspirone, cafergot, calcium channel blockers, caffeine, carbamazepine, cisapride, clozapine, cyclosporine, dapsone, diazepam, disopyramide, efavirenz, estradiol, fentanyl, HMG-CoA reductase inhibitors (lovastatin, simvastatin), indinavir, lidocaine, loratadine, lurasidone, methadone, midazolam, modafinil, nimodipine, pimozide, prednisone, progesterone, propafenone, quetiapine, quinidine, ritonavir, sildenafil, tacrolimus, testosterone, tertiary amine TCAs, triazolam, vinblastine, warfarin, zolpidem, zaleplon, ziprasidone
	Inhibitors	Antifungals, calcium channel blockers, cimetidine, efavirenz, indinavir, fluvoxamine, fluoxetine (norfluoxetine), grapefruit juice, macrolide antibiotics, mibefradil, nefazodone, ritonavir, verapamil, voriconazole
	Inducers	Armodafinil, carbamazepine, glucocorticoids, modafinil, oxcarbazepine, phenobarbital, phenytoin, pioglitazone, rifabutin, rifampin, ritonavir, St. John's wort, troglitazone

HMG-CoA, Hydroxymethylglutaryl coenzyme A; mCPP, m-chlorophenylpiperazine; NSAIDs, non-steroidal anti-inflammatory drugs; SSRIs, selective serotonin reuptake inhibitors; THC, tetrahydrocannabinol.

Excretion

Because most antidepressant, anxiolytic, and antipsychotic medications are largely eliminated by hepatic metabolism, factors that affect renal excretion (glomerular filtration, tubular reabsorption, and active tubular secretion) are generally far less important to the pharmacokinetics of these drugs than to lithium, for which such factors may have clinically-significant consequences. Conditions resulting in sodium deficiency (e.g., dehydration, sodium restriction, use of thiazide diuretics) are likely to result in increased proximal tubular reabsorption of lithium, resulting in increased lithium levels and potential toxicity. Lithium levels and clinical status must be monitored especially closely in the setting of vomiting, diarrhea, excessive evaporative losses, or polyuria. Factors, such as aging, that are associated with reduced renal blood flow and glomerular filtration rate (GFR) also reduce lithium excretion. For this reason, as well as for their reduced volume of distribution for lithium because of relative loss of total body water with aging, elderly patients typically require lower lithium doses than younger patients, and a low starting dose (i.e., 150 to 300 mg/day) is often prudent. Apparently separate from pharmacokinetic effects, however, elderly patients may also be more sensitive to the neurotoxic effects of lithium even at low therapeutic levels. Factors associated with an increased GFR, particularly pregnancy, may produce an increase in lithium clearance and a fall in lithium levels.

For other medications, renal excretion may sometimes be exploited in the treatment of a drug overdose. Acidification of the urine by ascorbic acid, ammonium chloride, or methenamine mandelate increases the rate of excretion of weak bases (such as the amphetamines and phencyclidine [PCP]). Therefore, such measures may be important in the emergency management of a patient with severe PCP or amphetamine intoxication. Conversely, alkalinization of the urine by administration of sodium bicarbonate or acetazolamide may hasten the excretion of weak acids (including long-acting barbiturates, such as phenobarbital).

ANTIPSYCHOTICS

Antipsychotic or neuroleptic drugs include the phenothiazines (e.g., chlorpromazine, fluphenazine, perphenazine, thioridazine, and trifluoperazine), butyrophenones (haloperidol), thioxanthenes (thiothixene), indolones (molindone), diphenylbutylpiperidines (pimozide), dibenzodiazepines (loxapine), and the newer atypical agents (clozapine, olanzapine, risperidone, quetiapine, ziprasidone, aripiprazole, iloperidone, paliperidone, asenapine, and lurasidone).[17] As a class, they are generally rapidly, if erratically, absorbed from the gastrointestinal tract after oral administration (peak plasma concentrations ranging from 30 minutes to 6 hours). They are highly lipophilic and distribute rapidly to body tissues with a large apparent volume of distribution. Protein-binding in the circulation ranges from approximately 90% to 98% except for molindone, paliperidone, and quetiapine, which are only moderately protein-bound. The antipsychotics generally undergo substantial first-pass hepatic metabolism (primarily oxidation and conjugation reactions), reducing their systemic bioavailability when given orally compared with intramuscular (IM) administration, the fractional absorption of which nearly approximates that of IV administration. Most of the individual antipsychotics have several pharmacologically active and inactive metabolites. Because of their propensity to sequester in body compartments, the elimination half-life of antipsychotics is quite variable, generally ranging from approximately 20 to 40 hours. For butyrophenones, however, elimination pharmacokinetics appear to be especially complex, and the disappearance of drug from the systemic circulation, and

even more so from brain, may take much longer, as it does for the newer agent, aripiprazole (and its active metabolite, dehydro-aripirazole), whose half-life may exceed 90 hours.

The lower-potency antipsychotics (including chlorpromazine, mesoridazine, thioridazine, and clozapine) are generally the most sedating and have the greatest anticholinergic, antihistaminic, and α_1-adrenergic antagonistic effects, whereas the higher-potency antipsychotics (including haloperidol, loxapine, molindone, and the piperazine phenothiazines, such as trifluoperazine), are more likely to be associated with an increased incidence of extrapyramidal symptoms (EPS), including akathisia, dystonia, and parkinsonism. The atypical antipsychotics generally have multiple receptor affinities, including antagonism at dopamine D_{1-4} receptors, serotonin 5-HT_1, 5-HT_5, and 5-HT_2 receptors, α_1- and α_2-adrenergic receptors, histamine-H_1 receptors, and cholinergic muscarinic receptors, with variations across agents; thus, for example, clozaril and olanzapine have notably greater affinity at the muscarinic receptors than the other agents and aripiprazole is a partial agonist at the D_2 receptor. Although the more complex pharmacological profile of these newer atypical agents, as well as the older low-potency antipsychotics, has generally been associated with a lower risk of EPS, the same broad range of receptor activity also poses greater risk of pharmacodynamic interactions.

Lower-potency drugs, as well as some atypical antipsychotics, can produce significant hypotension when combined with vasodilator or antihypertensive drugs related to α_1-adrenergic blockade (Table 11-3).[18,19] Hypotension can also occur when low-potency antipsychotics and atypical antidepressants are combined with tricyclic antidepressant (TCA) and MAOI antidepressants. Severe hypotension has been reported when chlorpromazine has been administered with the angiotensin-converting enzyme (ACE) inhibitor captopril. Paradoxical hypotension can develop when epinephrine is administered with low-potency antipsychotics. In this setting, the β-adrenergic stimulant effect of epinephrine, resulting in vasodilation, is thought to be unopposed by its usual pressor effect because α_1-adrenergic receptors are occupied by the antipsychotic. A similar effect may result if a low-potency neuroleptic is administered to a patient with a pheochromocytoma. Finally, hypotension may develop when low-potency antipsychotics are used in combination with a variety of anesthetics (such as halothane, enflurane, and isoflurane).

In addition, the low-potency antipsychotics have quinidine-like effects on cardiac conduction (and may prolong Q-T and P-R intervals).[20] Ziprasidone may also cause Q-T prolongation, although clinically-significant prolongation (QTc > 500 ms) appears to be infrequent when administered to otherwise healthy subjects. Significant depression of cardiac conduction, heart block, and life-threatening ventricular dysrhythmias may result from the co-administration of low-potency antipsychotics or ziprasidone with class I antiarrhythmics (e.g., quinidine, procainamide, disopyramide), as well as when administered with high doses of the TCAs, which have quinidine-like activity on cardiac conduction, and when administered in the context of other aggravating factors (including hypokalemia, hypomagnesemia, bradycardia, or congenital prolongation of the QTc). Pimozide also can depress cardiac conduction as a result of its calcium channel blocking action, and the combination of pimozide with other calcium channel blockers (e.g., nifedipine, diltiazem, verapamil) is contraindicated.

Another clinically-significant pharmacodynamic interaction arises when low-potency antipsychotics, as well as atypical antipsychotics, particularly clozapine or olanzapine, are administered with other drugs that have anticholinergic effects (including TCAs, benztropine, and diphenhydramine). When these drugs are combined, there is greater risk of urinary retention, constipation, blurred vision, impaired memory and

TABLE 11-3 Selected Drug Interactions with Antipsychotic Medications

Drug	Potential Interaction
Antacids (aluminum-magnesium containing), fruit juice	Interference with absorption of antipsychotic agents
Carbamazepine	Decreased antipsychotic drug plasma levels; additive risk of myelosuppression with clozapine
Cigarettes	Decreased antipsychotic drug plasma levels; reduced extrapyramidal symptoms
Rifampin	Decreased antipsychotic drug plasma levels
TCAs	Increased TCA and antipsychotic drug plasma levels; hypotension, depression of cardiac conduction (with low-potency antipsychotics)
SSRIs	Increased SSRI and antipsychotic drug plasma levels; arrhythmia risk with thioridine and pimozide
Bupropion, duloxetine	Increased antipsychotic drug plasma levels; arrhythmia risk with thioridazine
Fluvoxamine, nefazodone	Increased antipsychotic drug plasma levels; arrhythmia risk with pimozide; seizure risk with clozapine
β-Blockers (lipophilic)	Increased antipsychotic drug plasma levels; improved akathisia
Anticholinergic drugs	Additive anticholinergic toxicity; reduced extrapyramidal symptoms
Antihypertensive, vasodilator drugs	Hypotension (with low-potency antipsychotics and risperidone)
Guanethidine, clonidine	Blockade of antihypertensive effect
Epinephrine	Hypotension (with low-potency antipsychotics)
Class I antiarrhythmics	Depression of cardiac conduction; ventricular arrhythmias (with low-potency antipsychotics, ziprasidone)
Calcium channel blockers	Depression of cardiac conduction; ventricular arrhythmias (with pimozide)
Lithium	Idiosyncratic neurotoxicity

SSRIs, Selective serotonin reuptake inhibitors; TCAs, tricyclic antidepressants.

concentration, and increased intraocular pressure in the setting of narrow-angle glaucoma. With overdose, a severe anticholinergic syndrome can develop, including delirium, paralytic ileus, tachycardia, and dysrhythmias. Elderly patients are likely to be at increased risk for toxicity due to anticholinergic effects. The high-potency agents and non-anticholinergic atypical agents (e.g., risperidone) are indicated when anticholinergic effects need to be minimized.

The sedative effects of low-potency agents and atypical antidepressants are also often additive to those of the sedative-hypnotic medications and alcohol. In patients for whom sedative effects may be especially dangerous, including the elderly, the cautious selection and dosing of antipsychotics should always take into account the overall burden of sedation from their concurrent medications. For these patients, starting with a low, divided dose is often an appropriate first step.

Because dopamine receptor blockade is a property common to all antipsychotics, they are all likely to interfere, although to varying degrees, with the efficacy of levodopa and direct dopamine receptor agonists in the treatment of Parkinson's disease. When antipsychotic treatment is necessary in this setting, clozapine and the newer atypical agents, or the lower-potency conventional agents, have been preferred. Reciprocally, antipsychotics are likely to be less effective in the treatment of psychosis in the setting of levodopa, stimulants (e.g., dextroamphetamine), and direct agonists (e.g., ropinirole) that facilitate dopamine transmission. Nevertheless, these agents have been combined with antipsychotics in cautious, modestly successful efforts to treat the negative symptoms of schizophrenia (including blunted affect, paucity of thought and speech, and social withdrawal). In addition, elevated prolactin is common on antipsychotics, particularly higher-potency conventional agents and risperidone; it manifests with irregular menses, galactorrhea, diminished libido, or hirsutism. If these agents are necessary and other causes of hyperprolactinemia have been excluded, there is an appropriate role for concurrent, cautious use of dopamine agonists, particularly bromocriptine, to lower prolactin.

The risk of agranulocytosis, which occurs rarely with the low-potency antipsychotics, is much higher with clozapine, with an incidence as high as 1% to 3%. For this reason, the combination of clozapine with other medications associated with a risk of myelosuppression (e.g., carbamazepine) should be avoided. Similarly, as clozapine lowers the seizure threshold to a greater extent than other antipsychotics, co-administration with other medications that significantly lower the seizure threshold (e.g., maprotiline) should be avoided or combined use with an anticonvulsant should be considered.

The co-administration of lithium with antipsychotic agents (most notably haloperidol) has been associated, very rarely, with potentially irreversible neurotoxicity, characterized by mental status changes, EPS, and, perhaps in some cases, cerebellar signs and hyperthermia.[21] Related to this concern is the unconfirmed suggestion that lithium co-administration with an antipsychotic may increase the risk of neuroleptic malignant syndrome (NMS). Other clinical variables, including dehydration and poor nutrition, are likely to be of greater significance as putative risk factors for NMS. At present, the evidence is not sufficient to warrant avoidance of the widely used combination of lithium and neuroleptics. Such a possibility, however, should be considered when a patient receiving these medications has neuropsychiatric toxicity of unclear origin.

Pharmacokinetic drug interactions are common among the antipsychotic drugs.[18,19] Plasma levels of the neuroleptics, however, may vary as much as 10-fold to 20-fold between individuals even on monotherapy, and, as a class, antipsychotics fortunately have a relatively wide therapeutic index. Therefore, factors that alter antipsychotic drug metabolism may not have deleterious clinical consequences in many instances. Exceptions include those antipsychotic drugs linked to risk of arrhythmia, most notably thioridazine and pimozide. Related to cytochrome P450 isoenzyme inhibition, agents that interfere with P450 2D6 (such as fluoxetine, paroxetine, duloxetine, or bupropion) can greatly increase levels of low-potency agents, including thioridazine, and thus increase the risk of arrhythmia. Similarly, agents that interfere with P450 3A4 (such as erythromycin, fluvoxamine, or nefazodone) entail similar risk when combined with pimozide. These combinations are contraindicated. The concurrent administration of potent P450 3A4 inhibitors with ziprasidone may increase levels and theoretically increase QTc and risk of arrhythmias. Another exception has to do with patients who are maintained on antipsychotics carefully tapered to the lowest effective dose. In these patients, a small decrease in antipsychotic levels, as may occur with the introduction of a metabolic inducer or an agent that interferes with absorption, may bring them below the threshold for efficacy.

Antipsychotic drug levels may be lowered by aluminum-containing or magnesium-containing antacids, which reduce their absorption and are best given separately. Mixing liquid preparations of phenothiazines with beverages, such as fruit juices, presents the risk of causing insoluble precipitates and inefficient gastrointestinal absorption. Carbamazepine, known to be a potent inducer of hepatic enzymes, including P450 3A4 and others, has been associated with reduction of steady-state antipsychotic drug plasma levels by as much as 50%. This effect is especially important to bear in mind as a potential explanation when a neuroleptic-treated patient appears to deteriorate in the weeks following the introduction of carbamazepine. Oxcarbazepine may also induce antipsychotic drug metabolism, as can a variety of other anticonvulsants, including phenobarbital and phenytoin. Cigarette smoking may also be associated with a reduction in antipsychotic drug levels through enzyme metabolism. As inpatient units and community residential programs have widely become "smoke-free," there are often substantial differences in smoking frequency between inpatient and outpatient settings. Among patients who smoke heavily, consideration should be given to the impact of these changes in smoking habits on antipsychotic dose requirements.

When an antipsychotic drug is given together with a TCA, the plasma level of each agent may rise, presumably because of mutual inhibition of microsomal enzymes. Reciprocally, when a patient with psychotic depression is tapered off an antipsychotic, it is important to remember that the plasma level of TCAs may also decline. Selective serotonin reuptake inhibitors (SSRIs) and other antidepressants with inhibitory effects on cytochrome P450 isoenzymes may also produce an increase in the plasma levels of a concurrently administered antipsychotic agent (see Table 11-1). Thus, increases in clozapine, olanzapine, asenapine, and haloperidol plasma levels may occur when co-administered with fluvoxamine. Increases in risperidone, aripiprazole, iloperidone, and typical antipsychotic levels may follow initiation of fluoxetine, paroxetine, bupropion, duloxetine, or sertraline. Quetiapine, lurasidone, and ziprasidone levels may rise following addition of nefazodone, fluvoxamine, or fluoxetine. Phenothiazine drug levels may be increased when co-administered with propranolol, another inhibitor of hepatic microenzymes. Because propranolol is often an effective symptomatic treatment for neuroleptic-associated akathisia, the combined use of the β-blocker with an antipsychotic drug is common. When interactions present a problem, the use of a water-soluble β-blocker, such as atenolol, which is not likely to interfere with hepatic metabolism, provides a reasonable alternative.

MOOD STABILIZERS
Lithium

Lithium is absorbed completely from the gastrointestinal tract.[17] It distributes throughout total body water and, in contrast to most psychotropic drugs, does not bind to plasma proteins and is not metabolized in the liver. It is filtered and

TABLE 11-4 Selected Drug Interactions with Lithium

Drug	Potential Interaction
Aminophylline, theophylline, acetazolamide, mannitol, sodium bicarbonate, sodium chloride load	Decreased lithium levels
Thiazide diuretics	Increased lithium levels; reduction of lithium-associated polyuria
Non-steroidal anti-inflammatory drugs, COX-2 inhibitors, tetracycline, spectinomycin, metronidazole, angiotensin II receptor antagonists, angiotensin-converting enzyme inhibitors	Increased lithium levels
Neuromuscular blocking drugs (succinylcholine, pancuronium, decamethonium)	Prolonged muscle paralysis
Antithyroid drugs (propylthiouracil, thioamide, methimazole)	Enhanced antithyroid efficacy
Calcium channel blockers (verapamil, diltiazem)	Idiosyncratic neurotoxicity
Antipsychotic drugs	Idiosyncratic neurotoxicity

reabsorbed by the kidneys, and 95% of it is excreted in the urine. Lithium elimination is highly dependent on total body sodium and fluid balance; it competes with sodium for reabsorption in the proximal tubules. To a lesser extent, lithium is also reabsorbed in the loop of Henle but, in contrast to sodium, is not reabsorbed in the distal tubules. Its elimination half-life is approximately 24 hours; clearance is generally 20% of creatinine clearance but is diminished in elderly patients and in patients with renal disease. The risk of toxicity is increased in these patients, as well as in patients with cardiovascular disease, dehydration, or hypokalemia. The most common drug–drug interactions involving lithium are pharmacokinetic. Because lithium has a low therapeutic index, such interactions are likely to be clinically significant and potentially serious (Table 11-4).[22]

A number of medications are associated with decreased lithium excretion and therefore increased risk of lithium toxicity. Among the best studied of these interactions involve thiazide diuretics. These agents decrease lithium clearance and thereby steeply increase the risk of toxicity. Thiazide diuretics block sodium reabsorption at the distal tubule, producing sodium depletion, which, in turn, results in increased lithium reabsorption in the proximal tubule. Loop diuretics (e.g., furosemide, bumetanide) appear to interact to a lesser degree with lithium excretion, presumably because they block lithium reabsorption in the loop of Henle, potentially off-setting possible compensatory increases in reabsorption more proximally.[23,24] The potassium-sparing diuretics (e.g., amiloride, spironolactone, ethacrynic acid, triamterene) also appear to be somewhat less likely to cause an increase in lithium levels, but close monitoring is indicated when introduced. The potential impact of thiazide diuretics on lithium levels does not contraindicate their combined use, which has been particularly valuable in the treatment of lithium-associated polyuria. Potassium-sparing diuretics have also been used for this purpose. When a thiazide diuretic is used, a lithium dose reduction and frequent monitoring of lithium levels are required. Monitoring of serum electrolytes, particularly potassium, is also important when thiazides are introduced, because hypokalemia enhances the toxicity of lithium. Although not contraindicated with lithium, ACE inhibitors (e.g., captopril) and angiotensin II receptor antagonists (e.g., losartan) can elevate lithium levels, and close monitoring of levels is also required when these agents are introduced. Many of the non-steroidal anti-inflammatory drugs (NSAIDs) (including ibuprofen, indomethacin, naproxen, ketorolac, meloxicam, and piroxicam) have also been reported to increase serum lithium levels, potentially by as much as 50% to 60% when used at full prescription strength. This may occur by inhibition of renal clearance of lithium by interference with a prostaglandin-dependent mechanism in the renal tubule. The COX-2 inhibitors may also raise lithium levels. Limited available data suggest that aspirin is less likely to affect lithium levels.[25,26]

Finally, a number of antimicrobials are associated with increased lithium levels, including tetracycline, metronidazole, and parenteral spectinomycin. In the event that these agents are required, close monitoring of lithium levels and potential dose adjustment are recommended.

Conversely, a variety of agents can produce decreases in lithium levels, thereby increasing risk of psychiatric symptom breakthrough and relapse. The methylxanthines (e.g., aminophylline, theophylline) can cause a significant decrease in lithium levels by increasing renal clearance; close blood level monitoring is necessary when co-administration occurs. A reduction in lithium levels can also result from alkalinization of urine (e.g., with acetazolamide or sodium bicarbonate), osmotic diuretics (e.g., urea or mannitol), or from ingestion of a sodium chloride load, which also increases lithium excretion.

A probable pharmacodynamic interaction exists between lithium and agents (e.g., succinylcholine, pancuronium, decamethonium) used to produce neuromuscular blockade during anesthesia. Significant prolongation of muscle paralysis can occur when these agents are administered to the lithium-treated patient. Although the mechanism is unknown, the possible inhibition by lithium of acetylcholine synthesis and release at the neuromuscular junction is a potential basis for synergism.

Lithium interferes with the production of thyroid hormones through several mechanisms, including interference with iodine uptake, tyrosine iodination, and release of triiodothyronine (T_3) and thyroxine (T_4). Lithium may therefore enhance the efficacy of antithyroid medications (e.g., propylthiouracil, thioamide, methimazole) and has also been used preoperatively to help prevent thyroid storm in the surgical treatment of Graves' disease.

There are isolated reports of various forms of neurotoxicity, usually but not always reversible, when lithium has been combined with SSRIs, serotonin norepinephrine reuptake inhibitors (SNRIs), and other serotonergic agents, calcium channel blockers, antipsychotics, and anticonvulsants (such as carbamazepine). In some cases, features of the serotonin syndrome or NMS have been present. While it is worthwhile to bear this in mind when evaluating unexplained mental status changes in a lithium-treated patient, the combination of lithium with these classes of medication is neither contraindicated nor unusual.

Valproic Acid

Valproic acid is a simple branched-chain carboxylic acid that, like several other anticonvulsants, has mood-stabilizing properties. Valproic acid is 80% to 95% protein-bound and is rapidly metabolized primarily by hepatic microsomal glucuronidation and oxidation. It has a short elimination half-life of about 8 hours. Clearance is essentially unchanged in the elderly and in patients with renal disease, whereas it is significantly reduced in patients with primary liver disease.

In contrast to some other major anticonvulsants (such as carbamazepine and phenobarbital), valproate does not induce hepatic microsomes. Rather, it tends to act as an inhibitor of oxidation and glucuronidation reactions, thereby potentially

TABLE 11-5 Selected Drug Interactions with Valproate and Carbamazepine

Drug	Interaction with Valproate
Carbamazepine	Decreased valproate plasma levels; increased plasma levels of the epoxide metabolite of carbamazepine; variable effects on plasma levels of carbamazepine
Phenytoin	Decreased valproate plasma levels; variable effects on phenytoin plasma levels
Phenobarbital	Decreased valproate plasma levels; increased phenobarbital plasma levels
Oral contraceptives	Decreased valproate plasma levels
Carbapenem antibiotics	Decreased valproate plasma levels
Lamotrigine	Increased lamotrigine levels; hypersensitivity reaction
Aspirin	Increased unbound (active) fraction of valproate
Cimetidine Fluoxetine	Increased valproate plasma levels
Clonazepam	Rare absence seizures

Drug	Interaction with Carbamazepine
Phenytoin Phenobarbital Primidone	Decreased carbamazepine plasma levels
Macrolide antibiotics Isoniazid Fluoxetine Verapamil Diltiazem Danazol Propoxyphene	Increased carbamazepine plasma levels
Oral contraceptives Corticosteroids Thyroid hormones Warfarin Cyclosporine Phenytoin Ethosuximide Carbamazepine Valproate Lamotrigine Tetracycline Doxycycline Theophylline Methadone Benzodiazepines TCAs Antipsychotics Methylphenidate Modafinil	Induction of metabolism by carbamazepine
Thiazide diuretics Furosemide	Hyponatremia

TCAs, Tricyclic antidepressants.

increasing levels of co-administered hepatically-metabolized drugs, notably including lamotrigene as well as some TCAs, such as clomipramine, amitriptyline, and nortriptyline (Table 11-5).[27–29] A complex pharmacokinetic interaction occurs when valproic acid and carbamazepine are administered concurrently. Valproic acid not only inhibits the metabolism of carbamazepine and its active metabolite, carbamazepine-10,11-epoxide (CBZ-E), but also displaces both entities from protein-binding sites. Although the effect on plasma carbamazepine levels is variable, the levels of the unbound (active) epoxide metabolite are increased with a concomitant increased risk of carbamazepine neurotoxicity. Conversely, co-administration with carbamazepine results in a decrease in plasma valproic acid levels. Nevertheless, the combination of valproate and carbamazepine has been used successfully in the treatment of patients with bipolar disorder who were only partially responsive to either drug alone. Oral contraceptives as well as carbapanem antibiotics have also been associated with decreases in plasma valproic acid levels; enhanced monitoring of levels and valproate dose adjustments are recommended when these agents are used.

Cimetidine, a potent inhibitor of hepatic microsomal enzymes, is associated with decreased clearance of valproic acid resulting in increased levels. Dose reductions of valproic acid may be necessary in the patient starting cimetidine but not for other H_2-receptor antagonists. Elevated levels of valproic acid have also been reported sporadically with fluoxetine and other SSRIs. Aspirin and other salicylates may displace protein-binding of valproic acid, thereby increasing the unbound (free) fraction, which may increase risk of toxicity from valproate even though total serum levels are unchanged.

Absence seizures have been reported with the combination of clonazepam and valproate, although this is likely to be rare and limited to individuals with neurological disorders.

Lamotrigine

Lamotrigine is a phenyltriazine anticonvulsant that is moderately (50% to 60%) protein-bound and metabolized primarily by glucuronidation. Its most serious adverse effect is a life-threatening hypersensitivity reaction with rash, typically, but not always, occurring within the first 2 months of use. The incidence among individuals with bipolar disorder is estimated at 0.8 per 1,000 among patients on lamotrigine monotherapy and 1.3 per 1,000 among patients on lamotrigine in combination with other agents.

The risk of adverse effects including hypersensitivity reactions and tremor is increased when lamotrigine is combined with valproic acid. As much as a two-fold to three-fold increase in lamotrigine levels occurs when valproic acid is added, related to inhibition of glucuronidation of lamotrigine.[12,28] Accordingly, the *Physicians' Desk Reference* (PDR) provides guidelines for more gradual dose titration of lamotrigine and lower target doses when introduced in a patient already taking valproate. When valproate is added to lamotrigine, the dose of the latter should typically be reduced by one-half to two-thirds.

Conversely, lamotrigine levels can be decreased by as much as 50% when administered with metabolic inducers, particularly other anticonvulsants (including carbamazepine and phenobarbital). Guidelines have therefore been developed for the dosing of lamotrigine in the presence of these metabolic-inducing anticonvulsants. Of particular note, similar magnitude reductions in lamotrigine levels have been reported in patients on oral contraceptives, requiring an increase in the dose of lamotrigine.[30] Lamotrigine levels and symptom status should be monitored closely when oral contraceptives or metabolic-inducing anticonvulsants are started.

Carbamazepine

Carbamazepine is an iminostilbene anticonvulsant structurally related to the TCA imipramine. It is only moderately (60% to 85%) protein-bound. It is poorly soluble in gastrointestinal fluids, and as much as 15% to 25% of an oral dose is excreted unchanged in the feces. Its carbamazepine-10,11-epoxide (CBZ-E) metabolite is neuroactive. Carbamazepine, a potent inducer of hepatic metabolism, can also induce its own metabolism such that elimination half-life may fall from 18 to 55 hours to 5 to 20 hours over a matter of several weeks, generally reaching a plateau after 3 to 5 weeks.[17]

Most drug–drug interactions with carbamazepine occur by pharmacokinetic mechanisms.[29,31,32] The metabolism of a wide variety of drugs (e.g., valproic acid, phenytoin, ethosuximide, lamotrigine, alprazolam, clonazepam, TCAs, antipsychotics, methylphenidate, doxycycline, tetracycline, thyroid hormone, corticosteroids, oral contraceptives, methadone, theophylline, warfarin, oral hypoglycemics, cyclosporine) is induced by carbamazepine, thereby lowering drug levels and potentially leading to therapeutic failure or symptom relapse (see Table 11-5). Patients of childbearing potential on oral contraceptives must be advised to use an additional method of birth control.

Several drugs inhibit the metabolism of carbamazepine, including the macrolide antibiotics (e.g., erythromycin, clarithromycin, triacetyloleandomycin), isoniazid, fluoxetine, valproic acid, danazol, propoxyphene, and the calcium channel blockers verapamil and diltiazem. Because of its low therapeutic index, the risk of developing carbamazepine toxicity is significantly increased when these drugs are administered concurrently. Conversely, co-administration of phenytoin or phenobarbital, both microsomal enzyme inducers, can increase the metabolism of carbamazepine, potentially resulting in subtherapeutic plasma levels.

Carbamazepine has been associated with hyponatremia. The combination of carbamazepine with thiazide diuretics or furosemide has been associated with severe, symptomatic hyponatremia, suggesting the need for close monitoring of electrolytes when these medications are used concurrently. Carbamazepine has also been associated with bone marrow suppression, and its combination with other agents that interfere with blood cell production (including clozapine) should generally be avoided.

Oxcarbazepine appears to be a less potent metabolic inducer than carbamazepine, although it still may render certain important agents, particularly P450 3A4 substrates, less effective due to similar pharmacokinetic interactions. Women of childbearing potential should therefore receive guidance about supplementing oral contraceptives with a second non-hormonal form of birth control, as with carbamazepine. Similarly, like carbamazepine, oxcarbazepine is also associated with risk of hyponatremia.

ANTIDEPRESSANTS

The antidepressant drugs include the TCAs, the MAOIs, the SSRIs, the atypical agents (bupropion, trazodone, nefazodone, and mirtazapine), and the SNRIs (duloxetine, venlafaxine, and desvenlafaxine). Although the TCAs and MAOIs are used infrequently, they continue to serve a valuable role in the treatment of more severe, treatment-resistant depressive and anxiety disorders despite the wide range of drug–drug interactions they entail.

Selective Serotonin Reuptake Inhibitors and Other Newer Antidepressants

The SSRIs (fluoxetine, sertraline, paroxetine, fluvoxamine, citalopram, escitalopram, and vilazodone) share similar pharmacological actions, including minimal anticholinergic, antihistaminic, and α_1-adrenergic blocking effects, and potent pre-synaptic inhibition of serotonin reuptake. Vilazodone is also a partial agonist at the 5-HT$_{1A}$ receptor while vortioxetine is an antagonist, agonist or partial agonist at multiple serotonin receptor subtypes. There are important pharmacokinetic differences, which account for distinctions among them with respect to potential drug interactions (Table 11-6).[2,3,33] Nefazodone, similar to trazodone, is distinguished from classic SSRIs by its antagonism of the 5-HT$_2$ receptor (and differs from trazodone in its lesser antagonism of the α_1-adrenergic receptor). Mirtazapine also blocks the 5-HT$_2$ receptor, though it also blocks the 5-HT$_3$ receptor and α_2-adrenergic receptors. Venlafaxine,

TABLE 11-6 Potential Drug Interactions with the Selective Serotonin Reuptake Inhibitors and Other Newer Antidepressants

Drug	Potential Interaction
MAOIs	Serotonin syndrome
Secondary amine TCAs	Increased TCA levels when co-administered with fluoxetine, paroxetine, sertraline, bupropion, duloxetine
Tertiary amine TCAs	Increased TCA levels with fluvoxamine, paroxetine, sertraline, bupropion, duloxetine
Antipsychotics (typical) and risperidone, aripiprazole	Increased antipsychotic levels with fluoxetine, sertraline, paroxetine, bupropion, duloxetine
Thioridazine	Arrhythmia risk with P450 2D6 inhibitory antidepressants
Pimozide	Arrhythmia risk with P450 3A4 inhibitory antidepressants (nefazodone, fluvoxamine)
Clozapine and olanzapine	Increased antipsychotic levels with fluvoxamine
Diazepam	Increased benzodiazepine levels with fluoxetine, fluvoxamine, sertraline
Triazolobenzodiazepines (midazolam, alprazolam, triazolam)	Increased levels with fluvoxamine, nefazodone, sertraline
Carbamazepine	Increased carbamazepine levels with fluoxetine, fluvoxamine, nefazodone
Theophylline	Increased theophylline levels with fluvoxamine
Type 1C antiarrhythmics (encainide, flecainide, propafenone)	Increased antiarrhythmic levels with fluoxetine, paroxetine, sertraline, bupropion, duloxetine
β-Blockers (lipophilic)	Increased β-blocker levels with fluoxetine, paroxetine, sertraline, bupropion, duloxetine
Calcium channel blockers	Increased levels with fluoxetine, fluvoxamine, nefazodone

MAOIs, Monoamine oxidase inhibitors; TCAs, tricyclic antidepressants.

desvenlafaxine, levomilnacipran, and duloxetine, similar to TCAs, inhibit serotonin and norepinephrine reuptake but, in contrast to TCAs, are relatively devoid of post-synaptic anticholinergic, antihistaminic, and α_1-adrenergic activity. Milnacipran is also an SNRI, though FDA-approved only for fibromyalgia. While venlafaxine is predominantly serotonergic at low to moderate doses, duloxetine is a potent inhibitor of both the norepinephrine and serotonin transporters across its clinical dose range. Although not an approved antidepressant, the norepinephrine reuptake inhibitor atomoxetine, indicated for the treatment of attention-deficit/hyperactivity disorder (ADHD), may have a role in depression pharmacotherapy as single agent or as adjunctive treatment. It is neither a significant inhibitor nor an inducer of the P450 cytochrome system, but owing to its adrenergic effects, the risk of palpitations or pressor effects is likely to be greater than with serotonergic agents when combined with prescribed and OTC sympathomimetics, and its use with MAOIs is contraindicated.

All of the SSRIs, as well as nefazodone, are highly protein-bound (95% to 99%), with the exception of fluvoxamine (77%), citalopram (80%), and escitalopram (56%). Mirtazapine and bupropion are moderately protein-bound (85%). The SNRI duloxetine is highly protein-bound (90%), though venlafaxine, desvenlafaxine, and levomilnacipran are minimally protein-bound (15% to 30%). All of the antidepressants are hepatically metabolized, and all of them (except paroxetine and duloxetine) have active metabolites. The major metabolites of sertraline and citalopram, however, appear to be minimally active. Elimination half-lives range from 5 hours for venlafaxine and 11 hours for its metabolite, O-desmethylvenlafaxine, to 2 to 3 days for fluoxetine and 7 to 14 days for its metabolite, norfluoxetine. Nefazodone, similar to venlafaxine, has a short half-life (2 to 5 hours), with fluvoxamine, sertraline, paroxetine, citalopram, escitalopram, bupropion, mirtazapine, and duloxetine having half-lives in the intermediate range of 12 to 36 hours. Food may have variable effects on antidepressant bioavailability, including an increase for sertraline and vilazodone but a decrease for nefazodone, and no change for escitalopram.

The growing knowledge about the interaction of the newer antidepressants with the cytochrome P450 isoenzymes has revealed differences among them in their pattern of enzyme inhibition that are likely to be critical to the understanding and prediction of drug–drug interactions.

P450 2D6

Fluoxetine, norfluoxetine, paroxetine, bupropion, duloxetine, sertraline (to a moderate degree), and citalopram and escitalopram (to a minimal extent) inhibit P450 2D6, which accounts for their potential inhibitory effect on TCA clearance and the metabolism of other P450 2D6 substrates. Other drugs metabolized by P450 2D6 whose levels may rise in the setting of P450 2D6 inhibition include the type 1C antiarrhythmics (e.g., encainide, flecainide, propafenone), as well as lipophilic β-blockers (e.g., propranolol, timolol, metoprolol), antipsychotics (e.g., risperidone, haloperidol, aripiprazole, iloperidone, thioridazine, perphenazine), TCAs, and trazodone. P450 2D6 converts codeine and tramadol into their active form; hence the efficacy of these analgesics may be diminished when concurrently administered with a P450 2D6 inhibitor. So too, as P450 2D6 converts tamoxifen into its active N-desmethyl tamoxifen form for treatment of neoplasms, the use of inhibitors of 2D6 should be carefully re-evaluated during tamoxifen treatment. These observations underscore the need to exercise care and to closely monitor when prescribing these SSRIs, bupropion, or duloxetine in the setting of complex medical regimens. Plasma TCA levels do not routinely include levels of active or potentially toxic metabolites, which may be altered by virtue of shunting to other metabolic routes when P450 2D6 is inhibited. Therefore, particularly in the case of patients at risk for conduction delay, electrocardiography, as well as blood level monitoring, is recommended when combining TCAs with SSRIs, duloxetine, or bupropion.

P450 3A4

Fluoxetine's major metabolite (norfluoxetine), fluvoxamine, nefazodone, and, to a lesser extent, sertraline, desmethylsertraline, citalopram, and escitalopram inhibit P450 3A4. All of these agents have some potential therefore for elevating levels of pimozide and cisapride (arrhythmia risks), methadone, oxycodone, fentanyl (respiratory depression risks), calcium channel blockers, the "statins," carbamazepine, midazolam, and many other important and commonly prescribed substrates of this widely recruited P450 isoenzyme.

P450 2C

Serum concentrations of drugs metabolized by this subfamily may be increased by fluoxetine, sertraline, and fluvoxamine. Reported interactions include decreased clearance of diazepam on all three SSRIs, a small reduction in tolbutamide clearance on sertraline, and increased plasma phenytoin concentrations reflecting decreased clearance on fluoxetine. Warfarin is also metabolized by this subfamily, and levels may be increased by the inhibition of these enzymes. SSRIs may interact with warfarin and potentially increase bleeding diathesis by still other, probably pharmacodynamic, mechanisms (such as depletion of platelet serotonin). Although the combination is common, increased monitoring is recommended when SSRIs are prescribed with warfarin.

P450 1A

Among the SSRIs, only fluvoxamine appears to be a potent inhibitor of P450 1A2. Accordingly, increased serum concentrations of theophylline, haloperidol, clozapine, olanzapine, asenapine, and the tertiary amine TCAs (including clomipramine, amitriptyline, and imipramine) may occur when co-administered with this SSRI. Because theophylline and TCAs have a relatively narrow therapeutic index and because the degree of elevation of antipsychotic blood levels appears to be substantial (e.g., up to four-fold increases in haloperidol concentrations), additional monitoring and consideration of dose reductions of these substrates are necessary when fluvoxamine is co-administered.

Mirtazapine, although neither a potent inhibitor nor inducer of the P450 cytochrome isoenzymes, has numerous pharmacodynamic effects, including antagonism of the histamine-H_1, α_2-adrenergic, 5-HT_2 and 5-HT_3, and muscarinic receptors, creating the possibility of myriad pharmacodynamic interactions (including blockade of clonidine's antihypertensive activity) but also the possible benefit of attenuated nausea and sexual dysfunction that may occur with SSRIs.

The serotonin syndrome is a potentially life-threatening condition characterized by confusion, diaphoresis, hyperthermia, hyperreflexia, muscle rigidity, tachycardia, hypotension, and coma.[9,34] Although the serotonin syndrome may develop whenever an SSRI is combined with a serotonergic drug (e.g., L-tryptophan, clomipramine, venlafaxine, triptans) and drugs with serotonergic properties (e.g., lithium, mirtazapine, dextromethorphan, tramadol, meperidine, pentazocine), the greatest known risk is associated with the co-administration of an SSRI or SNRI with an MAOI, which constitutes an absolute contraindication. In view of the long elimination half-life of fluoxetine and norfluoxetine, at least 5 weeks must elapse after fluoxetine discontinuation before an MAOI can be safely introduced. With the other SSRIs and SNRIs, an interval of 2 weeks appears to be adequate. Because of the time required for the MAO enzymes to regenerate, at least 2 weeks must elapse after discontinuation of an MAOI before an SSRI or other potent serotonergic drug is introduced. The weak, reversible MAOI antimicrobial linezolid, used for treatment of multi-drug-resistant Gram-positive infections, has been implicated in a small number of post-marketing cases of serotonin syndrome in patients on serotonergic antidepressants, typically patients on SSRIs, as well as other medications (including narcotics).

Patients on serotonergic antidepressants receiving linezolid should be monitored for the occurrence of symptoms suggesting serotonin syndrome. The co-administration of SSRIs with other serotonergic agents is not contraindicated but should prompt immediate discontinuation in any patient on this combination of drugs who has mental status changes, fever, or hyperreflexia of unknown origin.

Tricyclic Antidepressants

TCAs are thought to exert their pharmacological action by inhibiting the pre-synaptic neuronal reuptake of norepinephrine and serotonin in the CNS with subsequent modulation of both pre-synaptic and post-synaptic β-adrenergic receptors. TCAs also have significant anticholinergic, antihistaminic, and α-adrenergic activity, as well as quinidine-like effects on cardiac condition, in these respects resembling the low-potency antipsychotic drugs that are structurally similar.

TCAs are well absorbed from the gastrointestinal tract and subject to significant first-pass liver metabolism before entry into the systemic circulation, where they are largely protein-bound, ranging from 85% (trimipramine) to 95% (amitriptyline). They are highly lipophilic with a large volume of distribution. TCAs are extensively metabolized by hepatic microsomal enzymes, and most have pharmacologically-active metabolites.

With two methyl groups on the terminal nitrogen of the TCA side-chain, imipramine, amitriptyline, trimipramine, doxepin, and clomipramine are called *tertiary amines*. The demethylation of imipramine, amitriptyline, and trimipramine yields the secondary amine TCAs, desipramine, nortriptyline, and protriptyline, which are generally less sedating and have less affinity for anticholinergic receptors. The demethylation of imipramine relies on cytochrome P450 isoenzymes 1A2 and 3A3/4, whereas that of amitriptyline appears to rely primarily on 1A2. These tertiary amines, as well as their secondary amine offspring, are then hydroxylated via cytochrome P450 2D6, a step sensitive to inhibition by a wide variety of other drugs. The hydroxymetabolites of the most commonly prescribed TCAs can be active. Furthermore, the hydroxymetabolite of nortriptyline may block the antidepressant effect of the parent drug, and some hydroxymetabolites of the TCAs may be cardiotoxic.

Additive anticholinergic effects can occur when the TCAs are co-administered with other drugs possessing anticholinergic properties (e.g., low-potency antipsychotics, antiparkinsonian drugs), potentially resulting in an anticholinergic syndrome. SSRIs, SNRIs, atypical antidepressants, and MAOIs are relatively devoid of anticholinergic activity, although the MAOIs may indirectly potentiate the anticholinergic properties of atropine and scopolamine. Additive sedative effects are not uncommon when TCAs are combined with sedative-hypnotics, anxiolytics, narcotics, or alcohol (Table 11-7).

TCAs possess class 1A antiarrhythmic activity and can lead to depression of cardiac conduction, potentially resulting in heart block or ventricular arrhythmias when combined with quinidine-like agents (including quinidine, procainamide, and disopyramide, as well as the low-potency antipsychotics).[35,36] The antiarrhythmics quinidine and propafenone, inhibitors of cytochrome P450 2D6, may additionally result in clinically significant elevations of the TCAs, thus increasing the risk of cardiotoxicity through both pharmacodynamic and pharmacokinetic mechanisms.

The arrhythmogenic risks of a TCA are enhanced in an individual with underlying coronary or valvular heart disease, recent myocardial infarction, or hypokalemia, and in a patient receiving sympathomimetic amines, such as dextroamphetamine.

TCAs also interact with several antihypertensive drugs. TCAs can antagonize the antihypertensive effects of

TABLE 11-7 Selected Drug Interactions with Tricyclic Antidepressants

Drug	Potential Interaction
Carbamazepine	Decreased TCA plasma levels
Phenobarbital	
Rifampin	
Isoniazid	
Antipsychotics	Increased TCA plasma levels
Methylphenidate	
SSRIs	
Quinidine	
Propafenone	
Antifungals	
Macrolide antibiotics	
Verapamil	
Diltiazem	
Cimetidine	
Class I antiarrhythmics	Depression of cardiac conduction; arrhythmias
Low-Potency Antipsychotics	
Guanethidine	Interference with antihypertensive effect
Clonidine	
Sympathomimetic amines (e.g., isoproterenol, epinephrine)	Arrhythmias, hypertension
Antihypertensives, vasodilator drugs	Hypotension
Anticholinergic drugs	Additive anticholinergic toxicity
MAOIs	Delirium, fever, convulsions
Sulfonylurea hypoglycemics	Hypoglycemia

MAOIs, Monoamine oxidase inhibitors; SSRIs, selective serotonin reuptake inhibitors; TCA, tricyclic antidepressant.

guanethidine, bethanidine, debrisoquine, or clonidine via interference with neuronal reuptake by noradrenergic neurons. Conversely, TCAs can cause or aggravate postural hypotension when co-administered with vasodilator drugs, antihypertensives, and low-potency neuroleptics.

Hypoglycemia has been observed on both secondary and tertiary TCAs, particularly in the presence of sulfonylurea hypoglycemic agents, suggesting the need for close monitoring.

Pharmacokinetic interactions involving the TCAs are often clinically important. The antipsychotic drugs (including haloperidol, chlorpromazine, thioridazine, and perphenazine) are known to increase TCA levels by 30% to 100%. Cimetidine can also raise tertiary TCA levels as predicted by microsomal enzyme inhibition, as can methylphenidate. The antifungals (e.g., ketoconazole), macrolide antibiotics (e.g., erythromycin), and calcium channel blockers (e.g., verapamil and diltiazem) as inhibitors of cytochrome P450 3A4 may also impair the clearance of tertiary amine TCAs, thereby requiring a TCA dose reduction. SSRIs, particularly fluoxetine, paroxetine, and, to a lesser extent, sertraline, have been associated with clinically-significant increases in TCA plasma levels, believed to be the result of inhibition primarily but not exclusively of cytochrome P450 2D6. Similar elevations in TCA levels would be expected with other potent P450 2D6 inhibitor antidepressants (including duloxetine and bupropion).

Inducers of P450 enzymes can increase the metabolism of TCAs. Thus, plasma levels of TCAs may be significantly reduced when carbamazepine, phenobarbital, rifampin, or isoniazid are co-administered or in the setting of chronic alcohol or cigarette use.

Monoamine Oxidase Inhibitors

Monoamine oxidase (MAO) is an enzyme located primarily on the outer mitochondrial membrane and is responsible for intracellular catabolism of the monoamines. It is found in high concentrations in brain, liver, intestines, and lung. In pre-synaptic nerve terminals, MAO metabolizes cytoplasmic monoamines. In liver and gut, MAO catabolizes ingested bioactive amines, thus protecting against absorption into the systemic circulation of potentially vasoactive substances, particularly tyramine. Two subtypes of MAO have been distinguished: intestinal MAO is predominantly MAO_A, whereas brain MAO is predominantly MAO_B. MAO_A preferentially metabolizes norepinephrine and serotonin. Both MAO subtypes metabolize dopamine and tyramine. The traditional MAOIs that have been used for treatment of depression—phenelzine, tranylcypromine, and isocarboxazid—are non-specific inhibitors of both MAO_A and MAO_B. More recently, selegiline, available in transdermal form, has been approved for treatment of depression. At low doses, selegiline is primarily an inhibitor of MAO_B, though it is a mixed MAO_A and MAO_B inhibitor at higher doses. When patients are using MAOIs, dietary[37,38] and medication restrictions must be closely followed to avoid serious interactions. The MAOIs are therefore generally reserved for use in responsible or supervised patients when adequate trials of other classes of antidepressants have failed.

The two major types of MAOI drug–drug interaction are the serotonin syndrome and the hypertensive (also called hyperadrenergic) crisis.[7,8,33] Hypertensive crisis is an emergency characterized by an abrupt elevation of blood pressure, severe headache, nausea, vomiting, and diaphoresis; intracranial hemorrhage or myocardial infarction can occur. Prompt intervention to reduce blood pressure with the α_1-adrenergic antagonist phentolamine or the calcium channel blocker nifedipine may be life-saving. Potentially catastrophic hypertension appears to be due to release of bound intraneuronal stores of norepinephrine and dopamine by indirect vasopressor substances. The reaction can therefore be precipitated by the concurrent administration of vasopressor amines, stimulants, anorexiants, and many OTC cough and cold preparations; these include L-dopa, dopamine, amphetamine, methylphenidate, phenylpropanolamine, phentermine, mephentermine, metaraminol, ephedrine, and pseudoephedrine. By contrast, direct sympathomimetic amines (e.g., norepinephrine, isoproterenol, epinephrine), which rely for their cardiovascular effects on direct stimulation of post-synaptic receptors, rather than on pre-synaptic release of stored catecholamines, may be somewhat safer when administered to individuals on MAOIs, although they are also contraindicated.

Hypertensive crises may also be triggered by ingestion of naturally-occurring sympathomimetic amines (particularly tyramine), which are present in various food products, including aged cheeses (e.g., stilton, cheddar, blue cheese, or camembert, rather than cream cheese, ricotta cheese, or cottage cheese), yeast extracts (e.g., marmite and brewer's yeast tablets), fava (broad) beans, over-ripened fruits (e.g., avocado), pickled herring, aged meats (e.g., salami, bologna, and many kinds of sausage), chicken liver, fermented bean curd, sauerkraut, many types of red wine and beer (particularly imported beer), and some white wines. Although gin, vodka, and whiskey appear to be free of tyramine, their use should be minimized during the course of MAOI treatment, as with other antidepressants, because of the risk of exaggerated side effects and reduced antidepressant efficacy. Other less stringent requirements include moderated intake of caffeine, chocolate, yogurt, and soy sauce. Because MAO activity may remain diminished for nearly 2 to 3 weeks following the discontinuation of MAOIs, a tyramine-free diet and appropriate medication restrictions should be continued for at least 14 days after an MAOI has been discontinued. The lowest dose available of transdermal selegiline has been shown to have minimal risks of hypertensive crisis on a normal diet and therefore does not require the same level of restriction; however, doses of 9 mg/24 hours and above carry the same dietary recommendations as oral MAOIs.

The serotonin syndrome, the other major drug–drug interaction involving the MAOIs, occurs when MAOIs and serotonergic agents are co-administered. Potentially fatal reactions most closely resembling the serotonin syndrome can also occur with other drugs with less selective serotonergic activity, most notably meperidine, as well as dextromethorphan, a widely available cough suppressant. Both of these medications, similar to the SSRIs, SNRIs, and clomipramine, are absolutely contraindicated when MAOIs are used. The 5-HT$_1$ agonist triptans, used in the treatment of migraine, have been implicated in serotonin syndrome when administered to patients on MAOIs. This may be a particular problem on the triptans that are metabolized in part through the MAO enzymes, including sumatriptan, rizatriptan, and zolmitriptan. Other serotonergic medications (e.g., buspirone and trazodone), although not absolutely contraindicated, should be used with care. Other narcotic analgesics (e.g., propoxyphene, codeine, oxycodone, morphine, alfentanil, or morphine) appear to be somewhat safer alternatives to meperidine, but, in conjunction with MAOIs, their analgesic and CNS depressant effects may be potentiated and rare serotonin syndrome–like presentations have been reported.[33,39] If opioid agents are necessary, they should be started at one-fifth to one-half of the standard doses and gradually titrated upward, with monitoring for untoward hemodynamic or mental status changes.

Extremely adverse, although reversible, symptoms of fever, delirium, convulsions, hypotension, and dyspnea were reported on the combination of imipramine and MAOIs. This has contributed to a general avoidance of the once popular TCA–MAOI combinations. Nevertheless, although incompletely studied, the regimen has been observed in some instances to be successful for exceptionally treatment-refractory patients. When combined, simultaneous initiation of a TCA–MAOI or initiation of the TCA before, but never after the MAOI has been recommended, although avoidance of the more serotonergic TCAs (including clomipramine, imipramine, and amitriptyline) is prudent.

The sedative effects of CNS depressants (including the benzodiazepines, barbiturates, and chloral hydrate) may be potentiated by MAOIs. MAOIs often cause postural hypotension, and severe additive effects have occurred when co-administered with vasodilator or antihypertensive medications or low-potency antipsychotics.

The MAOIs, similar to the TCAs, have also been observed to potentiate hypoglycemic agents, including insulin and sulfonylurea drugs, suggesting the need for more frequent glucose monitoring when MAOIs are co-administered with hypoglycemic medications.

Phenelzine has been associated with lowered serum pseudocholinesterase levels and prolonged neuromuscular blockade. The concurrent use of MAOIs is not a contraindication to surgery or electroconvulsive therapy (ECT), although it requires a detailed pre-procedure consultation with the anesthesiologist.

St. John's Wort

Although the efficacy of St. John's wort for depression has not been well established, it has emerged as one of the most carefully studied herbal preparation when it comes to drug–drug interactions. Initial concerns about the generally weak, though potentially variable, MAOI activity of this botanical and the associated risk of serotonin syndrome when combined with serotonergic agents have only been weakly borne out, with few cases of serotonin syndrome reported despite widespread concurrent use of St. John's wort with serotonergic antidepressants. However, both case reports and clinical trials indicate that some critical medications may be rendered less effective in some patients concurrently taking St. John's wort.[14,40] These medications include immunosuppressants (such as cyclosporine and tacrolimus), coumarin anticoagulants, antiretrovirals, theophylline, digoxin, amitriptyline, and oral contraceptives. Although the precise mechanisms and herbal constituents responsible for these effects remain to be elucidated, the primary focus has been on P450 3A4 and P-glycoprotein. A paucity of systematic information exists concerning potential drug interactions and adverse effects of other natural products, including a possible risk of increased bleeding in patients on *gingko biloba* and warfarin and of hepatoxicity in patients on certain kava preparations.[6]

BENZODIAZEPINES

The benzodiazepines are a class of widely-prescribed psychotropic drugs that have anxiolytic, sedative, muscle-relaxant, and anticonvulsant properties. Their rate of onset of action, duration of action, presence of active metabolites, and tendency to accumulate in the body vary considerably and can influence both side effects and the success of treatment.[17] Most benzodiazepines are well absorbed on an empty stomach, with peak plasma levels achieved generally between 1 and 3 hours, although with more rapid onset on some (e.g., diazepam, clorazepate) than others (e.g., oxazepam). Duration of action of a single dose of benzodiazepine generally depends more on distribution from systemic circulation to tissue than on subsequent elimination (e.g., more rapid for diazepam than lorazepam). With repeated doses, however, the volume of distribution is saturated, and elimination half-life becomes the more important parameter in determining duration of action (e.g., more rapid for lorazepam than diazepam). A benzodiazepine that is comparatively short-acting on acute administration may, therefore, become relatively long-acting on long-term dosing. Benzodiazepines are highly lipophilic and distribute readily to the CNS and to tissues. Plasma protein-binding ranges from approximately 70% (alprazolam) to 99% (diazepam).

Of the benzodiazepines, only lorazepam, oxazepam, and temazepam are not subject to phase I metabolism. Because phase II metabolism (glucuronide conjugation) does not produce active metabolites and is less affected than phase I metabolism by primary liver disease, aging, and concurrently used inducers or inhibitors of hepatic microsomal enzymes, the 3-hydroxy-substituted benzodiazepines are often preferred in older patients and patients with liver disease.

Perhaps the most common and clinically significant interactions involving benzodiazepines are the additive CNS-depressant effects, which can occur when a benzodiazepine is administered concurrently with barbiturates, narcotics, or ethanol. These interactions can be serious because of their potential to cause excessive sedation, cognitive and psychomotor impairment, and, at higher doses, potentially fatal respiratory depression. An interesting pharmacodynamic interaction exists between benzodiazepines and physostigmine, which can act as a competitive inhibitor at the benzodiazepine receptor, antagonizing benzodiazepine effects. The specific benzodiazepine antagonist flumazenil, however, is now more commonly the treatment of choice in managing a severe benzodiazepine overdose.

Pharmacokinetic interactions include a decreased rate, but not extent, of absorption of benzodiazepines in the presence of antacids or food. This is more likely to be a factor in determining the subjective effects accompanying the onset of benzodiazepine action for single-dose rather than the overall efficacy of repeated-dose administration. Carbamazepine, phenobarbital, and rifampin may induce metabolism, lowering levels of benzodiazepines that are oxidatively metabolized. In contrast, potential inhibitors of cytochrome P450 3A4 (including macrolide antibiotics, antifungals [e.g., ketoconazole, itraconazole], nefazodone, fluvoxamine, and cimetidine) may be associated with decreased clearance and therefore increased levels of the triazolobenzodiazepines, as well as the non-benzodiazepine sedative-hypnotics (zolpidem, zaleplon, and eszopiclone), which are metabolized through this pathway.[2] The metabolism of diazepam depends in part on cytochrome P450 2C19. Decreased diazepam clearance has been reported with concurrent administration of a variety of agents (including fluoxetine, sertraline, propranolol, metoprolol, omeprazole, disulfiram, low-dose estrogen containing oral contraceptives, and isoniazid).

PSYCHOSTIMULANTS AND MODAFINIL

A variety of miscellaneous drug–drug interactions involving the psychostimulants have been reported.[41] These include increased plasma levels of TCAs (and possibly other antidepressants); increased plasma levels of phenobarbital, primidone, and phenytoin; increased prothrombin time on coumarin anticoagulants; attenuation or reversal of the guanethidine antihypertensive effect; and increased pressor responses to vasopressor drugs. The risk of arrhythmias or hypertension should be considered when combining psychostimulants with TCAs. Although methylphenidate has been implicated in putative drug interactions more often than dextroamphetamine or mixed amphetamine salts, drug interactions involving psychostimulants have been insufficiently studied to draw firm conclusions about their comparative suitability for use among patients on complex medical regimens. Although contraindicated because of the risk of hypertensive crisis, the combination of psychostimulants and MAOIs has been cautiously used in patients with exceptionally treatment-refractory depression or in patients with limiting hypotension on MAOIs that proved resistant to other measures.[42,43] Urinary alkalinization (e.g., with sodium bicarbonate) may result in amphetamine toxicity, most likely because of increased tubular reabsorption of un-ionized amphetamine.

Modafinil and armodafinil interact with the P450 cytochrome isoenzymes as a minimal to moderate inducer of 1A2 and 3A4 and yet as an inhibitor of the 2C isoforms.[2] Modafinil and armodafinil may thereby engage in drug–drug interactions with common substrates, including oral contraceptives (whose levels may decrease) and lipophilic β-blockers, TCAs, clozapine, and warfarin (whose levels may increase), therefore requiring monitoring and patient education. It is important to advise use of a second non-hormonal form of contraception in modafinil and armodafinil-treated patients on oral contraceptives. Like St. John's wort, modafinil has also been implicated as a factor in lowered cyclosporine levels, presumably through P450 3A4 induction, and should be used with extreme care in patients on immunosuppressants that rely on this enzyme for metabolism. Although modafinil and armodafinil have been widely combined with SSRIs and other first-line antidepressants, its safety in combination with MAOIs is unknown.

Access the complete reference list and multiple choice questions (MCQs) online at https://expertconsult.inkling.com

KEY REFERENCES

1. Ciraulo DA, Shader RI, Greenblatt DJ, et al., editors: *Drug interactions in psychiatry*, ed 3, Baltimore, 2005, Williams & Wilkins.
2. Wynn GH, Cozza KL, Armstrong SC, et al. *Clinical manual of drug interaction principles for medical practice*, Washington, DC, 2008, American Psychiatric Publishing Inc.
3. Preskorn SH, Flockhart D. 2010 guide to psychiatric drug interactions. *Prim Psychiatry* 16(12):45–74, 2009.
4. Owen JA. Psychopharmacology. In Levenson JL, editor: *The American Psychiatric Publishing textbook of psychosomatic medicine: psychiatric care of the medically ill*, ed 2, Washington DC, 2011, American Psychiatric Publishing Inc.
5. Alpert JE. Drug-drug interactions in psychopharmacology. In Stern TA, Herman JB, Gorrindo T, editors: *Massachusetts General Hospital psychiatry update and board preparation*, ed 3, New York, 2012, McGraw-Hill, pp 401–409.
6. Mills E, Wu P, Johnston B, et al. Natural health product-drug interactions: a systematic review of clinical trials. *Ther Drug Monit* 27(5):549–557, 2005.
7. Livingston MG, Livingston HM. Monoamine oxidase inhibitors: an update on drug interactions. *Drug Saf* 14:219–227, 1997.
8. Flockhart DA. Dietary restrictions and drug interactions with monoamine oxidase inhibitors: an update. *J Clin Psychiatry* 73(Suppl. 1):17–24, 2012.
9. Boyer EW, Shannon M. Current concepts: the serotonin syndrome. *N Engl J Med* 352(11):1112–1120, 2005.
10. Wilkinson GR. Drug metabolism and variability among patients in drug response. *N Engl J Med* 352:2211–2221, 2005.
11. Buxton ILO, Benet LZ. Pharmacokinetics: the dynamics of drug absorption, distribution, and elimination. In Chabner BA, Knollman BC, editors: *Goodman and Gilman's the pharmacological basis of therapeutics*, ed 12, New York, 2011, McGraw-Hill.
12. Patsalos PN, Froscher W, Pisani F, et al. The importance of drug interactions in epilepsy therapy. *Epilepsia* 43(4):365–385, 2002.
13. Kahn AY, Preskorn SH. Pharmacokinetic principles and drug interactions. In Soares JC, Gershon S, editors: *Handbook of medical psychiatry*, New York, 2003, Marcel Dekker.
14. Zhou S, Chan E, Pan SQ, et al. Pharmacokinetic interactions of drugs with St. John's wort. *J Psychopharmacol* 18:262–276, 2004.
17. Rosenbaum JF, Arana GW, Hyman SE, et al. *Handbook of psychiatric drug therapy*, ed 5, Boston, 2005, Lippincott Williams & Wilkins.
18. Freudenreich O, Goff DC. Antipsychotics. In Ciraulo DA, Shader RI, Greenblatt DJ, et al., editors: *Drug interactions in psychiatry*, ed 3, Baltimore, 2005, Williams & Wilkins.
19. Spina E, de Leon J. Metabolic drug interactions with newer antipsychotics: a comparative review. *Basic Clin Pharmacol Toxicol* 100:4–22, 2007.
22. Sarid-Segal O, Creelman WL, Ciraulo DA, et al. Lithium. In Ciraulo DA, Shader RI, Greenblatt DJ, et al., editors: *Drug interactions in psychiatry*, ed 3, Baltimore, 2005, Williams & Wilkins.
27. DeVane CL. Pharmacokinetics, drug interactions, and tolerability of valproate. *Psychopharmacol Bull* 37(Suppl. 2):25–42, 2003.
28. Fleming J, Chetty M. Psychotropic drug interactions with valproate. *Clin Neuropharmacol* 28(2):96–101, 2005.
29. Ciraulo DA, Pacheco MN, Slattery M. Anticonvulsants. In Ciraulo DA, Shader RI, Greenblatt DJ, et al., editors: *Drug interactions in psychiatry*, ed 3, Baltimore, 2005, Williams & Wilkins.
33. Ciraulo DA, Creelman WL, Shader RI, et al. Antidepressants. In Ciraulo DA, Shader RI, Greenblatt DJ, et al., editors: *Drug interactions in psychiatry*, ed 3, Baltimore, 2005, Williams & Wilkins.
34. Keck PE, Arnold LM. The serotonin syndrome. *Psychiatr Ann* 30:333–343, 2000.
36. Witchel HJ, Hancok JC, Nutt DJ. Psychotropic drugs, cardiac arrhythmia and sudden death. *J Clin Psychopharmacol* 23:58–77, 2003.
41. Markowitz JS, Morrison SD, DeVane CL. Drug interactions with psychostimulants. *Int Clin Psychopharmacol* 14:1–18, 1999.

12 Side Effects of Psychotropic Medications

Jeff C. Huffman, MD, Scott R. Beach, MD, and Theodore A. Stern, MD

KEY POINTS

Background

- A systematic approach to side effects of medications should include consideration of the nature, severity, and timing of symptoms to facilitate optimal management of such side effects.

History

- Many medications (e.g., nefazodone) previously used in psychiatric disorders, but shown to have serious adverse side effects, have been removed from the market over the years.

Clinical and Research Challenges

- Rates of medication side effects may be difficult to quantify.
- Though some side effects may be class effects, others are specific to individual agents.
- It is difficult to predict who will suffer side effects; some side effects are idiosyncratic.

Practical Pointers

- Tricyclic antidepressants are associated with cardiac effects and can be dangerous in overdose.
- Use of monoamine oxidase inhibitors requires education about dietary limitations and drug–drug interactions.
- Selective serotonin reuptake inhibitors and other newer antidepressants are generally well tolerated and safer in overdose than older agents, but still may cause clinically significant side effects.
- Some selective norepinephrine (noradrenaline)-serotonin reuptake inhibitors have been associated with increased blood pressure (e.g., venlafaxine) and liver dysfunction (e.g., duloxetine).

- Bupropion is known to lower the seizure threshold and has also been associated with an increase in panic symptoms.
- Mirtazapine is associated most commonly with sedation and weight gain.
- Lithium and anticonvulsant mood stabilizers are associated with a variety of side effects, including cognitive slowing, weight gain, and neurological symptoms.
- Lamotrigine is the mood stabilizer most associated with the development of Stevens-Johnson syndrome, a rare but life-threatening skin disease.
- Typical antipsychotics are associated with tardive dyskinesia and, of them, the high-potency typical antipsychotics commonly cause extrapyramidal symptoms.
- Several atypical antipsychotics are linked to weight gain and metabolic side effects.
- Most antipsychotics can cause prolongation of the QTc interval, which may increase the risk for lethal ventricular arrhythmias.
- Stimulants have a propensity to cause increased heart rate and blood pressure, and their use is not recommended for patients with underlying ventricular arrhythmias.
- Benzodiazepines are associated with a variety of side effects (including falls, dizziness, and ataxia).
- Short-acting sedative-hypnotic agents, such as zolpidem, have been associated with various sleep-related behaviors, including eating and driving.

OVERVIEW

Side effects of psychotropics, which can range from minor nuisances to life-threatening conditions, can seriously affect the quality of a patient's life and his or her ability to comply with psychopharmacological treatments. For these reasons, it is important for clinicians who prescribe psychotropic medications to know their potential side effects and how such side effects can be managed.

Determining which medication is causing a specific side effect, and whether *any* medication is to blame for a given adverse effect, can be difficult. For example, more than half of all patients with untreated melancholic depression report headache, constipation, and sedation; these same symptoms are frequently attributed to side effects of antidepressant medications.[1] A stepwise approach to the assessment of a potential side effect can help to ensure that true side effects are quickly addressed, while knee-jerk reactions that result in the discontinuation of well-tolerated treatments can be avoided. This approach (Box 12-1) involves an assessment of the nature and severity of the effect, a thoughtful investigation into the

causality of the effect, and the appropriate management of the symptom.

In this chapter, the most common and most dangerous side effects of psychotropics will be discussed in an effort to guide clinicians to treatment decisions and management of adverse effects. For each agent or class of agents, we will review common initial side effects, frequent long-term side effects, severe but rare adverse events, consequences of overdose, and (where applicable) withdrawal symptoms.

ANTIDEPRESSANTS
Tricyclic Antidepressants

Tricyclic antidepressants (TCAs) have a number of common side effects that require careful management. Anticholinergic effects (including dry mouth, blurry vision, urinary hesitancy, constipation, tachycardia, and delirium) that result from the blockade of muscarinic cholinergic receptors can occur with use of TCAs. In addition, anticholinergic effects can also be dangerous to patients with pre-existing glaucoma (leading to

---

BOX 12-1 A Systematic Approach to Medication Side Effects

NATURE OF THE SIDE EFFECT

What exactly are the signs and symptoms? In some cases (e.g., drug rash) this can be easily ascertained, while in others (e.g., a severely demented patient with worsening agitation, possibly consistent with akathisia, restlessness, constipation) it may be difficult.

When did the symptom start?

Has this ever happened before?

Are there associated symptoms?

SEVERITY OF THE SIDE EFFECT

What subjective distress does the symptom cause?

What impact is it having on function and quality of life?

What medical dangers are associated with the side effect?

CAUSALITY OF THE SIDE EFFECT

Did the side effect start in the context of a new medication or a dosage change?

What other medications/remedies are being taken?

Have there been other changes in medication, medical issues, diet, environment, or psychiatric symptoms?

Are the current signs and symptoms consistent with known side effects of a given medication?

MANAGEMENT OF THE SIDE EFFECT

If it appears that a specific medication is causing the side effect, options for management include:

Discontinue the medication

Decrease the dose

Change the dosing schedule (e.g., splitting up dose, taking medication during meals)

Change the preparation (e.g., to longer-lasting formulation)

Add a new medication to treat the side effect (e.g., propranolol for akathisia)

BOX 12-2 Management of Antidepressant Side Effects

GENERAL PRINCIPLES

- Carefully consider whether the side effect is from the antidepressant.
- Consider the timing, dosing, and the nature of effect, as well as the impact of concomitant medications, environmental changes, and medical conditions.
- Consider drug–drug interactions as the cause of the adverse effects, rather than the effects of the antidepressant acting in isolation.
- If an antidepressant appears to be causing non-dangerous side effects, consider lowering the dose (temporarily or permanently), dividing the dose, or changing medications.

MANAGEMENT OF SPECIFIC SIDE EFFECTS

- Anticholinergic effects (e.g., dry mouth, urinary hesitancy, constipation): Symptomatic treatment (use hard candies for dry mouth, use laxatives for constipation); use bethanechol (25–50 mg/day) for refractory symptoms.
- Sedation: Move the dose to bedtime, divide the dose, or add a psychostimulant (e.g., methylphenidate, 5–15 mg each morning) or modafinil (100–200 mg each morning).
- Orthostatic hypotension: Increase fluid intake, divide the dose or move it to bedtime, or add a stimulant/mineralocorticoid.
- Gastrointestinal side effects: Divide the dose, take it with meals, give it at bedtime, or use an H_2 blocker (e.g., ranitidine 150 mg twice daily).
- Insomnia: Move the dose to the morning or add trazodone (25–100 mg), a sedative-hypnotic (e.g., zolpidem 5–10 mg), or another sedating agent.
- Weight gain: Use diet and exercise, and consider addition of an H_2 blocker, topiramate, or sibutramine.
- Sexual dysfunction: Options include switching to another agent (to bupropion, mirtazapine, or another agent not associated with sexual dysfunction), employing a drug holiday (often ineffective), or augmenting with a variety of agents (e.g., sildenafil, methylphenidate, bupropion, amantadine, buspirone, or yohimbine).

---

acute angle-closure glaucoma), benign prostatic hypertrophy (leading to acute urinary retention), and dementia (leading to acute confusional states). TCAs can also cause sedation that results from blockade of H_1 histamine receptors, and orthostatic hypotension, due to blockade of alpha$_1$ receptors on blood vessels. All three of these side-effect clusters are more common with tertiary amine TCAs (e.g., amitriptyline, doxepin, clomipramine, imipramine) than with secondary amine TCAs (e.g., nortriptyline, desipramine, protriptyline). TCAs may also cause increased sweating. Longer-term side effects of TCAs include weight gain (related to histamine receptor blockade) and sexual dysfunction. Box 12-2 describes the management of common side effects of TCAs and other antidepressants.

In addition to these common initial and long-term side effects, TCAs may have more serious but uncommon side effects; many of them are cardiac in nature. These agents are structurally similar to class I antiarrhythmics that are actually pro-arrhythmic in roughly 10% of the population; approximately 20% of patients with pre-existing conduction disturbances have cardiac complications while taking TCAs.[2] TCAs are associated with cardiac conduction disturbances and their use can lead to prolongation of the PR, QRS, and QT intervals on the electrocardiogram (ECG) and have been associated with all manner of heart block. Some have suggested that effects on cardiac conduction are most severe with desipramine, while other studies have found amitriptyline and maprotiline to be most associated with torsades de pointes.[3] Furthermore, these agents have been associated with an increased risk of

myocardial infarction (MI) when compared to selective serotonin reuptake inhibitors (SSRIs).[4] In addition to cardiac effects, other serious adverse events include the serotonin syndrome that occurs most often when TCAs are combined with other serotonergic agents, especially monoamine oxidase inhibitors (MAOIs). This syndrome can include confusion, agitation, and neuromuscular excitability (including seizures).

Adverse effects associated with TCA overdose include the exacerbation of standard side effects (e.g., severe sedation, hypotension, anticholinergic delirium). Ventricular arrhythmias and seizures can also result from TCA overdose. TCA overdose is frequently lethal, with death most often occurring via cardiovascular effects. Figure 12-1 shows an ECG (with characteristic QRS interval widening) of a patient following TCA overdose.[5] A withdrawal syndrome (manifested by malaise, nausea, muscle aches, chills, diaphoresis, and anxiety) can occur following abrupt discontinuation of TCAs; the syndrome is thought to result from cholinergic rebound.

Selective Serotonin Reuptake Inhibitors

Selective serotonin reuptake inhibitors (SSRIs) are generally well tolerated. The most common side effects of SSRIs include gastrointestinal side effects (e.g., nausea, diarrhea, heartburn) that likely result from interactions with serotonin receptors

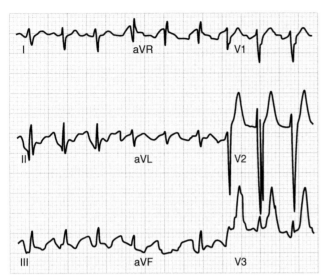

Figure 12-1. ECG showing findings consistent with tricyclic antidepressant poisoning, including sinus tachycardia with widened QRS complex (110 ms) and marked deviation of the terminal portion of the QRS complex in lead I (deep S wave) and aVR (large R wave). *(Re-drawn from Van Mieghem C, Sabbe M, Knockaert D, et al. The clinical value of the ECG in noncardiac conditions,* Chest *125:1561–1576, 2004.)*

(primarily 5-HT$_3$ that line the gut), central nervous system (CNS) activation (e.g., anxiety, restlessness, tremor, insomnia), and sedation that appear within the first few days of treatment. Gastrointestinal side effects may be most common with sertraline and fluvoxamine, CNS activation with fluoxetine, and sedation with paroxetine. Headache and dizziness can also occur early in treatment. These symptoms often improve or resolve within the first few weeks of treatment. Rarely, akathisia or other extrapyramidal symptoms (EPS) may occur (sertraline appears to be the most frequent offender due to its dopamine-blocking properties). Nausea, insomnia, and somnolence are adverse effects that most often lead to discontinuation of SSRIs. It is notable that the rate of discontinuation due to side effects is higher with fluvoxamine than with other SSRIs.

Longer-term side effects associated with SSRIs include sexual dysfunction, which occurs in 30% or more of SSRI-treated patients; SSRI-induced sexual dysfunction occurs in both men and women, affecting both libido and orgasms. Weight gain, fatigue, and apathy are infrequent long-term side effects; weight gain may occur more frequently with paroxetine. The syndrome of inappropriate antidiuretic hormone secretion (SIADH) can occur with all SSRIs, though it may be more frequent with fluoxetine.[6] Finally, SSRIs may increase the risk of bleeding, primarily due to the effects of these agents on serotonin receptors of platelets, resulting in decreased platelet activation and aggregation; it appears that the bleeding risk associated with use of SSRIs is similar to that of low-dose non-steroidal anti-inflammatory agents.[7] SSRIs are relatively safe in overdose. The serotonin syndrome can occur when these agents are combined with other serotonergic compounds, or, very rarely, when used alone.

SSRIs are generally considered safe in terms of cardiovascular side effects. Recently, concern has arisen regarding the possibility of SSRIs leading to prolongation of the QTc interval and increasing the risk for torsades de pointes, a potentially lethal ventricular arrhythmia. In fact, all SSRIs have been associated in case reports with QTc prolongation at therapeutic doses and in overdose.[8] In particular, citalopram has been

shown to have a modest QT-prolonging effect, which resulted in a recommendation from the Food and Drug Administration (FDA) in August 2011 to limit the maximum daily dose of citalopram to 40 mg (20 mg in patients with hepatic impairment or those older than 60 years) because of the increased risk of QTc prolongation at higher doses, and to declare its use contraindicated in patients with congenital long-QT syndrome. Less stringent recommendations were issued in March 2012, but citalopram remains not recommended for use at doses greater than 40 mg per day. No QTc-related recommendations have been issued for other SSRIs, though escitalopram appears to have a more modest, dose-dependent effect on prolongation of the QTc interval.[9]

Finally, abrupt withdrawal from SSRIs can lead to a withdrawal syndrome characterized by several somatic symptoms. The syndrome includes disequilibrium (dizziness, vertigo, and ataxia), flu-like symptoms (headache, lethargy, myalgias, rhinorrhea, and chills), gastrointestinal symptoms (nausea, vomiting, and diarrhea), sensory disturbances (paresthesias and sensations of electrical shock), and sleep disturbances (insomnia, fragmented sleep, and vivid, often frightening, dreams). In addition, a number of psychological symptoms (e.g., agitation, irritability, anxiety, crying spells) are associated with SSRI discontinuation.

Symptoms of the discontinuation syndrome typically begin 1 to 3 days after withdrawal of an SSRI, though when associated with a longer–half-life agent (fluoxetine in particular), symptoms may begin as long as 7 to 10 days after its discontinuation. Symptoms usually resolve within 2 weeks. If the original antidepressant is restarted, or another SSRI is substituted, the symptoms resolve, usually within 24 hours of re-initiation. This syndrome is most common with SSRIs with shorter half-lives (paroxetine and fluvoxamine); it rarely occurs with fluoxetine, whose metabolite has a half-life of more than 1 week. The syndrome is thought to result from diminished synaptic serotonin levels at serotonin receptors that have been desensitized in the context of serotonin reuptake inhibition.

Serotonin-Norepinephrine Reuptake Inhibitors

Venlafaxine

Venlafaxine's initial side effects are similar to those of the SSRIs. Nausea and CNS activation appear to occur somewhat more commonly than with the SSRIs; in addition, dry mouth and constipation may be associated with venlafaxine use despite lack of effects on muscarinic cholinergic receptors. Increased blood pressure, presumably related to effects on norepinephrine (noradrenaline), can occur with immediate-release venlafaxine, with 7% of patients taking 300 mg per day or less and 13% taking doses greater than 300 mg having elevation of blood pressure; this resolves spontaneously in approximately one-half of cases.[10] The extended-release (XR) formulation appears to be associated with lower rates of hypertension. Sexual dysfunction occurs at approximately the same rate as occurs with SSRIs. Venlafaxine does not appear to have substantial adverse effects on the cardiovascular system, though at least one study has suggested the possibility of QTc prolongation.[11] Among more serious side effects, SIADH and serotonin syndrome have been reported with venlafaxine.

Overdose of venlafaxine generally causes symptoms similar to those of SSRI overdose. However, venlafaxine, according to one large epidemiological study in the United Kingdom,[12] has been associated with a high rate of death in overdose (possibly via seizure and cardiovascular effects); other (smaller) studies have not found an increased lethality with overdose. Finally, due to the short half-life of venlafaxine, the discontinuation syndrome reported with SSRIs is common in patients who abruptly stop taking this antidepressant.[13]

Duloxetine

In general, duloxetine's common side effects are similar to those of SSRIs. Nausea, dizziness, headache, and insomnia may be somewhat more frequent than with SSRIs, but overall this agent is well tolerated.[14] Duloxetine does not appear to have significant effects on blood pressure or other cardiovascular parameters, including the QTc interval. Sexual dysfunction appears in concert with duloxetine use, but may be less common than with SSRIs such as paroxetine.[15] Duloxetine has not shown significant affinity for histaminic or cholinergic receptors, and thus sedation, weight gain, and anticholinergic effects are uncommon.

With respect to more severe adverse effects, SIADH has been reported with duloxetine use, and serotonin syndrome may develop with this agent because of its significant serotonin reuptake inhibition. Increased levels of hepatic transaminases develop in a small percentage of patients taking duloxetine; this is usually asymptomatic, but patients with chronic liver disease or cirrhosis have experienced elevated levels of bilirubin, alkaline phosphatase, and transaminases, and currently it is recommended that duloxetine should not be given to patients who consume substantial amounts of alcohol or who exhibit evidence of chronic liver disease.[16] Duloxetine does not appear to have increased rates of death in cases of overdose. A discontinuation syndrome similar to that seen with SSRIs and venlafaxine can occur with abrupt withdrawal of duloxetine,[17] though it is probably less likely than with venlafaxine or paroxetine due to its longer half-life.

Monoamine Oxidase Inhibitors

Tranylcypromine and phenelzine are the most commonly used oral MAOIs and are both irreversible inhibitors. Tranylcypromine is associated with anxiety, restlessness, insomnia, and tremor, while phenelzine is more associated with sedation, mild anticholinergic effects, and orthostatic hypotension (though this last effect can occur with both agents). Both agents are associated with headache, dry mouth, and gastrointestinal side effects. With regard to long-term side effects, weight gain and sexual dysfunction can occur with all MAOIs, though perhaps more commonly with phenelzine. MAOIs can result in symptoms of pyridoxine deficiency, including paresthesias and weakness. Finally, MAOIs have been associated with elevated liver transaminases, though true hepatotoxicity is exceedingly rare.

Hyperadrenergic crises, characterized by occipital headache, nausea, vomiting, diaphoresis, tachycardia, and severe hypertension, can occur in patients taking MAOIs. These most commonly occur when tyramine-containing foods are consumed or when adrenergic agonists (such as sympathomimetics) are taken in combination with MAOIs. Box 12-3 lists tyramine-containing foods that should be avoided by patients on MAOIs.[18] Serotonin syndrome can also occur with MAOIs when these agents are taken with SSRIs, TCAs, or other serotonergic agents (Box 12-4 lists medications that should be avoided by patients taking MAOIs). MAOI overdose is quite dangerous, with rates of death higher than those for SSRIs and other newer antidepressants[12]; with serotonin syndrome, neuromuscular excitability, seizures, arrhythmias, and cardiovascular collapse are all possible.

The transdermal MAOI (selegiline) patch does not require dietary modification at its lowest dose. At this lowest dose (6 mg/24 hours) transdermal selegiline appears to have an

---

BOX 12-3 Foods to Be Avoided by Patients Taking Monoamine Oxidase Inhibitors

- All matured or aged cheeses (fresh cottage, cream, ricotta, and processed cheese are tolerated)
- Pizza, lasagne, and other foods made with cheese
- Fermented/dried meat (e.g., pepperoni, salami, or summer sausage)
- Improperly stored meat and fish
- Fava or broad bean pods
- Banana peel (banana and other fruit are tolerated, but do not use more than ¼ pound of raspberries)
- All tap beer (two or less cans/bottles of beer or 4 oz glasses of wine per day)
- Sauerkraut
- Soy sauce and other soybean products (soy milk is acceptable)
- Marmite yeast extract (other yeast extract are acceptable)

Data from Gardner DM, Shulman KI, Walker SE, et al. The making of a user friendly MAOI diet, J Clin Psychiatry 57:99–104, 1996.

BOX 12-4 Medications to Be Avoided by Patients Taking Monoamine Oxidase Inhibitors

INCREASED RISK OF SEROTONIN SYNDROME
- SSRIs
- TCAs
- Mirtazapine
- Nefazodone
- Vilazodone
- Trazodone
- Buspirone
- Lithium
- Dextromethorphan
- Tramadol
- Methadone
- Carbamazepine
- Sumatriptan and related compounds
- Cocaine
- MDMA
- St. John's wort
- SAMe
- Linezolid

INCREASED RISK OF HYPERADRENERGIC CRISIS
- Dopamine
- L-dopa
- Psychostimulants
- Bupropion
- Amphetamine
- Cold remedies or weight loss products containing pseudoephedrine, phenylpropanolamine, phenylephrine, or ephedrine
- Other
- Meperidine (may cause seizures and delirium)

MDMA, 3,4-methylenedioxy-N-methylamphetamine; SAMe, S-adenosyl-methionine; SSRIs, selective serotonin reuptake inhibitors; TCAs, tricyclic antidepressants.

---

incidence of orthostatic hypotension, gastrointestinal side effects, weight gain, and sexual dysfunction that is greater than placebo, but lower than with orally-ingested MAOIs; skin irritation at the patch sites has been the most common adverse effect. At doses above 6 mg/24 hours, dietary modification is required, and at all doses concomitant medications that increase catecholamines or serotonin should be avoided as with the oral MAOIs.

Other Antidepressants

Bupropion

Bupropion, an agent that does not directly affect serotonin neurotransmission, has initial side effects that differ from those of SSRIs and dual-action agents. Its most common and important initial side effects include headache, dizziness, dry mouth, anxiety, restlessness, anorexia, nausea, and insomnia. Long-term side effects are rare; rates of sexual dysfunction and weight gain are equal to placebo (weight loss can occur in some patients), and this agent has minimal cardiovascular effects, even in overdose. The most serious side effect associated with bupropion use is seizure. The risk of seizure with the immediate-release preparation is 0.1% at doses less than 300 mg/day, and 0.4% at doses from 300 to 400 mg/day; the risk of seizure may be lower with longer-acting preparations, but guidelines to keep the total daily dose at or below 450 mg/day remain. In addition, maximum single doses should not exceed 150 mg for the immediate-release form and 200 mg for the sustained-release form. The longest-acting preparation, Wellbutrin XL, can be given as a single dose of up to 450 mg. Because of its increased risk of seizure, bupropion should not be used in those patients with a history of seizures, or in those at increased risk of seizures (e.g., those with eating disorders, head trauma, or alcohol abuse). Overdose is infrequently life-threatening, though seizures, arrhythmias, and death have occurred in overdose. There is no withdrawal syndrome associated with abrupt discontinuation of bupropion.

Mirtazapine

The most common initial side effects associated with mirtazapine include sedation and increased appetite due to histamine receptor blockade; sedation may be less prevalent at higher doses (i.e., 30 mg/day or greater) than at lower doses due to recruitment of noradrenergic effects at higher doses. Less frequently, dry mouth, constipation, and dizziness have been associated with mirtazapine use; orthostatic hypotension can occur occasionally. Gastrointestinal side effects, anxiety, insomnia, and headache are all less common than with use of most other antidepressants. Weight gain is the most common long-term side effect, and elevated lipids occur in approximately 15% of patients who use mirtazapine. Rare, but more serious, side effects have included an increase in liver transaminases (in approximately 2% of patients), and neutropenia (in 0.1%). Mirtazapine appears to be associated with less sexual dysfunction than the SSRIs and it has minimal cardiovascular effects; it has no withdrawal syndrome. There is also a low mortality rate in overdose.

Trazodone

Trazodone is associated with significant sedation. Other common initial side effects can include dry mouth, nausea, and dizziness; orthostasis is much more common than with nefazodone, with reports of syncope.[19] Weight gain and sexual dysfunction are rare, and trazodone is not associated with hepatotoxicity. Trazodone has, very infrequently, been associated with cardiac arrhythmias and QTc prolongation,[20] possibly due to effects on potassium channels, and it should be used with caution in patients with a propensity for, or a history of, arrhythmias. Priapism occurs in approximately 1 in 6,000 male patients who take trazodone; this effect usually occurs within the first month of treatment.[21] In overdose, sedation

and hypotension are the most common adverse effects; isolated trazodone overdose is rarely fatal. There is no discontinuation syndrome.

Vilazodone

Vilazodone, a newer antidepressant, has diarrhea, nausea, and headache as its most common side effects, all of which are typically transient. The dose is typically titrated incrementally to avoid gastrointestinal side effects. Dry mouth, dizziness, insomnia, and abnormal dreams have also been reported. Vilazodone has not been shown to have adverse cardiac effects and appears to have minimal effects on weight gain. Though purported to cause less sexual dysfunction than other antidepressants, the FDA reports that vilazodone does not meet the minimal criteria to make this claim.[22]

MOOD STABILIZERS
Lithium

Lithium has many associated adverse effects, summarized in Box 12-5. Gastrointestinal and neurological side effects (e.g., sedation, tremor), along with increased thirst, often occur early in therapy, while effects on thyroid and renal function occur more chronically. Box 12-6 summarizes potential treatments for lithium-induced side effects; change in dosing and formulation can reduce gastrointestinal side effects, while other side effects require additional therapies. Lithium has some effects on sino-atrial node transmission and (less commonly) an atrio-ventricular conduction. However, it has not been commonly associated with other effects on the cardiovascular system, and cardiac disease (aside from sick sinus syndrome) is not an absolute contraindication for lithium use. Lithium has a low therapeutic index and lithium toxicity (whether intentional or unintentional) can lead to a variety of symptoms, including neurological (e.g., severe sedation,

---

BOX 12-5 Common Adverse Effects of Lithium

NEUROLOGICAL
- Sedation
- Tremor (fine action tremor)
- Ataxia/incoordination
- Cognitive slowing

GASTROINTESTINAL
- Nausea and vomiting
- Diarrhea
- Abdominal pain
- Weight gain
- Renal
- Polydipsia/polyuria
- Nephrogenic diabetes insipidus
- Interstitial nephritis

DERMATOLOGICAL
- Acne
- Psoriasis
- Edema

CARDIOVASCULAR
- T-wave inversion on electrocardiogram
- Sinoatrial node slowing
- Atrioventricular blockade
- Other
- Hypothyroidism
- Leukocytosis
- Hypercalcemia

BOX 12-6 Management of Selected Lithium
Side Effects

TREMOR
- Propranolol (10–30 mg twice or three times daily); primidone is a second-line option (25–100 mg per day)
- Gastrointestinal
- Change the formulation to a longer-lasting oral preparation or lithium citrate syrup

POLYDIPSIA/POLYURIA
- Amiloride (5–20 mg/day); hydrochlorothiazide (50 mg/day) is a second-line option (halve the lithium dose and follow lithium levels closely)

EDEMA
- Spironolactone (25 mg/day); follow lithium levels closely

HYPOTHYROIDISM
- Treat with thyroid hormone and continue lithium therapy

---

tremor, dysarthria, delirium, anterograde amnesia, myoclonus, seizure), gastrointestinal (e.g., nausea, vomiting), and cardiovascular (e.g., arrhythmia) effects; renal function often is impaired, and dialysis may be required to treat lithium toxicity if supportive measures and intravenous (IV) normal saline to aid lithium excretion are ineffective. Lithium does not have a characteristic discontinuation syndrome, but rapid withdrawal of lithium therapy is associated with substantially higher rates of relapse than when lithium is tapered.[23]

Valproic Acid

Common initial side effects of valproate therapy include gastrointestinal side effects (nausea, vomiting, diarrhea, and abdominal cramps), sedation, tremor, and alopecia; gastrointestinal side effects are less frequent with divalproex sodium (Depakote) than with other preparations, and tremor can be treated with propranolol, as can lithium-induced tremor. Alopecia is sometimes transient and may be reduced by using a multivitamin with zinc and selenium. Longer-term side effects include weight gain and perhaps cognitive slowing. More serious adverse effects associated with valproic acid therapy include pancreatitis (occurring in approximately 1 in 3,000 patients), elevated transaminases (leading very rarely to liver failure), hyperammonemia (at times leading to confusion), thrombocytopenia, platelet dysfunction, and leukopenia. These effects are all quite rare, with the exception of elevated hepatic transaminase levels. There is some controversy regarding whether valproic acid is associated with polycystic ovarian syndrome (PCOS) in women[24]; some studies have suggested that this agent is associated with the development of PCOS, whereas other studies have indicated that bipolar disorder itself may be associated with menstrual irregularities. Practitioners are advised to watch for hirsutism, acne, menstrual irregularities, and weight gain in their female patients who take valproic acid and to initiate evaluation for PCOS if such symptoms arise. Valproate overdose can lead to CNS depression, but it is rarely fatal; dialysis has been used on occasion to aid removal of valproate. Abrupt withdrawal can theoretically increase the risk of seizure, especially in those patients on long-term therapy or with a seizure disorder, but there is no withdrawal syndrome.

Carbamazepine

Initial side effects of carbamazepine include gastrointestinal side effects (nausea, vomiting), neurological side effects (sedation, ataxia, vertigo, diplopia, and blurry vision), and rash. The rash is often benign (occurring in approximately 5% to 10% of patients), but the drug should be stopped if the rash is widespread, or if the rash is associated with systemic signs of illness, facial lesions, or mucous membrane involvement, as Stevens-Johnson syndrome has been reported with this agent. With respect to longer-term side effects, there is usually less weight gain than with use of either valproic acid or lithium. More serious side effects, in addition to Stevens-Johnson syndrome, can include hyponatremia (from SIADH), elevated liver transaminases (though less frequently than with valproic acid), and aplastic anemia and other blood dyscrasias (which occur in approximately 1 in 10,000 to 150,000 of treated patients). Carbamazepine also slows cardiac conduction and should be avoided in patients with high-grade atrioventricular block and sick sinus syndrome. Low free T_3 and T_4 values can occur with carbamazepine use; these levels are usually not of clinical significance, but hypothyroidism should be considered if refractory depression or clinical signs of hypothyroidism exist. Overdose of carbamazepine results in exacerbation of neurological side effects, the potential for high-grade atrio-ventricular (AV) block, and stupor/CNS depression; supportive care is required, and hemodialysis is ineffective. When possible, carbamazepine should be tapered rather than discontinued abruptly to minimize lowering of the seizure threshold.

Oxcarbazepine

Initial side effects from the related compound, oxcarbazepine, are very similar to those of carbamazepine, with gastrointestinal and neurological side effects being the most common. Rash is much less common with oxcarbazepine, but it does occur more frequently than with placebo. The neurological side effects (including cognitive difficulties, incoordination, visual changes, and sedation) associated with oxcarbazepine are reported to be less frequent than with carbamazepine but occur substantially more frequently than in patients who take placebo. Like carbamazepine, it appears to be associated with less weight gain than with lithium or valproic acid. With regard to more serious effects, oxcarbazepine can lead to elevation of transaminases, and it is thought to be associated with higher rates of hyponatremia than carbamazepine. Patients taking oxcarbazepine are at elevated risk of Stevens-Johnson syndrome and other serious dermatological syndromes; low T_4 values can also occur in isolation. However, oxcarbazepine has not been associated with blood dyscrasias. Overdose with oxcarbazepine has been managed supportively and symptomatically.

Lamotrigine

Initial side effects of lamotrigine include neurological side effects (such as dizziness, ataxia, visual changes [diplopia and blurred vision], sedation, and headache); nausea, vomiting, and uncomplicated rash may also occur. All of these initial effects, however, are uncommon, at least in part because of the slow dose escalation required to reduce the risk of dangerous dermatological conditions. Lamotrigine does not have significant long-term side effects; weight gain is rare, and neither hepatoxicity nor cardiovascular effects have been described at usual doses. However, the best-known and most important adverse effects associated with lamotrigine are dermatological conditions related to serious rash. Both Stevens-Johnson syndrome (Figure 12-2) and toxic epidermal necrolysis have occurred in association with lamotrigine use; the risk appears to be greater in pediatric patients, with rapid escalation of the dose, and with concomitant use of valproic acid (which inhibits lamotrigine metabolism). The risk of life-threatening rash appears to be between 0.1% and 0.3% (as opposed to an approximately 10% prevalence of benign rash), and it has been on the lower end of this continuum in trials of lamotrigine for psychiatric illness. Any patient who develops rash on lamotrigine should be promptly evaluated by a medical professional; furthermore, rash with significant facial involvement, mucous membrane involvement (e.g., dysuria, tongue/mouth lesions), or systemic symptoms (such as fever or lymphadenopathy) prompt great concern for life-threatening rash and require immediate emergency evaluation. Lamotrigine overdose can be fatal; the most common symptoms include stupor, convulsions, and intraventricular conduction delay, and treatment is largely supportive.

ANTIPSYCHOTICS
Typical Antipsychotics

Table 12-1 shows the relative frequencies of the common adverse effects of antipsychotics; chlorpromazine

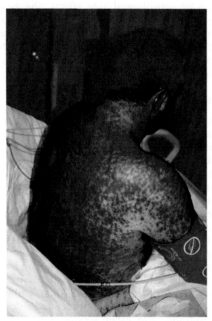

Figure 12-2. Stevens-Johnson syndrome. *(From The Stevens Johnson Syndrome Foundation, SJSmaleback1. Available at www.sjsupport.org.)*

(low-potency), perphenazine (mid-potency), and haloperidol (high-potency) are listed as the prototype agents in the classes of typical antipsychotics. Initial side effects of the low-potency typical agents are similar to those of the TCAs: sedation (due to H_1 receptor blockade), anticholinergic effects (dry mouth, urinary hesitancy, constipation, blurred vision, tachycardia, and risk of confusion, due to the blockade of muscarinic receptors), and orthostatic hypotension (due to alpha$_1$-receptor blockade); these effects can occur to a lesser degree with mid-potency agents and are relatively uncommon with high-potency agents. In contrast, EPS are common in patients taking high-potency typical antipsychotics, but their incidence decreases with decreasing potency (Box 12-7; see also Table 12-1). Common long-term side effects of typical antipsychotics include weight gain (greatest with low-potency agents), photosensitivity (perhaps greatest with chlorpromazine), sexual dysfunction (due to effects on alpha$_2$-receptors), and hyperprolactinemia (which can lead to amenorrhea, galactorrhea, infertility, and osteoporosis). Tardive dyskinesia (TD) (see Box 12-7) is another long-term potential side effect associated with use of all typical antipsychotics, occurring at a rate of approximately 5% per year.[25]

Rarer, but serious, side effects of low-potency antipsychotics include neuroleptic malignant syndrome (NMS; see Box 12-7), QTc prolongation, and torsades de pointes ventricular arrhythmias (especially with use of thioridazine, the antipsychotic most commonly associated with torsades de pointes, and IV haloperidol; Figure 12-3).[26] In addition, chlorpromazine has been associated with cholestatic jaundice (at a rate of approximately 0.1%) and thioridazine has been associated with irreversible pigmentary retinopathy (at doses > 800 mg/day) that can lead to blindness. Overdose of typical antipsychotics has been associated with lethargy, delirium, cardiac arrhythmias, hypotension, EPS, seizure, and death; symptomatic treatment is required and dialysis is not of benefit.

Atypical Antipsychotics

In general, most atypical antipsychotics have significantly lower rates of TD and EPS than do the typical antipsychotics, and (aside from clozapine) have relatively negligible anticholinergic effects; they are generally quite well tolerated. However, several of the atypical antipsychotics have been associated with significant weight gain and with metabolic side effects; these effects appear to be greatest with clozapine and olanzapine, moderate with iloperidone, risperidone,

TABLE 12-1 Selected Side Effects of Antipsychotic Medications

Agent	Sedation	Orthostasis	Ach	EPS	TD	Weight Gain	DM Risk	HyperPRL	QTc Prolongation
Chlorpromazine	Sev	Sev	Sev	Mod/Sev	Mod	Mod/Sev	Mild	Mild	Mod
Perphenazine	Mod	Mod	Mod	Mod	Mod	Mild	Mild	Mild	Mod
Haloperidol	Mild	0	0	Sev	Mod	Mild	0	Mod	Mod (PO form); Sev (IV form)
Risperidone	Mild	Mod/Sev	0	Mod/Sev	Mild	Mod	Mod	Sev	Mod
Ziprasidone	0	Mild	0	Mild[a]	Mild	Mild	Mild	Mild	Sev
Olanzapine	Mod	0	Mild	Mild	Mild	Sev	Sev	Mild	Mod
Aripiprazole	Mild	0	0	Mild[a]	Mild	Mild	Mild	0	0
Quetiapine	Mod	Mod	Mild	0/Mild	0	Mod	Mod	0	Mod
Clozapine	Sev	Mod/Sev	Sev	0	0	Sev	Sev	?	?
Iloperidone*	Mild	Sev	Mild	Mod	?	Mod/Sev	Mod/Sev	Mild	Mod/Sev
Paliperidone	Mild	Mod/Sev	0	Mod	Mild	Mod	Mod	Sev	Mild
Asenapine*	Mod	Mod/Sev	Mild	Mild[a]	?	Mild	Mild	Mild	Mod
Lurasidone*	Mild	Mild	0	Mod	?	Mild	Mild	Mod	0

Ach, Anticholinergic effects; DM, diabetes mellitus; EPS, extrapyramidal symptoms; HyperPRL, hyperprolactinemia; TD, tardive dyskinesia; 0, no effect; Mild, mild effect; Mod, moderate effect; Sev, severe effect; ?, insufficient data.
[a]Moderate frequency and intensity of akathisia.
*Newer agent; somewhat limited clinical experience available.

BOX 12-7 Extrapyramidal Symptoms

ACUTE DYSTONIA

Signs and Symptoms

Localized muscular contraction leading to jaw protrusion, torticollis, tongue protrusion, opisthotonos, extremity contraction, or a fixed upward gaze of the eyes (oculogyric crisis) with associated pain

Risk Factors

Age < 30, male gender, high-potency typical antipsychotics, intramuscular (IM) administration, increased dose, rapid titration of dose

Time Course

Usually occurs within the first several days of initiation or a dose increase

Treatment

Moderate-to-severe reaction: IM diphenhydramine (25–50 mg, repeat as needed) or benztropine (1–2 mg, repeat as needed)
Mild-to-moderate reaction: decrease of antipsychotic dose, addition of oral anticholinergic (e.g., benztropine 0.5–1 mg BID-TID, diphenhydramine 25 mg BID)

ANTIPSYCHOTIC-INDUCED PARKINSONISM

Signs and Symptoms

Muscular rigidity, bradykinesia, shuffling gait, masked facies, and resting (usually non–pill-rolling) tremor

Risk Factors

Female gender, advanced age, high-potency typical antipsychotics, and possibly increased dose

Time Course

Usually gradual in onset, occurs during first 3 months of treatment

Treatment

Decrease the dose or switch the agent; if this is ineffective or not feasible, the addition of an anticholinergic (diphenhydramine or benztropine) or amantadine can reduce symptoms; benzodiazepines or beta-blockers may be helpful in refractory cases

AKATHISIA

Signs and Symptoms

Internal, uncomfortable feeling of restlessness; frequent pacing, inability to remain seated

Risk Factors

High-potency typical antipsychotics (mid-potency typicals, risperidone, and aripiprazole to a lesser degree), higher dosage, rapid titration of dose; possibly advanced age, and diabetes mellitus

Time Course

Usually occurs within the first several days of initiation or a dose increase

Treatment

Reduction of dose (or change of agent); addition of propranolol (e.g., 10–20 mg BID-TID); benzodiazepines may be effective in refractory cases or when beta-blockers are contraindicated; anticholinergics are occasionally helpful, especially when other EPS also present

TARDIVE DYSKINESIA

Signs and Symptoms

Repetitive, involuntary, non-rhythmic movements, most frequently of the tongue and mouth, but potentially including facial (e.g., grimacing), extremity (e.g., repetitive hand gestures), truncal (e.g., opisthotonos), and ocular (e.g., oculogyric crisis) movements

Risk Factors

Typical antipsychotics (risperidone to a lesser degree), time of exposure, advanced age; possibly mood disorders, organic brain disease, and female gender

Time Course

Approximate incidence of 4% per year for first 5 years of treatment with typical antipsychotics; incidence may somewhat slow thereafter, but the prevalence continues to grow with increased time of exposure

Treatment

Few clear treatment options; change of agent, especially to clozapine, may lead to reduction of symptoms; other treatments (e.g., vitamin E, benzodiazepines, botulinum toxin, or reserpine) do not appear to be broadly effective

NEUROLEPTIC MALIGNANT SYNDROME (NMS)

Signs and Symptoms

Confusion, lethargy, rigidity, fever, autonomic instability (with abnormal laboratory values, including significantly increased creatine phosphokinase, elevated hepatic transaminases, and mild leukocytosis)

Risk Factors

Include dehydration, agitation, use of physical restraint, increased or titration of dose, high-potency typical antipsychotics (though NMS can appear with any antipsychotic), IM administration, and history of catatonia or NMS

Time Course

Usually occurs within the first several days of treatment

Treatment

Discontinuation of the offending agent and supportive care to prevent aspiration pneumonia, deep venous thrombosis, renal failure, and other complications in all cases of NMS; dopamine agonists (e.g., bromocriptine), muscle relaxants (e.g., dantrolene), benzodiazepines, and electroconvulsive therapy are all options in refractory or severe cases

---

paliperidone, and quetiapine, and low with aripiprazole, ziprasidone, asenapine and lurasidone (see Table 12-2 regarding weight gain and Table 12-3 regarding monitoring guidelines for metabolic side effects).[27-29] In addition, increased rates of cardiovascular events and death have been associated with the use of atypical antipsychotics among patients with dementia, with a 1.6- to 1.7-fold mortality rate increase in a pooled analysis of over 5,000 patients in 17 clinical trials.[30] These findings have led to a "black box warning" in the package inserts of these agents; of note, a larger analysis found

that the rate of stroke with atypical antipsychotics was not significantly greater than with typical antipsychotics among patients with dementia.[31] More information is needed to determine whether there is a differential risk between agents.

Risperidone

Common initial side effects of risperidone include dizziness and orthostatic hypotension (due to alpha$_1$ blockade), headache, and sedation, though sedation is less frequent with this

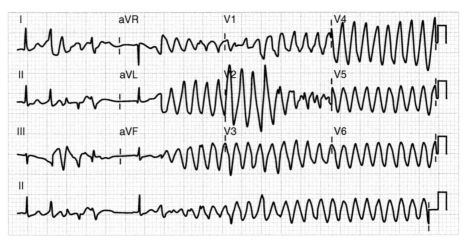

Figure 12-3. Torsades de pointes ventricular arrhythmia. *(Re-drawn from Khan IA. Twelve-lead electrocardiogram of torsades de pointes,* Tex Heart Inst J *28:69, 2001.)*

TABLE 12-2 Weight Gain Associated with 10 Weeks of Antipsychotic Treatment

Agent	Gain at 10 Weeks (kg) Estimated Weight	Estimated Weight Gain at 10 Weeks (lb)
Clozapine	4.45	9.8
Olanzapine*	4.15	9.1
Chlorpromazine	2.58	5.7
Risperidone*	2.10	4.6
Perphenazine	1.33	2.9
Haloperidol†	1.08	2.4
Ziprasidone†	0.04	0.1

*Weight gain associated with quetiapine appears to be intermediate between olanzapine and risperidone.
†Weight gain associated with aripiprazole appears to be intermediate between haloperidol and ziprasidone.
(Adapted from Allison DB et al. Antipsychotic-induced weight gain, Am J Psychiatry *156: 1686–1696, 1999.)*

TABLE 12-3 American Diabetes Association Guidelines for Monitoring Patients Taking Antipsychotics

Monitor	Baseline	4 Weeks	8 Weeks	12 Weeks	1 Year	5 Years
Weight	X	X	X	X*	X	X
Blood pressure	X			X	X†	
Lipid panel	X			X	X	X
Fasting glucose	X			X	X†	

*Weight should be monitored quarterly after 12 weeks.
†Blood pressure and glucose should be monitored yearly after 1 year.
(Adapted from ADA guidelines. American Diabetes Association, American Psychiatric Association, American Association of Clinical Endocrinologists, North American Association for the Study of Obesity: Consensus development conference on antipsychotic drugs and obesity and diabetes, Diabetes Care *27(2):596–601, 2004.)*

agent than with low- and mid-potency typical antipsychotics and many of the other atypicals. With respect to longer-term side effects, hyperprolactinemia is greatest with risperidone among all antipsychotics, and weight gain and risk of diabetes are intermediate between high-potency typical antipsychotics (low rates) and olanzapine and clozapine (very high rates). Risperidone also has one of the highest rates of EPS among atypicals. TD has been described with risperidone, at lower rates than with typical antipsychotics (0.6% per year versus 4.1% per year with haloperidol in one study),[32] but generally at higher rates than other atypicals when high doses of risperidone are used. NMS has also been reported in over 20 patients taking risperidone.[33] Risk of QTc prolongation appears to be intermediate compared with other atypicals.[29] Overdose with risperidone most commonly results in hypotension and sedation.

Paliperidone

Paliperidone is a metabolite of risperidone, and side effects are therefore similar. It is excreted primarily by the kidney and does not undergo processing by the liver. The most commonly reported side effects with paliperidone are headache, nausea, dizziness, insomnia, and dyspepsia. Sedation has been reported, though paliperidone appears to be less associated with sedation than many other atypicals.[29] Despite early claims that paliperidone was not as highly associated with EPS as risperidone, several studies have suggested rates of EPS of up to 20%.[34] Paliperidone has very high rates of hyperprolactinemia.[29] Paliperidone is thought to have effects on weight gain and metabolic parameters that are comparable to that of risperidone. Paliperidone has been associated with prolongation of the QTc interval, though less so than most other atypicals.

Iloperidone

Patients taking iloperidone have high rates of orthostasis, and the dose typically must be titrated very slowly to avoid this. Common side effects include dizziness, headache, dry mouth and insomnia. Weight gain with iloperidone is greater than with risperidone, and in a recent meta-analysis it appears that such weight gain may even approach rates seen with clozapine in the short-term, though longer-term studies are lacking.[29] EPS and hyperprolactinemia are less common than with risperidone. Iloperidone has been associated with QTc prolongation of 9.1 msec, which is similar in scope to that of ziprasidone and greater than is associated with oral haloperidol.[35]

Asenapine

Common side effects of asenapine include somnolence, dizziness and headache. These are likely due to prominent actions at histaminergic and alpha$_1$ receptors. Rates of somnolence are comparable to those seen with olanzapine. Oral hypoesthesia is a side effect seen in up to 7% of patients that appears to be unique to this agent.[36] Weight gain appears to be less common with asenapine than with risperidone, though long-term metabolic effects are unclear at this time. Up to 12% of patients report EPS, with akathisia being the most common manifestation. Hyperprolactinemia has also been reported, though appears to be uncommon. The effects of asenapine on the QTc interval appear comparable to those of risperidone, with a mean increase of 4.4 msec in one study.[36] Finally, serious hypersensitivity reactions have occurred following a single dose of asenapine.

Lurasidone

Sedation is the side effect most commonly reported with lurasidone. Alpha$_1$-antagonist properties also contribute to a risk of orthostatic hypotension and tachycardia. Other common side effects include headache, dry mouth and constipation. Lurasidone has been suggested to have higher rates of hyperprolactinemia and EPS, particularly akathisia and parkinsonism, than other atypical antipsychotics. As many as 13% of patients in a 6-week study experienced EPS, with 7% exhibiting parkinsonism and 8% exhibiting akathisia.[37] Weight gain and metabolic effects appear to be lower than with many other atypical antipsychotics. Lurasidone appears to be least associated with QTc prolongation.[29]

Ziprasidone

Neurological (dizziness, sedation, and headache) and gastrointestinal (nausea and dyspepsia) side effects are common with ziprasidone administration, but they are usually mild. Sedation with ziprasidone is equivalent to that seen with quetipaine. Akathisia is frequently reported, though some apparent akathisia may be a result of activating properties at lower doses. TD appears at much lower rates with ziprasidone than with typical antipsychotics, but can occur[38]; more long-term data are needed. Orthostasis can also uncommonly occur because of alpha$_1$ blockade. With respect to longer-term side effects, weight gain, risk of diabetes, and hyperprolactinemia appear to be lower with this agent. Risk for prolactin increase is moderate. Ziprasidone has been associated with QTc prolongation—greater than with other atypicals and oral haloperidol[39]—but in the clinical setting, this has not been a major issue (there has been a single report of torsades de pointes associated with ziprasidone monotherapy). Overdose with ziprasidone alone has appeared to be relatively safe; cardiotoxicity has not occurred, and the major symptoms have been sedation and dysarthria.

Aripiprazole

The most common initial side effects of aripiprazole include headache, anxiety, insomnia, akathisia, and gastrointestinal side effects (nausea, vomiting, and constipation). Sedation may also occur at higher doses, but is less common than with other atypicals. Akathisia is a common side effect of aripiprazole, and indeed aripiprazole may cause the most akathisia across all atypicals; other EPS are rare. As with ziprasidone, significant weight gain and glucose intolerance are less common with aripiprazole; furthermore, this agent appears to have no significant cardiovascular effects, including no prolongation of the QTc interval. Additionally, it is considered the only antipsychotic that does not cause hyperprolactinemia and may actually lower prolactin levels.[29] The risk of TD appears to be quite low. Aripiprazole overdose appears to be relatively safe, with the most common effects being sedation, vomiting, tremor, and orthostatic hypotension; however, more clinical experience is needed.

Olanzapine

Patients using olanzapine can initially experience sedation, dry mouth, constipation, increased appetite, dizziness (occasionally with orthostatic hypotension), and tremor. EPS occur more frequently than with placebo, but they are less frequent than with use of risperidone or high-potency typical antipsychotics. The major long-term side effects of olanzapine are metabolic. Weight gain occurs frequently with olanzapine; patients on average gain approximately 10 lb in the first 10 weeks of treatment (see Table 12-2) and they can continue to gain weight during ongoing treatment, with one-third to one-half of patients gaining significant weight (as defined by greater than 7% increase in body weight).[40] In addition, olanzapine has been associated with the development of diabetes mellitus; in one study the risk of developing diabetes was approximately six times greater than the risk of diabetes with placebo, and approximately four times the risk for patients on typical antipsychotics.[41] It appears that both insulin resistance and weight gain contribute to this increase in diabetes risk. Diabetic ketoacidosis (DKA) is rare but has been reported in patients taking olanzapine, often occurring within the first month of treatment. Hyperlipidemia, likely in the context of increased food intake and weight gain, is also common with long-term olanzapine therapy. The risks of these metabolic side effects are approximately equivalent to those associated with clozapine; greater than those for quetiapine, low-potency typical antipsychotics, and risperidone; and much greater than for use of the high-potency typicals. Given the risk of these side effects, the American Diabetes Association has developed guidelines for the monitoring of metabolic and cardiovascular parameters for patients taking antipsychotics (see Table 12-3).[27] Hyperprolactinemia is uncommon, but it can occur with olanzapine, especially at higher doses. TD and NMS can occur, but again are rare and less common than with use of typical antipsychotics; rates of TD are generally between 0.5% and 1% per year of treatment.[42] NMS with olanzapine manifests with fewer motor symptoms than with use of typical antipsychotics. Elevation of hepatic transaminases, without progression to liver failure, occurs in approximately 2% of patients; olanzapine has little effect on cardiac conduction. In overdose, olanzapine is relatively safe, with lethargy seen as the most common effect.

Clozapine

Clozapine has many initial side effects. Anticholinergic side effects, sedation, and orthostatic hypotension are common. Sialorrhea occurs frequently, especially at night, and it can be

TABLE 12-4 Monitoring Guidelines for Clozapine

Blood Count	Clozapine Administration	Monitoring
WBC > 3.5K	Continue	Obtain CBC weekly for first 6 months of treatment, then every other week throughout clozapine treatment
WBC between 3–3.5K, or drop of greater than 3K within 3 weeks	Continue	Repeat the value; if unchanged, obtain a CBC twice weekly until the WBC is > 3.5K; monitor for fever, sore throat, and other signs of infection
WBC between 2–3K or absolute neutrophil count (ANC) between 1–2K	Discontinue temporarily	Obtain a CBC daily until WBC is >3K and the ANC is > 2K; then check the WBC twice weekly until the WBC is > 3.5K; monitor for signs of infection
WBC < 2K or ANC less than 1K	Discontinue permanently	Daily CBC until the WBC is > 3.5K and the ANC is > 2K; monitor for infection

ANC, Absolute neutrophil count; CBC, complete blood count; WBC, white blood cell count.
(Adapted from Clozapine (Clozaril) package insert, East Hanover, NJ, January 2003, Novartis.)

quite upsetting to patients; clonidine, glycopyrrolate, or atropine drops administered on the tongue may reduce this symptom. Patients who take clozapine can also have drug-induced fever and tachycardia during the initial days of treatment. Long-term side effects are similar to those of olanzapine, with weight gain, development of diabetes, and hyperlipidemia all significantly prevalent; for both clozapine and olanzapine, weight gain is especially common among adolescents. Fortunately, TD does not seem to be associated with clozapine (with reports of TD improvement on switching to clozapine)[43]; this agent also appears to be prolactin-sparing.

There are several rare but serious adverse effects associated with clozapine. Agranulocytosis is the best-known adverse effect of clozapine; it was initially thought to occur in 1% to 2% of clozapine patients, but subsequent rates have been approximately 0.4% to 0.8%,[44,45] with the institution of mandatory weekly blood count monitoring for the first 6 months and twice-monthly monitoring for the remainder of treatment. Agranulocytosis occurs most frequently within the first 6 months of treatment, and appears to be more likely in women and in those of Ashkenazi Jewish descent; advanced age may also be a minor risk factor.[44] Specific guidelines (Table 12-4) serve to guide the clinician regarding when to stop treatment and when to check complete blood counts more frequently when leukocyte levels drop.[46] Seizures are another risk of clozapine treatment, and risk increases with increasing dose; 4% to 6% of patients treated with doses of 600 mg or more per day will have seizures. If clozapine is necessary, patients having seizures on clozapine can be re-started on the agent once adequate anticonvulsant treatment has been initiated. Uncommonly, cardiac complications occur and include myocarditis (characterized by chest pain, dyspnea, fatigue, and tachycardia, and occurring in approximately 0.2%) and cardiomyopathy (0.1% with long-term treatment). There have been more than 20 reports of NMS with clozapine, with classic symptoms aside from lack of rigidity. Hepatotoxicity can occur, though it is exceedingly rare.[47] Clozapine overdose can result in delirium, lethargy, tachycardia, hypotension, and respiratory failure. Cardiac arrhythmias and seizures have occurred in a minority of cases, and overdose can be fatal. Hemodialysis does not remove clozapine, and management is generally supportive and symptomatic.

ANTIANXIETY AND SLEEP AGENTS
Benzodiazepines

The most common initial side effects of benzodiazepines are sedation and associated daytime fatigue; these effects are frequently transitory and can be managed by lowering the dose or moving the dose to bedtime. Other potential side effects include dizziness, nausea, incoordination, ataxia, anterograde amnesia, and muscle weakness. Uncommon, but possible, psychological effects include increased irritability/hostility and paradoxical disinhibition. Cognitive effects appear to be greatest in the elderly, in those with dementia, and in delirious patients. Long-term side effects are uncommon; a minority of patients report increased depressive symptoms while taking benzodiazepines, and memory impairment and motor incoordination may persist. Furthermore, initial side effects can persist and occasionally worsen, especially with longer-acting agents (such as diazepam), or in patients with liver failure or otherwise impaired hepatic metabolism. Such effects may be less serious when using short-acting benzodiazepines and those agents (lorazepam, oxazepam, temazepam) that do not undergo hepatic oxidative metabolism.

Serious adverse events associated with benzodiazepine use include an increased risk of falls in the elderly, with one study finding an increased risk of hip fractures in the elderly, especially with use of higher doses of benzodiazepines.[48] Furthermore, patients who take benzodiazepines appear to be at higher risk for motor vehicle accidents and for accidental injuries, the risk of the latter being greatest during the initial period (2 weeks to 1 month) of therapy. Finally, respiratory depression can occur in the context of benzodiazepine use, especially in patients with pre-existing respiratory illness. Benzodiazepine overdose in isolation is usually non-fatal, with sedation, dysarthria, confusion, ataxia, and incoordination being common; however, respiratory depression, hypotension, and coma can occur, and deaths have resulted.

Benzodiazepines cause physiological dependence and have a characteristic and potentially dangerous withdrawal syndrome. The withdrawal syndrome usually appears within the first 12 to 48 hours of discontinuation of short-lasting benzodiazepines (such as lorazepam); it may not appear until 2 to 5 days after discontinuation in those patients taking longer-lasting agents (such as clonazepam or diazepam). Given this risk, benzodiazepines should be slowly tapered in all patients; short-lasting agents should be carefully tapered, and at times a switch to a longer-lasting agent (followed by taper of the longer-acting agent) may be required when taper of the shorter-acting agent proves problematic.[49] The withdrawal syndrome from benzodiazepines includes anxiety, tremor, diaphoresis, nausea, insomnia, and irritability; vital signs—especially blood pressure and heart rate—are often elevated in untreated benzodiazepine withdrawal. Generalized tonic-clonic seizures may result, usually early in the course of the syndrome. As withdrawal continues, delirium may result, characterized by more intense withdrawal symptoms, significant autonomic instability, and, frequently, psychotic symptoms. Delirium from benzodiazepine withdrawal is associated with significant risk of fall, congestive heart failure, aspiration, deep venous thrombosis, and other serious medical complications. For the vast majority of patients, development of benzodiazepine abuse is rare and significant dose escalation is uncommon; in fact, many patients who take benzodiazepines have residual symptoms that could benefit from additional therapy.[50] However, patients with ongoing substance use disorders have relatively high rates of benzodiazepine abuse,[51,52] and patients with prior substance use disorders appear to be at increased risk of abuse of prescribed benzodiazepines.

Short-acting Sedative-Hypnotic Sleep Agents (Zolpidem, Zaleplon, and Eszopiclone)

The initial side effects of these agents are similar to those of the benzodiazepines, though they appear to be less frequent. Sedation—their desired effect—is common and occasionally may result in daytime somnolence or fatigue. Dry mouth and headache are other common initial effects. Incoordination, memory disturbance, nausea, and dizziness are uncommon when these agents are used at standard doses in patients without impaired metabolism. An unpleasant taste has been reported by a minority of patients taking eszopiclone. Long-term side effects appear to be uncommon, though these agents have, for the most part, only been studied in short-term use. Tolerance and dose escalation are uncommon. Physiological dependence is also generally uncommon when used as prescribed, but withdrawal syndromes, similar to those seen with benzodiazepines, can occur occasionally when these agents are abruptly discontinued after long-term use; rates of withdrawal are much lower than with the short-lasting benzodiazepines.[53]

The one serious adverse effect that has been reported with zolpidem use involves sleep-associated behavior disorders, including somnambulism and night-eating disorder. These agents are relatively safe in isolated overdose, though respiratory and cardiovascular adverse effects can occur rarely. Treatment of overdose is generally supportive and symptomatic.

Ramelteon

Initial side effects associated with this melatonin receptor agonist are uncommon, but can include dizziness, sedation, nausea, and fatigue. Long-term and serious side effects appear to be rare. Overdose has not been reported, but ramelteon was administered in single doses up to 160 mg in an abuse liability trial, and no safety or tolerability concerns were seen. There is no characteristic withdrawal syndrome with discontinuation of ramelteon.

Buspirone

Buspirone is generally well tolerated. Headache, dizziness, and nausea are the most common side effects, and restlessness, insomnia, and increased anxiety may also occur. Sedation, incoordination, and cognitive effects do not appear to be associated with buspirone use. There are no known common long-term side effects, and there is no physiological dependence or withdrawal syndrome. There have been single case reports of the induction[54] and disappearance[55] of psychosis in the setting of buspirone initiation. Overdose with buspirone appears to be relatively safe, with dizziness, vomiting, and sedation among the most common effects; seizures occurred in the context of one buspirone overdose.[56]

Gabapentin

Gabapentin is frequently used to treat anxiety. Common initial side effects are similar to those of other anticonvulsants: sedation, dizziness, nausea, ataxia, headache, tremor, and visual changes. In general, these side effects are relatively mild and are often transient. Weight gain can occur as a long-term side effect, but it appears to be less common than with valproic acid. Gabapentin undergoes minimal hepatic metabolism and thus is not associated with hepatotoxicity; cardiovascular effects are few as well. In overdose, gabapentin is relatively safe, in part because of dose-limited absorption from the gut, but it is associated with sedation, ataxia, and diplopia; hemodialysis can be used if necessary.

OTHER AGENTS USED IN THE TREATMENT OF PSYCHIATRIC CONDITIONS
Beta-blockers

Initial side effects of the beta-blockers can include bradycardia, dizziness/orthostasis, fatigue, nausea, diarrhea, and insomnia. The effects of beta-blockers can affect a number of medical conditions (Table 12-5), including exacerbation or causation of bronchospasm in vulnerable individuals; in such patients a more β_1-selective agent (such as atenolol or metoprolol) may be required instead of less-selective agents (such as propranolol and pindolol) that act equally at β_1 and β_2 receptors. Patients who take beta-blockers for extended periods may develop sexual dysfunction or depressive symptoms. However, a large meta-analysis examining beta-blockers' link with fatigue, sexual dysfunction, and depression found that such associations were quite weak, with no significant associations between depression and the use of beta-blockers; furthermore, rates of fatigue (one additional report per 57 patient-years) and sexual dysfunction (one report per 1,999 patient-years) were very similar to placebo,[57] though idiosyncratic reactions can occur. Overdose of beta-blockers is serious and can cause bradycardia, hypotension, and more serious cardiac adverse events, up to and including cardiac arrest. Somnolence and lethargy are common in overdose, and propranolol has been associated with seizures in overdose. Abrupt withdrawal after pronged use of beta-blockers has, on occasion, led to angina, myocardial infarction, and, rarely, death in patients with (diagnosed or undiagnosed) coronary artery disease (CAD), and therefore these medications should be tapered after long-term use, especially in patients with CAD or with cardiac risk factors.

Clonidine

Dry mouth, sedation, fatigue, and dizziness are the most common side effects of clonidine. Hypotension (and

TABLE 12-5 Medical Conditions Adversely Affected by Use of Beta-blockers

Medical Condition	Beta-blockers' Effects Related to the Condition
Diabetes	May impair the adrenergic response (tachycardia, diaphoresis, and tremor) to hypoglycemia May inhibit glucose mobilization after hypoglycemia, preventing rapid recovery
Reactive airway disease (e.g., asthma)	Beta-blockers with β_2 activity produce bronchospasm and can lead to hypoxia and respiratory distress
Raynaud's syndrome	Increase the risk of peripheral vasoconstriction
Hypertension	May combine with patients' antihypertensive regimen to have additive effects on cardiac conduction and hypotension (especially true for calcium channel blockers)

orthostasis) can occur, especially among those patients taking other antihypertensive agents. Somewhat less common side effects include nausea, headache, restlessness, and irritability. Vivid dreams, nightmares and sexual dysfunction are infrequent, but have been reported among patients taking clonidine. In overdose, a variety of significant adverse events (including bradycardia, hypotension, respiratory depression, and lethargy) may occur, and in large overdoses, cardiac conduction defects, seizures, and coma can result. Abrupt withdrawal from clonidine has resulted in restlessness, agitation, tremor, and rebound hypertension, and has led rarely to hypertensive encephalopathy or cerebrovascular accidents.

Stimulants

Frequent side effects of the most commonly used psychostimulants (e.g., methylphenidate, dextroamphetamine, mixed amphetamine salts) include anxiety, insomnia, restlessness, and decreased appetite. Increased blood pressure and heart rate can occur in both children and adults, and these effects are generally dose-dependent. Stimulants have been associated with the development of tics; however, controlled studies, even those in children with co-morbid tic disorders, have not found elevated rates of tics among children who are taking psychostimulants.[58,59] In addition, there have been reports of growth retardation among children who receive psychostimulants; however, as with tics, controlled studies have not found a consistent association with growth retardation.[60] More serious adverse effects can include psychosis and disorientation, which are rare except in overdose. Overdose can also be characterized by hyperpyrexia, arrhythmias, seizures, and rhabdomyolysis. There is no characteristic withdrawal syndrome, though abrupt cessation of stimulants after long-term use can be associated with lethargy, dysphoria, irritability, and psychomotor slowing similar to that seen during withdrawal from illicit amphetamine use.

Modafinil

The most common side effects of modafinil include headache, nausea, anxiety, and insomnia. Hypertension and tachycardia occur infrequently (in less than 5% of patients), but have occurred more often than with placebo. This agent has not been extensively studied in patients with significant cardiac disease (such as patients with a history of MI). Modafinil has been associated with Stevens-Johnson syndrome, angioedema, and multi-organ hypersensitivity. Symptoms most commonly associated with modafinil overdose include restlessness, gastrointestinal symptoms, disorientation/confusion, and cardiovascular symptoms (tachycardia, hypertension, and chest pain); death has not occurred with modafinil overdose taken in isolation. There is no known withdrawal syndrome.

Atomoxetine

Initial side effects of atomoxetine include gastrointestinal side effects (decreased appetite, nausea, and vomiting), anticholinergic effects (e.g., urinary hesitancy/retention, dry mouth, constipation), dizziness, palpitations, and insomnia. Heart rate and blood pressure are elevated in a small percentage of patients; in pre-marketing trials, approximately 4% of pediatric patients had mean increases of heart rate of 25 or greater beats to a heart rate of 110 beats per minute. With regard to long-term effects, atomoxetine is associated with sexual dysfunction in both men and women. In addition, growth appears to initially slow in the first 9 months of treatment in pediatric patients, then appears to normalize over the course of 36 months of treatment. Rare, but more serious, side effects of atomoxetine include liver dysfunction, which has occurred in at least three patients since its release, all of whom have recovered after discontinuation of atomoxetine; systematic monitoring of liver function tests has not been recommended.[61] In addition, suicidal ideation emerged in a small percentage (approximately 4 in 1,000) of patients in pre-marketing trials; no suicide attempts were made. In overdose, fatalities have not been reported, and sedation/agitation, gastrointestinal symptoms, and tachycardia appear commonly. There appear to be no withdrawal symptoms associated with discontinuation of atomoxetine.

Anticholinergics

The most common side effects of anticholinergic medications (such as benztropine and diphenhydramine) include dry mouth, constipation, urinary hesitancy, tachycardia, thickening of secretions, and dry skin (related to effects on muscarinic cholinergic receptors). In addition, sedation is common, especially with diphenhydramine and related compounds, because of their effects on histaminic receptors. Dizziness, tremor, incoordination, dyspepsia, and hypotension can also occur, and these agents should not be used in patients with narrow-angle glaucoma or benign prostatic hypertrophy because of their potential to worsen the effects of these conditions. Long-term effects are generally extensions of the usual initial side effects. Anticholinergic medications can lead to daytime fatigue, slowed thinking, and frank delirium, especially in those with risk factors for the development of delirium (e.g., the elderly and those with dementia or another organic brain syndrome). Overdose of anticholinergic medications can lead to a variety of effects (including ataxia, disorientation/confusion, psychosis/hallucinations, agitation, tachycardia, a prolonged QTc interval, hypotension, cardiovascular collapse, seizure, and coma). In most cases, treatment is supportive; vasopressors can be used for hypotension. In patients with refractory symptoms, physostigmine can be used; this agent is often effective, but it can cause bradyarrthymias, asystole, seizures, and significant gastrointestinal effects, and it is contraindicated in patients with prolonged PR or QRS intervals. However, it is effective, and one study found physostigmine to be safer and more effective than benzodiazepines in the treatment of delirious patients with anticholinergic toxicity.[62]

Topiramate

The anticonvulsant topiramate is not an established mood stabilizer, but it has been used in the treatment of alcohol and cocaine use disorders. The most prominent initial side effects of topiramate are neurological side effects (including paresthesias, impaired memory and attention, dizziness, sedation, fatigue, anxiety, and impaired taste); insomnia and visual impairment are less common. Cognitive impairment occurs in up to one-third of patients. Gastrointestinal side effects (e.g., nausea, anorexia, dyspepsia, diarrhea) are also somewhat common with topiramate. Most of these effects—aside from decreased appetite, paresthesias, and cognitive slowing—tend to improve over time. Longer-term side effects include weight loss (in approximately 7% of patients who receive 200 to 400 mg/day).[63] Nephrolithiasis, resulting from inhibition of carbonic anhydrase, can also occur in about 1% of patients. One rare, but serious, adverse effect associated with topiramate is acute myopia with secondary angle-closure glaucoma; this syndrome causes bilateral ocular pain and blurred vision, and is a result of increased intraocular pressure. It usually occurs in the first month of treatment and resolves with discontinuation of topiramate. Metabolic acidosis can also occur, and it has been recommended that serum bicarbonate levels be checked intermittently during topiramate treatment. Topiramate does not have significant cardiac effects, and it has not been associated with liver failure when used alone. Overdose can lead to severe lethargy, confusion, impaired vision, and significant metabolic acidosis, though it is usually not fatal; hemodialysis can be used as needed.

Acamprosate

Acamprosate is used in the treatment of alcohol use disorder to reduce the risk of relapse. Diarrhea and GI upset are the most common side effects reported with acamprosate, causing discontinuation rates of up to 2%. Pruritus has also been reported with some frequency. Erythema multiforme has been noted as a complication in case reports, though it appears to be an extremely rare event. Acamprosate is contraindicated in patients with severe renal impairment, and dose adjustment must be made for patients with moderate renal impairment. Diarrhea is the most common manifestation of overdose; treatment is generally symptomatic and supportive.

Naltrexone

Naltrexone is used in the treatment of substance use disorders to reduce craving and improve abstinence rates. The most frequent side effects reported with naltrexone include nausea, dizziness, asthenia, and headache. Naltrexone is contraindicated in individuals with acute hepatitis or liver failure. Naltrexone has been associated with elevation of liver enzymes in some patients, and some clinicians may elect to monitor liver function tests prior to (and periodically after) initiation. Given its opioid receptor antagonism, it may precipitate acute withdrawal if given to patients who have used opioids in the past 7–10 days, and should be avoided in such patients. Overdose is generally managed supportively.

Buprenorphine

The partial opioid receptor agonist buprenorphine is used in patients with opioid use disorder both for management of acute withdrawal and as a maintenance treatment for relapse prevention. Naloxone is commonly added to buprenorphine in the sublingual formulation used to treat opioid use disorder to prevent IV injection of this agent. Side effects of buprenorphine parallel those of other opioids—sedation, nausea, dizziness, constipation, cognitive effects, and urinary retention—and respiratory depression, likewise, is possible with this agent, especially at high doses. However, respiratory depression is less likely than with full opioid agonists due to a ceiling effect.

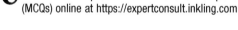 Access the complete reference list and multiple choice questions (MCQs) online at https://expertconsult.inkling.com

KEY REFERENCES

2. Roose SP, Laghrissi-Thode F, Kennedy JS, et al. Comparison of paroxetine and nortriptyline in depressed patients with ischemic heart disease. *JAMA* 279(4):287–291, 1998.
3. Vieweg WV, Wood MA. Tricyclic antidepressants, QT interval prolongation, and torsade de pointes. *Psychosomatics* 45(5):371–377, 2004.
7. Weinrieb RM, Auriacombe M, Lynch KG, et al. Selective serotonin re-uptake inhibitors and the risk of bleeding. *Expert Opin Drug Saf* 4(2):337–344, 2005.
8. Beach SR, Celano CM, Noseworthy PA, et al. QTc prolongation, torsades de pointes, and psychotropic medications. *Psychosomatics* 54(1):1–13, 2013.
9. Castro VM, Clements CC, Murphy SN, et al. QT interval and antidepressant use: a cross sectional study of electronic health records. *BMJ* 346:f288, 2013.
10. Thase ME. Effects of venlafaxine on blood pressure: a meta-analysis of original data from 3744 depressed patients. *J Clin Psychiatry* 59(10):502–508, 1998.

11. Waring WS, Graham A, Gray J, et al. Evaluation of a QT nomogram for risk assessment after antidepressant overdose. *Br J Clin Pharmacol* 70(6):881–885, 2010.
13. Haddad PM. Antidepressant discontinuation syndromes. *Drug Saf* 24(3):183–197, 2001.
15. Delgado PL, Brannan SK, Mallinckrodt CH, et al. Sexual functioning assessed in 4 double-blind placebo- and paroxetine-controlled trials of duloxetine for major depressive disorder. *J Clin Psychiatry* 66(6):686–692, 2005.
18. Gardner DM, Shulman KI, Walker SE, et al. The making of a user friendly MAOI diet. *J Clin Psychiatry* 57(3):99–104, 1996.
22. Laughren TP, Gobburu J, Temple RJ, et al. Vilazodone: clinical basis for the US Food and Drug Administration's approval of a new antidepressant. *J Clin Psychiatry* 72(9):1166–1173, 2011.
25. Latimer PR. Tardive dyskinesia: a review. *Can J Psychiatry* 40(7 Suppl. 2):S49–S54, 1995.
27. Allison DB, Mentore JL, Heo M, et al. Antipsychotic-induced weight gain: a comprehensive research synthesis. *Am J Psychiatry* 156(11):1686–1696, 1999.
28. American Diabetes Association, American Psychiatric Association, American Association of Clinical Endocrinologists, North American Association for the Study of Obesity. Consensus development conference on antipsychotic drugs and obesity and diabetes. *Diabetes Care* 27(2):596–601, 2004.
29. Leucht S, Cipriani A, Spineli L, et al. Comparative efficacy and tolerability of 15 antipsychotic drugs in schizophrenia: a multiple-treatments meta-analysis. *Lancet* 2013.
30. Schneider LS, Dagerman KS, Insel P. Risk of death with atypical antipsychotic drug treatment for dementia: meta-analysis of randomized placebo-controlled trials. *JAMA* 294(15):1934–1943, 2005.
31. Wang PS, Schneeweiss S, Avorn J, et al. Risk of death in elderly users of conventional vs. atypical antipsychotic medications. *N Engl J Med* 353(22):2335–2341, 2005.
34. Wang SM, Han C, Lee SJ, et al. Paliperidone: a review of clinical trial data and clinical implications. *Clin Drug Investig* 32(8):497–512, 2012.
35. Citrome L. Iloperidone: a clinical overview. *J Clin Psychiatry* 72(Suppl. 1):19–23, 2011.
36. Citrome L. Asenapine for schizophrenia and bipolar disorder: a review of the efficacy and safety profile for this newly approved sublingually absorbed second-generation antipsychotic. *Int J Clin Pract* 63(12):1762–1784, 2009.
37. Loebel A, Cucchiaro J, Sarma K, et al. Efficacy and safety of lurasidone 80 mg/day and 160 mg/day in the treatment of schizophrenia: a randomized, double-blind, placebo- and active-controlled trial. *Schizophr Res* 145(1–3):101–109, 2013.
41. Koro CE, Fedder DO, L'Italien GJ, et al. Assessment of independent effect of olanzapine and risperidone on risk of diabetes among patients with schizophrenia: population based nested case-control study. *BMJ* 325(7358):243, 2002.
44. Alvir JM, Lieberman JA, Safferman AZ, et al. Clozapine-induced agranulocytosis. Incidence and risk factors in the United States. *N Engl J Med* 329(3):162–167, 1993.
45. Honigfeld G. Effects of the clozapine national registry system on incidence of deaths related to agranulocytosis. *Psychiatr Serv* 47(1):52–56, 1996.
48. Wang PS, Bohn RL, Glynn RJ, et al. Hazardous benzodiazepine regimens in the elderly: effects of half-life, dosage, and duration on risk of hip fracture. *Am J Psychiatry* 158(6):892–898, 2001.
57. Ko DT, Hebert PR, Coffey CS, et al. Beta-blocker therapy and symptoms of depression, fatigue, and sexual dysfunction. *JAMA* 288(3):351–357, 2002.
58. Law SF, Schachar RJ. Do typical clinical doses of methylphenidate cause tics in children treated for attention-deficit hyperactivity disorder? *J Am Acad Child Adolesc Psychiatry* 38(8):944–951, 1999.
59. Tourette's Syndrome Study G. Treatment of ADHD in children with tics: a randomized controlled trial. *Neurology* 58(4):527–536, 2002.
61. Lim JR, Faught PR, Chalasani NP, et al. Severe liver injury after initiating therapy with atomoxetine in two children. *J Pediatrics* 148(6):831–834, 2006.
62. Burns MJ, Linden CH, Graudins A, et al. A comparison of physostigmine and benzodiazepines for the treatment of anticholinergic poisoning. *Ann Emerg Med* 35(4):374–381, 2000.

13 Natural Medications in Psychiatry

Felicia A. Smith, MD, and David Mischoulon, MD, PhD

KEY POINTS

- Complementary and alternative medical therapies are made up of a diverse spectrum of practices (including natural medications) that often overlap with more traditional medical practice.

- The use of natural medications is growing considerably in the US and around the world, and patients often do not report use of natural medications to their physicians.

- Historical lack of scientific research in this area has contributed to deficiencies in knowledge with respect to safety and efficacy of many of the natural remedies on the market today.

- Natural medications are used for the psychiatric indications of mood disorders, anxiety, insomnia, menstrual and menopausal symptoms, and dementia (among others).

OVERVIEW

Complementary and alternative medical therapies are made up of a diverse spectrum of practices and beliefs that often overlap with current medical practice. The National Institutes of Health (NIH) defines *complementary and alternative medicine (CAM)* as "healthcare practices outside the realm of conventional medicine, which are yet to be validated using scientific methods."[1] The National Center for Complementary and Alternative Medicine (NCCAM) is one of the NIH institutes and is the federal government's lead agency responsible for scientific research on complementary and alternative medicine. NCCAM distinguishes four domains within complementary medicine: mind–body medicine, energy medicine, manipulative and body-based practices, and biologically-based practices.[2] This chapter will focus on the biologically-based practices including natural medications. *Natural medications* are medications that are derived from natural products, and are not approved by the Food and Drug Administration (FDA) for their proposed indication.[3] Natural medications may include a wide variety of types of products such as hormones, vitamins, plants, herbs, fatty acids, amino acid derivatives, and homeopathic preparations. Natural medications have been used in Asia for thousands of years. Their use in the US has, however, been much more recent, with a dramatic increase over the past decade and a half. In fact, the National Health Interview Survey conducted in 2002 revealed that 62% of a randomly-sampled US population used some form of CAM, including prayer, for health reasons within the past year. When prayer was excluded, 36% of those sampled admitted to using some form of CAM.[4-6] Moreover, between 1990 and 1997 the prevalence of herbal remedy use increased by 380%, while high-dose vitamin use increased by 130%.[7] Between 1998 and 2002 CAM use doubled in the over-65 population.[6] Ethnic considerations also appear to be important, with African Americans being the group least likely in the US to try natural remedies and Hispanics being the most prone to their use.[8] Given the considerable portion of the US population trying natural remedies, it is clearly becoming increasingly important to be informed about these medications in order to provide comprehensive patient care. This chapter provides an overview of the use of natural medications in psychiatry. General safety and efficacy are discussed first. This is followed by an examination of some of the primary remedies used for psychiatric indications including mood disorders, anxiety and sleep disorders, menstrual disorders, and dementia.

EFFICACY AND SAFETY

Although both governmental agencies (including the NIH and NCCAM) and the pharmaceutical industry are sponsoring more clinical research involving natural medications, data regarding effectiveness still lag behind. The actual benefits of natural remedies are often unclear in a setting where relatively few systematic studies have adequately addressed the question of effectiveness.[9] The FDA does not routinely regulate natural medications, leaving questions of safety at the forefront. Consumers often believe that because a remedy is "natural," it is therefore safe. Moreover, since these remedies are most often purchased over the counter (OTC), there is no clear mechanism for reports of toxicity to reach those who use them. Another significant problem lies in the limited information regarding the safety and efficacy of combining natural medications with more conventional ones.[9] In cases where interactions are known, the psychiatrist faces the reality that patients frequently do not disclose their use of CAM therapies to their physicians. In one study, fewer than 40% of CAM therapies used were disclosed to a physician.[7] Asking very specific questions about a patient's use of both prescribed and OTC medications may improve disclosures in this regard. Finally, since natural medications are not regulated as more conventional ones are, significant variability exists among different preparations. Preparations often vary in purity, quality, potency, and efficacy while side effects may vary. The increase in government- and industry-sponsored studies may further clarify the potential uses, safety, and efficacy of these medications; until such results are available, caution should still be used in recommending those that are less well understood. The remainder of this chapter outlines the current understanding of some of the primary natural medications with potential psychiatric indications.

MOOD DISORDERS

Numerous natural medications have been used to treat mood disorders, including omega-3 fatty acids, St. John's wort (SJW), *S*-adenosylmethionine (SAMe), folic acid, vitamin B_{12}, and inositol (Table 13-1). Dehydroepiandrosterone (DHEA) may also have a role in the treatment of depression; however, further description of this adrenal steroid is reserved for the cognition and dementia section later in this chapter. The efficacy, possible mechanisms of action, dosing, adverse effects, and drug interactions of each of these medications are discussed in the following section.

TABLE 13-1 Natural Medications for Mood Disorders

Medication	Active Components	Possible Indications	Possible Mechanisms of Action	Suggested Doses	Adverse Events
Omega-3 fatty acids	Essential fatty acids (primarily EPA and DHA)	Depression, bipolar disorder, schizophrenia, ADHD	Effects on neurotransmitter signaling receptors; inhibition of inflammatory cytokines; lowering plasma norepinephrine (noradrenaline)	1,000–2,000 mg/day	Fishy taste and odor, GI upset, theoretical risk of bleeding
Folic acid	Vitamin	Depression, dementia	Neurotransmitter synthesis	400–800 mcg/day; 15 mg/day 5-MTHF (Deplin)	Masking of B_{12} deficiency, lowers seizure threshold in high doses, and adverse interactions with other drugs
Inositol	Six-carbon ring natural isomer of glucose	Depression, panic, OCD, and possibly bipolar disorder	Second messenger synthesis	12–18 g/day	Mild GI upset, headache, dizziness, sedation, and insomnia
SAMe	Biological compound involved in methylation reactions	Depression	Neurotransmitter synthesis	300–1,600 mg/day	Mild anxiety, agitation, insomnia, dry mouth, GI disturbance; also possible switch to mania and serotonin syndrome
St. John's wort (*Hypericum perforatum L.*)	Hypericin, hyperforin, polycyclic phenols, pseudohypericin	Depression	Inhibition of cytokines, decreased serotonin receptor density, decreased neurotransmitter reuptake, MAOI activity	900–1,800 mg/day	Dry mouth, dizziness, GI disturbance, and phototoxicity; also possible serotonin syndrome when taken with SSRIs and adverse interactions with other drugs
Vitamin B_{12}	Vitamin	Depression	Neurotransmitter synthesis	500–1,000 mcg/day	None

ADHD, Attention-deficit/hyperactivity disorder; DHA, docosahexaenoic acid; EPA, eicosapentaenoic acid; GI, gastrointestinal; MAOI, monoamine oxidase inhibitor; OCD, obsessive-compulsive disorder; SAMe, S-adenosylmethionine; SSRI, selective serotonin reuptake inhibitor.
(Adapted from Mischoulon D, Nierenberg AA. Natural medications in psychiatry. In Stern TA, Herman JB, editors: Psychiatry update and board preparation, ed 2, New York, 2004, McGraw-Hill.)

Omega-3 Fatty Acids

Omega-3 fatty acids are polyunsaturated lipids derived from fish oil and certain land-based plants (e.g., flax). Omega-3 fatty acids have been shown to have benefits in numerous medical conditions, including rheumatoid arthritis, Crohn's disease, ulcerative colitis, psoriasis, immunoglobulin A (IgA) nephropathy, systemic lupus erythematosus, multiple sclerosis, and migraine headache, among others.[10] Cardioprotective benefits have also been demonstrated,[11] although recent systematic reviews have been less supportive of their role as preventive agents for cardiovascular disease.[12-14] From a psychiatric standpoint, omega-3 fatty acids may have a role in the treatment of unipolar depression, post-partum depression, bipolar disorder, schizophrenia, and attention-deficit/hyperactivity disorder (ADHD).[15-19] The most promising data, however, are in the treatment of both bipolar disorder and unipolar depression; positive studies have been reported in each of these domains,[15,20-22] yet recent meta-analyses have also cast doubt on the degree of antidepressant efficacy of the omega-3s.[20-26] In countries with higher fish consumption, lower rates of depression and bipolar disorder provide a clue that omega-3 fatty acids may play a protective role in these disorders.[20] Although there are several types of omega-3 fatty acids, eicosapentaenoic acid (EPA) and docosahexaenoic acid (DHA) are thought to be psychotropically active.[3] While their mechanism of action is not completely clear, several have been proposed. These run the gamut from effects on membrane-bound receptors and enzymes that regulate neurotransmitter signaling, to the regulation of calcium ion influx through calcium channels, to the lowering of plasma norepinephrine (noradrenaline)

levels, or possibly to the inhibition of secretion of inflammatory cytokines that result in decreased corticosteroid release from the adrenal gland.[27-30] Omega-3 fatty acids may be consumed naturally from a variety of sources, including fatty fish (e.g., salmon), flax seeds, chia seeds, hemp seeds, and enriched eggs. Commercially available preparations of omega-3 fatty acids in pill form vary in composition, and the suggested ratio of EPA:DHA is at least 3:2 in favor of EPA.[25] Psychotropically-active doses are generally thought to be in the range of 1 to 2 g per day, with dose-related gastrointestinal (GI) distress being the major side effect. There is also a theoretical risk of increased bleeding, so concomitant use with high-dose non-steroidal anti-inflammatory drugs (NSAIDs) or anticoagulants is not recommended. There are thus far no known interactions with other mood stabilizers or antidepressants.

In sum, the use of omega-3 fatty acids remains promising, particularly given the range of potential benefits and the relatively low toxicity seen thus far. However, larger and more definitive studies are still needed.

St. John's Wort

St. John's wort (SJW) (*Hypericum perforatum*) is one of the biggest-selling natural medications on the market. It has been shown to be more effective than placebo in the treatment of mild-to-moderate depression.[31-34] Studies have further suggested that SJW is as effective as low-dose tricyclic antidepressants (TCAs) (e.g., imipramine 75 mg, maprotiline 75 mg, or amitriptyline 75 mg).[27,31] When compared with selective serotonin reuptake inhibitors (SSRIs), the efficacy of SJW has been comparable and better than placebo in some studies of mild depression. For example, SJW was shown to be as effective as sertraline and fluoxetine in the treatment of mild-to-moderate depression in at least two cases.[35,36] However, in other studies, SJW has not shown an advantage over placebo.[37,38] These mixed results may be explained by more severely depressed study populations in studies with negative outcomes.[27] *Hypericum* is thought to be the main antidepressant ingredient in SJW, while polycyclic phenols, pseudohypericin, and hyperforin are also thought to be active ingredients. As far as the mechanism of action of SJW is concerned, there are several proposed theories. These include the inhibition of cytokines, a decrease in serotonin (5-HT) receptor density, a decrease in reuptake of neurotransmitters, and monoamine oxidase inhibitor (MAOI) activity.[9,27] Since SJW has MAOI activity, it should not be combined with SSRIs because of the possible development of serotonin syndrome. Suggested doses range from 900 to 1,800 mg per day depending on the preparation, and adverse effects include dry mouth, dizziness, constipation, and phototoxicity. Care should be taken in patients with bipolar disorder due to the possibility of a switch to mania.[39] Finally, there are a number of important drug–drug interactions with SJW that are of particular note. Hyperforin is metabolized through the liver and induces cytochrome P-3A4 expression, which may reduce the therapeutic activity of a number of common medications, including warfarin, cyclosporine, oral contraceptives, theophylline, digoxin, and indinavir.[40,41] Transplant recipients should not use SJW since transplant rejections have been reported as a result of interactions between SJW and cyclosporine.[42] Individuals with human immunodeficiency virus (HIV) infection on protease inhibitors also should avoid SJW because of drug interactions.

In sum, SJW appears to be better than placebo and equivalent to low-dose TCAs for the treatment of mild depression. Emerging data also suggest that SJW may also compare favorably to SSRIs for mild depression. Data also seem to suggest that SJW may not be effective for more severe forms of depression. There are important drug–drug interactions that should be considered as outlined previously.

S-Adenosylmethionine

S-Adenosylmethionine (SAMe) is a compound found in all living cells that is involved in essential methyl group transfers. It is the principal methyl donor in the one-carbon cycle with SAMe levels depending on levels of the vitamins folate and B_{12} (Figure 13-1). SAMe is involved in the methylation of neurotransmitters, nucleic acids, proteins, hormones, and phospholipids—its role in the production of norepinephrine, serotonin, and dopamine may explain SAMe's antidepressant properties.[3,9,43,44] SAMe has been shown to elevate mood in depressed patients in doses of between 300 and 1,600 mg per day. Studies support antidepressant efficacy of SAMe when compared with placebo and TCAs.[44–46] Recent studies have demonstrated efficacy as augmentation for SSRI and SNRI partial responders.[47,48] Oral preparations of SAMe are somewhat unstable, making high doses required for adequate bioavailability. Since the medication is relatively expensive (and not covered by conventional medical insurance plans), the high cost may be prohibitive for many patients. Potential adverse effects are relatively minor and include anxiety, agitation, insomnia, dry mouth, bowel changes, and anorexia. Sweating, dizziness, palpitations, and headaches have also been reported. Psychiatrists should also watch for a potential switch to mania. Furthermore, suspected serotonin syndrome was reported when SAMe was combined with clomipramine in an elderly woman.[49] Finally, there have not yet been reports of significant drug–drug interactions or hepatotoxicity with SAMe.

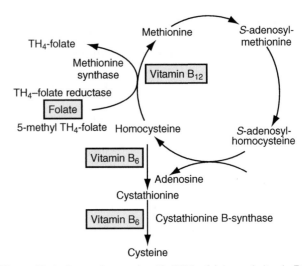

Figure 13-1. One-carbon cycle with SAMe, folate, and vitamin B_{12}. *(Redrawn from Dinavahi R, Bonita Falkner B. Relationship of homocysteine with cardiovascular disease and blood pressure,* J Clin Hypertens *6:495, 2004. © 2004 Le Jacq Communications, Inc.)*

SAMe therefore is a natural medication that appears to be relatively safe and shows promise as an antidepressant. Further study will help clarify its efficacy and safety.

Folate and Vitamin B_{12}

Folate and vitamin B_{12} are dietary vitamins that play a key role in one-carbon metabolism in which SAMe is formed[50] (see Figure 13-1). SAMe then donates methyl groups that are crucial for neurological function and play important roles in the synthesis of central nervous system (CNS) neurotransmitters (e.g., serotonin, dopamine, norepinephrine), as discussed previously. Folate and vitamin B_{12} deficiency states may cause or contribute to a variety of neuropsychiatric and general medical conditions (e.g., macrocytic anemia, neuropathy, cognitive dysfunction/dementia, depression). Folate deficiency, to start, has a number of potential etiologies. These include inadequate dietary intake, malabsorption, inborn errors of metabolism, or an increased demand (e.g., as seen with pregnancy, infancy, bacterial overgrowth, rapid cellular turnover). Drugs (such as anticonvulsants, oral contraceptives, sulfasalazine, methotrexate, triamterene, trimethoprim, pyrimethamine, and alcohol, among others) may also contribute to folate deficency.[51] Like folate, vitamin B_{12} deficiency may also be a result of inadequate dietary intake, malabsorption, impaired utilization, and interactions with certain drugs. Colchicine, H_2 blockers, metformin, nicotine, oral contraceptive pills, cholestyramine, K-Dur, and zidovudine are some examples of these.[40] From a psychiatric standpoint, deficiency of both folate and vitamin B_{12} has been linked with depression, though the association with folate seems to be greater.[50,52–54] Moreover, low folate levels have been associated with delayed onset of clinical improvement of depression in at least one study.[55] Studies suggest that folate deficiency may lessen antidepressant response,[52] and that folate supplementation may be a beneficial adjunct to SSRI-refractory depression.[56] A recent study on a prescription form of 5-methyl tetrahydrofolate (5-MTHF; Deplin) supports its efficacy as an augmenter of antidepressants at doses of 15 mg/day.[57] This form crosses the blood–brain barrier directly, without requiring enzymatic inter-conversion, and may theoretically deliver more active product to the brain. Metabolically significant vitamin B_{12} deficiency, in turn, has been shown to be associated with a two-fold risk of severe (not mild) depression in a population of geriatric women.[58] Low vitamin B_{12} levels have also been associated with poor cognitive status and psychotic depression in the geriatric population.[59,60] Although the data are somewhat mixed, folic acid and vitamin B_{12} supplementation in daily doses of 800 mcg and 1 mg, respectively, has been suggested to improve outcomes in depressed patients.[50] Adequate levels of each of these is thought to provide optimal neurotransmitter synthesis that may aid in reversing depression. One caveat is that supplementation with folate alone may "mask" vitamin B_{12} deficiency by correcting macrocytic anemia while neuropathy continues, so vitamin B_{12} levels should be routinely measured when high doses of folate are given. Folate may also reduce the effectiveness of other medications (e.g., phenytoin, methotrexate, and pheno-barbital) and has been reported to lower the seizure threshold since high doses disrupt the blood–brain barrier.[61,62]

In summary, correction of folate deficiency (and perhaps vitamin B_{12} deficiency) may improve depression or at least augment therapy with other medications. Folate (and maybe B_{12}) supplementation may also shorten the latency of response and enhance response in the treatment of depressed patients even with normal levels. While overall data are not conclusive, psychiatrists should at minimum be on the lookout for potential deficiency states as outlined here by checking serum levels in patients at risk of deficiencies or who have not responded to antidepressant treatment.

Inositol

Inositol is a natural isomer of glucose that is present in common foods. Inositols are cyclic carbohydrates with a six-carbon ring, with the isomer myo-inositol being the most common in the CNS of mammals (Figure 13-2). Myo-inositol is thought to modulate interactions between neurotransmitters, receptors, cell-signaling proteins, and drugs through its activity in the cell-signaling pathway, and is the putative target of the mood-stabilizing drug lithium.[63] There is also emerging evidence for a role of inositol in the mechanism of valproate and car-bamazepine.[64] Inositol has been found in various small studies to be effective in the treatment of depression, panic disorder, obsessive-compulsive disorder (OCD), and possibly bipolar depression.[65–69] While there are some promising findings, nega-tive monotherapy trials with inositol have also been seen in a variety of psychiatric illnesses, including schizophrenia, dementia, ADHD, premenstrual dysphoric disorder, autism, and electroconvulsive-therapy (ECT)-induced cognitive impair-ment.[9,68] Effective doses are thought to be in the range of 12 to 18 g/day. Adverse effects are generally mild and include GI upset, headache, dizziness, sedation, and insomnia. There is no apparent toxicity or known drug interactions at this time.[3,9]

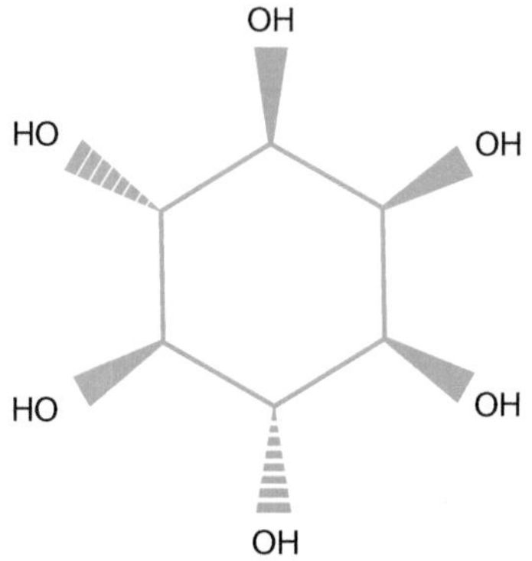

Figure 13-2. Myo-inositol (MI) cyclic carbohydrate with six-carbon ring.

In summary, treatment with inositol in the spectrum of illness treated with SSRIs and mood stabilizers as discussed previously appears to be safe and remains promising.

ANXIETY AND INSOMNIA
Valerian

Valerian (*Valeriana officinalis*) is a flowering plant extract that has been used to promote sleep and to reduce anxiety for over 2,000 years. Common names also include *all heal* and *garden heliotrope*. Typical preparations include capsules, liquid extracts, and teas made from roots and underground stems. A national survey of US adults in 2002 revealed that 1.1% of those surveyed had used valerian in the past week.[4] Since the data regarding valerian and sleep are much more substantial than that of valerian and anxiety,[70–73] sleep will be the focus of the rest of this section. Valerian is thought to promote natural sleep after several weeks of use by decreasing sleep latency and by improving overall sleep quality; however, methodological problems in the majority of studies con-ducted limit firm conclusions in this area.[71] A proposed mech-anism involves decreasing γ-aminobutyric acid (GABA) breakdown.[72,73] Sedative effects are dose-related with usual dosages in the range of 450 to 600 mg about 2 hours before bedtime. Dependence and daytime drowsiness have not been problems. Adverse effects, including blurry vision, GI symp-toms, and headache, seem to be uncommon. Although data are limited, valerian should probably be avoided in patients with liver dysfunction (due to potential hepatic toxicity). Major drug interactions have not been reported.

In summary, valerian has been used as a hypnotic for many years with relatively few reported adverse effects.

Melatonin

Melatonin is a hormone made in the pineal gland that has been shown to help travelers avoid jet lag and to decrease sleep latency for those suffering with insomnia. It may be particu-larly beneficial for night-shift workers as well. Melatonin is derived from serotonin (Figure 13-3) and is thought to play a role in the organization of circadian rhythms via interaction with the suprachiasmatic nucleus.[74,75] Low-dose melatonin treatment has been shown to increase circulating melatonin levels to those normally observed at night and thus to facilitate sleep onset and sleep maintenance without changing sleep architecture.[76] Melatonin generally facilitates falling asleep within 1 hour, independent of when it is taken. Optimal doses are not completely known, although they are thought to be in the range of 0.25 to 0.30 mg per day. Some preparations, however, contain as much as 5 mg of melatonin.[3,9] Higher doses have been noted to cause daytime sleepiness and confu-sion; other potential adverse effects include decreased sex drive, retinal damage, hypothermia, and fertility problems. Melatonin is contraindicated in pregnancy and in those who are immunocompromised.[3,9] There are few reports of drug–drug interactions.

Melatonin seems to be a relatively safe hypnotic and an organizer of circadian rhythms when taken in appropriate doses. Caution should be taken in at-risk populations and with use of higher doses (as discussed previously).

Kava

Kava (*Piper methysticum*) is derived from a root originating in the Polynesian Islands, where it is used as a social and ceremo-nial herb. Though it is thought to have mild anxiolytic and hypnotic effects, study results have been mixed. The mecha-nism of action is attributed to kavapyrones, which are central muscle relaxants that are thought to be involved in blockade of voltage-gated sodium ion channels, enhanced binding to $GABA_A$ receptors, diminished excitatory neurotransmitter release, reduced reuptake of norepinephrine, and reversible inhibition of MAO_B.[77] The suggested dose is 60 to 120 mg per day. Major side effects include GI upset, headaches, and dizziness.[3,9] Toxic reactions, including ataxia, hair loss, respiratory problems, yellowing of the skin, and vision problems, have been seen at high doses or with prolonged use. There have also been more than 70 published reports of severe hepatotoxicity worldwide,[78] including some that have required liver transplantation.[79] For this reason, several countries have pulled kava off the market. In the US, the FDA has issued a warning regarding the use of kava and NCCAM has suspended investigations involving kava since that warning.[80]

While kava appears to be somewhat efficacious in the treatment of mild anxiety, current concerns about safety make its use risky. Table 13-2 summarizes the natural medications discussed here for the treatment of insomnia and anxiety.

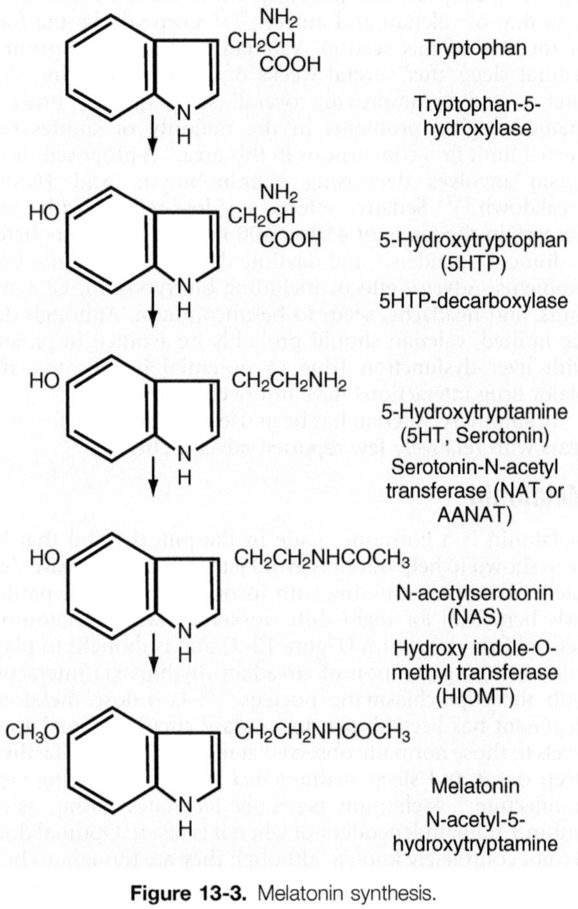

PREMENSTRUAL AND MENOPAUSAL SYMPTOMS
Black Cohosh

Black cohosh (*Cimicifuga racemosa*) is a member of the buttercup family native to the northeastern US. The available natural supplement, derived from the root of the plant, at a dose of 40 mg per day has been shown to reduce physical and psychological menopausal symptoms, as well as dysmenorrhea.[81,82] Active ingredients are thought to be triterpenoids, isoflavones, and aglycones, which may participate in suppression of luteinizing hormone in the pituitary gland,[3,9] though studies in humans have shown mixed results.[82] Effects on breast cancer proliferation are also inconsistent.[82] Headache, dizziness, GI upset, and weight gain are among the generally mild side effects reported. Limited data have not revealed specific toxicity or drug interactions. Black cohosh is not recommended for individuals who are pregnant or breast-feeding or who have heart disease or hypertension. Those with adverse reactions to aspirin should also avoid black cohosh since it contains salicylates. Beneficial effects and safety profiles will be further elucidated as more data are obtained.

Chaste Tree Berry

Chaste tree berry (*Vitex agnus castus*) is derived from the dried fruit of the chaste tree; it has been used since ancient Greece to help alleviate female reproductive complaints.[82] Its name comes from its earlier use to help monks keep their vow of chastity through decreasing the sex drive. The mechanism in both instances is thought to be via prolactin inhibition by binding dopamine receptors in the anterior pituitary,[82] though this remains under investigation. It is most commonly used to alleviate premenstrual syndrome (PMS) in suggested doses of 200 to 400 mg per day.[3,9] Side effects such as increased acne, increased menstrual flow, and GI disturbance seem to be minor. While there are no clear drug–drug interactions, there is a theoretical risk of decreased efficacy of birth control due to its effects on prolactin. Since it is thought to be a dopamine agonist, there may also be interactions with other dopamine agonists or antagonists.[82] A summary of the natural medica-

Figure 13-3. Melatonin synthesis.

TABLE 13-2 Natural Medications for Anxiety and Insomnia

Medication	Active Components	Possible Indications	Possible Mechanisms of Action	Suggested Doses	Adverse Events
Kava (*Piper methysticum*)	Kavapyrones	Anxiety	Central muscle relaxant, enhanced $GABA_A$ receptor binding, reversible inhibition of MAO_B	60–120 mg/day	Gastrointestinal disturbance, headaches, dizziness, ataxia, hair loss, visual problems, respiratory problems, rash, severe liver toxicity
Melatonin	Hormone made in pineal gland	Insomnia	Regulates circadian rhythm in suprachiasmatic nucleus	0.25–0.3 mg/day (may increase up to 5 mg/day if needed)	Sedation, confusion, hypothermia, retinal damage, decreased sex drive, infertility
Valerian (*Valeriana officinalis*)	Valepotriates (from roots and underground stems)	Insomnia	Decrease GABA breakdown	450–600 mg/day	Blurry vision, headache, and possible hepatotoxicity

GABA, γ-aminobutyric acid; MAO, monoamine oxidase.
Adapted from Mischoulon D, Nierenberg AA. Natural medications in psychiatry. In Stern TA, Herman JB, editors: Psychiatry update and board preparation, *ed 2, New York, 2004, McGraw-Hill.*

tions discussed here for premenstrual and menopausal symptoms is found in Table 13-3.

COGNITION AND DEMENTIA
Ginkgo biloba

Ginkgo biloba has been used in Chinese medicine for thousands of years. This natural medication comes from the seed of the gingko tree, and has generally been used for the treatment of impaired cognition and affective symptoms in dementing illnesses; however, a possible new role has also emerged in the management of antidepressant-induced sexual dysfunction.[83] As far as its role in cognition is concerned, target symptoms in patients with dementia include memory and abstract thinking. Studies have shown modest but significant improvements in both cognitive performance and social function with doses of 120 mg per day.[84-88] Evidence suggests that progression of disease may be delayed by 6 to 12 months, while those with mild dementia show greatest improvement and those with more severe disease may at most stabilize.[85] Recent studies have suggested that ginkgo may be effective in combination with registered nootropic agents, the cholinesterase inhibitors.[86] Furthermore, one study of healthy young volunteers taking *Ginkgo biloba* made significant improvements in speed of information processing, executive function, and working-memory, suggesting that gingko may also enhance learning capacity.[87] Flavonoids and terpene lactones are thought to be the active components, which may work by stimulating still functional nerve cells.[3,9] They may also play a role in protecting cells from pathological effects (such as hypoxia and ischemia). Since ginkgo has been shown to inhibit platelet-activating factor and has been associated with increased bleeding risk (though results are mixed), it should probably be avoided in those at high risk of bleeding until further data are available.[88] Other noted side effects include headache, GI distress, seizures in epileptics, and dizziness. The suggested dose of *Ginkgo biloba* is 120 to 240 mg per day, with a minimum 8-week course of treatment; however, it may take up to a year to appreciate the full benefit.

Ginkgo biloba appears to be a safe and efficacious cognition-enhancing medication. It may have an additional role in reducing antidepressant-induced sexual dysfunction. Further studies are needed to fully understand its complete and long-term effects.

Dehydroepiandrosterone

Dehydroepiandrosterone (DHEA) is an androgenic hormone synthesized primarily in the adrenal glands, and converted to testosterone and estrogen.[89] DHEA is thought to play a role in enhancing memory and in improving depressive symptoms, though studies in this regard have had mixed results.[89-91] Possible mechanisms of action may include modulation of *N*-methyl-D-aspartate (NMDA) receptors and GABA$_A$ receptor antagonism.[89] DHEA is available for purchase in a synthetic oral formulation and an intra-oral spray with doses ranging from 5 to 100 mg per day. Strength and purity are not regulated, as is the case with most other natural remedies. Side effects are principally hormonally driven with a risk of weight gain, hirsutism, menstrual irregularity, voice changes, and headache in women. Men may experience gynecomastia and prostatic hypertrophy. The effects on hormone-sensitive tumors are not known.[89] Larger studies will help flesh out the promising early data for DHEA use, and clarify risks versus benefits before it may be safely recommended. Table 13-4

TABLE 13-3 Natural Medications for Premenstrual and Menopausal Symptoms

Medication	Active Components	Possible Indications	Possible Mechanisms of Action	Suggested Doses	Adverse Events
Black cohosh (*Cimicifuga racemosa*)	Triterpenoids, isoflavones, aglycones	Menopausal and premenstrual symptoms	Suppression of luteinizing hormone (LH) in the pituitary gland	40 mg/day	Gastrointestinal upset, headache, weight gain, and dizziness, unclear effects on breast cancer proliferation
Chaste tree berry (*Vitex agnus castus*)	Unknown	Premenstrual symptoms	Prolactin inhibition by binding to dopaminergic receptors in the anterior pituitary	200–400 mg/day	Minor GI disturbance, increased acne, increased menstrual flow, possible decreased efficacy of birth control

GI, Gastrointestinal.
Adapted from Mischoulon D, Nierenberg AA. Natural medications in psychiatry. In Stern TA, Herman JB, editors: Psychiatry update and board preparation, ed 2, New York, 2004, McGraw-Hill.

TABLE 13-4 Natural Medications for Cognition and Dementia

Medication	Active Components	Possible Indications	Possible Mechanisms of Action	Suggested Doses	Adverse Events
Dehydroepiandrosterone (DHEA)	Androgenic hormone synthesized in adrenal glands	Depression and dementia	Modulation of NMDA receptors and GABA$_A$ receptor antagonism	5–100 mg/day	Weight gain, hirsutism, menstrual irregularity, voice changes in women, gynecomastia and prostatic hypertrophy in men
Ginkgo biloba	Flavonoids, terpene lactones	Dementia and sexual dysfunction	Nerve cell stimulation and protection and free radical scavenging	120–240 mg/day	Mild GI disturbance, headache, irritability, dizziness, seizures in epileptics

GABA, γ-aminobutyric acid; GI, gastrointestinal; NMDA, *N*-methyl-D-aspartate.
Adapted from Mischoulon D, Nierenberg AA. Natural medications in psychiatry. In Stern TA, Herman JB, editors: Psychiatry update and board preparation, ed 2, New York, 2004, McGraw-Hill.

outlines the natural medications described here for cognitive dysfunction and dementia.

CONCLUSION

Complementary and alternative medical therapies are becoming increasingly popular in the US and around the world. The spectrum of CAM therapies is quite diverse and may have significant overlap with more traditional medical practice. Lack of scientific research in this area historically has contributed to deficiencies in knowledge with respect to safety and efficacy of many of the natural remedies on the market today. This should be improved by a recent surge in funding by governmental and industry sources. Current knowledge about a few such therapies in the psychiatric realm has been outlined in this chapter; these include proposed treatments for mood disorders, anxiety and sleep disorders, menstrual disorders, and dementia. Many of these therapies may prove to be a valuable addition to the armamentarium of treatments available to psychiatrists in the future. There are also important drug–drug interactions and potential side effects as outlined in the prior sections. A general knowledge of these therapies and routine questioning about their use is an essential part of comprehensive care by the current psychiatrist.

Access the complete reference list and multiple choice questions (MCQs) online at https://expertconsult.inkling.com

KEY REFERENCES

3. Mischoulon D, Nierenberg AA. Natural medications in psychiatry. In Stern TA, Herman JB, Gorrindo T, editors: *Psychiatry update and board preparation*, ed 3, Boston, 2012, MGH Psychiatry Academy.

15. Freeman MP, Hibbeln JR, Wisner KL, et al. Omega-3 fatty acids: evidence basis for treatment and future research in psychiatry. *J Clin Psychiatry* 67(12):1954–1967, 2006.

23. Lin PY, Su KP. A meta-analytic review of double-blind, placebo-controlled trials of antidepressant efficacy of omega-3 fatty acids. *J Clin Psychiatry* 68(7):1056–1061, 2007.

24. Appleton KM, Rogers PJ, Ness AR. Updated systematic review and meta-analysis of the effects of n-3 long-chain polyunsaturated fatty acids on depressed mood. *Am J Clin Nutr* 91(3):757–770, 2010.

25. Sublette ME, Ellis SP, Geant AL, et al. Meta-analysis of the effects of eicosapentaenoic acid (EPA) in clinical trials in depression. *J Clin Psychiatry* 72(12):1577–1584, 2011.

26. Bloch MH, Hannestad J. Omega-3 fatty acids for the treatment of depression: systematic review and meta-analysis. *Mol Psychiatry* 17(12):1272–1282, 2012.

27. Mischoulon D. Update and critique of natural remedies as antidepressant treatments. *Psychiatr Clin North Am* 30(1):51–68, 2007.

33. Sarris J. St. John's wort for treatment of psychiatric disorders. *Psychiatry Clin North Am* 36(1):65–72, 2013.

38. Hypericum Depression Trial Study Group. Effect of *Hypericum perforatum* (St John's wort) in major depressive disorder: a randomized controlled trial. *JAMA* 287(14):1807–1814, 2002.

43. Mischoulon D, Fava M. Role of S-adenosyl-L-methionine in the treatment of depression: a review of the evidence. *Am J Clin Nutr* 76(5):1158S–1161S, 2002.

45. Papakostas GI, Alpert JE, Fava M. S-Adenosyl methionine in depression: a comprehensive review of the literature. *Curr Psychiatry Rep* 5:460–466, 2003.

46. Alpert JE, Papakostas G, Mischoulon D, et al. S-Adenosyl-L-methionine (SAMe) as an adjunct for resistant major depressive disorder: an open trial following partial or nonresponse to selective serotonin reuptake inhibitors or venlafaxine. *J Clin Psychopharmacol* 24(6):661–664, 2004.

47. Papakostas GI, Mischoulon D, Shyu I, et al. S-adenosyl methionine (SAMe) augmentation of serotonin reuptake inhibitors (SRIs) for SRI- non-responders with major depressive disorder: A double-blind, randomized clinical trial. *Am J Psychiatry* 167:942–948, 2010.

49. Coppen A, Bolander-Gouaille C. Treatment of depression: time to consider folic acid and vitamin B_{12}. *J Psychopharmacol* 9(1):59–65, 2005.

56. Papakostas GI, Shelton RC, Zajecka JM, et al. L-methylfolate as adjunctive therapy for SSRI-resistant major depression: Results of two randomized, double-blind, parallel-sequential trials. *Am J Psychiatry* 169:1267–1274, 2012.

65. Benjamin J, Agam G, Levine J, et al. Inositol treatment in psychiatry. *Psychopharmacol Bull* 31(1):167–175, 1995.

69. Mischoulon D. Herbal remedies for anxiety and insomnia: kava and valerian. In Mischoulon D, Rosenbaum J, editors: *Natural medications for psychiatric disorders: considering the alternatives*, ed 2, Philadelphia, 2008, Lippincott Williams & Wilkins.

72. Miyasaka LS, Atallah AN, Soares BG. Valerian for anxiety disorders. *Cochrane Database Syst Rev* 4:CD004515, 2006.

73. Zhdanova V, Friedman L. Melatonin for treatment of sleep and mood disorders. I: Mischoulon D, Rosenbaum J, editors: *Natural medications for psychiatric disorders: considering the alternatives*, ed 2, Philadelphia, 2008, Lippincott Williams & Wilkins.

81. Tesch BJ. Herbs commonly used by women: an evidence-based review. *Am J Obstet Gynecol* 188(5 Suppl.):S44–S55, 2002.

83. Le Bars PL, Katz MM, Berman N, et al. A placebo-controlled, double-blind, randomized trial of an extract of *Ginkgo biloba* for dementia: North American EGb Study Group. *JAMA* 278(16):1327–1332, 1997.

84. Le Bars PL, Velasco FM, Ferguson JM, et al. Influence of the severity of cognitive impairment on the effect of the *Ginkgo biloba* extract EGb 761 in Alzheimer's disease. *Neuropsychobiology* 45(1):19–26, 2002.

89. Wolkowitz OM, Reus VI, Roberts E, et al. Dehydroepiandrosterone (DHEA) treatment of depression. *Biol Psychiatry* 41(3):311–318, 1997.

90. Wolkowitz OM, Reus VI, Keebler A, et al. Double-blind treatment of major depression with dehydroepiandrosterone. *Am J Psychiatry* 156(4):646–649, 1999.

14 Dementia

Jennifer R. Gatchel, MD, PhD, Christopher I. Wright, MD, PhD, William E. Falk, MD, and Nhi-Ha Trinh, MD, MPH

KEY POINTS

Clinical Findings

- In the DSM-IV, dementia was defined as a syndrome with multiple etiologies and characterized by a disabling decline in memory as well as an impairment in at least one other higher cortical activity (e.g., with aphasia, apraxia, agnosia, or executive dysfunction).

- In the DSM-5, cognitive disorders are classified as "neurocognitive disorders" and exist on a spectrum of cognitive and functional impairment: delirium, mild neurocognitive disorder, major neurocognitive disorder, and their etiological subtypes.

- The term "dementia" is used to refer to certain etiological subtypes (e.g., Alzheimer's disease [AD], frontotemporal lobar dementia).

Differential Diagnoses

- An evaluation of a suspected dementia or major neurocognitive disorder must include a complete history; physical, neurological, and psychiatric examinations; evaluation of cognitive function; and appropriate laboratory testing.

Epidemiology

- AD accounts for 60%–80% of all dementias and afflicts at least 5 million Americans; however, other etiologies,

both common (e.g., vascular dementia, Lewy body dementia) and rare (e.g., frontotemporal dementia, progressive supranuclear palsy), must be considered during a comprehensive evaluation.

- Longevity is the greatest risk factor for AD, as well as for most other dementing disorders, but additional factors, such as genetic propensity (particularly in the rare cases of early-onset AD) and vascular pathology, as well as modifiable lifestyle factors can contribute to its prevalence.

Pathophysiology

- Animal models, structural and functional imaging studies, and recent advances in imaging and in biomarkers have led to a new working model of a continuum of neuropathological changes in dementing disorders and AD in particular, with increasing evidence of the pre-clinical or asymptomatic stage, when neuropathological changes may already be present.

Treatment Options

- With AD in particular, attention often focuses on primary and secondary prevention and on potential curative approaches that are based on our expanding knowledge.

OVERVIEW

The *Diagnostic and Statistical Manual of Mental Disorders, Fifth Edition* (DSM-5)[1] designates cognitive disorders on a spectrum of cognitive and functional decline: delirium, mild and major neurocognitive disorders, and their etiological subtypes. The term dementia is retained for consistency; it was used in the fourth edition (DSM-IV)[2] to describe a syndrome with a decline in memory, as well as an impairment of at least one other domain of higher cognitive function (e.g., aphasia [a difficulty with any aspect of language]; apraxia [the impaired ability to perform motor tasks despite intact motor function]; agnosia [an impairment in object recognition despite intact sensory function]; or executive dysfunction [such as difficulty in planning, organizing, sequencing, or abstracting]).

While dementia is encompassed by the term major neurocognitive disorder (MNCD), for a diagnosis of MNCD to be made there must be evidence of significant cognitive decline in one or more cognitive domains (complex attention, executive function, learning and memory, language, perceptual motor, or social cognition) based on concern of the individual, a knowledgeable informant, or the clinician, as well as by objective measures of substantial cognitive impairment on standardized neuropsychological testing or quantified clinical assessment. Several important qualifiers are included in the definition: i.e., the condition must represent a change from baseline, social or occupational function must be significantly impaired, and the impairment does not occur exclusively during an episode of delirium, or cannot be accounted for by another Axis I disorder, such as major depression.[2]

Many elderly adults complain of difficulties with their memory (e.g., with learning new information or names, or finding words). In most circumstances, such lapses are normal. The term *mild cognitive impairment* (MCI) was coined to recognize an intermediate category between the normal cognitive losses associated with aging and with dementia. While MCI was subsumed under cognitive disorder not otherwise specified in DSM-IV, this less severe level of cognitive impairment most closely corresponds with "mild neurocognitive disorder" in DSM-5.[2] Diagnostic criteria include evidence for a *modest* decline in cognition from a previous level of performance in one or more cognitive domains based on concern of the individual, a knowledgeable informant, or clinician, and based on objective evidence of cognitive decline. Important qualifiers include lack of interference with independence in everyday activities, and not exclusively occurring during an episode of delirium, and not accounted for by another Axis I disorder. MCI is characterized by a notable decline in memory or other cognitive functions as compared with age-matched controls. MCI is common among the elderly, although estimates vary widely depending on the diagnostic criteria used and the assessment methods employed; some, but not all, individuals with MCI progress to dementia. According to some studies, individuals with MCI may progress to Alzheimer's disease (AD) at a rate of 10%–15% per year. Risk factors for conversion from MCI to AD include carrier status of the E4 allele of the apolipoprotein E (*APOE*) gene, clinical severity, brain atrophy, specific patterns of CSF biomarkers and cerebral glucose metabolism, and AB deposition. Further identification of factors that place people at risk for progression of cognitive decline is an active area of research.[3]

EPIDEMIOLOGY OF DEMENTIA

The most common type of dementia (accounting for 60% to 80%) is AD.[4] Among the neurodegenerative dementias, Lewy body dementia is the next most common, followed by frontotemporal dementia (FTD). Vascular dementia (formerly known as multi-infarct dementia) can have a number of different etiologies; it can exist separately from AD, but the two frequently co-occur. Indeed, there is increasing awareness that AD is often mixed with other dementia causes. Dementias associated with Parkinson's disease (PD) and Creutzfeldt–Jakob disease (CJD) are much less common. Given the challenges of making an accurate diagnosis of dementia subtypes in epidemiological studies, and in light of neuropathological data suggesting that mixed pathologies are more common than discrete subtypes, the proportion of dementias attributed to different subtypes must be interpreted with caution.[5]

THE ROLE OF AGE OF ONSET

The onset of dementia is most common in the seventies and eighties, and is quite rare before age 40. Both the incidence (the number of new cases per year in the population) and the prevalence (the fraction of the population that has the disorder) rise steeply with age. This general pattern has been observed both for dementia overall, and for AD in particular, with the prevalence increasing exponentially with age, increasing from 3% among people age 65–74 years to nearly 50% in those >85 years.[6] Estimates of the prevalence of dementia vary to some extent depending on which diagnostic criteria are used. The incidence of dementia of almost all types increases with age such that it may affect 15% of all individuals over the age of 65 years, and up to 45% of those over age 80. However, the peak age of onset varies somewhat among the dementias, with FTD and vascular dementia tending to begin earlier (e.g., in the sixties) and AD somewhat later.

Dementia is the main cause of disability among older adults and not surprisingly the economic burden of dementia is enormous. Moreover, it is expected to rise steeply with anticipated demographic shifts. A substantial fraction of the increased burden will fall on developing countries, as a larger fraction of the population survives to old age. Indeed by one estimate, while there were 36.5 million people world-wide with dementia in 2010, the number of people living with dementia is expected to double every 20 years, with most of those living in low and middle income countries.[5] Because AD and many other neurodegenerative disorders have an insidious onset, the precise age of onset is indeterminate. However, the approximate age of onset (i.e., within 2 to 5 years) is critical from both the personal and the public health points of view. It may offer an important leverage on disease risk and morbidity. A sufficient delay in onset can be equivalent to prevention with a late-onset disorder. Later onset can also decrease the burden of disease by pushing it later into the life span. From the research perspective, age of onset shows a robust relationship to genetic risk factors, and may have value as an outcome in genetic and other causal models.

EVALUATION OF THE PATIENT WITH SUSPECTED DEMENTIA

The diagnostic criteria for dementia require that a number of confounding disorders have been ruled out, particularly delirium and depression. Of note, an underlying diagnosis of dementia may predispose a patient to delirium; thus, further evaluation of cognitive deficits is required once delirium has been treated successfully. Delirium may be differentiated from dementia in several important ways; the onset of delirium

---

BOX 14-1 Etiologies of Dementia, and of Mild and Major Neurocognitive Disorders

VASCULAR
Stroke, chronic subdural hemorrhages, post-anoxic injury, diffuse white matter disease

INFECTIOUS
Human immunodeficiency virus (HIV) infection, neurosyphilis, progressive multi-focal leukoencephalopathy (PMLE), Creutzfeldt–Jakob disease (CJD), tuberculosis (TB), sarcoidosis, Whipple's disease

NEOPLASTIC
Primary versus metastatic carcinoma, paraneoplastic syndrome

DEGENERATIVE
Alzheimer's disease (AD), frontotemporal dementia (FTD), dementia with Lewy bodies (DLB), Parkinson's disease (PD), progressive supranuclear palsy (PSP), multi-system degeneration, amyotrophic lateral sclerosis (ALS), corticobasal degeneration (CBD), multiple sclerosis (MS)

INFLAMMATORY
Vasculitis

ENDOCRINE
Hypothyroidism, adrenal insufficiency, Cushing's syndrome, hypoparathyroidism/hyperparathyroidism, renal failure, liver failure

METABOLIC
Thiamine deficiency (Wernicke's encephalopathy), vitamin B_{12} deficiency, inherited enzyme defects

TOXINS
Chronic alcoholism, drugs/medication effects, heavy metals, dialysis dementia (aluminum)

TRAUMA
Dementia pugilistica

OTHER
Normal pressure hydrocephalus (NPH), obstructive hydrocephalus

---

is typically acute or subacute, the course often has marked fluctuations, and level of consciousness and attention are impaired.

Depression also may be difficult to distinguish from dementia, particularly as the two diagnoses are often co-morbid. Further, depression alone may cause some cognitive impairment; in such cases it may precede AD by several years. Certain features (such as a more acute onset, poor motivation, prominent negativity, and a strong family history of a mood disorder) favor a diagnosis of depression.

Establishing a precise etiology of dementia (Box 14-1) whenever possible allows for more focused treatment and for an accurate assessment of prognosis. Although reversible causes will be found in less than 15% of new cases, a diagnosis may help a patient and his or her family to understand what the future holds for them and to make appropriate personal, medical, and financial plans.

History should never be obtained from the patient alone; family members or others who have observed the patient are essential informants for an accurate history. The patient often fails to report deficits, usually because the patient is unaware of them (anosognosia). Ideally, family members should be interviewed separately from the patient so that they can be as candid as possible.

When obtaining a history one should determine the nature of the initial presentation, the course of the illness, and the associated signs and symptoms (including those that are psychiatric or behavioral). These areas are important in determining disease etiology (e.g., recognizing the characteristic abrupt onset of vascular dementia as opposed to the gradual onset of AD).

Review of systems should be extensive and must include inquiry about gait and sleep disturbance, falls, sensory deficits, head trauma, and incontinence. Obtaining the full medical history may reveal risk factors for stroke or for other general medical or neurological causes of cognitive difficulties. The psychiatric history may suggest co-morbid illnesses (such as depression or alcohol abuse), particularly if prior episodes of psychiatric illness are elicited.

Up to one-third of cases of cognitive impairment may be at least partially caused by medication effects; common offenders include anticholinergics, antihypertensive agents, various psychotropics, sedative-hypnotics, and narcotics. Any drug is suspect if its first prescription and the onset of symptoms are temporally related.

Family history can be helpful in determining the type of dementia, as discussed later. A social and occupational history is useful when assessing pre-morbid intelligence and education, changes in the patient's level of function, and any environmental risk factors.

A general physical examination is essential with particular focus paid to the cardiovascular system. Physical findings can also suggest endocrine, inflammatory, and infectious causes. A complete neurological examination (including assessment of cranial nerves, sensory and motor functions, deep tendon reflexes, and cerebellar function) may reveal focal findings that suggest vascular dementia or another degenerative disorder, such as PD. Screening for acuity of vision and hearing is important because it may reveal losses that can masquerade as, or exacerbate, cognitive decline.

Psychiatric examination may reveal evidence of delirium, depression, or psychosis. On formal mental status testing, such as with the Folstein Mini-Mental State Examination,[7] and other cognitive tests (Table 14-1), documentation of particular findings, in addition to the overall score, allows cognitive functions to be followed over time.

Laboratory evaluation should include a complete blood count (CBC) and levels of vitamin B_{12} and folate, a sedimentation rate, electrolytes, glucose, homocysteine, blood urea nitrogen (BUN), and creatinine, as well as tests of thyroid function and liver function. Screening for cholesterol and triglyceride levels is also useful. Syphilis serology should also be included on an initial panel. A computed tomography (CT) scan of the brain, without contrast, can also be useful in identifying a subdural hematoma, hydrocephalus, stroke, or tumor.

Additional studies are indicated if the initial work-up is uninformative, if a particular diagnosis is suspected, or if the presentation is atypical (Table 14-2). Such investigations are particularly important in young patients with rapid progression of dementia or an unusual presentation. Neuropsychological testing may be quite useful, and is essential in cases where a patient's deficits are mild or difficult to characterize. Briefer screening tools, such as the MMSE, have poor sensitivity and specificity for dementia, particularly in highly educated or intelligent patients. Such tests also generally fail to assess executive function and praxis.

Other diagnostic tests can supplement initial assessment when indicated. Magnetic resonance imaging (MRI) of the brain is more sensitive for recent stroke and should be considered when focal findings are detected on the neurological examination; in addition, MRI scans can identify lesions not

TABLE 14-1 Supplemental Mental State Testing for Patients with Dementia

Area	Test
Memory	Recall name and address: "John Brown, 42 Market Street, Chicago"
	Recall three unusual words: "tulip, umbrella, fear"
Language	Naming parts: "lab coat: lapel, sleeve, cuff; watch: band, face, crystal"
	Complex commands: "Before pointing to the door, point to the ceiling"
	Word-list: "In one minute, name all the animals you can think of"
Praxis	"Show me how you would slice a loaf of bread"
	"Show me how you brush your teeth"
Visuospatial	"Draw a clock face with numbers, and mark the hands to ten after eleven"
Abstraction	"How is an apple like a banana?"
	"How is a canal different from a river?"
	Proverb interpretation

TABLE 14-2 Supplemental Laboratory Investigations

What	When	Why
Neuropsychological testing	Patient's deficits are mild or difficult to characterize	The sensitivity of the MMSE for dementia is poor, particularly in highly educated or intelligent patients (who can compensate for deficits)
Lumbar puncture (including routine studies and cytology)	Known or suspected cancer, immunosuppression, suspected CNS infection or vasculitis, hydrocephalus by CT, rapid or atypical courses	Look for infection, elevated pressure, abnormal proteins
MRI with gadolinium; EEG	Any atypical findings on neurological examination; suspected toxic-metabolic encephalopathy, complex partial seizures, Creutzfeldt–Jakob disease (CJD)	More sensitive than CT for tumor, stroke Look for diffuse slowing (encephalopathy) vs. focal seizure activity
HIV testing	Risk factors or opportunistic infections	Up to 20% of patients with HIV infection develop dementia, although it is unusual for dementia to be the initial sign
Heavy metal screening, screening for Wilson's disease or autoimmune disease	Suggested by history, physical examination, laboratory findings	May be reversible

CNS, Central nervous system; CT, computed tomography; EEG, electroencephalogram; MMSE, Mini-Mental State Examination; MRI, magnetic resonance imaging.

apparent on physical examination, so it should always be considered when the diagnosis is unclear. An electroencephalogram (EEG) may be used to identify toxic-metabolic encephalopathy, complex partial seizures, or CJD. A lumbar puncture (LP) may be indicated when cancer, infection of the central nervous system (CNS), hydrocephalus, or vasculitis is suspected. Testing for the human immunodeficiency virus (HIV) is indicated in a patient with appropriate risk factors, because up to 20% of patients with HIV infection develop dementia, although dementia is uncommon as an initial sign. Heavy metal screening, as well as tests for Lyme disease, Wilson's disease, and autoimmune diseases, should be reserved for patients in whom these etiologies are suspected.

ALZHEIMER'S DISEASE

Brief Description

AD is a progressive, irreversible brain disorder that robs those who have it of memory and overall mental and physical function; it eventually leads to death.

Epidemiology of Alzheimer's Disease

AD is the most common cause of dementia, affecting at least 5.3 million Americans and about 33.9 million people worldwide.[8,9] The prevalence of the disorder is expected to triple in the next 40 years given increases in life expectancies, and by 2050 the prevalence may reach more than 13.5 million cases in the US alone.[8] Currently, AD is the sixth leading cause of death for adults in the US. In 2013, the direct costs of caring for those with AD in the US is estimated to be $203 billion, and is projected to increase to $1.2 trillion in 2050 (in current dollars).[9] Female gender carries an increased risk, even when accounting for differences in longevity, but some of the difference is offset by a greater risk of vascular dementias in men. Many risk factors (except for male gender), including diabetes, atherosclerosis, hypertension, smoking, atrial fibrillation, and elevated cholesterol, increase the risk of AD, as well as vascular dementia, although the mechanisms are unclear.[10] A history of head trauma (severe, with loss of consciousness) also increases the risk of AD, while education, complexity of occupation, engaged lifestyle, and exercise have protective effects.[11] Indeed, many modifiable lifestyle factors may contribute to the development of AD and other dementias. Barnes and Yaffe,[8] in calculating the population-attributable risk of seven lifestyle factors, found that in the US, physical inactivity, depression, smoking, and mid-life hypertension had the highest correlation with AD risk. An additional modifiable risk factor is the effect of sleep-disordered breathing; women with sleep-disordered breathing have twice the risk of developing dementia as those without disordered breathing. The effect of diet, meanwhile, is more controversial; there is insufficient evidence to support the association of adherence to a particular diet and development of AD.[11]

Pathophysiology

In his initial 1907 case, Alois Alzheimer identified abnormal nerve cells and fiber clusters at autopsy in the cerebral cortex using what was then a new silver-staining method. These findings, considered to be the hallmark neuropathological lesions of AD, are known as neurofibrillary tangles (NFTs) and neuritic plaques (NPs) (Figure 14-1). Beta-amyloid protein, present in soluble form in the brain, but also a major component of plaques, is thought to play a central pathophysiological role in the disease, perhaps via direct neurotoxicity.[12] NFTs are found in neurons and are primarily composed of anomalous cytoskeletal proteins (such as hyperphosphorylated tau),

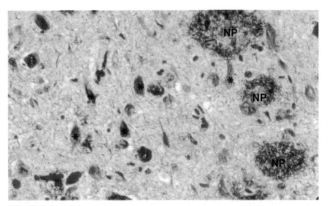

Figure 14-1. Plaques and tangles in Alzheimer's disease. NP, neuritic plaques; *, neurofibrillary tangles.

which may also be toxic to neurons and contribute to AD pathophysiology.[13,14]

However, the mechanisms by which changes in tau and beta-amyloid mediate neuronal death and dysfunction remain important unanswered questions and active areas of research. Two proposed methods of tau-mediated toxicity include NFT toxicity and conformational abnormalities of tangles, including a spreading process through multiple brain regions, in which abnormal tau can catalyze formation of abnormal tau in other cells through a prion-like process.[11] Soluble and diffusible beta-amyloid may cause cytotoxicity and synaptotoxicity, with amyloid plaques serving as reservoirs for sequestration of soluble oligmers.[11]

Genetics of Alzheimer's Disease

Before trying to identify specific genes, epidemiological approaches are used to look for evidence that genetic factors are involved in disease etiology. For AD, multiple lines of evidence support a role for genetic factors. First-degree relatives of AD patients have a twofold to threefold increased risk of developing AD, and often at a similar age, which can be reassuring for middle-aged individuals who care for elderly parents with AD. Examination of AD families generally reveals no clear pattern of inheritance, although some rare families—typically with an early onset—have an autosomal dominant inheritance, in which the disease is observed in approximately half the children in each generation, and an affected child typically has an affected parent. Twin studies are used to examine whether the increased risk in families is due to genetic factors. For AD, monozygotic twins (who share all their genes) typically show greater concordance than dizygotic twins (who share only half, like ordinary siblings). However, monozygotic twins do not uniformly share an AD diagnosis, and their age of onset may differ by 10 or more years.

In the context of genetic research, early-onset AD and late-onset AD are usually considered separately, divided by age of onset at 60 or sometimes 65 years. Early-onset AD is more likely to be familial; most autosomal dominant families have an early onset. However, late-onset AD also runs in families, and family and twin studies also support a role for genes in late-onset AD.[15] These family and twin findings hold, despite controlling for the known late-onset AD gene *APOE*.

Three genes have been identified as leading to early-onset AD in an autosomal dominant fashion. Although these genes have limited public health impact, they are devastating for affected families. These early-onset genes probably account for half of the cases of AD that occur before age 60. More critically, they have made a large contribution to our understanding of the pathophysiology of AD, and to the development of promising therapeutic strategies. Amyloid precursor protein (APP) on chromosome 21 was recognized first; there are 26 mutations that affect 72 families. The age of onset for these APP mutations varies, and it is modified by *APOE* genotype. Next discovered was presenilin 1 *(PSEN1)* on chromosome 14. There are 156 *PSEN1* mutations affecting 342 families; many have been found in a single family, often referred to as "genetically private." *PSEN1* mutations are associated with an age of onset in the forties and fifties; these mutations are not modified by the *APOE* genotype. Although overall quite rare, *PSEN1* accounts for the great majority of autosomal dominant early-onset AD. *PSEN1* mutations have also been observed in non-familial early-onset AD cases. The last early-onset gene is presenilin 2 *(PSEN2)* on chromosome 1. *PSEN2* has 10 reported mutations affecting 18 families. The age of onset is quite variable, extending into the late-onset AD range, and it is modified by *APOE* genotype.[16]

In addition to these genes, genetic factors that confer increased risk have been identified; the most powerful common risk gene is apolipoprotein E *(APOE)*. Rather than a deterministic gene like the other three, *APOE* is a susceptibility gene that increases the risk for AD without causing the disease and contributes to 40%–60% of cases. *APOE* has three alleles, 2, 3, and 4, which have a complex relationship to risk for both AD and cardiovascular disease, with the 2 allele decreasing risk of both disorders and increasing longevity, and the 4 allele increasing risk and decreasing longevity. The effect of *APOE-4* varies with age; it is most marked in the sixties, and falls substantially beyond age 80 or 90 years. *APOE* seems to act principally by modifying the age of onset, which is lowest in those with two copies of the risk allele, and intermediate in those with one. The *APOE* effect appears to be stronger in women and in Caucasians, which may relate to their lower risk of cardiovascular disease.

While APOE-4 remains the most important risk polymorphism, ten additional risk genes have been confirmed, including *PICALM* and *BIN1* (involved in protein sorting), *CLU* (the amyloid binding protein apolipoprotein J), *CR1* (a complement receptor), *CD2AP* (an adaptor gene) *TOMM40* (an outer mitochondrial membrane translocase) among others.[17] Future work utilizing whole genome exome sequencing as well as induced pluripotent stem cells derived from patients with familial or sporadic AD has promise in providing further insight into the molecular pathogenesis of AD.[17]

Patients frequently ask about their risk of AD based on their family history. Those with an autosomal dominant history are best referred for genetic counseling, ideally from an Alzheimer's Disease Research Center or a local genetic counselor. Genetic testing is commercially available for *PSEN1*, which is likely to be involved when there is an autosomal dominant family history and the age of onset is 50 or lower. It can be used both for confirmation of diagnosis and for the prediction of disease onset, but there are complex logistical and ethical issues.[18] Currently, genetic testing is only available for the remaining early-onset genes in research settings. Patients without such a history can be advised that there is an increased risk of AD in first-degree relatives. However, they should be made aware that this increase is modest and that age of onset tends to be correlated in families. Genetic testing for *APOE* can be used as an adjunct to diagnosis, but it contributes minimally. It is not recommended for the assessment of future risk because it lacks sufficient predictive value at the individual level. Many normal elderly carry an *APOE-4* allele, and many AD patients do not.

Clinical Features and Diagnosis

The typical clinical profile of AD is one of progressive memory loss. Other common cognitive clinical features include impairment of language, visuospatial ability, and executive function. Patients may be unaware of their cognitive deficits, but this is not uniformly the case. There may be evidence of forgetting conversations, having difficulty with household finances, being disoriented to time and place, and misplacing items frequently. In addition to its cognitive features, a number of neuropsychiatric symptoms are common in AD, even in its mildest clinical phases.[19] In particular, irritability, apathy, and depression are common early features, with psychosis (delusions and hallucinations) occurring more frequently later in the course of the disease.

According to original diagnostic criteria for AD, a definitive diagnosis required evidence of dementia and also rested on post-mortem findings of a specific distribution and number of its characteristic brain lesions (NFTs and NPs). Detailed clinical assessments (by psychiatry, neurology, and neuropsychology) in combination with structural and functional neuroimaging methods had a high concordance rate with autopsy-proven disease. Structural neuroimaging studies (such as MRI or CT) typically show atrophy in the medial temporal lobes, as well as in the parietal convexities bilaterally (Figure 14-2). Functional imaging studies of resting brain function or blood flow (i.e., positron emission tomography [PET] or single-photon emission computed tomography [SPECT]) display parietotemporal hypoperfusion or hypoactivity (Figure 14-3).

However, recent research advances in the areas of brain imaging and biomarkers have led to re-conceptualization of AD as existing on a continuum, with a progressive series of biological changes corresponding to pre-clinical and increasingly severe clinical stages of the disorder.[20] These changes,

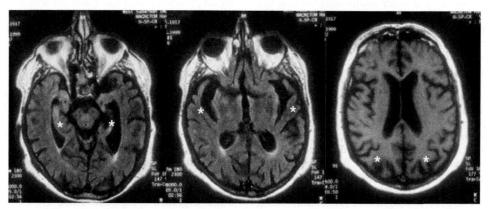

Figure 14-2. Axial MRI of atrophy in Alzheimer's disease. *, Temporal and parietal atrophy.

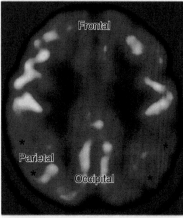
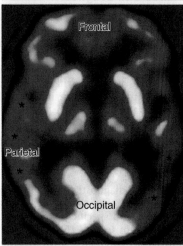

Figure 14-3. Parietotemporal hypoactivity in Alzheimer's disease. *, Regions of hypoactivity.

TABLE 14-3 FDA-Approved Pharmacotherapy for Alzheimer's Disease

Acetylcholinesterase inhibitors	Donepezil (Aricept)
	Rivastigmine (Exelon)
	Galantamine (Razadyne, formerly Reminyl)
Normalizes glutamate	Memantine (Namenda)

FDA, Food and Drug Administration.

progression to the clinical stages of AD while also evaluating promising AD treatment in pre-clinical stages when they may be most effective. Importantly, these research criteria as well as amyloid imaging and other AD biomarkers are not recommended for use in the clinical setting as of yet[20,21]; this may lie on the horizon, as these biomarkers are further evaluated in different populations over time.

Differential Diagnosis

For AD, like other dementias, it is important to exclude potentially arrestable or reversible causes of cognitive dysfunction, or of other brain diseases that could manifest as a dementia (see Box 14-1). Beyond this, the key features are insidious onset, gradual progression, and a characteristic pattern of deficits, particularly early prominent deficits in short-term memory.

Treatments

Behavioral strategies, including environmental cues, such as re-orientation to the environment with the addition of a clock and a calendar, can be reassuring to the patient. In addition, clear communication should be emphasized in this population, including keeping the content of communication simple and to the point, and speaking clearly and loudly enough, given that decreased hearing acuity is common in the elderly. For those patients who are easily distressed or are psychotic, reassurance and distraction are strategies that can be calming.

The re-conceptualization of AD on a continuum of neuropathological and clinical impairment and identification of pre-clinical AD through biomarker studies has led to a shift in focus toward intervention with potential disease-modifying treatments in the early stages of AD.[21] Such early intervention among asymptomatic individuals before clinical or biomarker changes develop is termed *primary prevention*, and has been effective for other chronic diseases.[22] Along these lines, general types of intervention include risk reduction for the general public, prevention in those with mutation or pre-clinical disease, and treatment aimed at delaying the progression of clinical signs and symptoms.[22] Possible preventive measures include weight control and exercise, as well as normalizing blood pressure, blood sugar, and cholesterol, which have been associated with risk for not only AD but also other major neurocognitive disorders.[10] Thus far, AD trials based on lowering specific risk factors, such as cholesterol, did not slow progression in the symptomatic stage of disease. However, this remains an active area of investigation.

Current pharmacotherapy in AD (Table 14-3) addresses both the symptoms and the pathogenesis of AD, and involves primarily cholinesterase inhibitors and NMDA receptor antagonists. AD has been linked to a deficiency of acetylcholine (ACh). Three of the four medications approved by the Food and Drug Administration (FDA) now in use for treatment of AD are designed to prevent the breakdown of ACh, thereby increasing concentrations of ACh in the hippocampus and neocortex, areas of the brain important for memory and for other cognitive symptoms. These cholinesterase inhibitors

some of which can be measured by AD biomarkers, begin in individuals who are cognitively normal, progress in those with MCI, and accumulate in dementia. Advances in CSF assays, neuroimaging, and other biomarkers now provide the ability to detect evidence of AD pathophysiology process *in vivo*.[21] Some promising biomarkers include MRI measurement of atrophy in the hippocampus and other AD-affected brain regions, PET measurements of glucose hypometabolism in AD-affected brain regions, PET measurements of fibrillar beta-amyloid deposition, and CSF measurements of beta-amyloid in combination with total tau and phosphorylated tau.[21] Indeed, increasing evidence from both genetically at-risk cohorts and clinically normal older adults suggests that the pathophysiology of AD begins years, if not decades before the diagnosis of clinical dementia.[20]

Based on these advances, the National Institute on Aging (NIA) International Working Group and Alzheimer's Association in 2011 proposed updated criteria for the diagnosis of AD and MCI, in addition to research criteria aimed at clarifying the pre-clinical stages of AD.[20] These new criteria reflect increasing knowledge of clinical course and pathophysiology: they take into account that memory impairment may not be a key clinical feature, other potential etiologies (dementia with Lewy bodies, vascular dementia, and frontotemporal dementia) as well as mixed pathology.[20] The new research criteria meanwhile focus on defining pre-clinical stages of disease based on biomarkers and genetic testing. The goals of research criteria are to provide insight into factors influencing include donepezil (Aricept), rivastigmine (Exelon), and galantamine (Razadyne). All have been shown to slow the progression of AD by stabilizing cognition and behavior, participation in activities of daily living (ADLs), and global function in mild-to-moderate AD, by improving cognition and behavior in moderate-to-severe patients with AD, by delaying nursing home placement, and by reducing both health care expenditures and caregiver burden for patients with AD.[23] However, the effects are modest, and they are not apparent in some individuals.

Certain pharmacokinetic properties should be kept in mind while prescribing these medications: donepezil and extended-release galantamine are given once daily, while both galantamine and rivastigmine are given twice daily; in particular, rivastigmine should be administered with meals to reduce gastrointestinal side effects. Common side effects include nausea, vomiting, diarrhea, insomnia or vivid dreams, fatigue, muscle cramps, incontinence, bradycardia, and syncope. Data also suggest that a cholinesterase inhibitor should be initiated as soon as a diagnosis of AD becomes apparent, and that treatment should be continued into the severe stages of the disease, provided that the medication is well tolerated.[24] Increasing numbers of studies are investigating the potential efficacy of introducing treatment at the stage of MCI; although studies to date have not been positive, interventions with these and other agents in pre-clinical AD and MCI remain active areas of investigation.

Another medication, memantine (Namenda), has been proven effective in patients with more severe forms of AD. Memantine normalizes levels of glutamate, a neurotransmitter involved in learning and memory, which in excessive quantities is thought to contribute to neurodegeneration. Memantine has been used in combination with cholinesterase inhibitors for greater effectiveness in slowing the progression of AD. Common side effects include dizziness, agitation, headache, and confusion. In patients with moderate-to-severe AD receiving donepezil, those assigned to continue donepezil had less cognitive decline than those assigned to discontinue the medication, and the combination of donepezil and memantine did not confer additional benefits above donepezil alone.[25]

Before the initiation of pharmacotherapy for behavioral and psychological symptoms of dementia (apathy, depression, anxiety, aggression/agitation, psychosis, sleep disturbance and disinhibition/perseveration), possible exacerbating medical (e.g., urinary infection) or environmental triggers should be carefully investigated and resolved. However, irritability and depressive symptoms have been treated effectively with antidepressant therapy (e.g., selective serotonin reuptake inhibitors [SSRIs]). The choice of agent is based principally on the side effects each particular medication produces.

There are no medications specifically FDA-approved for the neuropsychiatric manifestations of AD. However, in the course of the illness, neuropsychiatric symptoms (such as agitation, aggression, and psychosis) arise commonly and may require treatments with antipsychotic agents or mood stabilizers. Clinical experience suggests that second-generation (atypical) antipsychotics (such as olanzapine, quetiapine, risperidone, and aripiprazole) are preferred over the older conventional antipsychotics that are more likely to produce extrapyramidal side effects (EPS) (such as parkinsonism and dystonias). One recent review compared trials of atypical antipsychotics used for the treatment of neuropsychiatric symptoms in dementia and concluded that olanzapine and risperidone had the best evidence for efficacy, though effects were modest.[26] On the other hand, a recent clinical trial suggested that these and other atypical antipsychotics may be little better than placebo.[27]

Although these agents may work well if used judiciously, reports of a small but statistically significant increase in risk of cerebrovascular adverse events and death have led to an FDA warning for use of atypical antipsychotics in elderly with dementia. The potential for an increased risk of serious adverse events is of concern, and the risk/benefit ratio of antipsychotic medication use remains controversial; clinicians must weigh the risks against the potential benefits of these medications with patients and their families.

In general, such agents should be used only when necessary. Psychosis in particular does not require treatment unless it leads to dangerous behavior, causes distress to the patient, or is disruptive to the family or other caregivers. When such agents are used, choosing lower doses and titrating upward slowly is advised in this population. Once the target symptoms are controlled, it is then prudent to consider tapering off the medications after 2–3 months to determine whether longer-term treatment is necessary. Indeed, with longer-term treatment, benefits are less clear-cut and risks of severe adverse outcomes increase. Other treatment considerations involve optimizing behavioral interventions, removing deleterious medications, reducing excessive alcohol intake, and promoting restorative sleep by diagnosing and treating underlying sleep apnea.

Supportive and Long-term Care

Because AD is a chronic, progressive illness without an available disease-modifying therapy or cure, like all of the dementias described below, it creates significant burdens for the patient, his or her family, and the health care system. Giving early consideration for caregiving at home provides essential support to the patient and family. This may include a home health aide, meals-on-wheels, or a visiting nurse. Structured activities outside of the home, such as adult day care or exercise programs, are also important. Though difficult for the patient and family, it is crucial to think through the future care requirements while the patient is in early stages of the disease. This includes consideration of in-home and external care arrangements (e.g., assisted living, or a skilled nursing facility).[24]

Prognosis

Patients who live through the full course of the disease may survive for 10 to 20 years. However, many patients die in the early or middle stages of the illness.

Current AD treatments have not been found to increase survival or to definitively halt disease progression. However, several promising therapies for AD are on the horizon. These potential treatments involve targeting oxidative stress as well inhibiting enzymes (such as gamma secretase that produces beta-amyloid), or removing beta-amyloid from the brain (using immunological agents, such as beta-amyloid vaccinations or antibody infusions). Secretase inhibitors, in the initial stages of development, target secretase enzymes that are implicated in the creation of beta-amyloids.[28]

A vaccine that targets beta-amyloid protein has been in development for a number of years. Immunotherapy with the vaccine AN-1792 in an AD transgenic mouse model reduced amyloid plaques.[29] The clinical trial of this vaccine in patients with mild-to-moderate AD was halted when 6% of patients developed subacute meningoencephalitis.[30] Many passive immunization clinical trials involving anti-AB antibodies as well as IV Ig are currently underway, in addition to study of DNA-based vaccines. Ongoing antibody studies in AD include solanezumab in mild AD, crenezumab in mild-to-moderate AD, and BAN 2401 in MCI and mild AD.

Memory-consolidation compounds in development are designed to facilitate the creation of long-term memories. One approach increases levels of cyclic adenosine monophosphate (cAMP), which helps to establish long-term memories by carrying signals to proteins within brain cells. Another combats age-related forgetfulness through boosting levels of CRB, another protein that helps to establish long-term memories. Ampakines, now in phase II trials, have shown promise in normalizing the activity of glutamate by attaching to AMPA receptors, thus ramping up the voltage of electrical signals traveling between brain cells. In addition, they increase production of nerve growth factor (NGF), a naturally-occurring protein that is hypothesized to prevent brain cell death and to stimulate cell function in areas of the brain involved in memory. Additional strategies for anti-dementia drug development include nutraceuticals/medical foods, neurotransmitter-based therapies (as above), glial modulating drugs, metabolic and mitochondrial targets (antioxidants: vitamins E and C, coenzyme Q10), and tau-modulating, anti-tangle approaches (microtubule stabilizers, kinase inhibitors, and immunotherapies).

DEMENTIA WITH LEWY BODIES
Definition

Dementia with Lewy bodies (DLB) is a progressive brain disease that involves cognitive, behavioral, and motor system deterioration similar to that seen in PD.

Epidemiology and Risk Factors

DLB is arguably the second-leading cause of dementia in the elderly. Some researchers estimate that it accounts for up to 20% of dementia in the United States, afflicting 800,000 individuals. Slightly more men than women are affected. As with most dementias of adult-onset, advanced age is a main risk factor for DLB. Disease onset is usually in the seventh decade of life or later. DLB may cluster in families.

Pathophysiology

The main pathological features of DLB are proteinaceous deposits called Lewy bodies (Figure 14-4), named for Frederic H. Lewy, who first described them in the early 1900s. Among other proteins, Lewy bodies are composed of alpha-synuclein in the cortex and brainstem.[31] In PD, Lewy bodies are primarily restricted to the brainstem and dopaminergic cells of the substantia nigra. In DLB, Lewy bodies are found in the cortex and amygdala, as well as the brainstem. Triplication or mutations of the alpha-synuclein gene are rare causes of DLB. The mechanisms by which Lewy bodies cause neuronal dysfunction and eventual death are uncertain, but it is clear that both

the cholinergic and dopaminergic neurotransmitter systems are severely disrupted. Of note, Lewy body and AD pathology frequently co-occur.

Clinical Features and Diagnosis

The clinical features of DLB are similar to those of AD, and the diagnosis is challenging to make. DLB typically presents with cortical and subcortical cognitive impairments, and with visuospatial and executive dysfunction that is worse than that found in AD, with relatively spared language and memory function. A recent international consortium on DLB resulted in revised criteria for clinical and pathological diagnosis of DLB.[32] Core clinical features include fluctuating attention, recurrent visual hallucinations, and parkinsonism. Parkinsonian symptoms are also necessary for the diagnosis of DLB, with the motor symptoms occurring in most cases within about 1 year of the cognitive problems. Suggestive clinical features meanwhile include rapid eye movement (REM) behavior disorder, extreme sensitivity to neuroleptic medications, disorientation, and low dopamine transporter uptake on neuroimaging.[32] Other manifestations (such as apathy, irritability, depression, and agitation), repeated falls and syncope, autonomic dysfunction, delusions, hallucinations in other modalities, prominent slowing on electroencephalogram, and low uptake on MIBG myocardial scintography are considered supportive of the diagnosis, but not as specific.[32] While clinical features of the disease (e.g., hallucinations, fluctuations, visuospatial deficits, and REM behavior disorder) are helpful in the identification of possible cases of this disease, clinical-pathological concordance has not been great, and postmortem pathological findings of Lewy bodies in the cerebral cortex, amygdala, and brainstem are necessary to confirm the diagnosis.[33]

Structural imaging is typically not particularly helpful as atrophy may not be apparent early on in DLB (Figure 14-5, *left*). Sometimes pallor of the substantia nigra can be identified on MRI; as the disease progresses, there may be atrophy with a frontotemporal, insular, and visual cortex predominance. PET and SPECT may show evidence of decreased activity or perfusion in the occipitotemporal cortices (Figure 14-5, *right*) in early clinical disease stages. In later stages only the primary sensorimotor cortex may be spared.

Differential Diagnosis

As with AD, metabolic, inflammatory, infectious, vascular, medication-related, and structural causes for cognitive decline in the setting of parkinsonism should be excluded with testing. If the clinical picture is not highly consistent with DLB, other dementias with parkinsonism should be considered, including corticobasal degeneration (CBD), progressive supranuclear palsy (PSP), the "Parkinson's-plus" syndromes (e.g., multiple-system atrophy), and vascular parkinsonism with dementia. It is also sometimes difficult to distinguish between PD with dementia and DLB depending on the characteristics, severity, and presentation sequence of the cognitive and motor symptoms. This distinction is primarily based on whether or not parkinsonism precedes dementia for more than a year, as occurs in PD with dementia. Further, the motor symptoms of PD tend to respond better to dopaminergic therapies than they do in DLB.

Treatment

There are currently no FDA-approved treatments specific for DLB. Given the severe cholinergic losses that occur in DLB, the frequent co-occurrence of AD pathology, and several small

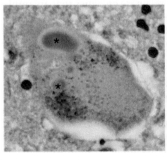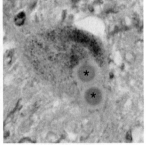

Figure 14-4. Lewy body pathology. *, Lewy bodies.

MRI   SPECT

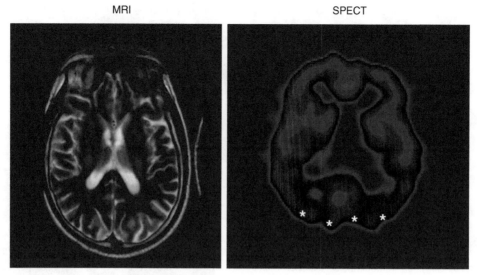

Figure 14-5. Lewy body dementia neuroimaging.

trials that suggest their effectiveness, cholinesterase inhibitors have been the off-label treatment of choice. Rivastigmine has been effective for cognitive deficits and behavioral problems in DLB as compared to placebo.[33] However, in a recent Cochrane Review summarizing the evidence from six trials investigating cholinesterase inhibitors in PD dementia, DLB, and MCI associated with PD, the authors concluded that efficacy of cholinesterase inhibitors in DLB remained unclear in contrast to their use in PDD.[34] While memantine may also be a logical choice because it enhances cognition in disorders with cholinergic deficits and it has dopaminergic effects that could benefit the parkinsonism in DLB, its efficacy has thus far been modest in two recent controlled trials.[35,36] Low dosages of levodopa/carbidopa (dopamine replacement) are sometimes helpful for the motor symptoms of DLB, although higher dosages of dopamine replacement therapy and direct dopamine agonists may exacerbate neuropsychiatric symptoms (e.g., hallucinations). Given that patients with DLB are sensitive to neuroleptics, typical antipsychotics and risperidone should be strictly avoided in patients with DLB, because even a single dose can lead to prolonged drug-induced akinesia and rigidity. Other atypical antipsychotics (such as quetiapine) may be very useful for management of DLB's behavioral symptoms, with fewer untoward motor side effects than typical antipsychotics. However, these agents pose other potential side effects (e.g., metabolic syndrome, weight gain, increased mortality risk). Tricyclic antidepressants or benzodiazepines may help with REM behavior disorder in DLB, but given their anticholinergic and sedative properties, they should be used with caution in the elderly with dementia.

Supportive Care and Long-term Management

These issues are similar as for AD, except that the neuropsychiatric features of DLB may be more severe than in AD, requiring additional supportive care. Greater levels of depression may occur in caregivers of patients with DLB versus caregivers of patients with AD; thus, early support for the patient and family is important.

Prognosis

The average duration of the disease is 5 to 7 years, though there may be substantial variability in the outcome of DLB.

The frequency of co-occurring AD and DLB pathologies in the same individual is greater than is anticipated by chance. Clinical syndromes with overlapping AD and DLB symptoms and the pathological findings have led to several diagnostic categories, such as AD with Lewy bodies or the Lewy body variant of AD. Future research in this area may elucidate the relationship and pathophysiology of both AD and DLB.

FRONTOTEMPORAL DEMENTIAS
Definition

Definitions of frontotemporal dementias (FTDs) are currently in flux. FTDs may be understood as a genetically and pathologically heterogenous group of neurodegenerative disorders that involve degeneration of different regions of the frontal and temporal lobes to differing extents. The clinical pictures and underlying pathologies are also heterogeneous. Currently subsumed under the term FTDs are Pick's disease, frontotemporal lobar degeneration, primary progressive aphasia, and semantic dementia.[37] Additionally, there can be significant overlap between FTD and motor amytrophic lateral sclerosis (FTD-ALS) as well as the atypical parkinsonian syndromes, PSP and corticobasal syndrome (CBS).[38]

Epidemiology and Genetic Risk Factors

FTD tends to manifest at younger ages than typical AD, with the majority of cases occurring in people under age 65, and it is the most common form of dementia with onset before 60 years of age, with most cases presenting between 45 and 64 years of age.[38] Unlike AD, onset after 75 years of age is rare. FTD sometimes runs in families. In fact, 25%–50% of patients with FTD have a first-degree relative with the disease, and autosomal dominant inheritance is frequently observed. Many of these families are found to harbor a mutation in *MATP*, the gene encoding the tau protein, which is found in neurofibrillary tangles. Patients with *MATP* mutations often have a motor syndrome, such as PD or PSP, along with their FTD. A total of 40 tau mutations have been reported across 113 families. In addition, FTD can sometimes be associated with mutations in *GRN*, *VCP*, *TARDBP PSEN1* and *CHMP2B*,[38,39] along with a recently identified C9ORF72 hexanucleotide repeat expansion.[39]

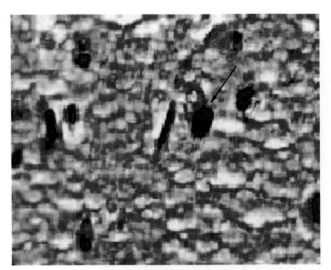

Figure 14-6. Neuropathology of frontotemporal disease: Pick's bodies.

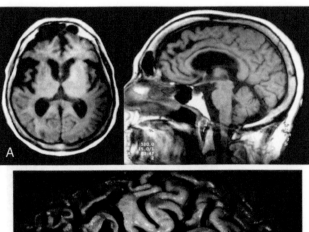

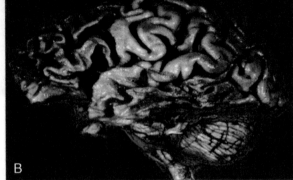

Figure 14-7. Frontotemporal atrophy (A) on MRI and (B) at autopsy.

Pathophysiology

The pathophysiology of FTD is poorly understood, and it likely represents a constellation of syndromes with different underlying causes. This notion is reflected in the variable pathologies that underlie the disease and somehow all lead to neuronal dysfunction and to death. Individuals with clinically-defined FTD may exhibit variable combinations of abnormal tau protein deposits, including tangles and Pick's bodies (as in Pick's disease, Figure 14-6); ubiquitin-positive inclusions; gliosis; non-specific spongiform degeneration; and prion-related spongiform changes. In some cases AD pathology distributed in the frontotemporal cortex can cause an FTD-like syndrome. Further, transactive response DNA-binding protein 43 (TDP-43) was identified in 2006 as the major inclusion protein in the majority of patients with amyotrophic lateral sclerosis (ALS) and in the most common subtype of FTD, frontotemporal lobar degeneration with TDP-43 pathology (FTLD-TDP).[39] Indeed, FTLD can be classified into three general categories based on the predominant neuropathological protein: microtubule-associated tau (FTLD-TAU); TAR DNA-binding protein 43 (FTLD-TDP), and fused in sarcoma protein (FTLD-FUS). Recently, the clinicopathologic overlap between ALS and FTD was supported by discovery of C9ORF72 repeat expansions, a GGGGCC hexanucleotide repeat in a non-coding region of C9ORF72 (chromosome 9 open reading frame 72), encoding an unknown C9ORF72 protein.[39] While genetic causes of FTD include tau mutations on chromosome 17 (FTD-17) (these cases often have associated symptoms of parkinsonism), currently repeat expansions in C9ORF72 are the most important genetic cause of familial ALS and FTD.[39]

Clinical Features, Diagnosis, and Differential Diagnosis

The classic hallmarks of FTD are behavioral and compartmental features out of proportion to amnesia. There is a generally slow onset followed by progressive loss of judgment, disinhibition, impulsivity, social misconduct, loss of awareness, and withdrawal. Other typical symptoms are stereotypies, excessive oral/manual exploration, hyperphagia, wanderlust, excessive joviality, sexually-provocative behaviors, and inappropriate words/actions.

In some cases, language is initially or primarily affected, and can remain as the relatively isolated deficit for years. In these cases there is often primarily left hemisphere pathology selectively involving the frontal or temporal lobes, or the perisylvian cortex. Depending on the localization of left hemisphere pathology, patients may exhibit different degrees of impairment of word-finding, object-naming, syntax, or word-comprehension abilities. Primary progressive aphasia (PPA) usually refers to symptomatic involvement of the frontal (or other perisylvian) language areas leading to a dysfluent aphasia with relatively preserved comprehension.[40] Semantic dementia is characterized by significant loss of word meaning (i.e., semantic losses) with relatively preserved fluency, which results from left anterior temporal lobe involvement. However, the definitions of these syndromes are in flux, and the clinicopathological correlates are not uniform.[41]

Clinical presentations of FTD vary based on the relative involvement of the hemisphere (right or left) or lobe (frontal or temporal) involved. Patients may initially have right greater than left temporal lobe involvement and exhibit primarily a behavioral syndrome with emotional distance, irritability, and disruption of sleep, appetite, and libido. With greater initial left than right temporal lobe involvement, patients exhibit more language-related problems, including anomia, word-finding difficulties, repetitive speech, and loss of semantic information (e.g., semantic dementia).[42] In some cases of FTD the frontal lobes may be involved to a greater extent than the temporal lobes. In these instances, patients exhibit symptoms of elation, disinhibition, apathy, and aberrant motor behavior. Depending on the combination of regions involved, patients with FTD exhibit specific cognitive and neuropsychiatric symptoms. As the disease progresses to involve greater expanses of the frontotemporal cortex, the clinical features become similar. The presumption is that the atrophy and underlying pathology that accompanies FTD is regionally specific, but it becomes more generalized as the disease progresses.

The evaluation and diagnosis of FTD is similar to that of the other dementias and should include clinical evaluation, laboratory studies, neuropsychological testing, and brain imaging (structural and functional imaging). Findings on CT or MRI

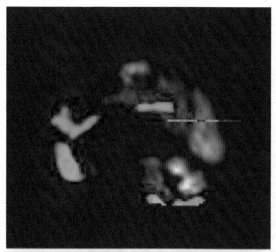

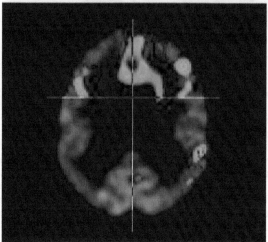

Figure 14-8. Regional hypoactivity in frontotemporal disease. Colored areas in sagittal (A) and horizontal (B) brain sections indicate activity 2 SD below the population mean. *(Courtesy of Keith Johnson.)*

scans may show frontotemporal atrophy (Figure 14-7, *A*), which can be quite striking at autopsy (Figure 14-7, *B*). Clinical findings of motor system or brainstem abnormalities should be investigated when considering the various diagnoses. For example, some cases of FTD are associated with parkinsonism (FTD-17) or motor neuron disease (e.g., amyotrophic lateral sclerosis [ALS]), with increasing evidence, as above, that ALS and FTD may be on a disease continuum with shared underlying pathogenesis. Other clinically-defined disorders may have features of FTD, but be distinguished by eye movement, sensory, or gait abnormalities (e.g., PSP, CBD, and NPH). Brain imaging studies of FTD may show focal atrophy in the frontotemporal cortices along with frontotemporal hypoperfusion or hypoactivity (Figure 14-8).

Treatment

There are no specific treatments or cures for FTD. The behavioral features are sometimes helped by SSRIs, and these are probably the best-studied treatments for these disorders. Cholinesterase inhibitors and memantine may exacerbate the neuropsychiatric symptoms. Antipsychotics (preferably atypical ones), mood stabilizers, and benzodiazepines are sometimes necessary to treat aggression and agitation, but they should be used sparingly.

Supportive Care and Long-term Management

As in the other dementias, supportive, long-term care is crucial for FTD, because it is often accompanied by loss of insight, lack of judgment, and severe behavioral symptoms.

Prognosis

There are no specific medical treatments for FTD. Across the disorders, the time between illness and death is typically about 7 years.

Although not all cases of FTD have the same underlying pathology, there is a developing notion that there is a group of associated dementias (including some instances clinically consistent with FTD) based on the presence of abnormal forms of the tau protein and TDP-43. These disorders cut across the regional neuroanatomic boundaries that typically characterize FTD and may exhibit features atypical for frontotemporal lobar degeneration. In particular, not only do some cases of clinically-defined FTD have tau pathology but also certain characteristic motor, sensory, and brainstem-related clinical features, as found in PSP, CBD, and FTD with parkinsonism or motor neuron disease. Other focal atrophies outside of the frontotemporal lobes may also reflect underlying tau pathology (such as progressive visuospatial and language dysfunction) that can occur in posterior (parietal) cortical atrophy.

VASCULAR DEMENTIA
Definition

Vascular dementia has become an overarching term that encompasses a variety of vascular-related causes of dementia, including multi-infarct dementia (MID) and small vessel disease. More recently the term "vascular cognitive impairment" has been used to take into account all forms of cognitive dysfunction caused by vascular disease, ranging from prodromal stages and mild cognitive dysfunction to dementia, or major neurocognitive impairment.

Epidemiology and Risk Factors

Various types of vascular dementia account for approximately 20% of all dementia cases, making it the second or third most common form of dementia. It is equally prevalent in males and females, but the frequency may be higher in males and in African Americans. Risk factors are similar to those for cardiovascular illness (including diabetes, hypercholesterolemia, hyperhomocysteinemia, hypertension, cigarette smoking, and physical inactivity). To the extent that these factors have familial or genetic bases, so does vascular dementia. Not all genetic risk factors have the same relevance for the different forms of vascular dementia. For example, it is uncertain whether an elevated cholesterol level is as crucial a risk factor as is hypertension for microvascular ischemic white matter disease; several large studies have failed to show a clinical benefit of decreased cholesterol for cognitive impairments even when rates of stroke and transient ischemic attacks (TIAs) are reduced.

Pathophysiology

There are several underlying causes of vascular dementia. Recurrent or specifically-localized embolic strokes (from sources such as the heart or carotid artery, or local thromboses of larger-caliber intracranial vessels) can lead to vascular dementia. These causes are most closely associated with the clinical entity of MID. Smaller subcortical strokes (e.g., lacunar

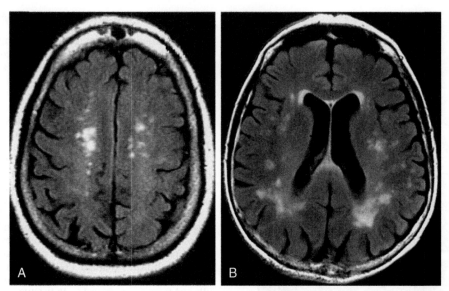

Figure 14-9. MRI of vascular dementia: small-vessel disease. (A) Coronal fluid attenuation inversion recovery (FLAIR) MRI image showing centrum semiovale ischemic white matter disease. (B) Coronal FLAIR MRI showing periventricular ischemic white matter disease.

infarctions) in gray and white matter structures may also lead to a form of vascular dementia.

White matter disease without clearly symptomatic strokes or gross tissue damage may cause insidiously-progressive cognitive decline (Figure 14-9). It is important to keep in mind that cerebral hemorrhages due to hypertension or amyloid angiopathy are possible mechanisms of vascular-induced cognitive impairment, but they require a different type of clinical management than does typical vascular occlusive disease. There are specific gene mutations (e.g., *notch 3*) that cause particular forms of vascular dementia (e.g., cerebral autosomal dominant arteriopathy with subcortical infarcts and leukoencephalopathy [CADASIL]), but these are extremely rare.

Clinical Features and Diagnosis

Vascular dementia has variable clinical features that are dependent on the localization of the vascular lesions. Overall, left hemisphere lesions tend to cause language problems, and right hemisphere lesions tend to cause visuospatial problems. Both the type of cognitive deficits and the time course of the cognitive changes are variable. Embolic or large-vessel stroke-related dementia may progress in a characteristic step-wise pattern, with intervening periods of stability punctuated by abrupt declines in cognitive function; the type of cognitive symptoms will be affected by the brain areas affected over time. This might be considered the classic presentation for vascular dementia associated with multiple infarcts, but may not be the most common presentation of vascular dementia.[43]

Multiple small subcortical infarcts may cause a more insidious decline, even in the absence of recognized stroke symptoms. However, small cortical infarcts at specific locations (e.g., the thalamus or caudate) can cause significant cognitive and motor symptoms. So-called small-vessel or microvascular ischemic disease preferentially involves the white matter, particularly in the centrum semiovale and periventricular regions (see Figure 14-9), and is also a common cause of vascular dementia. This has been called "leukoaraiosis." Symptoms in this case tend to develop in a gradual and insidious fashion and can be difficult to distinguish from AD. Memory or mood complaints are usually a presenting feature. Sometimes the memory disorder can be distinguished from that in AD.

Spontaneous recall is affected in both disorders, but recognition memory is often preserved in vascular dementia, which is not the case for AD. Presentations involving relatively isolated psychotic symptoms in the setting of preserved memory should also raise the possibility of vascular dementia. Likewise, apathy, executive dysfunction, and a relatively intact memory are suggestive of a small-vessel ischemic process. Vascular dementia is also often referable to altered frontal systems dysfunction by which there is disconnection or damage to white matter tracts that relay information to and from the region.

Differential Diagnosis

The main difficulty in diagnosing vascular dementia is distinguishing it from AD. Classically, vascular dementia is distinguished from AD based on an abrupt onset and a step-wise course. In addition, prominent executive dysfunction and preserved recognition memory are also suggestive of vascular dementia. However, in many cases the symptoms of vascular dementia overlap with those of AD. Further, autopsy studies show that the co-occurrence of AD and CNS vascular pathology is not infrequent; the interaction may cause cognitive impairment that might not otherwise occur if the same level of AD or vascular dementia pathology was present alone.

In addition, since the clinical features of vascular cognitive impairment may be variable, specific vascular lesions can mimic a variety of different dementias and even PD. The finding of focal features on examination or CNS vascular disease on structural imaging studies helps to determine the correct diagnosis.

Treatment

Treatment for vascular dementia involves control of vascular risk factors (e.g., hypercholesterolemia, hypertension, inactivity, diabetes, excess alcohol use, cigarette smoking, hyperhomocysteinemia). If strokes are found on brain imaging studies, a stroke work-up should be initiated to determine if surgery (e.g., for carotid stenosis), anticoagulation (for atrial fibrillation), or antiplatelet agents (e.g., for small-vessel strokes) are indicated. Such an evaluation may show hemorrhages from amyloid angiopathy or hypertension, in which case avoidance of anticoagulant or antiplatelet therapies may be prudent. In addition to treating these causes of CNS vascular disease, some literature indicates that symptomatic treatments (such as cholinesterase inhibitors or memantine) may be helpful for cognition.[44] However, there are no FDA-approved treatments for vascular dementia. Neuropsychiatric features (e.g., depression or psychosis) are common in vascular dementia and should be treated accordingly.

Recent work has highlighted a significant incidence of vascular-related cognitive impairment that does not reach clinical criteria for dementia. This is akin to the notion of MCI or prodromal AD. Although definitions for vascular-related cognitive impairment are currently under development, the idea highlights the importance of recognizing cognitive difficulties due to CNS vascular disease in their earliest stages so that vascular risk factors can be identified and treated.[45]

CORTICOBASAL DEGENERATION

Corticobasal degeneration (CBD) is a rare form of dementia that is related to FTD and typically involves specific motor and cognitive deficits. It usually occurs between ages 45 and 70 years, and may have a slight female predominance. It rarely runs in families, but may be associated with a specific tau gene haplotype. Pathologically, there are abnormal neuronal and glial tau accumulations in the cortex and basal ganglia, including the substantia nigra. Swollen, achromatic neurons are typical. The pathophysiology is unknown, and although thought to primarily relate to the toxic effects of the tau protein, it has been increasingly recognized to involve Tar-DNA binding protein-43 (TDP-43) positive inclusions as well as AD pathology.[46] Clinically, CBD is typically characterized by asymmetric sensorimotor symptoms involving one hemibody to a greater degree than the other, with features of cortical and basal ganglionic dysfunction. Patients tend to have problems performing complex sequenced movements and movements on command (i.e., apraxia). Dystonia and action- or stimulus-induced myoclonus are also not uncommon. One classic sensorimotor feature of CBD is the alien hand or limb phenomenon, in which a part of the body feels as if it is not one's own or like it is being moved by an external/alien force. Parkinsonian rigidity and walking problems may also develop in addition to these sensorimotor problems, as well as problems with language and memory, personality changes, and inappropriate behavior.

Structural imaging studies may show frontotemporal atrophy, asymmetric parietal atrophy, or both. Functional imaging studies may demonstrate asymmetric hypometabolism and hypoperfusion in the parietal cortex and basal ganglia with or without frontotemporal hypometabolism and hypoperfusion. In the setting of mild motor symptoms with more prominent cognitive or behavioral manifestations, CBD can be confused for AD or FTD or vascular dementia with vascular parkinsonism. Some studies indicate that up to 20% of clinically-diagnosed FTDs turn out to have the pathology of CBD. Because of the significant clinicopathologic heterogeneity, the term corticobasal syndrome (CBS) is sometimes used for patients with characteristic clinical features, while CBD is reserved for diagnosis based on neuropathological analysis.

There are no FDA-approved or other treatments specific for CBD. Treatment is therefore supportive or symptomatic based on the individual patient's specific disease manifestations.

PROGRESSIVE SUPRANUCLEAR PALSY

Progressive supranuclear palsy (PSP) is another dementia characterized by the presence of cognitive and behavioral features along with specific motor abnormalities. PSP tends to occur in middle age and is slightly more common in men than women. It is a rare and sporadic disease, but, like CBD, it has been associated with specific tau gene haplotypes. The pathology of PSP involves (usually) abnormal tau-reactive deposits in neurons and glia that are typically concentrated in various brainstem nuclei (including the substantia nigra), but sometimes also in the cortex. In addition to involvement of systems that coordinate somatic movement, the supranuclear systems that govern the cranial nerves are also affected.

The classic clinical features of the disease are progressive difficulties with balance and gait, resulting in frequent falls early in the disease, progressive loss of voluntary control of eye movements, and progressive cognitive and behavioral difficulties. Patients with PSP often have difficulties with the coordination of eyelid opening and closing, dysarthria, dysphagia, and fixed facial expression akin to surprise. Symptoms similar to those of PD are also present, particularly akinesia and axial rigidity. The cognitive and behavioral features are usually referable to frontal lobe dysfunction and may closely resemble those of FTD (such as executive dysfunction, apathy, and reduced processing speed). CT or MRI scans may show an atrophic brainstem with frontotemporal atrophy as the disease progresses.

There are no approved therapies or cures for PSP, and management is supportive or symptomatic. It is important to assess safety issues to reduce the risk of falls and injury. Swallowing evaluations help to determine diet modifications that delay aspiration from dysphagia.

NORMAL PRESSURE HYDROCEPHALUS

Normal pressure hydrocephalus (NPH) is a condition that involves enlargement of the ventricles leading to cognitive and motor difficulties. About 250,000 people in the United States suffer from this disease; it usually occurs in adults 55 years old or older. Intermittent pressure increases are thought to cause ventricular expansion over time, with damage to the adjacent white matter tracts that connect the frontal lobes. The main clinical features are gait disturbance, frontal systems dysfunction, and urinary incontinence.[47] Patients need not have all three symptoms to have NPH. There are no clear genetic causes. The main risk factors relate to conditions that adversely affect the function of the ventricular system for cerebrospinal fluid (CSF) egress, which include history of head trauma, intracranial hemorrhage, meningitis, or any inflammatory or structural process that might damage the meninges.

Evaluation usually includes structural brain imaging (MRI or CT) demonstrating the presence of ventricular enlargement out of proportion to atrophy. Reversal of CSF flow in the cerebral aqueduct or the presence of transependymal fluid on MRI may suggest NPH.

If NPH is suspected, it is prudent to remove CSF and to measure the CSF pressure, which can be done by a variety of techniques. It is most important to perform cognitive and motor testing before and after the removal of a large volume of CSF. LP, lumbar catheter insertion or CSF pressure, and outflow-resistance monitoring in combination with pre-procedure and post-procedure neuropsychological and motor testing can be very helpful in making a diagnosis and in estimating the likelihood of treatment success.[48] Placement of a CSF shunt is the treatment of choice and can arrest or even significantly improve a patient's condition.[49]

CREUTZFELDT–JAKOB DISEASE

Creutzfeldt–Jakob disease (CJD) is a rare disorder that causes a characteristic triad of progressive dementia, myoclonus, and distinctive periodic EEG complexes; cerebellar, pyramidal and extrapyramidal findings are also characteristic, as are psychiatric symptoms, which may be among the first signs of the disease. The typical age of onset is around 60 years. CJD is caused by prions, novel proteinaceous infective agents. Prion protein, PrP, an amyloid protein encoded on chromosome 20, is the major constituent of prions. PrP normally exists in a PrPc isoform; in a pathological state, it is transformed to the PrPSc isoform, which condenses in neurons and causes their death. As prion-induced changes accumulate, the cerebral cortex takes on the distinctive microscopic, vacuolar appearance of spongiform encephalopathy. The CSF in almost 90% of CJD cases contains traces of prion proteins detected by a routine LP. CJD is transmissible and can occur as three general forms: sporadic, familial or acquired, including a variant form of CJD. Treatment in these unfortunate cases is supportive, as it follows a characteristically rapid and fatal course over an average of 6 months.[50]

CONCLUSIONS

As the population ages, the number of people with dementing disorders is increasing dramatically; most have AD, vascular dementia, DLB or a combination of these disorders. Although none are curable, all have treatable components—whether they are reversible, static, or progressive. Further, the increasing recognition of the spectrum of cognitive impairment, in mild and major neurocognitive disorders and in pre-clinical stages of AD, has potential for identifying people at earlier stages of impairment and preventing progression. The role of a psychiatrist in the diagnosis and treatment of dementing disorders is extremely important, particularly in the identification of treatable psychiatric and behavioral symptoms, which are common sources of caregiver distress and institutionalization.

Family members are additional victims of all progressive dementias. They particularly appreciate the psychiatrist who communicates with them about the diagnosis and the expected course of the disorder. They can benefit from advice on how best to relate to the patient, how to restructure the home environment for safety and comfort, and how to seek out legal and financial guidance when appropriate. Family members should also be made aware of the assistance available to them through organizations such as the Alzheimer's Association.

Great advances have been made in our understanding of the pathophysiology, epidemiology, and genetics of various dementing disorders. The likelihood of having measures for early detection, prevention, and intervention in the near future is very promising.

Access the complete reference list and multiple choice questions (MCQs) online at https://expertconsult.inkling.com

KEY REFERENCES

3. Petersen RC. Mild cognitive impairment ten years later. *Arch Neurol* 66:1447–1455, 2009.
4. Mayeux R, Stern Y. Epidemiology of Alzheimer Disease. *Cold Spring Harbor Perspect Med* 2, 2012.
5. Sosa-Ortiz AL, Acosta-Castillo I, Prince MJ. Epidemiology of Alzheimer's Disease. *Arch Med Res* 43:600–608, 2012.
8. Barnes DE, Yaffee K. The projected effect of risk factor reduction on Alzheimer's disease prevalence. *Lancet Neurol* 10:819–828, 2011.

10. Reitz C, Brayne C, Mayeux R. Epidemiology of Alzheimer Disease. *Nat Rev Neurol* 7:137–152, 2011.
11. Carillo MC, Brashear HR, Logovinsky V, et al. Can we prevent Alzheimer's disease? secondary "prevention" trials. *Alzheimers Dement* 9:123–131, 2013.
17. Gandy S, DeKosky ST. Toward the treatment and prevention of Alzheimer's disease: rational strategies and recent progress. *Ann Rev Med* 64:367–383, 2013.
20. Sperling RA, Aisen PS, Beckett LA, et al. Toward defining the preclinical stages of Alzheimer's disease: recommendations from the National Institute on Aging-Alzheimer's Association workgroups on diagnostic guidelines for Alzheimer's disease. *Alzheimers Dement* 7:280–292, 2011.
21. Alzheimer's Disease. Implications of the updated diagnostic and research criteria. *J Clin Psychiatry* 72(9):1190–1196, 2011.
22. Pillai JA, Cummings JL. Clinical trials in predementia stages of Alzheimer Disease. *Med Clin North Am* 97(3):439–457, 2013.
25. Howard R, McShane R, Lindesay J, et al. Donepezil and memantine for moderate-to-severe Alzheimer's Disease. *N Engl J Med* 366(10):893–903, 2012.
26. Carson S, McDonagh MS, Peterson K. A systematic review of the efficacy and safety of atypical antipsychotics in patients with psychological and behavioral symptoms of dementia. *J Am Geriatr Soc* 54:354–361, 2006.
28. Selkoe DJ. Defining molecular targets to prevent Alzheimer disease. *Arch Neurol* 62(2):192–195, 2005.
30. Gilman S, Koller M, Black RS, et al. Clinical effects of Abeta immunization (AN1792) in patients with AD in an interrupted trial. *Neurology* 64(9):1553–1562, 2005.
31. Jellinger KA. Alpha-synuclein pathology in Parkinson's and Alzheimer's disease brain: incidence and topographic distribution—a pilot study. *Acta Neuropathol (Berl)* 106:191–201, 2003.
32. Weisman D, McKeith I. Dementia with Lewy bodies. *Semin Neurol* 27(1):42–47, 2007.
33. McKeith IG, Dickson DW, Lowe J, et al. Diagnosis and management of dementia with Lewy bodies: third report of the DLB consortium. *Neurology* 65:1863–1872, 2005.
34. Rolinski M, Fox C, Maidment I, et al. Cholinesterase inhibitors for dementia with Lewy bodies, Parkinson's disease dementia and cognitive impairment in Parkinson's disease. *Cochrane Database Syst Rev* 14(3):CD006504, 2012.
37. Forman MS, Farmer J, Johnson JK, et al. Frontotemporal dementia: clinicopathological correlations. *Ann Neurol* 59:952–962, 2006.
38. Seltman RE, Matthews BR. Frontotemporal lobar degeneration: epidemiology, pathology, diagnosis and management. *CNS Drugs* 26(10):841–870, 2012.
39. Van Blitterswijk M, DeJesus-Hernandez M, Rademakers R. How do C9ORF72 repeat expansions cause amyotrophic lateral sclerosis and frontotemporal dementia: can we learn from other non-coding repeat expansions disorders? *Curr Opin Neurol* 25(6):689–700, 2012.
40. Mesulam MM. Primary progressive aphasia—a language-based dementia. *N Engl J Med* 349:1535–1542, 2003.
44. Bowler JV. Acetylcholinesterase inhibitors for vascular dementia and Alzheimer's disease combined with cerebrovascular disease. *Stroke* 34:584–586, 2003.
45. Bowler JV. Vascular cognitive impairment. *J Neurol Neurosurg Psychiatry* 76(Suppl. 5):v35–v44, 2005.
46. Shelley BP, Hodges JR, Kipps CM, et al. Is the pathology of corticobasal syndrome predictable in life? *Mov Disord* 24(11):1593–1599, 2009.
48. Relkin N, Marmarou A, Klinge P, et al. Diagnosing idiopathic normal-pressure hydrocephalus. *Neurosurgery* 57:S4–S16, discussion ii–v, 2005.
50. Gencer AG, Pelin Z, Kucukali C, et al. Creutzfeldt-Jakob disease. *Psychogeriatrics* 11(2):119–124, 2011.

15 Alcohol-Related Disorders

John F. Kelly, PhD, and John A. Renner Jr., MD

KEY POINTS

Incidence

- Alcohol misuse is one of the leading causes of morbidity and mortality in the US.

Epidemiology

- The highest rates of alcohol use, heavy binge use, and alcohol use disorders occur between the ages of 18 and 29 years.

Pathophysiology

- Alcohol causes harm through three distinct, but related pathways: intoxication, toxicity, and alcohol use disorder.

Clinical Findings

- Alcohol use disorders are heterogeneous disorders that require assessment and an individualized clinical approach.
- It is possible to screen effectively and efficiently for the presence of an alcohol use disorder using brief, validated measures.

Differential Diagnoses

- Presentation of an alcohol use disorder is often complicated by the presence of co-morbid psychiatric symptoms and disorders that require assessment and monitoring, as well as an integrated treatment approach.

Treatment Options

- A number of effective pharmacological and psychosocial treatment approaches exist for alcohol use disorders that produce outcomes similar to, or better than, outcomes for other chronic illnesses.

Complications

- Heavy drinking can lead to accidents, violence, unwanted pregnancies, and overdoses.

OVERVIEW

Alcohol is an ambiguous molecule[1] often referred to as "man's oldest friend and oldest enemy".[2] Compared to more structurally complicated substances, such as cannabis ($C_{21}H_{30}O_2$), cocaine ($C_{17}H_{21}NO_4$), or heroin ($C_{21}H_{23}NO_5$), beverage alcohol (ethanol) possesses a simple chemical structure (C_2H_5OH) that belies the complexities of its medical, psychological, and social impact (Figure 15-1).

When the alcohol molecule reaches the human brain it is generally perceived as good news; pleasant subjective experiences of euphoria, disinhibition, anxiety reduction, and sedation, are the most likely outcomes. These are often encouraged and enhanced by social contexts and by culture-bound customs. If too high a dose is imbibed too rapidly, however, acute intoxication occurs, leading to a predictable sequence of behavioral disinhibition and cognitive and motor impairments. If a large quantity of alcohol is consumed, especially

if it is done rapidly,[3] alcohol-induced amnesia ("blackouts"), coma, and death, can occur.

Like several other drugs, alcohol causes harm in three distinct, but related, ways: through intoxication, toxicity, and alcohol use disorder.[4] As depicted in Figure 15-2, the acute intoxicating effects of alcohol produce physical and psychological impairments (e.g., ataxia, poor judgment, visuo-spatial deficits, sensory distortions) and disinhibition can lead to aggression, that can result in accidents and injuries (e.g., from car crashes, falls, fights). The toxic effects of alcohol, on the other hand, produce harm through the chronic deleterious action of alcohol on the human body that can result in liver damage, including cirrhosis, as well as damage to the brain, heart, and kidneys.[5] Because of the toxicity pathway to harm, it is possible for individuals who infrequently become intoxicated to, nevertheless, develop a variety of diseases associated with alcohol's *toxic* effects, such as cirrhosis of the liver or a variety of cancers (e.g., of the colon, rectum, breast, larynx, liver, esophagus, oral cavity, pharynx[6]; Figure 15-2). Somewhat paradoxically, cirrhosis is more common among individuals *without* alcohol addiction, since more florid manifestations of dependence are likely to result in more rapid remission, incarceration, or death, preventing the chronic damaging toxic effects associated with prolonged use of alcohol.[7] Alcohol use disorder (AUD) is the third pathway through which alcohol use causes harm. AUD contributes to a range of changes in the brain that often result in alcohol addiction. This can take a heavy toll on individuals' lives (with serious domestic and social problems, family disintegration, loss of employment and increased risk of mortality). Related to these pathways is the volume and frequency at which alcohol is consumed. Low-risk consumption is, for men, no more than 14 drinks per week and, for women, no more than 7 drinks in any given week. The *pattern* of consumption is also critical, however, for obvious reasons; 14 drinks in one sitting for some could constitute a lethal dose. Thus, to minimize harm from intoxication, and to reduce the risk from AUDs, no more than 2 drinks on any given day for men and no more than 1 for women is recommended[8] (Figure 15-3). It should be emphasized, however, that this pattern of consumption is "*low* risk" and *not* "*no* risk"; meta-analyses reveal even less than 1 drink a day is associated with an increased risk for a number of cancers (including breast cancer in women).[6] It is estimated that alcohol is responsible for about 20%–30% of esophageal cancers, liver cancer, cirrhosis of the liver, homicide, epileptic seizures, and motor vehicle accidents worldwide.[9] Excessive or risky alcohol consumption is the third leading cause of death in the US, accounting for approximately 100,000 deaths annually.[10] In terms of disability-adjusted life years (DALYs) lost, alcohol accounts for more disease, disability, and mortality combined in the United States than tobacco use, even though tobacco use accounts for a higher death rate. This is because alcohol causes more illness, impairment during the prime of individuals' lives, and death (e.g., alcohol is the leading risk factor for death among men 15–59 worldwide).[11] The economic burden attributed to alcohol-related problems in the US approaches $224 billion annually.[12,13]

Alcohol-related disorders are common in the general population, are prevalent among general medical patients, and are endemic among psychiatric patients. An awareness of the substantial roles that alcohol use, misuse, and associated disorders play in medicine and psychiatry will enhance the detection of these problems and lead to more efficient and effective targeting of clinical resources.

In this chapter we review pertinent clinical manifestations of heavy alcohol use and outline strategies for effective management of alcohol-related problems. The nature, etiology, epidemiology, and typologies of alcohol-related disorders are described, and optimal screening and assessment methods (to facilitate detection and appropriate intervention) are outlined. In the final sections, details of current knowledge regarding the mechanisms of action of heavy alcohol use are provided and effective psychosocial and pharmacological treatment approaches are reviewed.

DESCRIPTION AND DEFINITION

Alcohol-related disorders can be divided into two main groups: alcohol-induced disorders (such as alcohol intoxication, delirium, alcohol withdrawal, persisting alcohol-induced amnestic disorders, and fetal alcohol spectrum disorders), and alcohol use disorder (DSM-5[14], Box 15-1).

Heavy, chronic, alcohol use may also induce psychiatric symptoms and syndromes that mimic psychotic disorder, mood disorders, and anxiety disorders. Such syndromes most often remit with abstinence, but the diagnosis of an

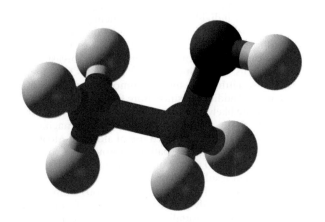

Figure 15-1. Molecular structure of beverage ethyl alcohol. *(From UCLA Chemistry, http://www.chem.ucla.edu/harding/IGOC/E/ethanol .html)*

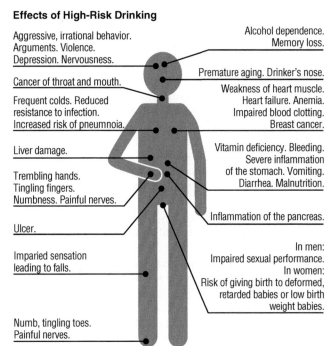

Figure 15-2. Alcohol-related disorders associated with high-risk drinking. *(From Rehm J, Room R, Monteiro M, et al. Alcohol use. In Ezzati M, Lopez AD, Rodgers A, Murray CJL, editors: Comparative quantification of health risks: global and regional burden of disease attributable to selected major risk factors. Geneva, 2004, World Health Organization.)*

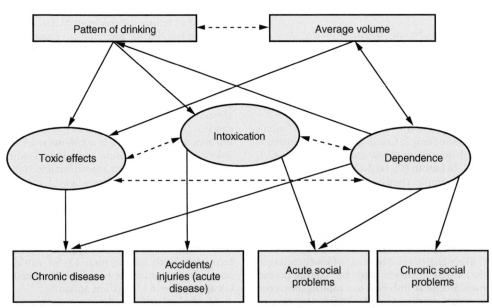

Figure 15-3. Patterns of drinking and pathways to harm. *(From Babor TF, Caetano R, Casswell S, et al. Alcohol: no ordinary commodity-research and public policy. ed 2. Oxford, UK, 2010, Oxford University Press.)*

BOX 15-1 The DSM-5 Diagnostic Criteria: Alcohol Use Disorder[14]

A. A problematic pattern of alcohol use leading to clinically significant impairment or distress, as manifested by at least two of the following, occurring within a 12-month period:

1. Alcohol is often taken in larger amounts or over a longer period than was intended.
2. There is a persistent desire or unsuccessful efforts to cut down or control alcohol use.
3. A great deal of time is spent in activities necessary to obtain alcohol, use alcohol, or recovery from its effects.
4. Craving, or a strong desire or urge to use alcohol.
5. Recurrent alcohol use resulting in a failure to fulfill major role obligations at work, school, or home.
6. Continued alcohol use despite having persistent or recurrent social or interpersonal problems caused or exacerbated by the effects of alcohol
7. Important social, occupational, or recreational activities are given up or reduced because of alcohol use.
8. Recurrent alcohol use in situations in which it is physically hazardous.
9. Alcohol use is continued despite knowledge of having a persistent or recurrent physical or psychological problem that is likely to have been caused or exacerbated by alcohol.
10. Tolerance, as defined by either of the following:
    a. A need for markedly increased amounts of alcohol to achieve intoxication or desired effect.
    b. A markedly diminished effect with continued use of the same amount of alcohol.
11. Withdrawal, as manifested by either of the following:
    a. The characteristic withdrawal syndrome for alcohol
    b. Alcohol (or a closely related substance, such as a benzodiazepine) is taken to relieve or avoid withdrawal symptoms.

Specify if:

In early remission: After full criteria for alcohol use disorder were previously met, none of the criteria for alcohol use disorder have

been met for at least 3 months but for less than 12 months (with the exception that Criterion A4, "Craving, or a strong desire or urge to use alcohol," may be met).

In sustained remission: After full criteria for alcohol use disorder were previously met, none of the criteria for alcohol use disorder have been met at any time during a period of 12 months or longer (with the exception that Criterion A4, "Craving, or a strong desire or urge to use alcohol," may be met).

Specify if:

In a controlled environment: This additional specifier is used if the individual is in an environment where access to alcohol is restricted.

• **Coding note** based on current severity, for ICD-10-CM codes: If an alcohol intoxication, alcohol withdrawal, or another alcohol-induced mental disorder is also present, do not use the codes below for alcohol use disorder. Instead, the comorbid alcohol use disorder is indicated in the 4th character of the alcohol-induced disorder code (see the coding note for alcohol intoxication, alcohol withdrawal, or a specific alcohol-induced mental disorder). For example, if there is comorbid alcohol intoxication and alcohol use disorder, only the alcohol intoxication code is given, with the 4th character indicating whether the comorbid alcohol use disorder is mild, moderate, or severe: F10.129 for mild alcohol use disorder with alcohol intoxication or F10.229 for a moderate or severe alcohol use disorder with alcohol intoxication.

Specify current severity:

305.00 (F10.10) Mild: Presence of 2–3 symptoms.
303.90 (F10.20) Moderate: Presence of 4–5 symptoms.
303.90 (F10.20) Severe: Presence of 6 or more symptoms.

Reprinted with permission from the Diagnostic and statistical manual of mental disorders, *ed 5, (Copyright 2013). American Psychiatric Association.*

independent co-occurring psychiatric disorder is difficult to discern in an individual who is actively drinking. At least 4 weeks of sobriety is recommended to establish the diagnosis of an independent psychiatric disorder. The next sections describe alcohol-induced disorders and AUDs.

ALCOHOL-INDUCED DISORDERS
Alcohol Intoxication

The action of alcohol on the brain is complex. Low blood alcohol concentrations (BACs) produce activation and disinhibition, whereas higher BACs produce sedation. Behavioral disinhibition is mediated by alcohol's action as a γ-aminobutyric acid (GABA) agonist, and its interactions with the serotonin system may account for its association with violent behavior. The GABA, N-methyl-D-aspartate (NMDA), and serotonin systems have all been implicated in the escalation to violence.[15,16] Blood alcohol concentrations (BACs, measured as the percentage of alcohol in the blood) from 0.19% to 29% may impair memory or lead to an alcoholic blackout, with argumentativeness or assaultiveness developing at levels of 0.10%–0.19% and coma or death occurring at 0.40%–0.50%. Yet, chronic alcoholics may be fully alert with a BAC of more than 0.40%, owing to tolerance. Resolution of intoxication follows steady-state kinetics, so that a 70-kg man metabolizes

approximately 10 ml of absolute ethanol (or 1.5 to 2 drink equivalents; 1 standard drink = 0.5 oz of whiskey, 4 oz of wine, or 12 oz of beer) per hour (Figure 15-4).

Treatment

If it becomes necessary to sedate an intoxicated individual, one should begin with a smaller-than-usual dose of a benzodiazepine to avoid cumulative effects of alcohol and other sedative-hypnotics. Once the individual's tolerance has been established, a specific dose can be safely determined. Lorazepam (Ativan) (1 to 2 mg) is effectively absorbed via oral (PO), intramuscular (IM), or intravenous (IV) administration. Diazepam (Valium) and chlordiazepoxide (Librium) are erratically and slowly absorbed after IM administration unless they are given in large, well-perfused sites. When incoordination suggests that the additive effect of a benzodiazepine has produced excessive sedation, it may be advantageous to use haloperidol 5 to 10 mg PO or IM. The initial dose should be followed by a delay of 0.5 to 1 hour before the next dose. If there is no risk of withdrawal, the patient can safely be referred to an outpatient program. Inpatient detoxification is preferable to outpatient care if the patient is psychosocially unstable; has serious medical, neurological, or psychiatric co-morbidity; has previously suffered from complications of withdrawal (such as seizures or delirium tremens [DTs]); or is undergoing

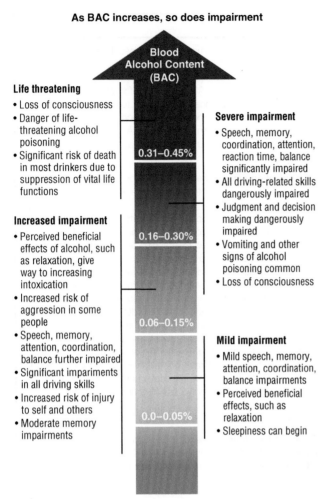

As BAC increases, so does impairment

Blood Alcohol Content (BAC)

Life threatening
- Loss of consciousness
- Danger of life-threatening alcohol poisoning
- Significant risk of death in most drinkers due to suppression of vital life functions

0.31–0.45%

Increased impairment
- Perceived beneficial effects of alcohol, such as relaxation, give way to increasing intoxication
- Increased risk of aggression in some people
- Speech, memory, attention, coordination, balance further impaired
- Significant impariments in all driving skills
- Increased risk of injury to self and others
- Moderate memory impairments

0.16–0.30%

0.06–0.15%

0.0–0.05%

Severe impairment
- Speech, memory, coordination, attention, reaction time, balance significantly impaired
- All driving-related skills dangerously impaired
- Judgment and decision making dangerously impaired
- Vomiting and other signs of alcohol poisoning common
- Loss of consciousness

Mild impairment
- Mild speech, memory, attention, coordination, balance impairments
- Perceived beneficial effects, such as relaxation
- Sleepiness can begin

Figure 15-4. Impairment as a result of increased blood alcohol content (BAC). *(From National Institute on Alcohol Abuse and Alcoholism (NIAAA). Alcohol overdose: the dangers of drinking too much. NIAAA Brochures and Fact Sheets, 2013. http://pubs.niaaa.nih.gov/publications/AlcoholOverdoseFactsheet/Overdosefact.htm)*

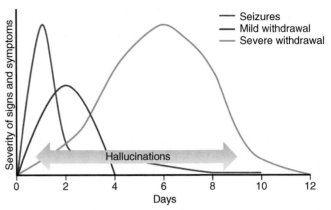

Figure 15-5. Progress of alcohol withdrawal syndrome. *(From Frank L, Pead J. New concepts in drug withdrawal: a resource handbook. Melbourne, 1995, University of Melbourne.)*

his or her first episode of treatment.[17] Repeatedly undertreated withdrawal may place the patient at subsequent risk for withdrawal seizures and for other neurological sequelae through "kindling," an electrophysiological effect[18] that may be mediated, similar to other neurodegenerative effects of ethanol, via the glutamate excitatory neurotransmitter system.[19]

Alcohol-induced Coma

Alcohol-induced coma, although rare, is a medical emergency. It occurs when extraordinary amounts of alcohol are consumed, and it can occur in conjunction with use of other drugs. Young adults/college-age youth may be particularly susceptible when goaded into drinking contests. This age group is also at significantly higher risk for alcohol-related injuries. A 2002 study by the federally supported Task Force on College Drinking estimated that 1,400 college students in the US are killed each year in alcohol-related accidents.

Alcohol Withdrawal Syndrome

The syndrome of alcohol withdrawal can range from mild discomfort (that requires no medication) to multi-organ failure (that requires intensive care). Uncomplicated

withdrawal is surprisingly common and is frequently missed. Although more than 90% of alcoholics in withdrawal need nothing more than supportive treatment, those hospitalized with co-morbid medical conditions have a higher rate of complications.[20] The most common features of uncomplicated alcohol withdrawal emerge within hours and resolve after 3 to 5 days. Early features (loss of appetite, irritability, and tremor) of uncomplicated withdrawal symptoms are predictable. A hallmark of alcohol withdrawal is generalized tremor (fast in frequency and more pronounced when the patient is under stress). This tremor may involve the tongue to such an extent that the patient cannot talk. The lower extremities may tremble so much that the patient cannot walk. The hands and arms may shake so violently that a drinking glass cannot be held without spilling the contents. Typically, the patient is hypervigilant, has a pronounced startle response, and complains of insomnia.

Less commonly, patients experience hallucinations (without delirium) or seizures associated with alcohol withdrawal. Illusions and hallucinations may appear and produce vague uneasiness. These symptoms may persist for as long as 2 weeks and then clear without the development of delirium. Grand mal seizures ("rum fits") may occur, usually within the first 2 days. More than one out of every three patients who suffer seizures develops subsequent DTs (Figure 15-5).

Treatment

Rigid adherence to a single protocol for all cases of alcohol withdrawal is unrealistic. Symptom-triggered dosing, in which dosages are individualized and only administered on the appearance of early symptoms, is often recommended. Assessment of the severity of alcohol withdrawal's signs and symptoms is best accomplished with the use of standardized alcohol withdrawal scales, such as the CIWA-Ar.[21] This reduces use of medication doses by a factor of four, substantially shortens the length of treatment, and shortens symptom duration by a factor of six,[17,22] although the benefits may be less dramatic in medically ill inpatients.[23] Chlordiazepoxide (50 to 100 mg PO) can be given initially, and be followed by 50 to 100 mg every 1 to 2 hours until the patient is sedated and the vital signs are within normal limits. Alternatively, diazepam (10 to 20 mg) may be given initially, and then repeated every 1 to 2 hours until sedation is achieved. Often a first day's dose of a long-acting benzodiazepine is sufficient for the entire detoxification process because of the self-tapering effect and slow elimination.[24] Patients with impaired liver function, the elderly, or individuals with co-occurring medical or psychiatric conditions are often better managed with a shorter-acting agent, such as lorazepam 1 to 4 mg PO or IM, or 0.5 mg/min slow IV infusion in severe withdrawal, repeated after 1 to 2 hours, with dose tapering by 25% per day over the subsequent 3 to 6 days.

The α2-agonist dexmedetomidine is sometimes used in cases of alcohol withdrawal, especially when patients require escalating doses of benzodiazepines and additional intubation and mechanical ventilation to protect airways, which can lead to complications and prolonged hospital stays.[25] Similarly, phenobarbital is used to augment benzodiazepine-assisted alcohol withdrawal to prevent the need for intubation and ICU admission. A prospective, randomized, double-blind, placebo-controlled study with 102 patients, half of whom received either a single dose of IV phenobarbital (10 mg/kg in 100 ml of normal saline) or placebo (100 ml of normal saline) in addition to a symptom-guided lorazepam-based alcohol withdrawal protocol, found that patients who received phenobarbital had fewer ICU admissions (8% vs. 25%), and there were no differences in adverse events.[26]

Alcohol Withdrawal Seizures

Withdrawal seizures occur in roughly 1% of unmedicated alcoholics undergoing withdrawal, although the prevalence is increased in individuals with inadequately treated prior episodes of alcohol withdrawal, prior alcohol withdrawal seizures, seizure disorders, and previous brain injuries. Although brain imaging may not be necessary in patients with their first episode,[27] seizures during alcohol withdrawal require careful evaluation for other causes. Indications for imaging include neurological and other physical findings suggestive of focal lesions, meningitis, or subarachnoid hemorrhage—all of which may occur in a patient with a history of alcohol withdrawal seizures. Multiple prior detoxifications predispose patients to withdrawal seizures more than the quantity or duration of a drinking history, implying a kindling cause.[28] Seizures may occur following a rapid drop in the BAC or during the 6 to 24 hours after drinking cessation. Generalized seizures typically occur (i.e., in 75% of cases) in the absence of focal findings, and in individuals with otherwise unremarkable electroencephalogram (EEG) findings. Repeated seizures may occur over a 24-hour period; however, status epilepticus occurs in less than 10% of those who seize.

Treatment

In patients without a prior seizure disorder, diphenylhydantoin offers no benefit over placebo, and given the potential for side effects, diphenylhydantoin is therefore not recommended.[28] Also, given that loading with carbamazepine or valproate may not address the rapid time course of withdrawal seizures, the most parsimonious approach remains effective treatment with benzodiazepines. Prompt treatment of early withdrawal symptoms, as described below, is the most effective measure to prevent the development of seizures. In cases where there is a known seizure disorder, however, conventional management with an anticonvulsant is in order.

Alcohol Withdrawal Delirium

Delirium tremens, or "DTs," the major acute complication of alcohol withdrawal, was renamed "alcohol withdrawal delirium" in the *Diagnostic and Statistical Manual of Mental Disorders*, ed 4 (DSM-IV).[29] Until open-heart procedures spawned new postoperative deliria, DTs were by far the most frequently encountered delirium in general hospitals, reportedly occurring in 5% of hospitalized alcoholics. Although it was first described in the medical literature more than 150 years ago and it has been frequently observed ever since, DTs still go undiagnosed in a large number of cases. It is missed because physicians tend to forget that alcoholism is rampant among people of all backgrounds and appearances.[30] Because deaths have occurred in 10% of patients with untreated alcohol withdrawal delirium and in 25% of those patients with medical or concomitant surgical complications, it is imperative to be on the alert for this life-threatening condition.

It is difficult to predict who will develop DTs. Until a decade ago, DTs rarely developed in patients younger than 30 years of age. This is no longer true. Today the condition is frequently observed in young patients who may have had a decade or more of chronic heavy alcohol consumption. The mechanisms may involve NMDA-glutamate receptor supersensitivity.[18] Although delirium is regarded as a withdrawal syndrome, some heavy drinkers fail to develop delirium after sudden withdrawal of ethanol. Infection, head trauma, and poor nutrition are potentially contributing factors to delirium. A history of DTs is the most obvious predictor of future DTs.[31]

The incidence of DTs is approximately 5% among hospitalized alcoholics and about 33% in patients with alcohol withdrawal seizures. If DTs do occur, they generally do so between 24 and 72 hours after abstinence begins. There have been reports, however, of cases in which the clinical picture of DTs did not emerge until 7 days after the last drink. The principal features are disorientation (to time, place, or person), tremor, hyperactivity, marked wakefulness, fever, increased autonomic tone, and hallucinations. Hallucinations are generally visual, but they may be tactile (in which case they are probably associated with a peripheral neuritis), olfactory, or auditory. Vestibular disturbances are common and often hallucinatory. The patient may complain of the floor moving or of being on an elevator. The hallucinatory experience is almost always frightening, such as seeing spiders and snakes that may have additional characteristics (e.g., more vivid colors and mice or insects sensed on the skin). Once the condition manifests itself, DTs usually last 2 to 3 days, often resolving suddenly after a night of sound sleep. Should it persist, an infection or subdural hematoma may be the cause. There are, however, a small number of individuals whose course is characterized by relapses with intervals of complete lucidity. These patients offer the clinician the most challenging diagnostic opportunities. As a rule of thumb, it is always wise to include DTs in the list of diagnoses considered whenever delirium appears. Even skilled clinicians are apt to miss the diagnosis of DTs when the patient's manner, social position, or reputation belies a preconceived and distorted stereotype of an "alcoholic." The clinician is also frequently misled when the delirium is intermittent and the patient is examined during a lucid stage. Although a course of intermittent episodes is highly atypical for DTs, it can occur.

The prognosis for DTs is reasonably good if the patient is aggressively medicated, but death can occur as the syndrome progresses through convulsions to coma and death. Death can also result from heart failure, an infection (chiefly pneumonia), or injuries sustained during the restless period. In a small proportion of patients the delirium may merge into Wernicke-Korsakoff syndrome, in which case the patient may not regain full mentation. This is more apt to happen in those with closely spaced episodes of DTs and in the elderly, but it should be assessed and continually monitored.[32]

Treatment

Prevention is the key. Symptom-triggered dosing for alcohol withdrawal has been shown to reduce DTs more than use of standing doses of benzodiazepine in medically ill inpatients.[23]

As in the treatment of any delirium, the prime concern must be round-the-clock monitoring so that the patient cannot harm himself or herself or others. Although not necessarily suicidal, delirious patients take unpremeditated risks. Falling out of windows, slipping down stairs, and walking into objects are common examples. Restraints should be used only when necessary. When four-point restraint is used, the patient must be closely observed, and relief must be provided every hour. Usually, use of physical restraints can be avoided with aggressive pharmacotherapy.

The delayed onset of this hyperarousal may reflect alcohol's broad effects across multiple neurotransmitter systems, chief among which may be the NMDA-glutamate system.[19] Adrenergic hyperarousal alone appears to be an insufficient explanation, so that α-adrenergic agonists (e.g., clonidine, lofexidine) alone are not sufficient. Benzodiazepines alone may not suffice. In rare cases, doses of diazepam in excess of 500 mg/day may prove insufficient. Haloperidol 5 to 10 mg PO or IM may be added and repeated after 1 to 2 hours when psychosis or agitation is present. Propofol may be used in those cases of severe DTs unresponsive to other medications.[33]

Because the B vitamins are known to help prevent peripheral neuropathy and the Wernicke–Korsakoff syndrome, their use is *vital*. Thiamine (100 mg IV) should be given immediately, and 100 mg should be given IM for at least 3 days until a normal diet is resumed. A smaller amount of thiamine may be added to infusions for IV use. Folic acid 1 to 5 mg PO or IM each day should be included to prevent megaloblastic anemia and peripheral neuropathy. A high-carbohydrate soft diet containing 3,000 to 4,000 calories a day should be given with multivitamins.

Wernicke–Korsakoff Syndrome

Victor and colleagues,[34] in their classic monograph *The Wernicke–Korsakoff Syndrome*, state that "Wernicke's encephalopathy and Korsakoff's syndrome in the alcoholic, nutritionally deprived patient may be regarded as two facets of the same disease. Patients evidence specific central nervous system pathology with resultant profound mental changes." Although perhaps 5% of alcoholics have this disorder, in 80% of these cases, the diagnosis is missed.[32] In all of the cases reported by Victor and colleagues,[34] alcoholism was a serious problem and was almost invariably accompanied by malnutrition. Malnutrition, particularly thiamine deficiency, has been shown to be the essential factor.

Wernicke's Encephalopathy

Wernicke's encephalopathy appears suddenly and is characterized by ophthalmoplegia and ataxia followed by mental disturbance. The ocular disturbance, which occurs in only 17% of cases, consists of paresis or paralysis of the external recti, with nystagmus, and a disturbance in conjugate gaze. A globally confused state consists of disorientation, unresponsiveness, and derangement of perception and memory. Exhaustion, apathy, dehydration, and profound lethargy are also part of the picture. The patient is apt to be somnolent, confused, and slow to reply, and may fall asleep in mid-sentence. Once treatment with thiamine is started for Wernicke's encephalopathy, improvement is often evident in the ocular palsies within hours. Recovery from ocular muscle paralysis is complete within days or weeks. According to Victor and colleagues,[34] approximately one-third recovered from the state of global confusion within 6 days of treatment, another third within 1 month, and the remainder within 2 months. The state of global confusion is almost always reversible, in marked contrast to the memory impairment of Korsakoff's psychosis.

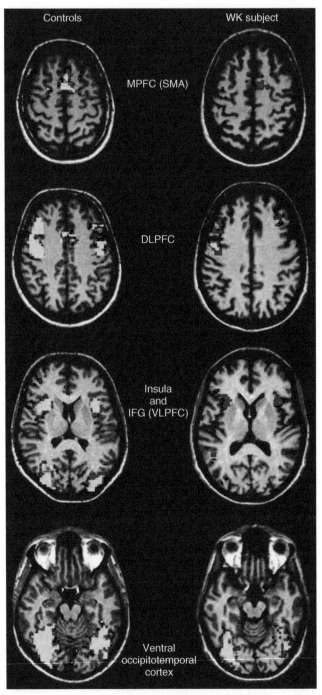

Figure 15-6. Brain activation in Wernicke–Korsakoff (WK) patients compared to controls. VLPFC, ventro lateral pre-frontal cortex; IFG, inferior frontal gyrus. *(From Caulo M, Van Hecke J, Toma L, et al. Functional MRI study of diencephalic amnesia in Wernicke–Korsakoff syndrome. Brain 128(Pt 7):1584–1594, 2005.)*

Functional magnetic resonance imaging (fMRI) studies show substantially diminished global activation in the brain among Wernicke–Korsakoff's patients compared to normal controls (Figure 15-6).

Treatment

Administration of the B vitamin thiamine (IM or IV) should be routine for *all* suspected cases of alcohol intoxication and dependence.[35] The treatment for Wernicke's encephalopathy and Korsakoff's psychosis is identical, and both are *medical emergencies*. Because subclinical cognitive impairments can occur even in apparently well-nourished patients, routine management should include thiamine, folic acid, and multi-vitamins with minerals, particularly zinc. Prompt use of vitamins, particularly thiamine, prevents advancement of the disease and reverses at least a portion of the lesions where permanent damage has not yet been done. The response to treatment is therefore an important diagnostic aid. In patients who show only ocular and ataxic signs, the prompt administration of thiamine is crucial in preventing the development of an irreversible and incapacitating amnestic disorder. Treatment consists of 100 mg of thiamine and 1 mg of folic acid (given IV) immediately and 100 mg IM of thiamine each day until a normal diet is resumed, followed by oral doses for 30 days. Parenteral feedings and the administration of B-complex vitamins become necessary if the patient cannot eat. If a rapid heart rate, feeble heart sounds, pulmonary edema, or other signs of myocardial weakness appear, the patient may require digitalis. Because these patients have impaired mental function, nursing personnel should be alerted to the patient's tendency to wander, to be forgetful, and to become obstreperously psychotic.

Korsakoff's Psychosis (Alcohol-induced Persisting Amnestic Disorder)

Korsakoff's psychosis, also referred to as confabulatory psychosis and alcohol-induced persisting amnestic disorder,[29] is characterized by impaired memory in an otherwise alert and responsive individual. This condition is slow to start and may be the end stage of a lengthy alcohol-dependence process. Hallucinations and delusions are rarely encountered. Curiously, confabulation, long regarded as the hallmark of Korsakoff's psychosis, was exhibited in only a limited number of cases in the large series collected and studied by Victor and colleagues.[34] Most of these patients have diminished spontaneous verbal output, have a limited understanding of the extent of their memory loss, and lack insight into the nature of their illness.

The memory loss is bipartite. The retrograde component is the inability to recall the past, and the anterograde component is the lack of capacity for retention of new information. In the acute stage of Korsakoff's psychosis, the memory gap is so blatant that the patient cannot recall simple items (such as the examiner's name, the day, or the time) even though the patient is given this information several times. As memory improves, usually within weeks to months, simple problems can be solved, limited always by the patient's span of recall.

Patients with Korsakoff's psychosis tend to improve with time.[36] Among Victor and colleagues' patients,[34] 21% recovered more or less completely, 26% showed no recovery, and the rest recovered partially.[29] During the acute stage, however, there is no way of predicting who will improve and who will not. The EEG may be unremarkable or may show diffuse slowing, and magnetic resonance imaging (MRI) may show changes in the periaqueductal area and medial thalamus.[18] The specific memory structures affected in Korsakoff's psychosis are the medial dorsal nucleus of the thalamus and the hippocampal formations.

Fetal Alcohol Spectrum Disorder

Fetal alcohol spectrum disorder (FASD) is an umbrella term that describes the range of effects that can occur in an individual whose mother drank alcohol during pregnancy. These effects may include physical, mental, behavioral, or learning disabilities with possible life-long implications.[37] Formerly

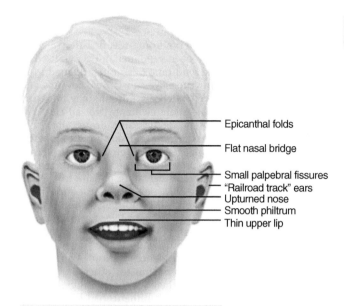

Figure 15-7. Characteristics of fetal alcohol spectrum disorder. *(From Wattendorf DJ, Muenke M. Fetal alcohol spectrum disorders. Am Fam Physician 72(2):279–282, 285, 2005.)*

known as "fetal alcohol syndrome," these disorders can include a set of birth defects caused by alcohol during pregnancy.[38] Children with this condition typically have facial deformities, a mis-proportioned head, mental retardation, and behavioral problems (Figure 15-7).

However, even when these abnormalities are not evident, brain damage may still have occurred. Approximately 30%–40% of all women who drink heavily during pregnancy will have a baby with some degree of FASD. It is the leading cause of preventable mental retardation in the Western Hemisphere. Studies using MRI to view the brains of children with FASD show that brain areas that regulate movement and cognitive processes related to attention, perception, thinking, and memory are particularly sensitive to pre-natal alcohol exposure, and that brain size is reduced.[39]

The minimum amount of alcohol needed to produce harmful effects in exposed children is not known. Thus, the safest approach is to completely avoid alcohol during pregnancy. People with pre-natal alcohol exposure have a high risk of learning and mental disabilities, school dropout, delinquency, alcohol and other drug use disorders, mental illness, and poor psychosocial function. Education, screening, and early intervention are critical.

ALCOHOL USE DISORDERS

Alcohol use disorder has been re-classified in DSM-5 into a single, 11-item, category of "alcohol use disorder" which was constructed by combining three of the four former "abuse" criteria (repeated legal consequences was dropped) with the seven "alcohol dependence" criteria specified in DSM-IV, and by adding a new "craving" criterion. The other major classification system, the International Classification of Diseases, Version 10 (ICD-10), however, has maintained its distinction between "alcohol dependence" and "harmful use". Importantly, both systems delineate "polythetic" classifications of AUD, since only two from a list of 11 symptoms are required to meet a diagnostic threshold in DSM-5 and three in ICD-10 for a "dependence" diagnosis. This highlights a degree of heterogeneity within the syndrome that has typological and clinical implications for detecting and treating the disorder. The DSM-5 criteria can be seen in Box 15-1.

The alcohol dependence syndrome was first described in the 1970s[40] and has since been validated and generalized to describe the dependence syndrome (also often referred to as "addiction") across all psychoactive substances. Edwards and Gross[40] noted that the dependence syndrome may be recognized by the clustering of certain elements. Not all elements need be present or present to the same degree, but with increasing intensity the syndrome is likely to show logical consistency. It is conceptualized as an integration of physiological and psychological processes that leads to a pattern of heavy alcohol use that is increasingly unresponsive to external circumstances or to adverse consequences. Furthermore, they viewed the syndrome not as an all-or-nothing dichotomy, but as occurring with graded intensity, and its presentation as being influenced by personality, as well as by social and cultural contexts. Their conceptualization also introduced a "bi-axial" model with the dependence syndrome constituting one axis and alcohol-related problems the other.

In the US before DSM-III[41] there was only a single descriptive category, "alcoholism," which hitherto had been viewed as a personality disorder. DSM-III was influenced by the syndrome and bi-axial concepts of Edwards and Gross[40] and, consequently, introduced a distinction between "dependence" and "abuse." DSM-III was the first diagnostic manual of mental disorders in the US to introduce actual itemized criteria, increasing the reliability of these diagnoses.[42]

The term *alcoholism* was originally coined to describe alcohol dependence/addiction and is often still used as an alternative to *dependence*. However, it is often used more broadly to describe alcohol dependence as well as harmful/hazardous use, sometimes without explicit mention of the fact. "Dependence" has also been used to differentiate physiological dependence on a drug (e.g., on opiates following pain management after surgery) from "addiction", which may or may not include physiological dependence, but is a syndrome that involves drug-seeking behavior and a great deal of time seeking, using, and getting over the effects of the drug. These variations in usage can be confusing.[43] It may also lead to errors in clinical and scientific communication as it has implications for inferences that are drawn from clinical data and may ultimately affect treatment policy decisions.[43] Thus, we believe care should be taken in choosing descriptive terms and in using them accurately and consistently.[44-46]

As described in Box 15-1, AUD is characterized by the broad elements of neuroadaptation (tolerance and withdrawal) and an impaired ability to alter or to stop alcohol consumption for very long, despite the personal suffering it causes (impaired control over use). As a construct, assessment of AUD has been shown to be reliable and to possess good construct and predictive validity. Furthermore, The AUD construct has demonstrated construct and predictive validity and can be reliably measured.

ETIOLOGY AND EPIDEMIOLOGY
Etiology

Knowledge about the onset and course of AUDs provides valuable information for the tailoring and timing of assessments, as well as for prevention and intervention strategies. Alcohol dependence is considered a *complex* disorder with many pathways that lead to its development. Genetic and other biological factors, along with temperament, cognitive, behavioral, psychological, and sociocultural factors, are involved in the emergence of AUD.[47] Genes confer at least four separate domains of risk: alcohol metabolizing enzymes (e.g., the functional genetic variants of alcohol dehydrogenase that demonstrate high alcohol oxidizing activity, and the genetic variant of aldehyde dehydrogenase that has low acetaldehyde oxidizing activity, protect against heavy drinking and alcoholism[48]); impulsivity and disinhibition (e.g., dopinergic *DRD2* genes[49]), psychiatric disorders (e.g., the miRNA biogenesis pathway[50] and individuals' level of response to alcohol[47,51]), although the latter be reflect differences in alcohol-metabolizing genes.

The relative contributions of genetic and environmental factors to the manifestation of AUDs can be expressed as the population-attributable risk percent, meaning the percentage of disease incidence that would be eliminated if the risk factor were removed. A genetic heritability estimate for alcohol dependence is sometimes estimated at approximately 50%, with the other 50% (equaling "100%") attributable to "environmental causes." However, these estimates are misleading since the attributable risks for a complex disease, such as alcohol dependence, can add to well over 100% because the disorder can be avoided in many different ways and can be increased by many different genetic variants. These additional percentages can be described as interactions among the various risk factors (e.g., gene–environment interactions). For example, a genetic abnormality may be necessary for a disease to occur, but the disease will not occur without the presence of an environmental risk factor. Thus, the attributable risks for the genetic aberration and the environmental factor would both be 100%. Phenylketonuria is an example of this: the disease can be avoided either by not having the genetic abnormality or by eliminating phenylalanine from the diet.[52] Similarly, regardless of an individual's high genetic risk for AUD, the disorder can be completely avoided if the individual chooses to abstain, or if there is no access to alcohol in the environment. AUDs are heterogeneous disorders. Heritable genetic factors increase the risk for developing alcohol dependence, but it should be remembered that many individuals without any family history of AUDs may still meet criteria for alcohol dependence.

Factors that influence the initiation of alcohol consumption should be distinguished from those that affect patterns of consumption once drinking is initiated. Studies of adolescent twins have demonstrated that initiation of drinking is primarily influenced by the drinking status of parents, siblings, and friends as well as by environmental variation across geographical regions where adolescent twins reside. Several cross-national studies, including studies in the US, indicate that initiation of alcohol use during adolescence is influenced chiefly by cultural rather than genetic factors.[53-55] The influence of genetic factors is negligible. Conversely, once initiated, alcohol use topography is strongly influenced by genetic factors. However, these influences are modulated also by sibling and peer-context effects (e.g., college settings) and by regional environmental variation.[56]

Pedigree, twin, and adoption studies all point to an increased risk for alcohol dependence in offspring when there is a history of such disorders in the family.[57] For example, family studies indicate a four-fold increased risk for dependence among relatives of individuals with alcohol dependence, with higher vulnerabilities for those with a greater number (higher density) of alcohol-dependent close relatives.[58] These genes influence a variety of characteristics or endophenotypes (such as impulsivity, disinhibition, and sensation seeking), enzymes (such as alcohol and aldehyde dehydrogenases), and a low level of response to alcohol's effects. These characteristics then correlate with and interact with environmental events to increase the risk for the condition.[58-60] Hence, genetic predispositions are not deterministic. AUDs are caused by a combination of interacting factors. These consist of genetic, biological, and environmental factors.

Epidemiology

Rates of alcohol use and AUD vary along several dimensions. Some of the most important among these are gender, life-stage, ethnicity, geographic location, and psychiatric co-morbidity.

In general, just over half of all Americans report alcohol consumption in the prior month.[61] Among drinkers, the lifetime prevalence for an AUD is about 14.6%. Surveys assessing past-year prevalence of these disorders indicate that nearly 8.5% (18 million) of American adults meet standard diagnostic criteria for DSM-5 AUD.[14,62] The rates of AUD in the general population vary by gender, with men having higher rates (12.4%) than women (4.9%). Highest rates of past year AUD occur among 18–29 year olds (16.2%) and the lowest among individuals age 65 years and older (1.5%). When translated into the impact AUDs have on families in the US, surveys show that more than half of all families report at least one close relative as having a drinking problem. As alluded to above, rates of heavy alcohol use and AUD among adolescents, young adults, and adults vary by geographic location, due to subcultural differences across regions. The differences may be reflected in varying proscriptions against intoxication and/or differences in alcohol policy (Figures 15-8–15-10).[63]

The highest rates of alcohol use, heavy/binge use, and AUDs occur between the ages 18 and 29.[61] Under-age drinking is a major public health problem in its own right, with about 11 million under-age persons aged 12 to 20 years (28.7%) reporting alcohol use in the past month, with the vast majority of these (10 million) drinking heavily or binging on alcohol. More males than females aged 12 to 20 years report binge drinking (22.1% versus 17.0%) and heavy drinking (8.2% versus 4.3%). Heavy drinking in this age group can lead to accidents, violence, unwanted pregnancies, and overdosing. Among populations seen in specialty psychiatric settings, rates of heavy use are likely to be even more prevalent and screening for alcohol use should be routine.[63,64] Early exposure to alcohol is also a significant independent risk factor for developing DSM-IV alcohol dependence. In the National Epidemiologic Survey on Alcohol and Related Conditions (NESARC), among individuals who began drinking before age 14, 47% were alcohol-dependent at some point in their life, and 13% were dependent in the prior year, compared to just 9% and 2%, respectively, who began drinking after age 20.[65]

In the US, there are differences among racial groups in the use of alcohol. Caucasians and persons reporting two or more races are typically more likely than are other racial/ethnic groups to report current use.[61] An estimated 55% of Caucasians and 52% of persons reporting two or more races used alcohol in the past month, whereas the rates were 40% for Hispanics, 37% for Asians, 37% for African Americans, and 36% for American Indians or Alaska Natives. Young non–African American males are almost twice as likely as young African American males to have an AUD. While disorders generally decline with age, they increase among African American women aged 30–44 years. In terms of AUD, there are marked differences across ethnic groups in the US. Among 12–17 year olds, for example, rates are highest for Hispanics (6%) and Native Americans and Alaskans (5.7%) relative to Whites (5%), African Americans (1.8%), and Asian and Pacific Islanders (1.6%). Among adults, the 12-month prevalence of AUD is greatest among Native Americans and Alaska Natives (12.1%) than among Whites (8.9%), Hispanics (7.9%), African Americans (6.9%), and Asian and Pacific Islanders (4.5%) (Figure 15-11).

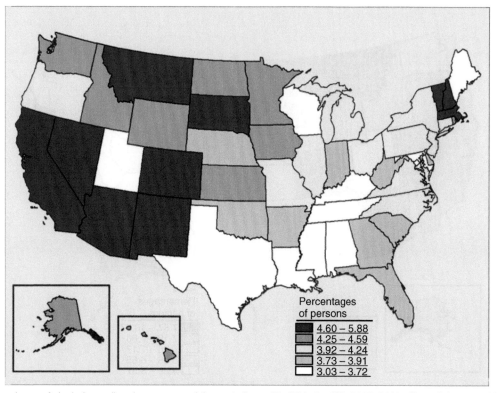

Figure 15-8. Prevalence of alcohol use disorders among adolescents (ages 12–17) in the US, 2010–2011. *(From Substance Abuse and Mental Health Services Administration. Results from the 2010 National Survey on Drug Use and Health: Summary of National Findings. Rockville, MD, 2011, Substance Abuse and Mental Health Services Administration.)*

Percentages of persons
- 4.60 – 5.88
- 4.25 – 4.59
- 3.92 – 4.24
- 3.73 – 3.91
- 3.03 – 3.72

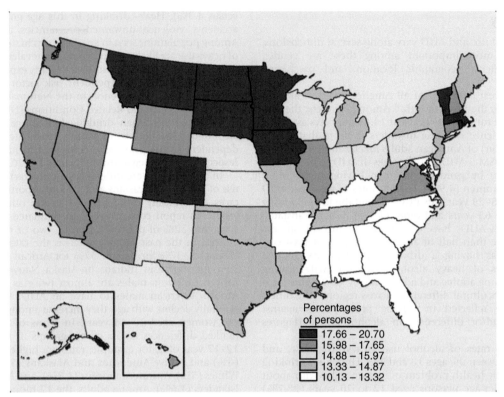

Figure 15-9. Prevalence of alcohol use disorder among young adults (ages 18–25) in the US, 2010–2011. *(From Addiction Treatment Strategies. Finger tapping study shows alcoholics may recruit other brain regions. 2012; http://www.addictionts.com/2012/08/17/finger-tapping-study-shows-alcoholics-may-recruit-other-brain-regions/, 2013.)*

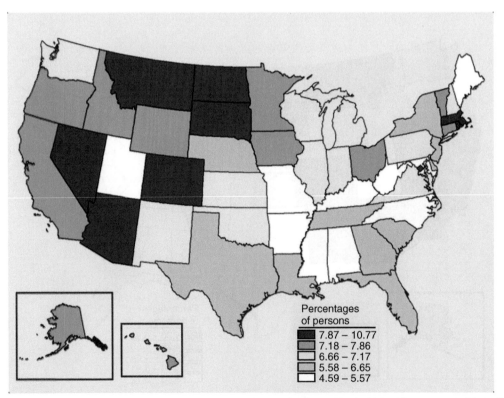

Figure 15-10. Prevalence of alcohol use disorder among persons aged 12 and older and in the United States, 2010–2011. *(From Substance Abuse and Mental Health Services Administration. Results from the 2010 National Survey on Drug Use and Health: Summary of National Findings. Rockville, MD, 2011, Substance Abuse and Mental Health Services Administration.)*

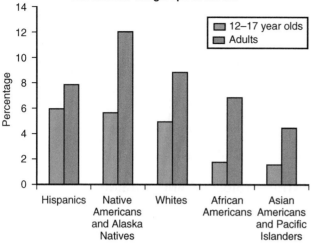

Figure 15-11. Twelve-month prevalence of alcohol use disorders across race/ethnic subgroups of the US. *(From Substance Abuse and Mental Health Services Administration.* Results from the 2010 National Survey on Drug Use and Health: Summary of National Findings. *Rockville, MD, 2011, Substance Abuse and Mental Health Services Administration.)*

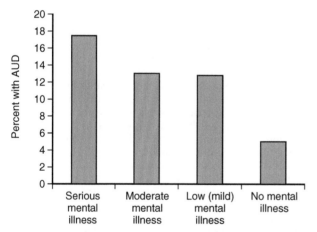

Figure 15-12. Past year alcohol use disorder among adults aged 18 or older, by level of mental illness: 2011. *(From Substance Abuse and Mental Health Services Administration.* Results from the 2010 National Survey on Drug Use and Health: Summary of National Findings. *Rockville, MD, 2011, Substance Abuse and Mental Health Services Administration.)*

ALCOHOL USE DISORDERS AND CO-OCCURRING PSYCHIATRIC ILLNESS

The co-occurrence of AUDs with other psychiatric disorders has been widely recognized.[66] Large-scale epidemiological surveys on co-morbidity in the US have been completed in the general household population. The most common life-time occurrences of psychiatric disorders for individuals with alcohol dependence are anxiety disorders (47%), other drug use disorders (43%), and affective disorders (41%); these are followed by conduct (32%) and antisocial personality disorder (13%). As shown in Figure 15-12, there is a moderately

strong correlation between the severity of mental illness and the prevalence of AUD.[66]

There are several possible explanations for these co-occurrences. Both conditions may be due to a common pathway (e.g., a genetic predisposition). One disorder may substantially influence the onset of the other, such as when an individual begins to use alcohol to cope with psychiatric distress (e.g., social anxiety), or when there are methodological determinants (e.g., unmeasured common causes or selection biases in some clinical studies).

These co-morbidities can be regarded clinically in two ways: a patient may present with an AUD, perhaps in an addiction-treatment setting, and also a co-occurring psychiatric illness; and a patient may present with a psychiatric disorder, perhaps in a mental health clinic, and an additional AUD. Among patients with AUDs seen in addiction-treatment settings, more than half will have at least a life-time history of another co-occurring DSM psychiatric disorder, and many will have a continuing psychiatric disturbance in one of these other areas in addition to their alcohol use. The job of the discerning clinician will be to patiently and carefully determine the presence of non–substance-induced syndromes that may persist perniciously with abstinence. The "dual diagnosis" patient can be challenging as he or she may not respond as well to standard addiction treatment, and may have greater rates of relapse, attrition, and re-admissions. However, if a co-morbid psychiatric disorder is observed or detected, determining the relative onset of the two disorders may have clinical significance, since primary disorders (i.e., those emerging first) tend to be of greater long-term clinical significance. For instance, patients whose bipolar disorder precedes the onset of their alcohol dependence tend to have better alcohol outcomes (and worse bipolar outcomes) than those whose alcohol dependence occurred first; these patients tend to have worse alcohol outcomes and better bipolar outcomes.[67] Nevertheless, both disorders will need to be attended to simultaneously for optimum results.[68,69]

For patients entering primary mental health settings, AUDs often go undetected. Left unnoticed, these disorders can undermine the salutary effects of psychotropic and psychosocial interventions aimed at ameliorating the symptoms of psychiatric illness. It is important to note that any generalizations about "dual diagnosis" patients should be made with caution. The term obviously covers an immense amount of clinical territory, since it not only covers the presence of an alcohol or other drug use disorder, which in themselves are heterogeneous and vary greatly in severity, but also a vast array of psychopathological disturbances, each with its own sub-variations and degrees of severity. Thus, the specific type, severity, and relative clinical significance of the co-morbid psychiatric disorder on the patient's presentation and future function should always be considered when approaching these dual problems. If a generalization can be made it is that both types of disorders should always be assessed and psychiatric symptoms monitored for continued and independent influence in the context of sustained abstinence from alcohol (or another drug).[70,71] If present, these conditions should be treated in an integrated fashion.[69]

Typologies

AUDs are complex and heterogeneous. Hence, attempts have been made to try to identify more homogeneous subtypes. Various typologies, some formal and others less formal, have been proposed during the past 50 years. Early typologies relied more on theoretically-framed, clinical observations. More recently, data-driven, multi-variate sub-classifications have been derived that have etiological significance and predictive validity, and may have clinical utility.

One of the first and most well-known was Jellinek's typology consisting of five subspecies of alcoholism simply labeled using the first five letters of the Greek alphabet: alpha, beta, delta, gamma, epsilon.[72] Jellinek's very broad definition of alcoholism as any use that causes harm yielded a similarly broad typology. Jellinek's typology was not successfully validated, but it did highlight the important topic of heterogeneity and it sparked further interest and efforts to identify particular subtypes of individuals suffering from alcoholism for the purposes of tailoring treatments.

During the past 25 years, multi-variate typologies have been investigated with the use of more complex data extraction methods (e.g., cluster and factor analysis). Cloninger's Type I or Type II and Babor's Type A or B were the first of these. Cloninger and colleagues[73] identified two separate forms of alcoholism based on differences in alcohol-related symptoms, patterns of transmission, and personality characteristics using data derived from a cross-fostering study of Swedish adoptees. Type I was characterized by either mild or severe alcohol use in the probands and no criminality in the fathers. These Type I alcoholics came from relatively high socioeconomic backgrounds and were frequently associated with maternal alcohol use. Type I alcoholics were thought to be more responsive to environmental influence, to have relatively mild alcohol-related problems, and to have a late age of onset (older than 25 years). On the other hand, Cloninger's Type II alcoholism is characterized as being associated with a family history, having severe alcohol problems, having other drug use, and having an early onset (before age 25). Although multi-variate statistical methods were used to identify subtypes, Cloninger's types of alcoholism have been criticized due to the small sample sizes (less than 200), sample selection methods, and indirect assessment of family variables.[74]

A second typology was proposed by Babor and colleagues[75] based on a sample of 321 alcoholic inpatients. Babor's Type A resembled Cloninger's Type 1, and was characterized by a later age of onset, fewer childhood behavior problems, and less psychopathology. Type B resembled Type II alcoholism and was defined by a high prevalence of childhood behavior problems, familial alcoholism, early onset of alcohol problems, more psychopathology, more life stress, and a more chronic treatment history.

A broad distinction of early-onset versus late-onset alcohol dependence may have some clinical matching utility, although evidence is limited. For example, use of selective serotonin reuptake inhibitors (SSRIs) has produced modest drinking reductions that may be more apparent in men with depression and late-onset type alcoholism.[76,77] Also, double-blind placebo-controlled studies of anti-craving medications (e.g., ondansetron) have shown efficacy for early-onset alcoholics, as have others (e.g., topiramate) for a broad range of unselected alcoholic patients.

Later studies examining typologies have found more than two subtypes that have clinical and etiological significance, particularly regarding gender, and internalizing/externalizing disorders, in addition to family history and age of onset. For example, several multi-variate, multi-dimensional analyses have revealed that there may be as many as four general, homogeneous subtypes of alcohol dependence[78,79]: chronic/severe, depressed/anxious, mildly affected, and antisocial.[80] These four subtypes of alcohol dependence are found within both genders and across different ethnic subgroups, but more prospective research is needed to examine their relative clinical course and responsiveness to various pharmacological and psychosocial interventions. These approaches to AUD typologies have employed either empirical or clinical/observational strategies using data derived principally from treatment samples. However, only about one-fourth of those who meet criteria for alcohol addiction actually receive treatment.[81] Thus, the majority of individuals suffering from alcohol addiction are missed, biasing our knowledge to only those alcohol-dependent cases that seek treatment—a phenomenon known as "Berkson' bias." Consequently, using data from the National Epidemiological Survey on Alcohol and Related Conditions (NESARC), Moss, Chen, and Yi[82] discovered five subtypes of alcohol dependence, distinguished by family history, age of dependence onset, endorsement of DSM-IV AUD criteria, and the presence of co-morbid psychiatric and substance use disorders. These general population-derived subtypes await further study, but they may enhance our understanding of the etiology and natural history of AUD, and lead to improved and more targeted treatment interventions.

PATHOPHYSIOLOGY AND IMAGING

The deleterious effect of alcohol is diffuse. However, the impact on the brain is central to the development of AUDs and related conditions. Of the approximately 18 million individuals with an AUD in the US, approximately one-half to two-thirds develop some sort of impairment in cognitive and/or motor processes and up to 2 million people suffer enough alcohol-induced damage to require life-long care.[83] These conditions, such as alcohol-induced persisting amnestic disorder (i.e., Wernicke–Korsakoff syndrome) and dementia, seriously affect memory, reasoning, language, and problem-solving abilities.

Importantly, many individuals with a history of alcohol dependence and neuropsychological impairments show some improvement in function within a year of abstinence, but others take considerably longer.[84-87] Unfortunately, little is known about the rate and extent to which people recover specific structures and functions once abstinence has been achieved, but the rate of recovery will likely co-vary with the topography and chronicity of alcohol use, dietary factors, and individual variables related to family history and biological vulnerability. The cerebral cortex (dorsolateral and orbitofrontal cortex),[88] and subcortical areas, such as the limbic system (e.g., amygdala), the thalamus (involved with communications within the brain), the hypothalamus (involved with hormones that affect sexual function and behavior, as well as reproduction), and the basal forebrain (involved with learning and memory) are the key brain regions susceptible to alcohol-related damage.[89] Areas that influence posture and movement, such as the cerebellum, also seem to be affected.[86] MRI and diffusion tensor imaging (DTI) can be used in combination to assess a patient's brain when he or she first stops drinking and again after long periods of sobriety, to monitor brain changes and to detect correlates of relapse.

MRI and DTI studies reveal a loss of brain tissue, and neuropsychological tests show cognitive impairments in individuals who either have an AUD or are heavy drinkers.[90] Abnormalities on scans have been reported in 50% or more of individuals with chronic alcohol dependence. These abnormalities can occur in individuals in whom there is neither clinical nor neuropsychological test evidence of cognitive defects. In individuals with binge drinking and chronic alcohol dependence, MRI has demonstrated accelerated gray matter loss,[91] which is to some extent reversible with abstinence, suggesting that some of these changes are secondary to changes in brain tissue hydration.[92]

The frontal areas of the brain are particularly susceptible to alcohol-related damage despite the fact that alcohol has diffuse bilateral cortical effects.[86,89,93] The prefrontal cortex has been shown to be important in cognitive and emotional function and interpersonal behavior. Because the prefrontal cortex is necessary for planning and for regulation of behavior, good judgment, and problem-solving, damage in these brain regions may relate to impulsivity and susceptibility to alcohol relapse and may be particularly negatively affected by alcohol.[94-96]

Positron emission tomography (PET) has been used to analyze alcohol's effects on various neurotransmitter systems, as well as on brain cell metabolism and blood flow within the brain. These studies in alcoholics have detected deficits, particularly in the frontal lobes (which are responsible for numerous functions associated with learning and memory), as well as in the cerebellum (which controls movement and coordination).[97-99]

Effects on Neurotransmitters

The typical subjective effects from alcohol include euphoria, disinhibition, anxiety reduction, sedation, and sleep. These effects are mediated by a variety of neurotransmitters including GABA, glutamate, serotonin, endorphins, and dopamine. Alcohol effects neurotransmitter systems by causing either neuronal excitation or inhibition.[100] If alcohol is consumed over extended periods (e.g., several days or weeks), receptors adapt to its presence, producing neurotransmitter imbalances that can result in sedation, agitation, depression, and other mood and behavior disorders, as well as seizures.

The results of neuropsychological testing reveal that short-term memory, performance on complex memory tasks, visual-motor coordination, visual-spatial performance, abstract reasoning, and psychomotor dexterity are the areas most seriously damaged. Intelligence scores often do not change, and verbal skills and long-term memory often remain intact. As a consequence, it is possible for individuals to appear cognitively intact unless they are administered neuropsychological tests.

Glutamate is the major excitatory neurotransmitter in the brain and it is significantly effected by alcohol. Alcohol influences the action of glutamate, and research has shown that chronic, heavy alcohol consumption increases glutamate receptor sites in the hippocampus that can effect the consolidation of memory and may account for "blackout" phenomena. Contrary to popular belief, blackouts are much more common among social drinkers than previously assumed. In a large sample of college student drinkers, more than half (51%) reported blacking out at some point in their lives, and 40% reported experiencing a blackout in the prior

year.[101] Hence, blackouts should be viewed as a potential consequence of acute intoxication and not specific to alcohol dependence.

Glutamate receptors adapt to the presence of alcohol and thus become overactive during alcohol withdrawal; this process can lead to stroke and seizure.[102] Deficiencies of thiamine caused by malnutrition, common among individuals with alcohol dependence, may exacerbate this potentially destructive overactivity.[103]

GABA is also affected by alcohol use. It is the major inhibitory neurotransmitter in the brain, and alcohol appears to increase GABA's effects (i.e., increases inhibition and sedation). However, chronic, intense alcohol use leads to a gradual reduction of GABA receptors. Thus, when an individual suddenly ceases alcohol use, the decrease in inhibitory effects in combination with fewer GABA receptors and increased glutamatergic discharge contributes to over-excitation and possible withdrawal seizures. It is likely that both GABA and glutamate systems interact in this process.[104] The effects of chronic alcohol use are influenced by adaptations in $GABA_A$ receptor function and expression, and subcellular localization that contribute to tolerance, dependence, and withdrawal hyperexcitability (Figure 15-13).[105] Patients with alcohol dependence should be assessed and monitored for signs of alcohol withdrawal and signs of other associated problems.

Alcohol also directly stimulates release of other neurotransmitters, such as serotonin,[106,107] as well as endorphins[108] and dopamine (DA),[109] which contribute to the subjective euphoria and rewarding effects associated with alcohol.[100] Research findings regarding acetylcholine and other neurotransmitters are mixed and effects are currently not as well understood.

Intense, chronic use of alcohol has wide-ranging deleterious effects on the brain. These can lead to lasting, sometimes life-long, impairments in function that result in prodigious familial, social, and fiscal costs. Consequently, education, prevention, and early detection and intervention are keys to minimizing the impact on individuals and their loved ones.

SCREENING AND ASSESSMENT

Given the regrettable impact that a failure to detect and intervene with alcohol problems can have, routine screening for alcohol misuse should be standard in all clinical settings. There are brief and effective screening measures that can yield

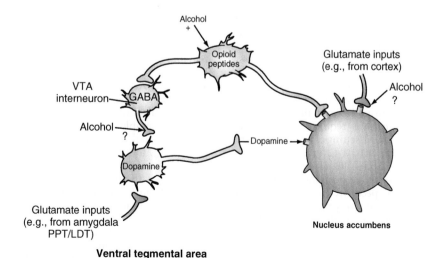

Figure 15-13. Alcohol's effect on neurotransmitter systems. VTA, ventral tegmental area; PPT, pedunculopontine tegmental nucleus; LDT, laterodorsal tegmental nucleus *(From Gilpin NW, Koob GF. Neurobiology of alcohol dependence: focus on motivational mechanisms. National Institute on Alcohol Abuse and Alcoholism (NIAAA).)*

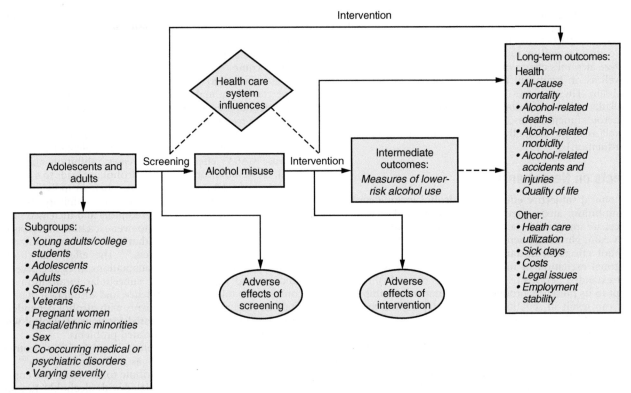

Figure 15-14. Screening and assessment process. *(From Jonas DE, Garbutt JC, Brown JM, et al. Screening, behavioral counseling, and referral in primary care to reduce alcohol use. Rockville, 2012, Agency for Health Research and Quality.)*

high rates of detection of these pervasive and debilitating disorders. Controlled studies reveal that even a brief, detailed discussion by a clinician can yield measurable reductions in the consequences from alcohol misuse (Figure 15-14).[110,111]

The National Institute on Alcohol Abuse and Alcoholism (NIAAA) has recommended either the use of a single alcohol screening question (SASQ) or administration of the Alcohol Use Disorders Identification Test (AUDIT) self-report questionnaire as standard screening procedures for the detection of alcohol-related problems. The AUDIT (Table 15-1) and manual are available for free, in English and in Spanish; the AUDIT has been validated across a variety of cultural and ethnic groups. When using the SASQ clinicians are advised to ask if an individual has consumed five or more standard drinks (for a man) on one occasion during the last year (four drinks for women). A positive response may indicate an alcohol-related problem and requires more detailed assessment.[63] A more traditional alternative screening interview is captured by the CAGE acronym,[112] although this has less sensitivity to detect harmful and hazardous patterns of alcohol use, and has not been validated in adolescents, the elderly, and women. When even more brevity is required due to time constraints, such as in busy clinical settings, a shorter 3-item version of the AUDIT called the AUDIT-C, includes only the first three AUDIT items (i.e., the three "Consumption" items; hence the "C"). This shorter version has been shown to possess about as much sensitivity and specificity as the full 10-item AUDIT[113] and can be used efficiently in primary care settings with a cut-off score of 4 or more for a man and 3 or more for a woman.[114] In psychiatric settings, a cut-off score 4 or more is recommended.

Compared to the SASQ or the AUDIT and AUDIT-C, the CAGE lacks sensitivity to detect hazardous/problem drinking. Similar to the CAGE interview, the TWEAK interview (i.e., "Tolerance," others "Worried" about your drinking, "Eye-opener," "Amnesia," ever wanted to/tried to "Cut down"), is brief and has good psychometric properties, but similar to the CAGE is a "life-time" measure and lacks sensitivity to detect hazardous drinking. The Michigan Alcoholism Screening Test (MAST) is another self-report measure with good psychometric properties, but is longer than the AUDIT.

For adolescents the CRAFFT screen is recommended, which is the acronym for having ever ridden in a CAR driven by someone (including yourself) who was "high" or had been using alcohol or drugs; ever used alcohol or drugs to RELAX, feel better about yourself, or fit in; ever use alcohol or drugs while ALONE; ever FORGOT things while using alcohol or drugs; FAMILY or FRIENDS ever recommend cutting down on drinking or drug use; ever gotten into TROUBLE while using alcohol or drugs. These questions have excellent sensitivity and specificity.[115] One point is given for each positively endorsed item and a score of 2 or more is indicative of a potential AUD that requires further assessment. Figure 15-15 shows the probability of an AUD based on derived screening score.

Medical biomarker screens may also be useful. Screening for recent alcohol use can be a carried out with a Breathalyzer or a sample of urine or saliva. For more chronic use, laboratory markers, such as the serum γ-glutamyl transpeptidase (GGT), the mean corpuscular volume (MCV),[20] and the percent carbohydrate-deficient transferrin (% CDT) can be used. CDT is the newest alcohol biomarker approved by the Food and Drug Administration (FDA) in 2001.[116] It is the only laboratory test approved specifically for the detection of heavy drinking.[117] An average daily consumption of 60 g of alcohol or more (i.e., approximately 5 standard drinks in the US) for at least the previous 2 weeks causes a higher percentage of transferrin. CDT, quantified as a percent of total serum transferring, rather than the absolute level of CDT, is recommended as it corrects for individual variations in transferrin levels. Laboratory test results of more than 2.5% suggest heavy

TABLE 15-1 The AUDIT/AUDIT-C (IN BOX) for Alcohol Screening[113,114]

PATIENT: Because alcohol use can affect your health and can interfere with certain medications and treatments, it is important that we ask some questions about your use of alcohol. Your answers will remain confidential so please be honest. Place an X in one box that best describes your answer to each question.

Questions	0	1	2	3	4	Score
How often do you have a drink containing alcohol?	Never	Monthly or less	2 to 4 times a month	2 to 3 times a week	4 or more times a week	
How many drinks containing alcohol do you have on a typical day when you are drinking?	1 or 2	3 or 4	5 or 6	7 to 9	10 or more	
How often do you have five or more drinks on one occasion?	Never	Less than monthly	Monthly	Weekly	Daily or almost daily	
How often during the last year have you found that you were not able to stop drinking once you had started?	Never	Less than monthly	Monthly	Weekly	Daily or almost daily	
How often during the last year have you failed to do what was normally expected of you because of drinking?	Never	Less than monthly	Monthly	Weekly	Daily or almost daily	
How often during the last year have you needed a first drink in the morning to get yourself going after a heavy drinking session?	Never	Less than monthly	Monthly	Weekly	Daily or almost daily	
How often during the last year have you had a feeling of guilt or remorse after drinking?	Never	Less than monthly	Monthly	Weekly	Daily or almost daily	
How often during the last year have you been unable to remember what happened the night before because of your drinking?	Never	Less than monthly	Monthly	Weekly	Daily or almost daily	
Have you or someone else been injured because of your drinking?	No		Yes, but not in the last year		Yes, during the last year	
Has a relative, friend, doctor, or other health care worker been concerned about your drinking or suggested you cut down?	No		Yes, but not in the last year		Yes, during the last year	
Total:						

NOTE: This self-report questionnaire (the Alcohol Use Disorders Identification Test [AUDIT]) is from the World Health Organization. To reflect standard drink sizes in the United States, the number of drinks in question 3 was changed from 6 to 5. A free AUDIT manual with guidelines for use in primary care is available online at http://www.who.org.

Information from Reinert DF, Allen JP. The alcohol use disorders identification test: an update of research findings. Alcohol Clin Exp Res 31(2):185–199, 2007, and Bradley KA, DeBenedetti AF, Volk RJ, Williams EC, Frank D, Kivlahan DR. AUDIT-C as a brief screen for alcohol misuse in primary care. Alcohol Clin Exp Res 31(7):1208–1217, 2007.

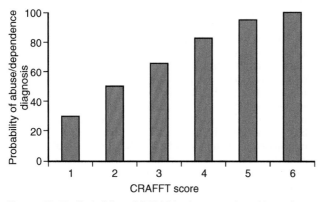

Figure 15-15. Probability of DSM-IV substance abuse/dependence diagnosis based on CRAFFT adolescent screening score. *(From Center for Adolescent Substance Abuse Research. The CRAFFT Screening Interview. Boston, 2009, Children's Hospital Boston.)*

drinking. Regarding specificity, other than heavy alcohol use, only end-stage liver disease, biliary cirrhosis, and a rare genetic variability will elevate CDT. Ethyl glucuronide (EtG) is a newer biomarker and is a direct metabolite of alcohol. It has been evaluated as a biomarker test for alcohol use and to monitor abstinence (e.g., among health care professionals, attorneys, airline pilots in recovery from addiction). EtG can be detected in urine up to 7 days and in hair for months after alcohol has left the body.[118] A disadvantage of EtG is that it can yield false positives from incidental exposure, from things such as mouthwash, foods, and over-the-counter medications.

Many of these biomarker measures lack sensitivity, but can be helpful if used in combination (e.g., CDT and GGT) and especially when used with other screening measures, such as the AUDIT. Screening for alcohol problems has been shown to be very cost-effective.[119]

Screening for alcohol withdrawal is also critical since, as mentioned previously, alcohol withdrawal can be life-threatening. The Clinical Institute Withdrawal Assessment for Alcohol Revised (CIWA-Ar)[21] is a semi-structured, 5-minute interview used to assess and quantify severity of withdrawal from alcohol. It is easy to administer and possesses very good psychometric properties. It is thus an efficient and reliable method that can prevent serious or life-threatening problems and is useful to help clinicians determine levels of care.[21] Recent evidence suggests, however, that this scale may under-estimate symptoms of alcohol withdrawal in certain ethnic groups, such as Native Americans.[120]

There are several measures that can be employed to assess the presence of an AUD and the degree of dependence and impairment. The choice of each may depend on the time demands and specialization of the clinical setting. For clinical diagnostic purposes, the Structured Clinical Interview for Diagnosis (SCID), Substance Use Disorders module, can be used. This is a valid and reliable, semi-structured, assessment tool that will give life-time and current diagnoses for AUD and can be completed in approximately 20 minutes.[121] Also, as detailed more below in the section on Brief Interventions, the Alcohol Use Disorders Identification Test (AUDIT)[122] can be used as a screening tool and to help determine treatment recommendations.

The Addiction Severity Index (ASI) is a semi-structured interview that assesses multiple domains of function (e.g., legal, work, and psychiatric, as well as alcohol and drug use) and is widely used in clinical and research settings. It has adequate psychometrics and can be completed in approximately 30 to 40 minutes. The Alcohol Dependence Scale (ADS) is a self-report measure that focuses on the core dependence syndrome. It contains 25 items and takes approximately 5 minutes to complete. It assesses past-year symptoms, with a score of 9 or more indicative of alcohol dependence. The Leeds Dependence Questionnaire (LDQ)[123,124] is a brief 10-item self-report measure that measures severity of addiction across multiple substances, including alcohol. The Drinker Inventory of Consequences (DRINC) is a 50-item, multi-dimensional self-report that takes about 5 minutes to complete. It is a validated measure of drinking consequences with good psychometric properties. There are a variety of other assessment tools available that assess drinking topography, chronicity, and impact.[125,126] Many of these measures have clinical utility as they can elucidate the drinking topography, chronicity, addiction severity, and degree of impairment that can inform the type and level of treatment intensity.[127] Also, these may become increasingly important as health systems move to performance-based payments.[128]

TREATMENT FOR ALCOHOL USE DISORDERS

As with most difficulties that individuals encounter during their lives, individuals suffering from AUDs first try to resolve their problems without help. They may mobilize their own skills and, through a process of trial and error, learn ways to minimize or resolve these problems. Successful resolution of an alcohol problem without formal intervention is often called "natural recovery".[129] Others use informal resources, such as a member of the clergy, a friend, or a family member, or access Alcoholics Anonymous (AA) or another mutual-help group. When these resources are realized to be insufficient to cope with the magnitude of the problem, individuals often seek formal treatment, although informal resources (e.g., AA) may continue to be used as effective adjuncts.[130,131]

Given the variability in the demographic and drinking patterns of patients, and the addiction severity and impact that alcohol use has had in their lives, a number of treatment options should be available to help patients.[2] The National Institute of Alcohol Abuse and Alcoholism (NIAAA) was founded in 1970. This began a federally supported public health initiative that increased research efforts to develop, test, and implement effective interventions for risky alcohol use, as well as for abuse and dependence. Numerous reviews of the treatment literature[132–135] indicate that a wide array of empirically-based, effective treatments can be brought to bear on these problems. These range from brief interventions to more intensive and extensive individual and group-based psychosocial interventions and, increasingly, pharmacological interventions.[134]

Brief Intervention

A concerned and focused assessment with brief advice by a health care provider can make a positive difference to drinking problems. Brief interventions are generally recommended for those who drink to excess, but are generally not showing signs of addiction. Thus, its goal may be moderate drinking rather than abstinence.[135–137] Brief interventions are generally restricted to four or fewer sessions, lasting from a few minutes to 1 hour each, designed to be conducted by clinicians, not necessarily specialized in addiction.[138]

Research indicates that brief interventions for alcohol problems are more effective than no intervention[139–142] and, in some cases, can be as effective as more extensive intervention.[135,143] Capitalizing on these findings, and in order to expand access to treatment for alcohol-related problems, the Center for Substance Abuse Treatment (CSAT) has devised an initiative known as "Screening, Brief Intervention, Referral, and Treatment" (SBIRT). The goal of the initiative is intended to shift the emphasis to alcohol users whom the traditional system has largely ignored—the large number of individuals who consume more than the medically-accepted limits but are not yet dependent. Rejecting the notion that only people with very heavy alcohol use levels or who are alcohol dependent need targeted interventions, SBIRT assumes that everyone, regardless of current level of alcohol consumption, can benefit from learning the facts about safe alcohol consumption and knowing how their own usage compares to accepted limits. Using the AUDIT/AUDIT-C as a screening device, front-line clinicians in any setting can assess for alcohol-related problems quickly and easily. SBIRT triage guidelines provide recommendations along the lines of an individual's alcohol involvement. Simple clinical advice to cut down or stop is recommended if someone scores between 7 and 16 on the AUDIT; multiple sessions of brief treatment and monitoring are recommended if an individual scores between 16 and 19 (or has consumed alcohol to intoxication five or more days per month, as disclosed on screening interview); and if an individual has an AUDIT score of 20 or more a referral for more intensive assessment and treatment is recommended.[144]

What is it about brief interventions that make them effective? After reviewing the key ingredients in a variety of brief intervention protocols, Miller and Sanchez[145] proposed six critical elements that they summarized with the acronym FRAMES: Feedback, Responsibility, Advice, Menu, Empathy, and Self-efficacy. The clinician completes some assessment and provides Feedback on the patient's alcohol-related problems ("Your results show. …"), stresses the patient's Responsibility to address the problem ("It's your choice. …"), gives clear Advice to change drinking behavior ("I would recommend that you cut down or stop. …"), provides a Menu of treatment strategies ("There a number of different things you might do. …"), expresses Empathy for the patient's problem ("This can be difficult to hear and making changes is not always easy, but. …"), and stresses Self-efficacy ("However, it is quite possible for you to achieve this. …")—the expectation is that the patient has the skills needed to successfully resolve his or her drinking problems. Additional components of goal-setting, follow-up, and timing also have been identified as important to the effectiveness of brief interventions.[136,146] Even brief contact with an addiction specialist has been shown to yield improvement in 30% to 50% of patients. However, brief interventions are more effective with those who have no prior psychiatric illness or history of addiction treatment and good social function and resources.[147] Although non-specialist clinicians, such as primary care providers, can have an impact on heavy or at-risk drinking through appropriate brief intervention, patients with alcohol dependence tend to experience better outcomes when seen by addiction specialists (e.g., counselors, social workers, and addiction-trained nurses, or physicians with specialized addiction training) than general practitioners,[148,149] perhaps due to their more specific education and training on addiction. For example, compared with general consultation psychiatrists, specialist addiction nurse consultants were found to double the rate of patient follow-through and completion in rehabilitation.[150]

Intensive-Extensive Interventions

Three broad elements are important in recovery from AUDs: deconditioning, skills training, and cognitive re-structuring.[151] There is a broad array of evidence-based interventions for AUDs that address these critical elements.[132,133,152] Some of these include Twelve-Step Facilitation (TSF), a professional therapy designed to engage patients and support long-term involvement in the fellowship of AA; motivational enhancement therapy (MET), an intervention based on the principles of motivational interviewing[146,153]; a variety of cognitive-behavioral approaches, such as the Community Reinforcement Approach (CRA), designed to engage multiple therapeutic elements in the community; interpersonal system-based interventions, such as behavioral marital therapy (BMT) and family therapies; and pharmacotherapies (e.g., naltrexone/depot natrexone, acamprosate, or disulfiram).

Although most interventions are directly focused on the primary sufferer (the individual with the AUD), it is clear that loved ones also suffer greatly as a result of the AUD. Community Reinforcement and Family Training (CRAFT) is a validated approach based on the concept that a supportive environment "community" will help the alcohol-dependent person achieve recovery. CRAFT targets individuals who refuse to participate in treatment through their loved ones. It provides specific, contingency-based strategies that support family members and friends in their efforts to help their loved one become engaged in treatment. It has been shown also to substantially reduce psychological distress and symptoms among the family members themselves.[154]

Despite vastly differing theoretical assumptions regarding the specifics of treatment content, and for how long, at what intensity, and by whom the treatment should be delivered, comparisons of the relative efficacy of active treatments reveal surprisingly similar effects, suggesting that they may all mobilize common change processes.[155] However, it seems clear that it is the *duration and continuity* of care that is linked to treatment outcome rather than amount or intensity.[46,155-157] Consequently, there have been recent shifts from intensive inpatient services to "extensive" outpatient models of addiction recovery management and ongoing assessment and re-intervention that match the chronic relapse-prone nature of addictive disorders (e.g., telephone case monitoring and long-term outpatient treatment).[158-160]

In recent years, there has tended to be an almost exclusive focus on high-fidelity delivery of manualized treatment content rather than a focus on the characteristics of the clinician who delivers the content and how it is delivered. The issue of therapeutic alliance and successfully gaining the patient's trust is often fundamental to the success of treatment, yet is seldom specifically addressed. A respectful, empathic, patient-centered approach appears to be most helpful, and a harsh, confrontational approach may increase the patient's resistance.[132] The principles and practices of motivational

TABLE 15-2 Motivational Interviewing Processes

Engaging	Establishing a helpful connection and working relationship
Focusing	Developing and maintaining specific direction in the conversation about change
Evoking	Eliciting the patients' own motives about change
Planning	Developing commitment to change and forming a specific action plan to change

From Miller WR, Rollnick S. Motivational interviewing: helping people change, ed 3. New York, 2012, Guilford Press.

interviewing[153] are a particularly useful framework in this regard and have strong empirical support for use among individuals with AUDs (Table 15-2). The main principles here are to avoid arguing with a patient, to "roll with resistance" (e.g., try to understand the patients' frame of reference), to develop discrepancies between the patient's values and his or her behavior, to support the patient's self-efficacy/confidence to achieve the desired outcome, and to be empathic. There are four main processes of MI: engaging (establishing a helpful connection and working relationship), focusing (developing and maintaining specific direction in the conversation about change), evoking (eliciting the patients' own motives about change), and planning (developing commitment to change and forming a specific action plan to change).[146]

Emanating from the brief intervention literature and humanistic psychology, motivational interviewing has been shown to be an important and effective way to interact with patients with a range of alcohol problems, including dependence. It has been defined as a patient-centered, yet directive, method for enhancing intrinsic motivation to change by exploring and resolving patient ambivalence.[153] This approach has been shown to be helpful for many patients.[161-163] It can be used as a stand-alone intervention but can also be an effective way to communicate with patients while providing other interventions.

Studies of treatment outcome show that patients treated for addiction have similar rates of improvement as patients treated for other chronic medical diseases.[164] For example, between 40% and 60% of patients treated for addiction to alcohol remain abstinent after a year and another 15% maintain clinically meaningful improvement in their alcohol use problems. Similarly, during the course of a year, 60% of patients with high blood pressure or asthma and 70% of diabetics maintain improvements in their symptoms.[39,165] While full remission and recovery can take many years to achieve following initial attempts to stop,[166] full sustained remission is the most likely ultimate outcome.[167] Consequently, AUD can be considered a good prognosis disorder with adequate extensive monitoring, management, and re-intervention when necessary.[46]

Engaging and retaining individuals in treatment for at least 90 days is associated with better long-term treatment outcomes.[168] Individual or group counseling and other behavioral therapies are critical components of effective treatment for alcohol addiction. Behavioral therapy also facilitates interpersonal relationships and the individual's ability to function in the family and community contexts. In therapy, issues of motivation can be addressed, and assertiveness, goal-setting skills, and problem-solving strategies can be learned along with new ways to replace alcohol-related activities with other constructive and rewarding activities.

Pharmacological Interventions

Three medications have been approved by the FDA for the treatment of alcohol dependence: disulfiram (approved in 1947), intended to prevent any drinking through the

TABLE 15-3 Pharmacological Treatments for Alcoholism

Drug (Trade Name)	Pharmacokinetics/Pharmacodynamics	Effects
Disulfiram (Antabuse)	Inhibits acetaldehyde dehydrogenase, leading to a build-up of acetaldehyde	Produces undesirable consequences when alcohol is consumed, including flushing, palpitations, nausea, vomiting, and headache
Naltrexone (ReVia, Long acting = Vivitrol)	μ-opioid receptor antagonist	Reduces the reinforcement/euphoria produced by alcohol
Acamprosate	Antagonist at glutamatergic N-methyl-D-aspartate (NMDA) receptors and agonist at gamma-aminobutyric acid (GABA) type A receptors	Reduces alcohol cravings

anticipated threat of the very unpleasant reaction caused by the alcohol–disulfiram interaction; naltrexone (approved as an oral formulation in 1994 with the long-acting injectable formulation approved in 2006), intended to reduce the reinforcing effect of alcohol and to reduce the severity of relapse and the extent of heavy drinking; and acamprosate (approved in 2004), intended to reduce the probability of any drinking by reducing symptoms associated with postacute withdrawal/craving following initial detoxification (Table 15-3).

Disulfiram inhibits acetaldehyde dehydrogenase, leading to a build-up of the ethanol metabolite acetaldehyde. It has been shown to reduce drinking days in alcohol-dependent persons by approximately 50%.[169] If a patient drinks alcohol after taking disulfiram, the build-up of acetaldehyde produces flushing, hypotension, headache, nausea, and vomiting (Table 15-3). Treatment of severe disulfiram–ethanol reactions may require a modified Trendelenburg position, an anticholinergic agent for bradycardia, and ascorbic acid 1 mg IV every 1 to 2 hours. The effectiveness of disulfiram is compromised by poor compliance. However, if a spouse or significant other is willing to participate and to observe and monitor the compliance with the medication, effectiveness increases substantially. A written contract in this regard between spouse and partner, which is often done in behavioral marital therapy (BMT), enhances compliance and outcomes.[170-172]

The opiate antagonist naltrexone which has no specific adverse reaction with alcohol has produced reductions in drinking-days presumably through diminished reward from alcohol secondary to actions on central brain reward pathways.[173,174] The recent FDA-approval for a long-acting IM formulation of naltrexone in April 2006 significantly expands pharmacotherapy options. Best results have been reported in patients able to sustain a week of abstinence before their first injection. Naltrexone also appears to be most effective in patients with a strong family history of alcoholism. Because both naltrexone and disulfiram have a slight risk for hepatotoxicity, liver function studies are recommended at baseline and then at 1, 3, and every 6 months thereafter. Also, pharmacogenetic research suggests that individuals with the *OPRM1* genotype may respond particularly well to naltrexone.[175]

Acamprosate is another drug that has been approved for relapse-prevention among individuals suffering from alcohol addiction. It is thought to act primarily at glutamate-NMDA receptors by moderating symptoms related to prolonged alcohol withdrawal (i.e., post-acute withdrawal), and is thus most effective in patients who have recently completed detoxification. It is preferred for patients with liver damage since acamprosate is metabolized through the kidneys and not the liver. Meta-analyses suggest that, in keeping with the purported mechanisms of action of naltrexone and acamprosate, naltrexone has stronger effects on reducing heavy drinking (presumably through diminishing alcohol's mu opioid receptor-mediated rewarding effects), while acamprosate is better at increasing complete abstinence (presumably through attenuating rebound glutamate-NMDA mediated excitation).

SSRIs have produced only modest drinking reductions—independent of antidepressant effects—through an anti-craving effect. This effect may be more apparent in men with depression and late-onset alcoholism.[76,77] The SSRIs do not appear to have any relapse-prevention effect in women. Recent double-blind placebo-controlled studies have shown efficacy for ondansetron in early-onset alcoholics and topiramate has shown promise as an effective pharmacotherapy for alcohol dependence in a broad range of alcohol-dependent individuals.[176,177] All of these agents are gaining renewed interest as adjuncts to a comprehensive psychosocial recovery program and should be considered in the treatment of all individuals with AUD.

Substance-induced psychiatric symptoms are common before admission for detoxification and may persist for 2–4 weeks after detoxification.[70,71] If symptoms continue for longer than 4 weeks, it suggests the existence of an independent co-occurring psychiatric disorder. In these situations, a specific psychiatric treatment plan is required to address the co-occurring disorder. Studies support initiation of an SSRI for co-occurring major depression, mood stabilizers for bipolar illness, buspirone for generalized anxiety, and second-generation antipsychotics for a psychotic illness.[178] The best outcomes are seen when treatment for any co-occurring psychiatric disorder is integrated into the addiction recovery program.[69,179]

Alcoholics Anonymous and Long-term Support

As with other chronic illnesses, relapses to alcohol use can occur during or after successful treatment episodes. Hence, addicted individuals often require prolonged treatment and multiple episodes of care to achieve long-term abstinence and fully restored function. Participation in mutual-help organizations, such as AA, during and following treatment is often also helpful and cost-effective in helping patients achieve and maintain recovery.[180-186] Other organizations such as SMART Recovery, Secular Organization for Sobriety, and Women for Sobriety are also likely to be helpful to many patients, but are less available and little is known about their effectiveness.[181,184,185,187] A recent randomized comparative trial, found benefit for problem-drinkers who were randomized to receive either an on-line cognitive-behavioral intervention featuring the elements of SMART Recovery, attendance at SMART Recovery meetings, or both, and found that all groups improved significantly across the 3-month follow-up.[188]

AA possesses several elements that make it attractive as an ongoing adjunct to formal AUD treatment. It is accessible and flexible, with meetings held several times a day in many communities, and patients can self-select meetings that seem like a good fit. AA members also often make themselves available "on demand" (e.g., by telephone), providing a degree of flexibility not available in professional settings. This degree of availability means that AA is self-adaptive: patients can access these resources at times of high relapse risk (e.g., unstructured

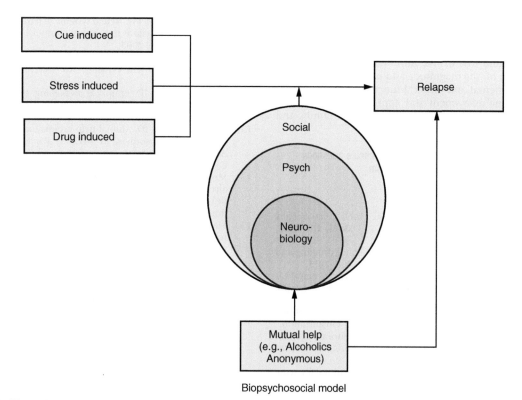

Biopsychosocial model

Figure 15-16. Biopsychosocial model of how mutual help organizations, such as Alcoholics Anonymous may attenuate relapse risk over time. *(From Kelly JF, Yeterian JD. Mutual-help groups for alcohol and other substance use disorders. In McCrady BS, Epstein EE, editors:* Addictions: a comprehensive guidebook. *ed 2. New York, 2013, Oxford University Press.)*[131]

time; evenings/weekends) or whenever they feel they need it. Furthermore, it provides recovery-specific experience and support, with members serving as role models. AA meeting formats also provide continuing reminders of past negative experiences and the positive benefits of staying sober that help maintain and enhance recovery momentum.[189] AA also possesses a low threshold for entry, with no paperwork or third-party insurance approval, and AA can be attended free of charge for as long as individuals desire, making it a highly cost-effective public health resource.[185] Studies with adults[182,183] and adolescents[190] reveal that participation in AA can enhance recovery outcomes and remission rates while simultaneously and substantially reducing health care costs.

In theory, the influence of common precursors to alcohol relapse (i.e., stress-related, cue-related, and drug-related) may be attenuated by participation in groups like AA through AA's ability to mobilize salutary changes in individuals' social networks as well in several psychological domains. Figure 15-16 illustrates the relationship between common high-risk precursors to relapse and how mutual-help organizations (MHOs), like AA might attenuate this risk through facilitating changes in social networks, psychological factors (e.g., enhancing coping, abstinence self-efficacy, motivation for abstinence), and bio/neurobiological factors.[131,191]

Empirically, there has now been rigorous scientific studies conducted on how exactly MHOs, like AA, confer recovery benefits. These studies suggest that the main ways that AA aids remission and recovery is through facilitating changes in the social networks of attendees and by boosting abstinence self-efficacy, coping, and by maintaining abstinence motivation.[192,193] Evidence suggests too that these broad benefits may depend on severity of dependence[191] and also gender,[194] whereby for more severely addicted individuals, in addition to facilitating important social network changes, AA may also

aid recovery by reducing negative affect and increasing spiritual practices.

AA and similar approaches that examine broader character, lifestyle, and spiritual issues are popular in the US and in many other countries.[195] In the US, AA is the most commonly sought-after source of help for an alcohol problem,[196] with 1.3 million members, and 60,000 meetings held weekly,[197] and it has been shown empirically to be helpful in achieving and maintaining abstinence for many different types of patients (including men and women, those with religious/spiritual and non-religious/non-spiritual backgrounds, and those who are dually diagnosed).[185,198–202]

When encouraging AA participation and making AA referrals, greatest success is achieved if clinicians use empirically-supported methods. For example, Twelve-Step Facilitation (TSF)[203] is an empirically-supported therapy for helping patients become actively involved in AA, and manuals can be obtained free of charge through the NIAAA website (www.niaaa.nih.gov). TSF approaches involve educating patients about the content, format, and structure of mutual-help groups early during treatment, and then continuing to monitor patients' reactions and responses to meeting attendance.[189] Also, substantially more effective referrals to AA can be made if clinicians assist patients in making personal contact with existing members whenever possible to facilitate fellowship integration.[201,204–210] Interventions that incorporate or employ TSF have been shown to enhance patients' outcomes by approximately 10%–20% over and above outcomes achieved with standard CBT.[208]

CONCLUSIONS

Alcohol misuse and related disorders permeate virtually every aspect of psychiatry and medicine. Preventing early exposure to alcohol among youth, minimizing heavy use, and screening for the presence of alcohol-induced, and alcohol use, disorders can help prevent an array of acute and chronic debilitating morbidities and loss of life. An enhanced sensitivity for, and appreciation of, the magnitude and pervasiveness of alcohol's effects on mental and physical function should advance the use of routine assessment and appropriate intervention that can lead to similarly widespread individual, family, and societal benefits.

⊗ Access the complete reference list and multiple choice questions (MCQs) online at https://expertconsult.inkling.com

KEY REFERENCES

4. Babor TF, Caetano R, Casswell S, et al. *Alcohol: no ordinary commodity-research and public policy*, ed 2, Oxford, UK, 2010, Oxford University Press.

6. Bagnardi V, Rota M, Botteri E, et al. Light alcohol drinking and cancer: a meta-analysis. *Ann Oncol* 24(2):301–308, 2013.

8. U.S. Department of Health and Human Services and U.S. Department of Agriculture. *Dietary Guidelines for Americans, 2005*, Washington, DC, 2005, HHS and USDA.

11. World Health Organization. *Global status report on alcohol and health*, Geneva, Switzerland, 2011, World Health Organization.

12. Bouchery EE, Harwood HJ, Sacks JJ, et al. Economic costs of excessive alcohol consumption in the U.S. 2006. *Am J Prev Med* 41(5):516–524, 2011.

26. Rosenson J, Clements C, Simon B, et al. Phenobarbital for acute alcohol withdrawal: a prospective randomized double-blind placebo-controlled study. *J Emerg Med* 44(3):592–598, e592, 2013.

32. Isenberg-Grzeda E, Kutner HE, Nicolson SE. Wernicke–Korsakoff-syndrome: under-recognized and under-treated. *Psychosomatics* 53(6):507–516, 2012.

45. Kelly JF, Westerhoff CM. Does it matter how we refer to individuals with substance-related conditions? A randomized study of two commonly used terms. *Int J Drug Policy* 21:202–207, 2010.

46. Kelly JF, White WL, eds. Addiction Recovery Management. In Rosenbaum JF, editor: *Current clinical psychiatry*, New York, 2011, Springer.

47. Schuckit MA. An overview of genetic influences in alcoholism. *J Subst Abuse Treat* 36(1):S5–S14, 2009.

57. Urbanoski KA, Kelly JF. Understanding genetic risk for substance use and addiction: a guide for non-geneticists. *Clin Psychol Rev* 32(1):60–70, 2012.

58. Schuckit MA. *Vulnerability factors for alcoholism*, Baltimore, 2002, Lippincott Williams & Wilkins.

63. National Institute on Alcohol Abuse and Alcoholism (NIAAA). *Helping patients who drink too much: a clinician's guide and related professional support services: National Institute on Alcohol and Alcoholism*, Washington, DC, 2005, USDHHS.

81. Dawson DA, Grant BF, Stinson FS, et al. Recovery from DSM-IV alcohol dependence: United States, 2001–2002. *Addiction* 100(3):281–292, 2005.

94. Everitt BJ, Robbins TW. Neural systems of reinforcement for drug addiction: from actions to habits to compulsion. *Nature Neurosci* 8(11):1481–1489, 2005.

110. Fleming MF. Brief interventions and the treatment of alcohol use disorders: current evidence. *Rec Dev Alcohol* 16:375–390, 2003.

130. Kelly JF, Yeterian JD. Empirical awakening: the new science on mutual help and implications for cost containment under health care reform. *Subst Abus* 33(2):85–91, 2012.

131. Kelly JF, Yeterian JD. Mutual-help groups for alcohol and other substance use disorders. In McCrady BS, Epstein EE, editors: *Addictions: A comprehensive guidebook*, ed 2, New York, 2013, Oxford University Press.

133. Moyer A, Finney JW, Swearingen CE, et al. Brief interventions for alcohol problems: a meta-analytic review of controlled investigations in treatment-seeking and non-treatment-seeking populations. *Addiction* 97(3):279–292, 2002.

134. Maisel NC, Blodgett JC, Wilbourne PL, et al. Meta-analysis of naltrexone and acamprosate for treating alcohol use disorders: when are these medications most helpful? *Addiction* 108(2):275–293, 2013.

138. Madras BK, Compton WM, Avula D, et al. Screening, brief interventions, referral to treatment (SBIRT) for illicit drug and alcohol use at multiple healthcare sites: comparison at intake and 6 months later. *Drug Alcohol Depend* 99(1–3):280–295, 2009.

157. White WL. *Recovery management and recovery-oriented systems of care: scientific rationale and promising practices*, 2008, Northeast Addiction Technology Transfer Center, Great Lakes Addiction Technology Transfer Center, Philadelphia Department of Behavioral Health/Mental Retardation Services.

158. Dennis ML, Scott CK. Four-year outcomes from the Early Re-Intervention (ERI) experiment using Recovery Management Checkups (RMCs). *Drug Alcohol Depend* 121(1–2):10–17, 2012.

164. McClellan A, Lewis D, O'Brien C, et al. Drug dependence, a chronic medical illness: implications for treatment, insurance, and outcomes evaluation. *JAMA* 284(13):1689–1695, 2000.

167. White WL. *Recovery/remission from substance use disorders: An analysis of reported outcomes in 415 scientific reports, 1868–2011*, 2012, Philadelphia Department of Behavioral Health and Intellectual disability Services, Great Lakes Addiction Technology Transfer Center.

181. Humphreys K. *Circles of recovery: self-help organizations for addictions*, Cambridge, UK, 2004, Cambridge University Press.

187. Kelly JF, White W. Broadening the base of addiction recovery mutual aid. *J Groups Addict Recover* 7(2–4):82–101, 2012.

192. Kelly JF, Magill M, Stout RL. How do people recover from alcohol dependence? A systematic review of the research on mechanisms of behavior change in Alcoholics Anonymous. *Addict Res Theory* 17(3):236–259, 2009.

194. Kelly JF, Hoeppner B. Does Alcoholics Anonymous work differently for men and women? A moderated multiple-mediation analysis in a large clinical sample. *Drug Alcohol Depend* 130(1–3):186–193, 2013.

16 Drug Addiction

John A. Renner, Jr., MD, and E. Nalan Ward, MD

KEY POINTS

Incidence

- Depending on the drug used and the clinical setting, up to 50% of patients in mental-health treatment will have a co-occurring substance-use disorder.

Epidemiology

- Substance abuse is a major public health problem that affects a large number of psychiatric patients.
- Screening for substance use and abuse should be a routine part of all mental-health evaluations.
- The problem is particularly severe in public sector treatment settings.

Prognosis

- Research has demonstrated that integrated treatment delivered in settings that are skilled in the management of both mental-health and substance-use disorders will significantly improve outcome.

Treatment Options

- Brief interventions, motivational-enhancement therapy, cognitive-behavioral therapy, and pharmacotherapy with methadone and buprenorphine are each efficacious for addictions.
- Psychiatrists need to become adept in the use of evidence-based treatment for substance-use disorders.
- The availability of effective psychotherapies and pharmacotherapies for addictive disorders makes it possible to successfully manage patients (in outpatient settings) who are addicted to opiates and cocaine.

Complications

- Unrecognized and untreated substance-use disorders are associated with poor outcomes and treatment failure for co-occurring mental health disorders.

OVERVIEW

The chronic, relapsing nature of substance abuse is inappropriately thought to imply that substance-abuse treatment is not helpful. This leads clinicians to ignore multiple opportunities to intervene in the disease process. Most clinicians fail to appreciate that the relapse rate of other common chronic medical disorders (e.g., diabetes, hypertension, asthma) exceeds that for substance-use disorders.[1] Problems related to substance abuse should always be addressed with the same degree of compassion and persistence that is directed to other common relapsing medical disorders.

Among individuals who abuse drugs, 53% have a co-occurring psychiatric disorder. Successful treatment of this expanding group of patients requires that clinicians improve their skills in the management of patients with substance-use disorders and co-occurring psychiatric disorders.

The National Survey on Drug Use and Health (NSDUH) findings in 2011 showed that 22.5 million Americans, or 8.7% of the population ≥ age 12, used an illicit drug in the past month.[2] Marijuana continues to be the most commonly-abused illicit drug, followed by non-medical use of prescribed or over-the-counter (OTC) medication abuse (Figure 16-1).

During the last decade, the number of patients treated for substance abuse–related problems in the US has grown steadily. Between 2004 and 2011, the number of emergency department (ED) visits for drug-related events increased by 100%.[3] In the same period, the number of drug-related suicide attempts rose by 41%. Adolescents and young adults were the most vulnerable to the adverse effects of drug use. The majority of ED visits for those in these age groups were the result of medical emergencies related to drug misuse/abuse (Figure 16-2).

In 2011, cocaine and marijuana were the most commonly-used illicit drugs that led to ED visits.[3] Non-medical use of prescription drug or OTC medication–related ED visits increased by 132% between 2004 and 2011, with opiate/opioid involvement rising by 183%.[3]

These results are not surprising in that they reflect the extent of the prescription pain-reliever addiction epidemic in the US. About 4.5 million individuals reported current non-medical use of pain relievers in 2011.[2]

In recent years, the liberal prescription of potent opioid medications, as well as their increased availability and diversion in communities, have played a significant role in the development of this public health problem.[4] More than half of those who use illicit pain relievers reported that they had obtained the pain relievers from family or friends[2] (Figure 16-3).

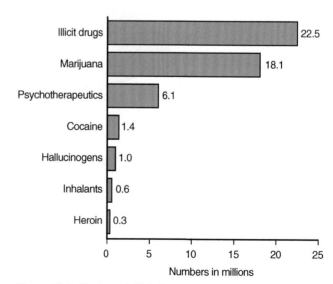

Figure 16-1. Past month illicit drug use among persons aged 12 or older: 2011. *(Findings from National Survey on Drug Use and Health, 2011: Summary of National Findings, NSDUH Series H-44, HHS Publication No. (SMA) 12-4713. Rockville, MD: Substance Abuse and Mental Health Services Administration, 2012.)*

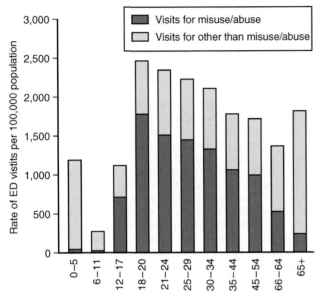

Figure 16-2. Rates of drug-related ED visits per 100,000 population, by age group, 2011. *(From Substance Abuse and Mental Health Services Administration, Center for Behavioral Health Statistics and Quality. Drug Abuse Warning Network, 2008: National Estimates of Drug-Related Emergency Department Visits. HHS Publication No. SMA 11-4618. Rockville, MD, 2011, HHS.)*

THE NEUROBIOLOGY OF ADDICTION

Disruption of the endogenous reward systems in the brain is a common feature of drug abuse; most addictive drugs act by disrupting central nervous system (CNS) dopamine circuits. Acutely, synaptic dopamine increases and circuits that mediate motivation and drive, conditioned learning, and inhibitory controls are disrupted (Figure 16-4). This enhancement of synaptic dopamine is particularly rewarding for individuals with abnormally low density of the D_2 dopamine receptor (D_2DR). Normal individuals (with normal D_2DR levels) find this experience too intense and aversive and thus may be shielded from the risk of addiction. Low D_2DR availability is associated with an increased risk for abuse of cocaine, heroin, methamphetamine, alcohol, and methylphenidate. Chronic drug use produces long-lasting and significant decreases in dopamine brain function, manifested by decreases in both the D_2DR and dopamine cell activity. These decreases are also associated with dysfunction in the prefrontal cortex, including the orbitofrontal cortex (which is involved in salience attribution) and the cingulated gyrus (which is involved in inhibitory control and mood regulation). Low baseline levels of beta-plasma endorphins are associated with a higher endorphin response to alcohol and an increased risk for alcohol dependence; it is less clear whether this abnormality also increases the risk for opiate dependence. Table 16-1 lists the major drugs of abuse and the associated disruption of CNS neurotransmitter systems.

COCAINE
Abuse

The percent of persons with cocaine dependence or abuse decreased between 2006 and 2011 from 0.7 to 0.3 %.[2] In 2011,

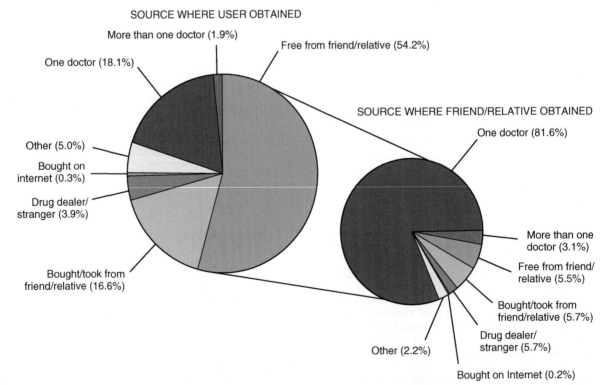

Figure 16-3. Source where pain relievers were obtained for most recent non-medical use among past year users aged 12 or older: 2010–2011. The Other category includes the sources "Wrote Fake Prescription," "Stole from Doctor's Office/Clinic/Hospital/Pharmacy," and "Some Other Way." *(Findings from National Survey on Drug Use and Health: Summary of National Findings, NSDUH Series H-44, HHS Publication No. (SMA) 12-4713. Rockville, MD: Substance Abuse and Mental Health Services Administration, 2012.)*

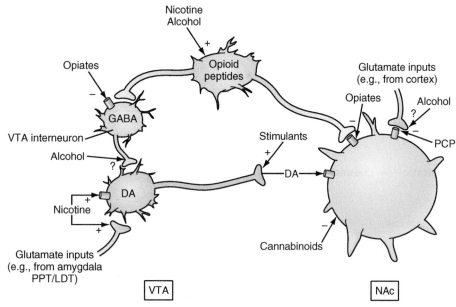

Figure 16-4. Converging acute actions of drugs of abuse on the ventral tegmental area and nucleus accumbens. DA, dopamine; GABA, γ-aminobutyric acid; LDT, laterodorsal tegmentum; NAc, nucleus accumbens; PCP, phencyclidine; PPT, pedunculopontine tegmentum; VTA, ventral tegmental area. *(Redrawn from Nestler EJ. Is there a common molecular pathway for addiction? Nat Neurosci 8(11):1445–1449, 2005.)*

TABLE 16-1 Neurobiology of Drug Reinforcement

Drug Type	Mechanism of Reinforcement
Cocaine	Mesolimbic dopamine system
Amphetamines	
Nicotine	
Opioids	Mesolimbic dopamine system
Alcohol	GABA and glutamate
	Dopamine and serotonin
	Opioid peptide systems
Cannabinoids	Dopamine in the nucleus accumbens

GABA, γ-aminobutyric acid.

the number of persons with cocaine dependence or abuse was roughly 821,000. Despite the downward trend, cocaine, after alcohol, remained the leading substance of abuse related to frequent ED contacts, general hospital admissions, family violence, and other social problems.[3] Cocaine use resulted in 40% of all illicit drug-related ED visits in 2011. Even individuals with normal psychological profiles are vulnerable to compulsive cocaine use. Acute use leads to intense euphoria that is often associated with increased sexual desire and with improved sexual function. These rewards are often followed by a moderate-to-severe post–cocaine use depression that stimulates a strong incentive for further cocaine use. These responses are primarily mediated by disruptions of synaptic dopamine. The initial cocaine response is a function of elevated dopamine generated by blockade of the dopamine reuptake transporter (DAT) and the inhibition of the reuptake of synaptic dopamine. Chronic cocaine use leads to downregulation of dopamine receptors and ultimately to depletion of synaptic dopamine, which is thought to be the cause of post–cocaine use depression (Figure 16-5). Like other stimulants, cocaine also disrupts the synthesis and reuptake of serotonin. Other receptors affected include norepinephrine, N-methyl-D-aspartate (NMDA), gamma-aminobutyric acid (GABA), and opioid receptors. Plasma cholinesterases rapidly convert cocaine into benzoylecognine (BE), an inactive metabolite that can be detected in the urine for 3 days. When alcohol is taken in conjunction with cocaine, liver esterases produce cocaethylene, an active metabolite that has a longer half-life (2–4-hours) and is more cardiotoxic than cocaine. The combination of cocaine and marijuana also produces more intense euphoria, higher plasma levels, and more cardiotoxicity than does cocaine alone.

The signs and the symptoms of acute cocaine intoxication are similar to those of amphetamine abuse. Typical complaints associated with intoxication include anorexia, insomnia, anxiety, hyperactivity, and rapid speech and thought processes ("speeding"). Signs of adrenergic hyperactivity (such as hyperreflexia, tachycardia, diaphoresis, and dilated pupils responsive to light) may also be seen. More severe symptoms (e.g., hyperpyrexia, hypertension, cocaine-induced vasospastic events [e.g., stroke or myocardial infarction]) are relatively rare among users, but are fairly common in those seen in hospital EDs. Patients may also manifest stereotyped movements of the mouth, face, or extremities. Snorting the drug may produce rhinitis or sinusitis and, rarely, perforations of the nasal septum. Free-basing (inhalation of cocaine alkaloid vapors) may produce bronchitis. Grand mal seizures are another infrequent complication. Patients also describe "snowlights" (i.e., flashes of light usually seen at the periphery of the visual field). Crack is a highly addictive free-base form of cocaine that is sold in crystals and can be smoked.

The most serious psychiatric problem associated with chronic cocaine use is a cocaine-induced psychosis (manifest by visual and auditory hallucinations and paranoid delusions often associated with violent behavior). Tactile hallucinations (called "coke bugs") involve the perception that something is crawling under the skin. A cocaine psychosis may be indistinguishable from an amphetamine psychosis, but it usually does not last as long. High doses of stimulants can also cause a state of excitation and mental confusion known as "stimulant delirium."

Management

Cocaine abuse became common among affluent young people in the early to mid-1980s, but with the availability of packaged smokable cocaine, or crack, in low-cost doses, all classes and racial groups have become potential users. Occasional cocaine

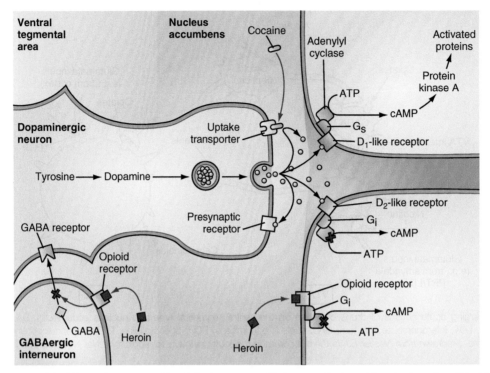

Figure 16-5. Schematic of the effects of cocaine and heroin in the synapse. *(Redrawn and adapted from Leshner A and the US National Institute on Drug Abuse.* New understandings of drug addiction, Hospital Practice Special Report, *1997. New York, 1997, McGraw-Hill.)*

use does not require specific treatment except in the case of a life-threatening overdose. Most potentially lethal doses are metabolized within 1 hour. In the interim, intubation and assisted breathing with oxygen may be necessary. Stroke has been reported, and death can be caused by ventricular fibrillation or myocardial infarction. The cardiac status should therefore be monitored closely. High doses of benzodiazepines are recommended for management of stimulant-induced delirium and agitation. Neuroleptics should be avoided because of the risk of potentially fatal hyperthermia. Intravenous (IV) diazepam should be used to control convulsions.

Chronic cocaine use produces tolerance, severe psychological dependency, and physiological dependence (marked by irritability, anhedonia, low mood, insomnia or hypersomnia, and anxiety).[5] Dependent users typically follow a cyclical pattern of 2 or 3 days of heavy binge use, followed by a withdrawal "crash." Use is resumed again in 3 to 4 days, depending on the availability of cash and the drug. A gradual reduction in use of the drug is almost never possible. Detoxification is accomplished by the abrupt cessation of all cocaine use, usually through restricted access (e.g., a loss of funds or contacts, or incarceration). Symptoms of withdrawal begin to resolve within 7 days; the value of medication treatment for withdrawal symptoms has yet to be confirmed. Drugs that enhance CNS catecholamine function may reduce craving, although they are of limited clinical benefit and they have not been proven effective in double-blind placebo-controlled trials. There is some indication that amantadine (an indirect dopamine agonist) and propranolol may be helpful to individuals with severe withdrawal symptoms. The major complication of withdrawal is a severe depression with suicidal ideation.[6] If this occurs, the patient typically requires psychiatric hospitalization. The need for inpatient care may be time-limited, since suicidal ideation usually clears promptly with the cessation of cocaine use. A less severe anhedonic state may persist for 2 to 3 months and is thought to reflect a more persistent state of dopamine depletion.

For the cocaine addict, the compulsion to use is overwhelming. For this reason, a hospitalized, cocaine-dependent patient should be monitored closely and should have a drug screen performed after behavioral change, particularly after departures from the floor or receiving visitors. Urine should be examined for cocaine metabolites and, preferably, for all drugs of abuse.

Once compulsive cocaine use has begun, it is almost impossible for the user to return to a pattern of occasional, controlled use. Such individuals are also likely to develop problems with alcohol and other drugs. For that reason, the goal of treatment should be abstinence from cocaine and all other drugs. All cocaine abusers should be referred for individual or group counseling, and participation in 12-step self-help programs should be strongly recommended. Manual-guided cognitive-behavioral therapy (CBT) has been efficacious in the treatment of cocaine dependence.[7] Twelve-step facilitation and CBT appear to be helpful, particularly in individuals with more severe dependence and in those with co-morbid disorders.[8] Family members or significant others should be referred separately to Al-Anon because they will gain insights that may help them eliminate systemic support for the patient's drug use. There is no Food and Drug Administration (FDA)–approved pharmacotherapy for cocaine dependence. Trials with desipramine, fluoxetine, bupropion, amantadine, and carbamazepine have had inconsistent results. Positive responses have been reported in trials with topiramate, baclofen, and modafinil, but these drugs require further investigation. Several trials with disulfiram have shown benefit, with reduced craving and use, and a reported increase in the aversive effects of cocaine should the patient relapse. These reactions are thought to be mediated by the inhibitory effect of disulfiram on dopamine beta-hydroxylase. This action will elevate depleted plasma dopamine levels in chronic users and will produce abnormally high dopamine levels if cocaine is ingested; this results in a dysphoric experience for most users.

AMPHETAMINES

Abuse

In 2011, roughly 970,000 persons ≥ 12 years were active non-medical users of prescription stimulants.[2] Between 2004 and 2011, prescription CNS stimulants led to a striking 307% increase in ED visits. Among these agents, the ADHD drug amphetamine-dextroamphetamine (e.g., Adderall®) showed a 650% increase during that period.[3]

Illicitly-produced methamphetamine fueled an epidemic of abuse on the West Coast and in much of the Midwest in the 1990s. Since then, the number of methamphetamine abusers had declined as a result of stricter federal controls on the production and distribution of certain medications.

The primary action of these drugs is an increase in synaptic dopamine via the release of dopamine into the synapse; methamphetamine also blocks the DAT. This produces a dopamine "high" that is both more intense and longer lasting than results from cocaine, lasting anywhere from 8 to 24 hours. Methamphetamine, invented for military use by the Japanese in World War I, is currently a schedule II drug, that can be taken orally ("speed"), taken anally, smoked ("crystal"), snorted, or injected. It has been approved for the treatment of ADHD and obesity. Long-term use of amphetamines can cause cognitive impairment (including dulled awareness, decreased intellectual capacity, memory impairment, and motor retardation). Positive positron emission tomography (PET) scans show loss of DAT in the caudate and the putamen, and magnetic resonance imaging (MRI) studies show decreased perfusion in the putaman and the frontal cortex as well as loss of volume in both the amygdala and the hippocampus. Routine medical evaluation may uncover the most common type of amphetamine abuse seen in clinical settings (involving use of amphetamines to control obesity and that later led to chronic amphetamine abuse). Amphetamine abusers quickly develop tolerance and may use 100 mg each day in an unsuccessful effort to control weight. This type of amphetamine abuse can be treated by abruptly discontinuing the drug or by gradually tapering the dose. In either case, the patient should be given a more appropriate program for weight control.

A more serious problem involves the patient who develops a severe psychological dependence on amphetamines and who may have the same symptoms seen in younger street-drug users and abusers. Illicit amphetamine and methamphetamine (speed) use accounted for 12.8 % of all illicit-drug-use-related ED visits in 2011.[3]

The signs and symptoms of acute amphetamine intoxication are similar to those of cocaine abuse. Long-term effects include depression, brain dysfunction, and weight loss. In addition, either with acute or chronic amphetamine intoxication a paranoid psychosis without delirium can develop. Although typically seen in young people who use IV methamphetamine hydrochloride, paranoia can also occur in chronic users of dextroamphetamine or other amphetamines. A paranoid psychosis may also occur with or without other manifestations of amphetamine intoxication. The absence of disorientation distinguishes this condition from most other toxic psychoses. This syndrome is clinically indistinguishable from an acute schizophrenic episode of the paranoid type, and the correct diagnosis is often made in retrospect, based on a history of amphetamine use and a urine test that is positive for amphetamines. Use of haloperidol or low-dose atypical antipsychotics is often effective in the acute management of this type of substance-induced psychosis.

Other distinctive features of chronic stimulant abuse include dental problems (e.g., caries, missing teeth, bleeding and infected gums), muscle cramps (related to dehydration and low levels of magnesium and potassium), constipation (due to dehydration), nasal perforations, and excoriated skin lesions (speed bumps) (Figure 16-6). The urine may have a stale smell due to ammonia constituents used in the illicit manufacture of methamphetamine.

Treatment

Amphetamines can be withdrawn abruptly. If the intoxication is mild, the patient's agitation can be handled by reassurance alone. The patient can be "talked down," much as one might handle an adverse D-lysergic acid diethylamide (LSD) reaction. If sedation is necessary, benzodiazepines are the drugs of choice. Phenothiazines should be avoided because they may heighten dysphoria and increase the patient's agitation. Hypertension will usually respond to sedation with benzodiazepines. When severe hypertension arises, phentolamine is recommended for vasodilation. Beta- or mixed alpha- and beta-adrenergic blockers (such as propranolol or labetalol) are to

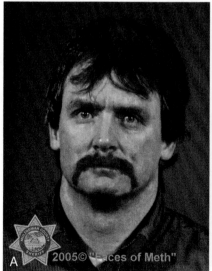 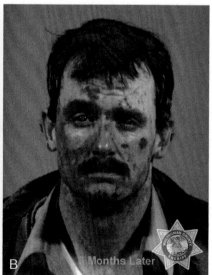

Figure 16-6. Face of a patient with chronic methamphetamine abuse. Before use (A) and after 3 months of use (B). *(From the Faces of Meth educational program. Copyright 2005 Multnomah County [Oregon] Sheriff's Office, Portland, Oregon.)*

be avoided because they may exacerbate stimulant-induced cardiovascular toxicity.

Most signs of intoxication clear in 2 to 4 days. The major problem is management of depression upon discontinuation of amphetamine use. In mild cases, this depression can be manifest by lethargy, as well as by the temptation to use amphetamines for energy. In more serious cases, the patient may become suicidal and require inpatient psychiatric treatment. The efficacy of antidepressants in such cases has not been adequately documented. Even with support and psychotherapy, most patients experience symptoms of depression for 3 to 6 months following the cessation of chronic amphetamine abuse. CBT has been helpful, but it may need to be adapted to allow for the cognitive impairment associated with long-term methamphetamine use.

CLUB DRUGS

During the 1990s the abuse of "club drugs," primarily 3,4-methylenedioxy-methamphetamine (MDMA, or "ecstasy"), γ-hydroxybutyrate (GHB), and ketamine steadily increased. This trend was reversed between 1998 and 2001 when the Monitoring the Future Survey (MFS) reported a steep decline in the use of ecstasy. The drop has been attributed to a general recognition of the dangers associated with the use of this drug. In 2012, MFS reported a 1.5% past-year use of club drugs among 12th graders.[9]

MDMA has both amphetamine-like and hallucinogenic effects. Its primary mechanism of action is via indirect serotonin agonism, but it also affects dopamine and other neurotransmitter systems. These club drugs increase synaptic dopamine and alter serotonergic neurotransmission. MDMA was initially used experimentally to facilitate psychotherapy, but its use was banned after it was found to be neurotoxic to animals. The intense feelings of empathy experienced by users may be a result of the flooding of the serotonin system. In toxic amounts, it produces distorted perceptions, confusion, hypertension, hyperactivity, and potentially fatal hyperthermia. With chronic use, serotonin stores are depleted and subsequent doses produce a less robust high and more unpleasant side effects (such as teeth gnashing and restlessness). Frequent users learn to anticipate these effects and tend to limit their long-term consumption of the drug.

GHB (sodium oxybate) is structurally similar to GABA and it acts as a CNS depressant. It has been approved by the FDA as a schedule III controlled substance for the treatment of narcolepsy. GHB has a relatively low therapeutic index; as little as twice the dose that produces euphoria can cause CNS depression. In overdose it can produce a potentially fatal coma; it has also been identified as a "date rape" drug. Ketamine ("Special K," "Super K," or "K") is a non-competitive NMDA antagonist that is classified as a dissociative anesthetic. It is currently used as a veterinary anesthetic and it can produce delirium, amnesia, and respiratory depression when abused. Ketamine, like phencyclidine (PCP), binds to the NMDA receptor site and blocks the action of excitatory neurotransmission; it affects perceptions, memory, and cognition. More recently, studies suggest it can rapidly reverse treatment-refractory depression.

The treatment for overdoses of all of these drugs is primarily symptomatic.

OPIOIDS

While abuse of all major drug classes increased during the 1990s, the most dramatic increase was seen among new abusers of prescription pain relievers. In 2011, an estimated 4.5 million (1.7%) individuals were active non-medical users of pain relievers.[2] In the US, prescription pain reliever-abuse is considered an epidemic. Many public health problems have been associated with this particular type of drug abuse. The perception of prescription drugs as being less harmful than illicit drugs likely contributed to the problem.[2]

Due to frequency of prescription pain relievers, they are considered an "entry drug" after illicit marijuana. According to the 2012 MFS, 1 out of every 12 high school seniors reported taking prescription pain relievers for non-medical use within the last year.[9] Unfortunately, with the progression of the abuse, many individuals turn to heroin. The latest NSDUH data estimated a significant increase in heroin use in 2007 (373,000) to 2011 (620,000).[2] The major health concerns with increased heroin use are intravenous (IV)-related medical complications.

Nearly one-third (31%) of individuals with acquired immunodeficiency syndrome (AIDS) in the US are related to injection drug use.[10] An estimated 70% to 80% of the new hepatitis C infections occurring in the US each year are among IV drug users. Other public health problems that have emerged over the last decade include increased ED visits and deaths due to overdoses. Specifically, prescription methadone, oxycodone and hydrocodone-related ED visits quadrupled between 2004 and 2008[11] (Figure 16-7).

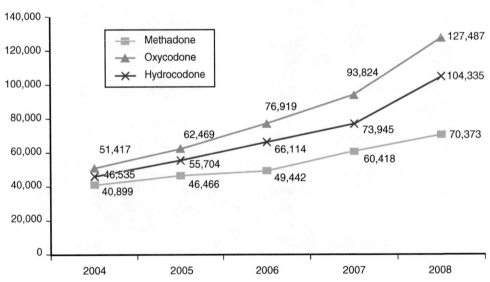

Figure 16-7. Emergency department visits related to methadone, oxycodone and hydrocodone: 2004–2008. DAWN 2008.

Death rates
Deaths per 100,000 population

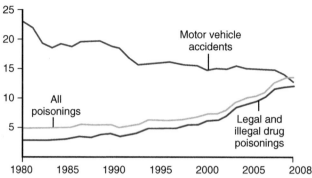

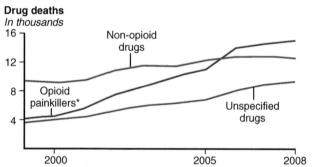

*Note: morphine, hydrocodone, oxycodone, methadone, fentanyl and others

Figure 16-8. Overdose death rates. *(Warner M, Chen LH, Makuc DM, Anderson RN, Miniño AM. Drug poisoning deaths in the United States, 1980–2008. NCHS data brief, no 81. Hyattsville, MD, 2011, National Center for Health Statistics.)*

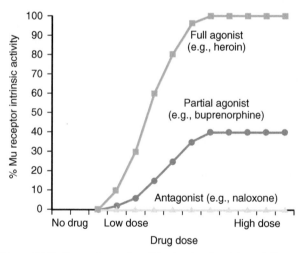

Figure 16-9. Comparison of activity levels of opiates at the mu receptor.

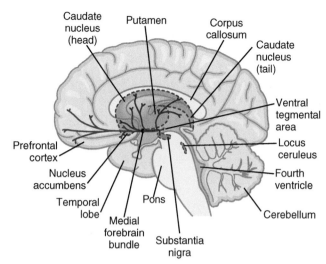

Figure 16-10. Schematic of reward pathways in the brain. *(Redrawn and adapted from Leshner A and the US National Institute on Drug Abuse.* New understandings of drug addiction, Hospital Practice Special Report, *April 1997. New York, 1997, McGraw-Hill.)*

TABLE 16-2 Opioid Agonist Drug Effects	
Acute-use effects	Euphoria
	Vomiting
	Constricted pupils
	Depressed respiration
	Drowsiness
	Decreased pain sensation
	Decreased awareness
	Decreased consciousness
Large-dose acute-use effects	Non-responsiveness
	Pin-point pupils
	If severe anoxia, pupils may dilate
	Bradycardia and hypotension
	Skin cyanotic
	Skeletal muscle flaccid
	Pulmonary edema in approximately 50%
	Slow or absent respiration
Chronic-use effects	Physical dependence
	Psychological dependence
	Lethargy and indifference
	Reduction in bowel movement

In 2008, there were more poisoning-related deaths than deaths caused by motor vehicle accidents (Figure 16-8). In 2011, pain relievers accounted for 46% of all medical emergencies associated with non-medical use of pharmaceuticals. Since 2007, there were more overdose deaths with prescription pain relievers than there were with heroin and cocaine combined.[12]

Opiates act by binding to the mu opioid receptor (Figure 16-9). Binding to receptors in the ventral tegmental area stimulates the release of dopamine (Figure 16-10), which activates brain reward centers in the nucleus accumbens. Opiates produce a wide range of effects (including analgesia, euphoria,

sedation, decreased secretions, nausea, vomiting, constipation, miosis, urinary hesitation, and hypotension [Table 16-2]). The classic signs of opiate withdrawal are easily recognized and usually begin 8 to 12 hours after the last dose (of a short-lasting agent) (Box 16-1). The patient generally admits the need for drugs and shows sweating, yawning, lacrimation, tremor, rhinorrhea, marked irritability, dilated pupils, piloerection ("gooseflesh"), and an increased respiratory rate. More severe signs of withdrawal occur 24 to 36 hours after the last dose and include tachycardia, hypertension, insomnia, nausea, vomiting, and abdominal cramps. Untreated, the syndrome subsides in 3 to 7 days. Withdrawal symptoms are similar in patients addicted to methadone, but they may not appear until 24 to 36 hours after the last dose (because of methadone's longer half-life) and abate over 2 to 4 weeks. Patients addicted to oxycodone may present with a particularly severe and prolonged withdrawal syndrome and may require high doses of opiates for adequate control.

As the treatment of opioid dependence becomes more commonplace on medical and surgical floors of general hospitals, physicians are challenged to provide proper management, necessitating up-to-date knowledge of FDA regulations

---

BOX 16-1 Signs and Symptoms of Opiate Withdrawal

- Dysphoric mood
- Nausea ± vomiting
- Body aches
- Lacrimation
- Rhinorrhea
- Pupillary dilation
- Sweating
- Piloerection
- Diarrhea
- Yawning
- Mild fever
- Insomnia
- Irritability
- Opioid craving

---

and community treatment resources, as well as competence in the management of detoxification and opiate substitution therapy.

Opiate Substitution Therapy

FDA regulations define opiate substitution therapy (with either methadone, levo-alpha-acetylmethadol [LAAM], or buprenorphine) as treatment with an approved opiate that extends beyond 30 days. An addicted individual cannot be placed into a methadone maintenance treatment unless he or she manifests physiological evidence of current addiction (withdrawal signs) and can document a 1-year history of addiction. The only exceptions to this rule are being pregnant and addicted; being addicted and hospitalized for the treatment of a medical, surgical, or obstetric condition; and having been addicted and recently released from incarceration. In the methadone clinic setting, initiation of maintenance treatment begins with an oral dose of 20 to 30 mg per day. Increases are made daily in increments of 10 mg until a dose is achieved that eliminates withdrawal symptoms and blocks craving. More rapid dose escalation runs the risk of excessive sedation and prolongation of the QTc interval. Doses in the range of 80 to 120 mg per day are required to stabilize most addicts and to block the euphoric effect of illicit opiates. Success in methadone maintenance treatment has been associated with higher doses (range 60 to 120 mg daily), long-term treatment, and the provision of comprehensive counseling and rehabilitation services.

In addition to methadone, FDA-approved medications for opiate substitution therapy include LAAM (a synthetic opiate with a duration of action of 48 to 72 hours) and buprenorphine (a long-acting partial opiate agonist). Patients on LAAM must be monitored for evidence of a prolonged QTc interval. Buprenorphine, a partial opioid agonist, produces a milder state of opiate dependence. Because it only partially activates opiate receptors, buprenorphine does not suppress brainstem function and it is relatively safe in overdose (Figure 16-8). Buprenorphine has a high affinity for opiate receptors and is slowly dissociated from the receptor. It will displace most other opiates from the receptor and may precipitate opiate withdrawal in dependent individuals if other opiates are present. To avoid this problem, the initial buprenorphine dose should not be administered until the patient demonstrates mild-to-moderate symptoms of withdrawal.

Buprenorphine can be used in the treatment of patients who meet *Diagnostic and Statistical Manual of Mental Disorders, Fifth Edition* (DSM-5), criteria for opioid dependence.[13] Unlike methadone, treatment with buprenorphine does not require documentation of a 1-year history of addiction. When sublingual (SL) buprenorphine is dispensed in a combination tablet (with naloxone), it has minimal potential for IV abuse and has been effective for maintenance treatment.[14] Buprenorphine has been approved for use in the office-based treatment of opiate dependence and it provides an attractive alternative to methadone treatment for higher-functioning individuals and for those with shorter histories of opiate dependence. To initiate buprenorphine treatment, a patient should be instructed to refrain from the use of heroin, or any other opiate, for at least 24 hours. Once opiate withdrawal is documented (and monitored with an opiate withdrawal scale, such as the Clinical Opiate Withdrawal Scale [COWS]), treatment should begin with 4 mg/1 mg of SL buprenorphine/naloxone. The patient should be observed for 1–4 hours after the initial dose for any signs of precipitated withdrawal. Additional doses of 4 mg/1 mg can be given every 2–4 hours as needed to stabilize the patient. Most clinicians do not prescribe more than 8–12 mg/2–3 mg on the first day. Should precipitated withdrawal occur, more aggressive dosing is recommended to manage the withdrawal symptoms. Most patients can be maintained on SL doses in the range of 12 to 16 mg/day; an adequate stabilizing dose can usually be achieved within 2 to 3 days.

If a patient on methadone maintenance is to be switched to buprenorphine, the methadone dose should be gradually reduced to 30 mg per day. The patient should be maintained on that dose for 1–2 weeks before being transferred to buprenorphine. To avoid precipitated withdrawal, the first buprenorphine dose should not be administered until a mild level of opiate withdrawal is evident (in the range of 5 to 13 on the COWS). Most patients will usually need to wait 24 to 48 hours after their last methadone dose before buprenorphine can be safely administered. The dosing procedure is similar to that described previously for patients using heroin. Long-term methadone patients usually require higher buprenorphine doses (in the range of 16 to 24 mg for stabilization). Because of the ceiling effect seen with partial opiate agonists, there is no pharmacological benefit from doses higher than 32 mg/day. Extensive research has shown that opiate substitution therapy is highly effective. It reduces illicit drug use, the mortality rate, criminal behavior, and transmission of hepatitis and human immunodeficiency virus (HIV) infection, and permits many of those with addictions to attain normal levels of social function.[15] Evaluations conducted under the Drug Addiction Treatment Act of 2000 demonstrated a very positive response to the introduction of buprenorphine treatment for opiate dependence. Of the more than 104,600 individuals that had been treated, approximately 35% had never been in treatment before and 60% were new to treatment with medication[16] (Figure 16-11). Compared to patients on methadone, patients attracted to buprenorphine treatment are more likely to be white, female, better educated, and employed (Figure 16-12).

Opiate Antagonist Therapy

Naltrexone is an opioid receptor antagonist which has been available as an oral agent for many years. It fully occupies the opioid receptor and prevents the euphoric effects of opioid agonists such as heroin, oxycodone etc. Therefore, patients taking naltrexone would not get the reinforcing "high" feeling and that would result in decrease in use pattern. Medication should be given 7–10 days after last opioid use to prevent precipitated withdrawal symptoms. Oral naltrexone has been documented to have better outcomes among motivated health care professionals and within the criminal justice system population.

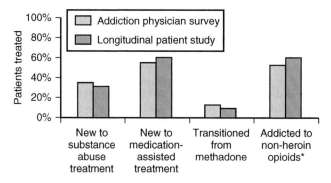

* Inpatient study, drug of abuse

Figure 16-11. Characteristics of patients treated under the buprenorphine waiver program.

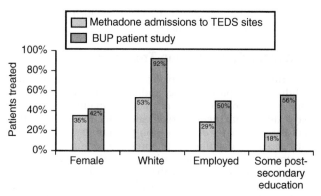

Figure 16-12. Methadone patients and buprenorphine (BUP) patients study sample: demographic differences. (The Treatment Episode Data Set [TEDS] reports primarily on admissions to facilities receiving public funding. Admissions to private facilities are underrepresented.)

In 2010, an injectable form of naltrexone has been approved by FDA. Injectable form of naltrexone (Vivitrol) appears to be a safe and effective alternative in increasing patient compliance and reduce relapse rates.[37]

Managing the Opiate-addicted Hospitalized Patient

If a patient is already receiving opiate substitution treatment before admission to the hospital, the methadone, LAAM, or buprenorphine dose should be confirmed by inpatient staff and should not be changed without consultation with the physician responsible for the patient's outpatient treatment. Under current FDA regulations, hospital-based physicians may prescribe methadone, LAAM, or buprenorphine to any addicted hospitalized person without a specialized treatment waiver or an opioid treatment program registration, as long as the patient was admitted for treatment of a condition other than opiate dependence. The patient should not be withdrawn from opiate substitution therapy unless there is full agreement among the patient, the hospital-based physician, and the outpatient treatment staff on this course of action. Such detoxification is rarely successful, particularly if the patient is under stress from a co-morbid medical or surgical condition. Withdrawal from drugs may complicate the management of the primary illness. The option of detoxification should not be considered until the patient has fully recovered from the condition that required hospitalization. Maintenance treatment should be continued until the individual has fully recovered

from the presenting illness and been referred to an opiate substitution treatment program.

Patients on long-term methadone therapy should continue to receive daily oral methadone treatment while hospitalized. If a switch to parenteral medication is necessary, methadone can be given in IM doses of 5 or 10 mg every 8 hours. This regimen should keep the patient comfortable regardless of the previous oral dose. An alternative method is to give one-third of the daily oral dose intramuscularly every 12 hours. As soon as oral medication can be tolerated, the original oral dose should be re-instated.[17]

Establishing the appropriate dose of methadone for a street addict is a trial-and-error process. Because the quality of street heroin is never certain, the addict's description of the size of the current habit is of minimal value. The safest guide to dosage is to monitor the patient's pulse, respiration, and pupillary size and to use opiate withdrawal scales (such as the COWS). After withdrawal is documented, the patient should receive 10 to 20 mg of methadone orally. Only if the patient is well known as a heavy user should a dose of 30 mg be started. A relatively young patient or a patient who reports a small habit can begin treatment with 10 mg given orally. If vital signs have not stabilized or if withdrawal signs reappear after 2 hours, an additional 5 or 10 mg can be given orally. It is rare for the patient to require more than 40 mg during the first 24 hours. Successful long-term outpatient maintenance treatment generally uses daily doses in the range of 80 to 120 mg, although lower doses may be adequate to control withdrawal symptoms in the inpatient setting. A patient with opioid addiction should be maintained on a single daily oral dose that keeps him or her comfortable and that keeps heart rate and respiratory rate within the normal range. The dose should be reduced by 5 or 10 mg if the patient appears lethargic.

Inpatient Detoxification

If the patient is to be withdrawn from drugs immediately, withdrawal symptoms should first be controlled with methadone. The methadone dose can then be reduced by 10% to 20% each day. If the patient has been maintained on methadone in the hospital for 2 or more weeks or if the patient has been on methadone treatment before admission, detoxification should proceed more slowly. The dose can be reduced by 5 to 10 mg/day until 20 mg/day is reached. Further dosage reduction should occur more gradually, particularly if the patient experiences significant cravings or withdrawal symptoms. Symptoms of chronic pain and anxiety disorders, particularly panic disorder, may also intensify during detoxification. Symptomatic treatment should be provided as needed.

Clonidine, an alpha2-adrenergic agonist, suppresses the noradrenergic symptoms of withdrawal and can be used as an alternative medication for withdrawal. The patient should first be stabilized on methadone. Clonidine should not be substituted for methadone until the methadone dose has been reduced to 20 mg/day. After an initial oral dose of 0.2 mg of clonidine, patients usually require doses in the range of 0.1 to 0.2 mg every 4–6 hours. The total dose should not exceed 1.2 mg/day. Patients on clonidine should be monitored closely for side effects (particularly hypotension and sedation). Clonidine doses should be withheld for a systolic blood pressure below 90 mm Hg, or a diastolic blood pressure below 60 mm Hg. In an inpatient setting, clonidine can be tapered and discontinued over 3–4 days.[18,19] A transdermal clonidine patch is often applied on the third day. Supplemental doses of lorazepam can also be used to moderate withdrawal-related anxiety. Because clonidine does not adequately suppress the subjective symptoms of withdrawal, as does methadone and buprenorphine, and is relatively ineffective for the treatment of muscle aches and insomnia, it is not acceptable for many opioid-dependent patients.

Buprenorphine has also been effective for the short-term inpatient detoxification of opiate addicts. Patients can usually be detoxified over 3 to 5 days. After a patient shows signs of opiate withdrawal, he or she can be dosed up to buprenorphine/ naloxone 8 mg/2 mg on day 1, and increased to 12 mg/3 mg on day 2. The dose can be cut to 6 mg/1.5 mg on day 3, with additional 2 mg cuts on each of the following days, if required. Opioid-addicted patients usually report that a buprenorphine detoxification is more comfortable than a detoxification with either methadone or clonidine. Rates for successful completion of opiate detoxification with buprenorphine are almost 65% higher than those reported for clonidine.[20]

Chances for successful treatment of withdrawal are enhanced if the patient is aware of the dose and is able to choose a withdrawal schedule within the limits established by the physician. By involving the patient in the treatment process and by using a flexible withdrawal schedule, the physician can keep withdrawal symptoms to a tolerable level. Rigid adherence to a fixed-dosing schedule is less likely to achieve success, and it may lead to premature termination of treatment.

Other techniques can be used for rapid inpatient detoxification from opiates, but they require more intensive medical management. The patient is first stabilized on clonidine as described previously, and 12.5 mg of naltrexone is added orally. Over the next 3 days, clonidine is gradually reduced, while naltrexone is gradually increased (up to a single dose of 150 mg) by the fourth day. A supplemental benzodiazepine is also given for agitation and insomnia. At the end of 5 days, there are no further withdrawal symptoms and the patient can be discharged directly to an outpatient naltrexone program.[19,21] Serious side effects have been reported with this procedure, including a 25% incidence of delirium that has necessitated termination of treatment.[22] A more rapid experimental protocol using high doses of opiate antagonists given under general anesthesia permits completion of detoxification in 48 hours.[23] This approach has not been adequately evaluated in randomized clinical trials, and it cannot be recommended at this time.

Although techniques that permit a safe, rapid, and medically effective detoxification from opiates seem highly attractive in an era of managed care, clinicians must recognize that detoxification alone is rarely successful as a treatment for any addiction. Unless an opiate addict is directly transferred to a long-term residential treatment program, relapse rates following detoxification are extremely high. The resulting costs to the patient, to society, and to the health care system far outweigh any saving realized from a rapid "cost-effective" detoxification protocol.

Discharge planning should be initiated as quickly as possible after admission. For patients who are not already in treatment, several weeks may be required to arrange admission to a drug-free residential program or to an opiate substitution therapy program. Physicians able to provide office-based buprenorphine treatment can be identified via the "physician locator" at the SAMHSA website (http://www.buprenorphine .samhsa.gov) or at the website maintained by the National Alliance of Advocates for Buprenorphine Treatment (www .naabt.com). Because a serious medical illness usually causes a patient with opioid addiction to re-examine his or her behavior and possibly to choose rehabilitation, the treating physician should always emphasize the need for long-term treatment. No individual should be discharged while still receiving methadone unless he or she is returning to a maintenance program or specifically refuses detoxification. Even

when a physician discharges a patient for disciplinary reasons, medical ethics necessitate that the patient be withdrawn from methadone before discharge.

According to federal regulations, hospital-based physicians can treat patients' withdrawal symptoms for detoxification purposes with methadone or buprenorphine as long as the opioid-dependence diagnosis is incidental for that inpatient admission. Similarly, if a patient who has been maintained on methadone by a methadone program, or buprenorphine by an outpatient provider, gets admitted for medical reasons, the hospital-based physicians can keep patients on methadone or buprenorphine for opioid dependence after the treatment team confirms the dose with the outside provider or the methadone program.[24]

Regardless of the form of opiate substitution therapy employed, all patients require supplemental counseling and rehabilitation services; these should include educational and vocational services as needed. CBT has been shown to be much more effective than drug counseling alone. Contingency management has also helped to reduce illicit drug use in patients on maintenance therapy.

Outpatient Detoxification Treatment

The primary purpose of detoxification treatment is to control withdrawal symptoms while gradually reducing the dose of opiates. According to FDA regulations, maintenance clinics may extend outpatient detoxification treatment from 30 to 180 days if a briefer detoxification program is not successful. The procedures described in the previous section can be easily adapted to the outpatient setting. The primary advantage of outpatient detoxification is that a more gradual procedure greatly reduces the severity of withdrawal symptoms. While the procedures previously described for detoxification with clonidine can be used on an outpatient basis, the risks associated with hypotension and sedation have generally limited the use of clonidine to inpatient settings.

With the approval of SL buprenorphine for the treatment of opiate dependence in office-based settings, clinicians have reported success with this drug for outpatient detoxification. Withdrawal symptoms can be adequately controlled within 48 hours using the dosing-induction procedure described for inpatient detoxification. It is rare for patients to require more than 16 mg/4 mg buprenorphine/naloxone to suppress symptoms. Protocols for dose reduction have ranged from 3 to 28 days, with no general consensus on the optimal duration of treatment. All of these protocols have been reported to produce satisfactory results, either equal to, or superior to, methadone, and consistently superior to clonidine. While those who are addicted almost uniformly prefer buprenorphine detoxification to either methadone or clonidine, it is important to remember that there are few data to support the long-term efficacy of any detoxification treatment. For even the most motivated patients, 12-month relapse rates generally exceed 82%.[15]

Pain Management for Patients Receiving Opiate Substitution

Determining the appropriate dosage of pain medications for a patient receiving opiate substitution therapy is a common clinical problem. The analgesic effect of methadone is minimal in maintenance patients, and, at best, lasts only 6 to 8 hours. If pain control is required, an addicted person should be given standard doses of other narcotics in addition to his or her maintenance dose of methadone. Because of cross-tolerance, a patient on maintenance narcotic therapy metabolizes other narcotics more rapidly and may therefore require more frequent administration of analgesics than might a non-addicted patient. Pentazocine and other partial opiate agonists are contraindicated for such patients. Because of their narcotic antagonist effects, these analgesics produce withdrawal symptoms in opiate addicts. If a patient is maintained on the buprenorphine/naloxone combination tablet and requires additional narcotic analgesia treatment, supplemental 2 mg/0.5 mg SL doses of buprenorphine/naloxone every 4–6 hours can be added to the patient's daily maintenance dose. Similar to methadone, buprenorphine will provide more effective analgesia if the daily maintenance dose is divided and administered on a TID schedule. If the patient requires treatment for severe pain, higher-than-usual narcotic doses may be required to overcome the partial antagonist action of buprenorphine. As long as the supplemental opiate is added following the daily buprenorphine dose, there will be no risk of precipitated withdrawal. Dispensing the other opiate before giving the daily buprenorphine dose must be avoided since buprenorphine will displace the other opiate at the receptor and will precipitate withdrawal. Pain in buprenorphine-maintained patients can also be managed with non-opiate analgesics, regional analgesia, or conscious sedation.[25] Alternatively, such patients can be switched to methadone and can be managed as described previously.

Overdose Prevention and Reversal

Opiate overdoses are medical emergencies and they require immediate attention to the maintenance of airway, breathing, and circulation (i.e., ABCs of resuscitation). Opiate-induced respiratory depression can be treated with 0.4 mg/ml of IV or IM naloxone. This medication can be repeated every 2 minutes, as needed (up to a total dose of 2 mg). If the patient does not respond after 20 minutes, he or she should be treated for a combined drug overdose. Because of the long duration of action of methadone and LAAM, overdoses of these drugs often require an IV naloxone drip.

As a response to the prescription pain-reliever epidemic, many states have implemented intranasal Narcan *overdose-prevention programs*. Practitioners caring for those who abuse, or are addicted to, prescription opioids or heroin are advised to educate their patients, as well as family and friends, about the risk of overdose. Intranasal Narcan can be provided free by state public health agencies or prescribed to such high-risk individuals as well as to household members. Between 2007 and 2011, intranasal Narcan reversed more than 1,000 opiate overdoses in Massachusetts.[26]

BENZODIAZEPINES

In 2011, DAWN estimated 357,836 ED visits for non-medical use of prescription benzodiazepines.[3] Benzodiazepines account for 28.7% of all prescription medication-related ED visits, the second highest following narcotic pain-relievers in this category.

Neurobiology

Benzodiazepines, classified as GABA agonists, bind to a subunit of the GABA receptor; of note, GABA is the major inhibitory neurotransmitter in the CNS. Attachment to the receptor opens chloride ion channels and increases the electric gradient across the cell membrane, thus making the neuron less excitable. Their primary clinical effects are sedation, a reduction in anxiety, and an increase in the seizure threshold. Long-term binding to the GABA receptor can alter the number of receptors or change the affinity of the ligand for the receptor.

BOX 16-2 Sedative-hypnotic Withdrawal Symptoms (DSM-IV Diagnostic Criteria)

- Autonomic hyperactivity (sweating or pulse rate over 100)
- Increased hand tremor
- Insomnia
- Nausea or vomiting
- Transient visual, tactile, or auditory hallucinations or illusions
- Psychomotor agitation
- Anxiety
- Grand mal seizures

BOX 16-3 DSM-5 Diagnostic Criteria: Sedative, Hypnotic, or Anxiolytic Intoxication

A. Recent use of a sedative, hypnotic, or anxiolytic.
B. Clinically significant maladaptive behavioral or psychological changes (e.g., inappropriate sexual or aggressive behavior, mood lability, impaired judgment) that developed during, or shortly after, sedative, hypnotic, or anxiolytic use.
C. One (or more) of the following signs or symptoms developing during, or shortly after, sedative, hypnotic, or anxiolytic use:
   1. Slurred speech
   2. Incoordination
   3. Unsteady gait
   4. Nystagmus
   5. Impairment in cognition (e.g., attention, memory)
   6. Stupor or coma.
D. The signs or symptoms are not attributable to another medical condition and are not better explained by another mental disorder, including intoxication with another substance.

Reprinted with permission from the Diagnostic and statistical manual of mental disorders, *ed 5, (Copyright 2013). American Psychiatric Association.*

Patterns of Chronic Use versus Abuse

Benzodiazepines can produce dependence, especially when used in high doses or for prolonged periods. Up to 45% of patients receiving stable, long-term doses show evidence of physiological withdrawal. Withdrawal symptoms, which are usually the same in both high-dose and low-dose patients, include anxiety, insomnia, irritability, depression, tremor, nausea, vomiting, and anorexia. Seizures and psychotic reactions have also been reported. The more common symptoms are similar to those seen during withdrawal from all of the sedative-hypnotic drugs, and they may be difficult to distinguish from the symptoms for which the benzodiazepine was originally prescribed (Box 16-2 contains DSM-IV diagnostic criteria; refer to Box 16.3 for DSM-5 criteria). In general, withdrawal symptoms abate within 2 weeks.

Benzodiazepines (such as diazepam and alprazolam) with a rapid onset of action seem to be sought out by drug abusers and are generally presumed to have a greater potential for abuse than benzodiazepines with a slower onset of action (e.g., oxazepam). Nonetheless, there is relatively little evidence for the abuse of benzodiazepines when they are prescribed for legitimate medical conditions. Ciraulo and collagues[27] found that the use patterns of benzodiazepines, even among former alcoholics, were similar to those of other psychiatric patients. A study of alcoholics conducted at the Addiction Research Foundation of Ontario found that 40% were recent users of benzodiazepines and that there was a 20% life-time incidence of anxiolytic abuse or dependence.[28] Although these studies suggest that concerns about the abuse of benzodiazepines by alcoholics can be exaggerated, the problem can occur in some patients. Anxiolytics may be prescribed to this population, but they should never be a first-line treatment, and patients must always be carefully monitored for signs of abuse. There is no evidence that anxiolytics are effective as a primary treatment for alcoholism or for drug dependence.

It is important to distinguish between a drug abuser who uses benzodiazepines primarily to get high, often deliberately mixing them with alcohol and other drugs of abuse, and an individual who takes benzodiazepines appropriately under medical supervision. In both cases, the user may develop physiological and psychological dependence. Such dependence, in and of itself, is not evidence of addiction or drug abuse. Unless there is evidence of dose escalation, the deliberate use to produce a high, or dangerous states of intoxication, there is no reason to assume that chronic benzodiazepine users are abusers. Even though clonazepam is the only benzodiazepine with an indication for long-term use, common medical practice supports the merit of the continued use of benzodiazepines in some individuals with chronic medical and psychiatric conditions.

Overdose

Flumazenil, a specific benzodiazepine antagonist, reverses the life-threatening effects of a benzodiazepine overdose. An initial IV dose of 0.2 mg should be given over 30 seconds, followed by a second 0.2 mg IV dose if there is no response after 45 seconds. This procedure can be repeated at 1-minute intervals (up to a cumulative dose of 5 mg). This treatment is contraindicated in individuals dependent on benzodiazepines or those taking tricyclic antidepressants (TCAs), because flumazenil may precipitate seizures in these patients.[29,30] When flumazenil is contraindicated, benzodiazepine overdoses should be handled similarly to other sedative-hypnotic overdoses (see the following section).

Withdrawal

In cases in which there is clear evidence of benzodiazepine abuse or when the patient desires to stop using these medications, it is important that detoxification occurs under medical supervision. During the withdrawal process, patients should be warned about a temporary increase in anxiety symptoms. The simplest approach to detoxification is a gradual reduction in dose that may be extended over several weeks or months; under no circumstances should benzodiazepines be stopped abruptly. When a more rapid detoxification is desired, inpatient dosage reduction can be completed within 2 weeks. For some patients, this rapid withdrawal process produces an unacceptable level of subjective distress. An alternative approach is to switch to a high-potency, long-acting benzodiazepine (such as clonazepam). Most patients seem to tolerate detoxification on clonazepam quite well. Because of the prolonged self-taper after completion of detoxification with clonazepam, patients experience a smoother course of withdrawal with a minimum of rebound anxiety.[31,32] An alternative approach for inpatient detoxification is a 3- to 4-day taper using anticonvulsants. Carbamazepine and valproate are the best-studied medications for this purpose, though topiramate and gabapentin are probably effective.

Withdrawal from the high-potency, short-acting benzodiazepines (such as alprazolam) has been particularly problematic. A rapid tapering of these drugs is often poorly tolerated by patients, and a switch to equivalent doses of a long-acting benzodiazepine often allows acute withdrawal symptoms to emerge. In general, clonazepam is substituted for alprazolam, at a dose ratio of 0.5 mg of clonazepam for each 1 mg of alprazolam. Clonazepam should then be continued for 1 to 3 weeks. A drug taper is not always required, although abrupt discontinuation of even a long-acting agent (such as clonazepam) can be associated with a withdrawal syndrome that includes seizures, but it tends to occur several days after discontinuation. A 2- to 3-week taper is usually adequate.

Supplemental medication is of little use during benzodiazepine withdrawal; beta-adrenergic blockers (e.g., propranolol) and alpha-adrenergic agonists (e.g., clonidine) offer no advantage over detoxification using benzodiazepines alone. Although they tend to moderate the severity of physiological symptoms, they are ineffective in controlling the patient's subjective sense of anxiety, and they do not prevent withdrawal seizures or delirium. Buspirone has no cross-tolerance for the benzodiazepines and does not control withdrawal symptoms from this class of drugs.

SEDATIVE-HYPNOTICS
Abuse

Use of CNS depressants accounts for high rates of ED visits related to suicidal attempts and accidental overdoses (consequent to recreational use and self-medication). Although benzodiazepines have become the most commonly abused sedative-hypnotics in the US, there are still areas where the non-medical use of barbiturates (such as butalbital [Fiorinal and Esgic]), carisoprodol (Soma), and other sedative-hypnotics (such as methaqualone, glutethimide) causes serious clinical problems. More recently, a significant increase with zolpidem-related ED visits has been noted.[33]

Clinical Syndromes

A person intoxicated on a CNS depressant typically has many of the same diagnostic features associated with alcohol intoxication. Slurred speech, unsteady gait, and sustained vertical or horizontal nystagmus that occur in the absence of the odor of alcohol on the breath suggest the diagnosis. Unfortunately, since drug abusers frequently combine alcohol with other sedative-hypnotics, the clinician may be misled by the odor of alcohol. The diagnosis of mixed alcohol–barbiturate intoxication can be missed unless a careful history is taken and blood and urine samples are analyzed for toxic drugs. The behavioral effects of barbiturate intoxication can vary widely, even in the same person, and may change significantly depending on the surroundings and on the expectations of the user. Individuals using barbiturates primarily to control anxiety or stress may appear sleepy or mildly confused as a result of an overdose. In young adults seeking to get high, a similar dose may produce excitement, loud boisterous behavior, and loss of inhibitions. The aggressive and even violent behavior commonly associated with alcohol intoxication may follow. The prescribed regimen for managing an angry alcohol abuser can also be used for the disinhibited abuser of sedative-hypnotics.

As tolerance to barbiturates develops, there is no concomitant increase in the lethal dose, as occurs in opiate dependence. Although the opiate addict may be able to double his or her regular dose and still avoid fatal respiratory depression, as little as a 10%–25% increase over the usual daily dosage may be fatal to the barbiturate addict. Thus, a barbiturate overdose should always be considered potentially life-threatening, especially in a drug abuser.

In overdose, a variety of signs and symptoms may be observed, depending on the drug or the combination of drugs used, the amount of time since ingestion, and the presence of complicating medical conditions (e.g., pneumonia, hepatitis, diabetes, heart disease, renal failure, or head injury). Initially the patient appears lethargic or semi-comatose. The pulse rate is slow, but other vital functions are often normal. As the level of intoxication increases, the patient becomes unresponsive to painful stimuli, reflexes disappear, and there is a gradual depression of the respiratory rate; eventually cardiovascular collapse ensues. Pupillary size is not changed by barbiturate intoxication, but secondary anoxia may cause fixed, dilated pupils. In persons who have adequate respiratory function, pin-point pupils usually indicate an opiate overdose or the combined ingestion of barbiturates and opiates. Such patients should be observed carefully for increased lethargy and for progressive respiratory depression. Appropriate measures for treating overdoses should be instituted as necessary. Patients should not be left unattended until all signs of intoxication have cleared.

Because there is no cross-tolerance between narcotics and barbiturates, special problems are presented by patients receiving methadone or buprenorphine maintenance who continue to abuse sedative-hypnotics. If a barbiturate overdose is suspected, the opiate-dependent patient should be given a narcotic antagonist to counteract any respiratory depression caused by the opiate. Naloxone hydrochloride (Narcan) 0.4 mg is given IM or IV because it is a pure narcotic antagonist and it has no respiratory depressant effect, even in large doses. If respiratory depression does not improve after treatment with naloxone, the patient should be treated for a pure barbiturate overdose. Supportive measures include maintenance of adequate airway, mechanic ventilation, alkalinization of the urine, correction of acid–base disorders, and diuresis with furosemide or mannitol. Severe overdose cases may require dialysis or charcoal resin hemoperfusion.[30]

Withdrawal

Withdrawal from sedative-hypnotics can present with a wide variety of signs and symptoms (including anxiety, insomnia, hyperreflexia, diaphoresis, nausea, and vomiting), or sometimes delirium and convulsions. As a general rule, individuals who ingest 600 to 800 mg/day of secobarbital for more than 45 days develop physiological addiction and show symptoms after taper or discontinuation. Minor withdrawal symptoms usually begin within 24–36 hours after the last dose. Pulse and respiration rates are usually elevated, pupil size is normal, and there may be postural hypotension. Fever may develop, and dangerous hyperpyrexia can occur in severe cases. Major withdrawal symptoms (such as convulsions and delirium) indicate addiction to large doses (more than 900 mg/day of secobarbital).

Because of the danger of convulsions, barbiturate withdrawal should be carried out only on an inpatient basis. Grand mal seizures, if they occur, are usually seen between the third and seventh days, although there have been cases reported of convulsions occurring as late as 14 days after the completion of a medically controlled detoxification. Withdrawal seizures are thought to be related to a rapid drop in the blood barbiturate level. Treatment should therefore be carefully controlled so that barbiturates are withdrawn gradually, with minimal fluctuation in the blood barbiturate level. Theoretically, this should decrease the danger of convulsions. Treatment with phenytoin does not prevent convulsions caused by barbiturate withdrawal, although it controls convulsions caused by epilepsy.

Withdrawal delirium occurs less frequently than do convulsions, and it rarely appears unless preceded by convulsions. It usually begins between the fourth and sixth days after drug use is stopped and is characterized by both visual and auditory hallucinations, delusions, and fluctuating level of consciousness. The presence of confusion, hyperreflexia, and fever helps distinguish this syndrome from schizophrenia and other nontoxic psychoses.

Treatment for Withdrawal

Several techniques are available for the management of barbiturate withdrawal. The basic principle is to withdraw the addicting agent slowly to avoid convulsions. First, the daily dosage that produces mild toxicity must be established. Because barbiturate addicts tend to underestimate their drug use, it is dangerous to accept the patient's history as completely accurate. Treatment should begin with an oral test dose of 200 mg of pentobarbital, a short-acting barbiturate. If no physical changes occur after 1 hour, the patient's habit probably exceeds 1,200 mg of pentobarbital per day. If the patient shows only nystagmus and no other signs of intoxication, the habit is probably about 800 mg/day. Evidence of slurred speech and intoxication, but not sleep, suggests a habit of 400 to 600 mg/day. The patient can then be given the estimated daily requirement divided into four equal doses administered orally every 6 hours. Should signs of withdrawal appear, the estimated daily dosage can be increased by 25% following an additional dose of 200 mg of pentobarbital given intramuscularly. After a daily dose that produces only mild toxicity has been established, phenobarbital is substituted for pentobarbital (30 mg phenobarbital equals 100 mg pentobarbital) and then withdrawn at a rate of 30 to 60 mg/day[34] (Table 16-3).

The long-acting barbiturate phenobarbital is the drug of choice for managing detoxification for drugs in this class. Cross-tolerance with benzodiazepines is incomplete. A dose of 30 mg of phenobarbital can be substituted for each 100 mg of other barbiturates, or 200 mg of meprobamate or 400 mg of carisoprodol (Soma). An alternative method is to treat emerging withdrawal symptoms orally with 30 to 60 mg of phenobarbital hourly, as needed, for 2–7 days. After the patient has received similar 24-hour doses for 2 consecutive days, the 24-hour stabilizing dose is given in divided doses every 3 to 6 hours. A gradual taper is then instituted as described previously. This latter method is recommended because the use of a long-acting barbiturate produces fewer variations in the blood barbiturate level and should produce a smoother withdrawal.

TABLE 16-3 Equivalent Doses of Common Sedative-Hypnotics

Generic Name	Dose (mg)
BARBITURATES	
Phenobarbital	30
Secobarbital	100
Pentobarbital	100
BENZODIAZEPINES	
Alprazolam	1
Diazepam	10
Chlordiazepoxide	25
Lorazepam	2
Clonazepam	0.5–1
OTHERS	
Meprobamate	400

Inpatient Management and Referral

Those addicted to sedative-hypnotic drugs can present with a variety of psychological management problems. Effective treatment requires a thorough evaluation of the patient's psychiatric problems and the development of long-term treatment plans before discharge. Treatment for withdrawal or overdose presents an opportunity for effective intervention for the addict's self-destructive lifestyle. Drug abuse patients have a reputation for deceit, manipulation, and hostility. They frequently sign out against medical advice. It is rarely acknowledged that these problems are sometimes caused by clinicians who fail to give appropriate attention to the patient's psychological problems. Most of these difficulties can be eliminated by effective medical and psychiatric management. The patient's lack of cooperation and frequent demands for additional drugs are often the result of anxiety and the fear of withdrawal seizures. This anxiety is greatly relieved if the physician thoroughly explains the withdrawal procedure and assures the patient that the staff members know how to handle withdrawal and that convulsions will be avoided if the patient cooperates with a schedule of medically supervised withdrawal.

Physicians sometimes fail to realize that the patient's tough, demanding behavior is a defense against a strong sense of personal inadequacy and a fear of rejection. Addicts have been conditioned to expect rejection and hostility from medical personnel. The trust and cooperation necessary for successful treatment cannot be established unless physicians show by their behavior that they are both genuinely concerned about the patient and medically competent to treat withdrawal. Physicians can expect an initial period of defensive hostility and testing behavior and should not take this behavior personally. Patients need to be reassured that their physician is sincerely concerned about them.

If the patient manifests signs of a character disorder and has a history of severe drug abuse, the setting of firm limits is necessary to ensure successful treatment. Visitors must be limited to those individuals of known reliability. This may mean excluding spouses and other relatives. Urine should be monitored periodically for use of illicit drugs. Family counseling should be started during hospitalization and should focus on the family's role in helping the patient develop a successful long-term treatment program. Hospital passes should not be granted until detoxification is completed; however, passes with staff members as escorts should be used as much as possible. An active program of recreational and physical therapy is necessary to keep young, easily-bored patients occupied. Keys to successful inpatient treatment are summarized in Box 16-4.

Because treatment for detoxification or for an overdose rarely cures an addict, referrals for long-term outpatient or residential care should be made early in the treatment process. Ideally, the patient should meet the future therapist before discharge. Alcoholics Anonymous and Narcotics Anonymous are useful adjuncts to any outpatient treatment program. If transferring to a halfway house or residential program, the patient should move there directly from the hospital. Addicts are not likely to execute plans for follow-up care without strong encouragement and support.

Bath Salts

Since 2010 there has been a rapid increase in the number of reports of the abuse of various synthetic derivatives of methcathinone, either mephedrone or methylenedioxypyrovalerone (MDPV).[35] These compounds are DEA schedule I substances that are considered illegal only if intended for human consumption. Typically they have been sold legally and labeled "plant food or bath salts, not for human consumption," though it is apparent that they were never intended for use as bath salts. In 2011, the DEA, using its emergency scheduling authority, made sale and possession of these substances illegal in the US. These substances are derived from Khat (or qat; *Catha edulis*), a flowering plant from East Africa. They contain cathione, an amphetamine analogue and they have been chewed in some African cultures for centuries. Recently, cathinone has been isolated from the Khat plant and has been transformed into the more potent methcathinone (ephedrine).[36] It is sold as a white or tan crystalline powder that can be ingested orally, or administered nasally, rectally, IM, or IV. The average dose is 5 to 20 mg; psychoactive effects begin at 3 to 5 mg. The typical package contains 500 mg, thus creating a high risk for overdose. Consumption increases intracellular dopamine and serotonin by their effects on dopamine and serotonin reuptake transporters. Prolonged exposure leads to addictive patterns of use. Subjective effects include euphoria, empathic mood, sexual stimulation, greater mental focus, and enhanced energy (users typically report feelings similar to those produced by MDMA). The peak "rush" occurs at 90 minutes, with effects lasting for 3–4 hours. The total experience lasts for 6–8 hours and it is often followed by a crash. More intense psychic effects can include panic attacks, agitation, paranoia, hallucinations, psychosis, and aggressive, violent, or bizarre self-destructive behavior; use may also lead to anorexia, delirium, and depression. Physical effects included tachycardia, hypertension, mydriasis, arrhythmias, hyperthermia, sweating, rhabdomyolysis, seizures, stroke, cerebral edema, myocardial infarction, cardiovascular collapse, and death. The differential diagnosis includes abuse of cocaine, amphetamines, LSD or PCP, as well as serotonin syndrome, neuroleptic malignant syndrome, or anticholinergic toxicity. Bath salts will not be detected by routine toxic screens. Clinical management usually involves benzodiazepines for acute agitation; antipsychotics should be used with caution because of the risk of rhabdomyolysis, arrhythmias, seizures, and NMS. Cardiac monitoring, and IV fluids are recommended; autonomic instability may require monitoring in an ICU.

MIXED-DRUG ADDICTION

Increasing numbers of patients are addicted to varying combinations of drugs, including benzodiazepines, cocaine, alcohol, and opiates. Accurate diagnosis is difficult because of confusing, inconsistent physical findings and unreliable histories. Blood and urine tests for drugs are required to confirm the diagnosis. A patient who is addicted to both opiates and sedative-hypnotics should be maintained on

---

BOX 16-4 Inpatient Management and Referral: Keys to Successful Inpatient Treatment

- Perform a psychiatric evaluation
- Develop a long-term treatment plan
- Demonstrate explicit concern and expertise
- Expect testing behavior
- Set appropriate limits
- Limit and monitor visitors
- Supervise passes
- Monitor urine for illicit drug use
- Encourage ward activities and recreation
- Initiate family/network therapy
- Treat with respect

TABLE 16-4 Equivalent Doses of Narcotic Pain Medications

Generic Name	Parenteral Dose (mg)
Morphine	10
Oxycodone (Percocet, OxyContin)	5–10
Hydrocodone (Vicodin, Lortab)	10
Meperidine (Demerol)	100
Hydromorphone (Dilaudid)	2.5
Methadone	5
Heroin	10

methadone or buprenorphine while the barbiturate or other sedative-hypnotic is withdrawn. Then the methadone or buprenorphine can be withdrawn in the usual manner. Dose equivalents of narcotics are provided in Table 16-4.

Behavioral problems should be dealt with as previously described. Firm limit-setting is essential to the success of any effective psychological treatment program. Some patients who overdose or have medical problems secondary to drug abuse (such as subacute bacterial endocarditis and hepatitis) are not physiologically addicted to any drug despite a history of multiple-drug abuse. Their drug abuse behavior is usually associated with severe psychopathology. These patients should receive a thorough psychiatric evaluation and may require long-term treatment.

 Access a list of MCQs for this chapter at https://expertconsult .inkling.com

REFERENCES

1. O'Brien CP, McLellan AT. Myths about the treatment of addiction. *Lancet* 347:237–240, 1996.
2. Substance Abuse and Mental Health Services Administration. *Results from the 2011 National Survey on Drug Use and Health: Summary of National Findings*, NSDUH Series H-44, HHS Publication No. (SMA) 12-4713, Rockville, MD, 2012, Substance Abuse and Mental Health Services Administration.
3. Substance Abuse and Mental Health Services Administration. *Drug Abuse Warning Network, 2011: National Estimates of Drug-Related Emergency Department Visits*, HHS Publication No. (SMA) 13-4760, DAWN Series D-39, Rockville, MD, 2013, Substance Abuse and Mental Health Services Administration.
4. Boscarino J, Rukstalis M, Hoffman S. Prevalence of prescription opioid-use disorder among chronic pain patients: Comparison of the DSM-5 vs. DSM-4 diagnostic criteria. *J Addict Dis* 30(3):185–194, 2011.
5. Volkow ND, Fowler JS, Wang GJ. The addicted human brain: insights from imaging studies. *J Clin Invest* 111:1444–1451, 2003.
6. Gawin F, Kleber H. Abstinence symptomatology and psychiatric diagnosis in cocaine abusers. *Arch Gen Psychiatry* 43:107–113, 1986.
7. Carroll KM. Relapse prevention as a psychosocial treatment approach: a review of controlled clinical trials. *Exp Clin Psychopharmacol* 4:46–54, 1996.
8. American Psychiatric Association. Practice guidelines: treatment of patients with substance use disorders. *Am J Psychiatry* 163(Suppl.):8, 2006.
9. Johnston LD, O'Malley PM, Bachman JG, et al. *Monitoring the Future national results on drug use: 2012 Overview, Key Findings on Adolescent Drug Use*, Ann Arbor, 2013, Institute for Social Research, The University of Michigan.
10. Centers for Disease Control and Prevention. Reported US AIDS cases by HIV-exposure category—1994. *MMWR* 44:4, 1995.
11. Substance Abuse and Mental Health Services Administration, Center for Behavioral Health Statistics and Quality. *Drug Abuse Warning Network, 2008: National Estimates of Drug-Related Emergency Department Visits*, HHS Publication No. SMA 11–4618, Rockville, MD, 2011, HHS.
12. CDC. Vital Signs: Overdoses of Prescription Opioid Pain Relievers—United States, 1999–2008. *MMWR* 60:1–6, 2011.
13. American Psychiatric Association. *Diagnostic and statistical manual of mental disorders*, ed 5, Washington, DC, 2013, American Psychiatric Association.
14. Ling W, Charuvastra C, Collins JF, et al. Buprenorphine maintenance treatment of opiate dependence: a multicenter, randomized clinical trial. *Addiction* 93:475–486, 1998.
15. Ball JC, Ross A. *The effectiveness of methadone maintenance treatment*, New York, 1991, Springer-Verlag.
16. US Department of Health and Human Services, Substance Abuse and Mental Health Services Administration, Center for Substance Abuse Treatment. *Evaluation of the buprenorphine waiver program*, Presented at American Society of Addiction Medicine. San Diego, May 5, 2006.
17. Fultz JM, Senay EC. Guidelines for the management of hospitalized narcotics addicts. *Ann Intern Med* 82:815–818, 1975.
18. Charney DS, Sternberg DE, Kleber HD, et al. The clinical use of clonidine in abrupt withdrawal from methadone. *Arch Gen Psychiatry* 38:1273–1277, 1981.
19. Jaffe JH, Kleber HD. Opioids: general issues and detoxification. In American Psychiatric Association: *Treatment of psychiatric disorders: a task force report of the American Psychiatric Association*, vol. 2, Washington, DC, 1989, American Psychiatric Association.
20. Fingerhood MI, Thompson MR, Jasinski DR. A comparison of clonidine and buprenorphine in the outpatient treatment of opiate withdrawal. *Subst Abus* 22:193–199, 2001.
21. O'Connor PG, Waugh ME, Carrol KM, et al. Primary care-based ambulatory opioid detoxification. *J Gen Intern Med* 10:255–260, 1995.
22. Golden SA, Sakhrani DL. Unexpected delirium during rapid opioid detoxification (ROD). *Addict Dis* 23(1):65–75, 2004.
23. Legarda JJ, Gossop M. A 24-h inpatient detoxification treatment for heroin addicts: a preliminary investigation. *Drug Alcohol Depend* 35:91–95, 1994.
24. Code of Federal Regulations, Chapter II, Drug Enforcement Administration, Department of Justice (4-1-04 Edition). § 1306.07 Administering or dispensing of narcotic drugs.
25. Alford DP, Compton P, Samet JH. Acute pain management for patients receiving maintenance methadone or buprenorphine therapy. *Ann Intern Med* 144:127–134, 2006.
26. Massachusetts Department of Public Health (MDPH). Overdose Education and Naloxone Distribution (OEND) Program Data, 2011.
27. Ciraulo D, Sands B, Shader R. Critical review of liability for benzodiazepine abuse among alcoholics. *Am J Psychiatry* 145:1501–1506, 1988.
28. Ross HE. Benzodiazepine use and anxiolytic abuse and dependence in treated alcoholics. *Addiction* 88:209–218, 1993.
29. Weinbroum A, Halpern P, Geller E. The use of flumazenil in the management of acute drug poisoning: a review. *Intensive Care Med* 17(Suppl. 1):S32–S38, 1991.
30. Wiviott SD, Wiviott-Tishler L, Hyman SE. Sedative-hypnotics and anxiolytics. In Friedman L, Fleming NF, Roberts DH, et al., editors: *Source book of substance abuse and addiction*, Baltimore, 1996, Williams & Wilkins.
31. Herman JB, Rosenbaum JF, Brotman AN. The alprazolam to clonazepam switch for the treatment of panic disorder. *J Clin Psychopharmacol* 7:175–178, 1987.
32. Patterson JF. Withdrawal from alprazolam dependency using clonazepam: clinical observations. *J Clin Psychiatry* 51:47–49, 1990.
33. SAMHSA, Center For Behavioral Health Statistics and Quality. The Dawn Report. *Emergency department visits for adverse reactions involving the insomnia medication Zolpidem*, Rockville, MD, 2013, SAMHSA.
34. Smith DE, Wesson DR. Phenobarbital technique for treatment of barbiturate dependence. *Arch Gen Psychiatry* 24:56–60, 1971.
35. Ross EA, Watson M, Goldberger B. "Bath salts" intoxication. *N Engl J Med* 365(10):967–968, 2011.
36. Coppola M, Mondola R. Synthetic cathinones: Chemistry, pharmacology and toxicology of a new class of designer drugs of abuse marketed as "bath salts" or "plant food". *Toxicol Lett* 211(2):144–149, 2012.
37. Syed YY, Keating GM. Extended-release intramuscular naltrexone (VIVITROL®): a review of its use in the prevention of relapse to opioid dependence in detoxified patients. *CNS Drugs* 27(10):851–861, 2013.

SUGGESTED READING

Carroll KM. *A cognitive-behavioral approach: treating cocaine addiction. NIDA therapy manuals for drug addiction series (DHHS pub no ADM 98–4308)*, Rockville, MD, 1998, National Institute on Drug Abuse.

Galanter M, Kleber HD, editors: *The American Psychiatric Publishing textbook of substance abuse treatment*, ed 3, Washington, DC, 2004, American Psychiatric Publishing, Inc.

Graham AW, Schultz TK, Mayo-Smith MF, et al., editors: *Principles of addiction medicine*, ed 3, Chevy Chase, MD, 2007, American Society of Addiction Medicine.

Kranzler HR, Ciraulo DA. *Clinical manual of addiction psychopharmacology*, Washington, DC, 2005, American Psychiatric Publishing, Inc.

McNicholas L, Howell EF. *Buprenorphine clinical practice guidelines*, Rockville, MD, 2000, Substance Abuse Mental Health Services Administration, Center for Substance Abuse Treatment. Available at: <http://www.buprenorphine.samhsa.gov>.

Miller WR, Rollnick S. *Motivational interviewing: preparing people for change*, ed 2, New York, 2002, Guilford Press.

Smith DE, Wesson DR. *Diagnosis and treatment of adverse reactions to sedative-hypnotics*, (DHHS pub no ADM 75–144), Rockville, MD, 1974, National Institute on Drug Abuse.

17 Pathophysiology, Psychiatric Co-morbidity, and Treatment of Pain

Ajay D. Wasan, MD, MSc, Menekse Alpay, MD, and Shamim H. Nejad, MD

KEY POINTS

- There is a high rate of psychiatric co-morbidity in patients with pain syndromes.
- Specific terminology is used to characterize pain and pain syndromes.
- Pain is transmitted in pathways involving the peripheral and central nervous systems.
- Psychiatric treatment can be effective for pain and the psychiatric co-morbidities of pain.
- Multimodal and multidisciplinary treatment facilitates provision of the highest-quality care for chronic pain.

OVERVIEW

Pain, as determined by the International Association for the Study of Pain (IASP), is "an unpleasant sensory and emotional experience associated with actual or potential tissue damage or described in terms of such damage."[1] This chapter will describe the physiological aspects of pain transmission, pain terminology, and pain assessment; discuss the major classes of medications used to relieve pain; and outline the diagnosis and treatment of psychiatric conditions that often affect patients with chronic pain.

EPIDEMIOLOGY

Psychiatric co-morbidity (e.g., anxiety, depression, personality disorders, and substance use disorders [SUDs]) afflicts those with both non-cancer-related and cancer-related pain. Epidemiological studies indicate that roughly 30% of those in the general population with chronic musculoskeletal pain also have depression or an anxiety disorder.[2] Similar rates exist in those with cancer pain.[3] In clinic populations, 50%–80% of pain patients have co-morbid psychopathology, including problematic personality traits. The personality (i.e., the characterological or temperamental) component of negative affect has been termed *neuroticism*, which may be best described as "a general personality maladjustment in which patients experience anger, disgust, sadness, anxiety, and a variety of other negative emotions."[4] Frequently, in pain clinics, maladaptive expressions of depression, anxiety, and anger are grouped together as disorders of negative affect, which have an adverse impact on the response to pain.[5]

Rates of substance dependence in chronic pain patients are also elevated relative to the general population, and several studies have found that 15%–26% of chronic pain patients have an SUD, including illicit drugs or prescription medications.[6] Prescription opiate addiction is a growing problem that affects approximately 5% of those who have been prescribed opiates for chronic pain, although good epidemiology studies are lacking. This chapter will concentrate on those with

affective disorders and somatoform disorders in the setting of chronic pain.

While many chronic pain patients experience somatization and have difficulty adapting to pain, a *Diagnostic and Statistical Manual of Mental Disorders*, ed 4, Text Revision (DSM-IV-TR) diagnosis of somatization disorder, *per se*, is less frequently encountered by those who treat patients with chronic pain. The DSM-IV-TR accounts for this distinction by classifying the somatoform component of a pain disorder into several categories (such as pain disorder associated with psychological factors, pain disorder associated with psychological factors and a general medical condition, and somatization disorder). With some degree of controversy, in DSM-5, some individuals with chronic pain would be diagnosed as having somatic symptom disorder, with predominant pain. For others, psychological factors affecting other medical conditions or an adjustment disorder would be more appropriate.

PATHOPHYSIOLOGY OF PAIN TRANSMISSION

Detection of noxious stimuli (i.e., nociception) starts with the activation of peripheral nociceptors (resulting in somatic pain) or with the activation of nociceptors in bodily organs (leading to visceral pain).

Tissue injury stimulates the nociceptors by the liberation of adenosine triphosphate (ATP), protons, kinins, and arachidonic acid from the injured cells; histamine, serotonin, prostaglandins, and bradykinin from the mast cells; and cytokines and nerve growth factor from the macrophages. These substances and decreased pH cause a decrease in the threshold for activation of the nociceptors, a process called *peripheral sensitization*. Subsequently, axons transmit the pain signal to the spinal cord, and to cell bodies in the dorsal root ganglia (Figure 17-1). Three different types of axons are involved in the transmission of pain from the skin to the dorsal horn. A-β fibers are the largest and most heavily myelinated fibers that transmit awareness of light touch. A-Δ fibers and C fibers are the primary nociceptive afferents. A-Δ fibers are 2 to 5 μcm in diameter and are thinly myelinated. They conduct "first pain," which is immediate, rapid, and sharp, with a velocity of 20 m/sec. C fibers are 0.2 to 1.5 μcm in diameter and are unmyelinated. They conduct "second pain," which is prolonged, burning, and unpleasant, at a speed of 0.5 m/sec.

A-Δ and C fibers enter the dorsal root and ascend or descend one to three segments before synapsing with neurons in the lateral spinothalamic tract (in the substantia gelatinosa in the gray matter) (see Figure 17-1). Second pain transmitted with C fibers is integrally related to chronic pain states. Repetitive C-fiber stimulation can result in a progressive increase of electrical discharges from second-order neurons in the spinal cord. NMDA receptors play a role when prolonged activation occurs. This pain amplification is related to a temporal summation of second pain or "wind-up." This hyperexcitability of neurons in the dorsal horn contributes to central sensitization, which can occur as an immediate or as a delayed phenomenon. In addition to wind-up, central sensitization involves several factors: activation of A-β fibers and lowered firing thresholds for spinal cord cells that modulate pain (i.e., they trigger pain

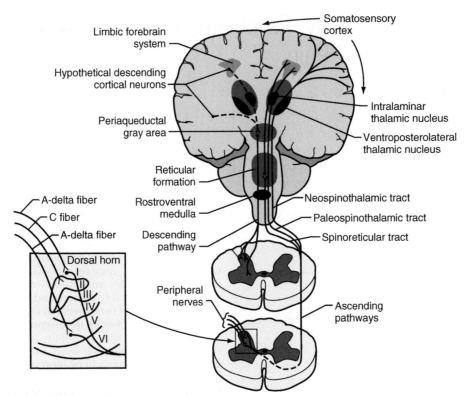

Figure 17-1. Schematic diagram of neurological pathways for pain perception. *(From Hyman SH, Cassem NH. Pain. In Rubenstein E, Fedeman DD, editors: Scientific American medicine: current topics in medicine, subsection II, New York, 1989, Scientific American. Originally from Stern TA, Herman JB, editors.* Psychiatry update and board preparation, *New York, 2004, McGraw-Hill.)*

more easily); neuroplasticity (a result of functional changes, including recruitment of a wide range of cells in the spinal cord so that touch or movement causes pain); convergence of cutaneous, vascular, muscle, and joint inputs (where one tissue refers pain to another); or aberrant connections (electrical short-circuits between the sympathetic and sensory nerves that produce causalgia). Inhibition of nociception in the dorsal horn is functionally quite important. Stimulation of the A-Δ fibers not only excites some neurons but also inhibits others. This inhibition of nociception through A-Δ fiber stimulation may explain the effects of acupuncture and transcutaneous electrical nerve stimulation (TENS).

The lateral spinothalamic tract crosses the midline and ascends toward the thalamus. At the level of the brainstem, more than half of this tract synapses in the reticular activating system (in an area called the spinoreticular tract), in the limbic system, and in other brainstem regions (including centers of the autonomic nervous system). Another site of projections at this level is the periaqueductal gray (PAG) (Figure 17-2), which plays an important role in the brain's system of endogenous analgesia. After synapsing in the thalamic nuclei, pain fibers project to the somatosensory cortex, located posterior to the Sylvian fissure in the parietal lobe, in Brodmann's areas 1, 2, and 3. Endogenous analgesic systems involve endogenous peptides with opioid-like activity in the central nervous system (CNS) (e.g., endorphins, enkephalins, and dynorphins). Different opioid receptors (mu, kappa, and delta receptors) are involved in different effects of opiates. The centers involved in endogenous analgesia include the PAG, the anterior cingulate cortex (ACC), the amygdala, the parabrachial plexus (in the pons), and the rostral ventromedial medulla.

The descending analgesic pain pathway starts in the PAG (which is rich in endogenous opiates), projects to the rostral

ventral medulla, and from there descends through the dorsolateral funiculus of the spinal cord to the dorsal horn. The neurons in the rostral ventral medulla use serotonin to activate endogenous analgesics (enkephalins) in the dorsal horn. This effect inhibits nociception at the level of the dorsal horn since neurons that contain enkephalins synapse with spinothalamic neurons. Additionally, there are noradrenergic neurons that project from the locus coeruleus (the main noradrenergic center in the CNS) to the dorsal horn and inhibit the response of dorsal horn neurons to nociceptive stimuli. The analgesic effect of tricyclic antidepressants (TCAs) and the serotonin-norepinephrine reuptake inhibitors (SNRIs) is thought to be related to an increase in serotonin and norepinephrine (noradrenaline) that inhibits nociception at the level of the dorsal horn, through their effects on enhancing descending pain inhibition from above.

CORTICAL SUBSTRATES FOR PAIN AND AFFECT

Advances in neuroimaging have linked the function of multiple areas in the brain with pain and affect. These areas (e.g., the ACC, the insula, and the dorsolateral prefrontal cortex [DLPFC]) form functional units through which psychiatric co-morbidity may amplify pain and disability (see Figure 17-2). These areas are part of the spinolimbic (also known as the medial) pain pathway,[7] which runs parallel to the spinothalamic tract and receives direct input from the dorsal horn of the spinal cord. The interactions among the function of these areas, pain perception, and psychiatric illness are still being investigated. The spinolimbic pathway is involved in descending pain inhibition (which includes cortical and subcortical structures), whose function may be negatively affected by the presence of psychopathology. This, in turn, could lead to heightened pain perception. Coghill and colleagues[8] have shown that differences in

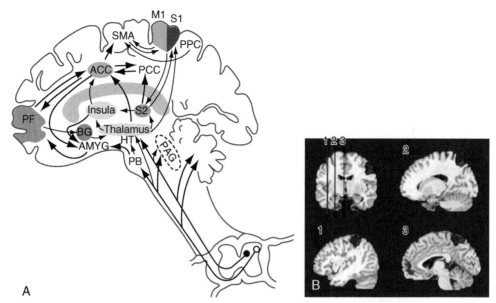

Figure 17-2. Pain processing in the brain. Locations of brain regions involved in pain perception are color-coded in a schematic A and in an example magnetic resonance imaging (MRI) scan B. (A) Schematic shows the regions, their inter-connectivity, and afferent pathways. (B) The areas corresponding to those in part A are shown in an anatomical MRI, on a coronal slice, and on three sagittal slices as indicated on the coronal slice. The six areas used in meta-analysis are primary and secondary somatosensory cortices (S1 and S2, red and orange), anterior cingulated (ACC, green), insula (blue), thalamus (yellow), and prefrontal cortex (PF, purple) Other regions indicated include primary and supplementary motor cortices (M1 and SMA), posterior parietal cortex (PPC), posterior cingulated (PCC), basal ganglia (BG, pink), hypothalamic (HT), amygdala (AMYG), parabrachial nuclei (PB), and periaqueductal gray (PAG). *(Redrawn from Apkarian AV, Bushnell MC, Treede RD, Zubieta JK. Human brain mechanisms of pain perception and regulation in health and disease,* Eur J Pain *9:463–484, 2005.)*

pain sensitivity between patients can be correlated with differences in activation patterns in the ACC, the insula, and the DLPFC. The anticipation of pain is also modulated by these areas, suggesting a mechanism by which anxiety about pain can amplify pain perception. The disruption or alteration of descending pain inhibition is a mechanism of neuropathic pain, which can be described as *central sensitization* that occurs at the level of the brain, a concept supported by recent neuroimaging studies of pain processing in the brains of patients with fibromyalgia.[9] The ACC, the insula, and the DLPFC are also laden with opioid receptors, which are less responsive to endogenous opioids in pain-free subjects with high negative affect.[10] Thus, negative affect may diminish the effectiveness of endogenous and exogenous opioids through direct effects on supraspinal opioid binding.

INTERACTIONS BETWEEN PAIN AND PSYCHOPATHOLOGY

The majority of patients with chronic pain and a psychiatric condition have an organic or physical basis for their pain. However, the perception of pain is amplified by co-morbid psychiatric disorders, which predispose patients to develop a chronic pain syndrome. This is commonly referred to as the *diathesis-stress model,* in which the combination of physical, social, and psychological stresses associated with a pain syndrome induces significant psychiatric co-morbidity.[5] This can occur in patients with or without a pre-existing vulnerability to psychiatric illness (e.g., a genetic or temperamental risk factor). Regardless of the order of onset of psychopathology, patients with chronic pain and psychopathology report greater pain intensity, more pain-related disability, and a larger affective component to their pain than those without psychopathology. As a whole, studies indicate that it is not the specific qualities or symptomatology of depression, anxiety, or neuroticism, but the overall levels of psychiatric symptoms that are predictive of

poor outcome.[11] Depression, anxiety, and neuroticism are the psychiatric conditions that most often co-occur in patients with chronic pain, and those with a combination of pathologies are predisposed to the worst outcomes.

PAIN TERMINOLOGY

Acute pain is usually related to an identifiable injury or to a disease; it is self-limited, and resolves over hours to days or in a time frame that is associated with injury and healing. Acute pain is usually associated with objective autonomic features (e.g., tachycardia, hypertension, diaphoresis, mydriasis, or pallor).

Chronic pain (i.e., pain that persists beyond the normal time of healing or lasts longer than 6 months) involves different mechanisms in local, spinal, and supraspinal levels. Characteristic features include vague descriptions of pain and an inability to describe the pain's timing and localization. It is usually helpful to determine the presence of a dermatomal pattern (Figure 17-3), to determine the presence of neuropathic pain, and to assess pain behavior.

Neuropathic pain is a disorder of neuromodulation. It is caused by an injured or dysfunctional central or peripheral nervous system; it is manifest by spontaneous, sharp, shooting, or burning pain, which may be distributed along dermatomes. Deafferentation pain, phantom limb pain, complex regional pain syndrome, diabetic neuropathy, central pain syndrome, trigeminal neuralgia, and postherpetic neuralgia are examples of neuropathic pain. Qualities of neuropathic pain include hyperalgesia (an increased response to stimuli that are normally painful); hyperesthesia (an exaggerated pain response to noxious stimuli [e.g., pressure or heat]); allodynia (pain with a stimulus not normally painful [e.g., light touch or cool air]); and hyperpathia (pain from a painful stimulus with a delay and a persistence that is distributed beyond the area of stimulation). Both acute and chronic pain conditions

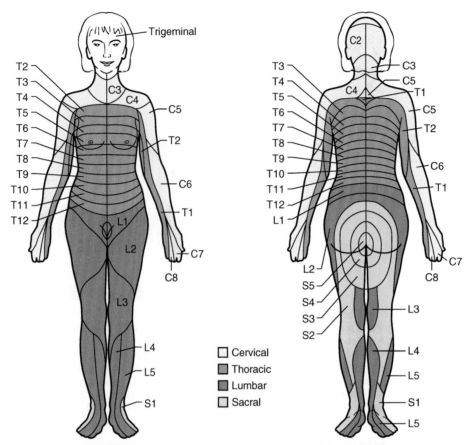

Figure 17-3. Schematic diagram of segmental neuronal innervation by dermatomes. *(From Hyman SH, Cassem NH. Pain. In Rubenstein E, Fedeman DD, editors: Scientific American medicine: current topics in medicine, subsection II, New York, 1989, Scientific American. Originally from Stern TA, Herman JB, editors. Psychiatry update and board preparation, New York, 2004, McGraw-Hill.)*

can involve neuropathic processes in addition to nociceptive causes of pain.

Idiopathic pain, previously referred to as *psychogenic pain*, is poorly understood. The presence of pain does not imply or exclude a psychological component. Typically, there is no evidence of an associated organic etiology or an anatomical pattern consistent with symptoms. Symptoms are often grossly out of proportion to an identifiable organic pathology.

Myofascial pain can arise from one or several of the following problems: hypertonic muscles, myofascial trigger points, arthralgias, and fatigue with muscle weakness. Myofascial pain is generally used to describe pain from muscles and connective tissue. Myofascial pain results from a primary diagnosis (e.g., fibromyalgia) or, as more often is the case, a co-morbid diagnosis (e.g., with vascular headache or with a psychiatric diagnosis).

ASSESSMENT OF PAIN

The evaluation of pain focuses first on five questions: (1) Is the pain intractable because of nociceptive stimuli (e.g., from the skin, bones, muscles, or blood vessels)? (2) Is the pain maintained by non-nociceptive mechanisms (i.e., have the spinal cord, brainstem, limbic system, and cortex been recruited as reverberating pain circuits)? (3) Is the complaint of pain primary (as occurs in disorders such as major depression or delusional disorder)? (4) Is there a more efficacious pharmacological treatment? (5) Have pain behavior and disability become more important than the pain itself? Answering these questions allows the mechanism(s) of the pain and suffering to be pursued. A psychiatrist's physical examination

of the pain patient typically includes examination of the painful area, muscles, and response to pinprick and light touch (Table 17-1).

The experience of pain is always subjective. However, several sensitive and reliable clinical instruments for the measurement of pain are available. These include the following:

1. The *pain drawing* involves having the patient draw the anatomical distribution of the pain as it is felt in his or her body.
2. The *Visual Analog Scale* and *Numerical Rating Scales* employ a visual analog scale from "no pain" to "pain as bad as it could possibly be" on a 10 cm baseline, or a 0 to 10 scale where the patient can rate pain on a scale of 1 to 10. It is also exquisitely sensitive to change; consequently, the patient can mark this scale once a day or even hourly during treatment trials, if desired.
3. The *Pain Intensity Scale* is a categorical rating scale that consists of three to six categories for the ranking of pain severity (e.g., no pain, mild pain, moderate pain, severe pain, very severe pain, worst pain possible).

CORE PSYCHOPATHOLOGY AND PAIN-RELATED PSYCHOLOGICAL SYMPTOMS

In patients with chronic pain, heightened emotional distress, negative affect, and elevated pain-related psychological symptoms (i.e., those that are a direct result of chronic pain, and when the pain is eliminated, the symptoms disappear) can all be considered as forms of psychopathology and psychiatric co-morbidity, since they represent impairments in mental

TABLE 17-1 General Physical Examination of Pain by the Psychiatrist

Physical Finding	Purpose of Examination
Motor deficits	Does the patient give-way when checking strength? Does the person try? Is there a pseudoparesis, astasia-abasia, or involuntary movement that suggests a somatoform disorder?
Trigger points in head, neck, shoulder, and back muscles	Are common myofascial trigger points present that suggest myofascial pain? Is there evoked pain (such as allodynia, hyperpathia, or anesthesia) that suggests neuropathic pain?
Evanescent, changeable pain, weakness, and numbness	Does the psychological complaint pre-empt the physical?
Abnormal sensory findings	Does lateral anesthesia to pinprick end sharply at the midline? Is there topographical confusion? Is there a non-dermatomal distribution of pain and sensation that suggests either a somatoform or CNS pain disorder? Is there an abnormal sensation that suggests neuropathy or CNS pain?
Sympathetic or vascular dysfunction	Is there swelling, skin discoloration, or changes in sweating or temperature that suggests a vascular or sympathetic element to the pain?
Uncooperativeness, erratic responses to the physical examination	Is there an interpersonal aspect to the pain, causing abnormal pain behavior, as in somatoform disease?

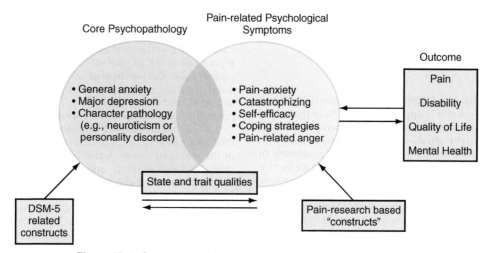

Figure 17-4. Common psychiatric symptoms in patients with chronic pain.

health and involve maladaptive psychological responses to medical illness (Figure 17-4). This approach combines methods of classification from psychiatry and behavioral medicine to describe the scope of psychiatric disturbances in patients with chronic pain. In pain patients the most common manifestations of psychiatric co-morbidity involve one or more core psychopathologies in combination with pain-related psychological symptoms. Unfortunately, not all patients and their symptoms fit precisely into DSM categories of illness.

Pain-related anxiety which includes state and trait anxiety related to pain is the form of anxiety most germane to pain.[12] Elevated levels of pain-related anxiety, such as fear of pain, also meet DSM-5 criteria for an anxiety disorder due to a general medical condition. Since anxiety is present in both domains of core psychopathology and pain-related psychological symptoms, the assessment of anxiety in a patient with chronic pain (as detailed below) must include a review of manifestations of generalized anxiety as well as pain-specific anxiety symptoms (e.g., physiological changes associated with the anticipation of pain).

Limited coping skills are often linked with pain-related psychological symptoms and behaviors including passive responses to chronic pain (e.g., remaining bed-bound), catastrophization (including cognitive distortions centered around pain and mistakenly assuming chronic pain is indicative of

ongoing tissue damage), and low self-efficacy (i.e., with a low estimate by the patient of what he or she is capable of doing).[13] Patients with decreased coping mechanisms employ few self-management strategies (such as using ice, heat, or relaxation strategies). A tendency to catastrophize often predicts poor outcome and disability, independent of other psychopathology, such as major depression. The duration of chronic pain and psychiatric co-morbidity are each an independent predictor of pain intensity and disability. High levels of anger, which tend to occur more often in men, can also explain a significant variance in pain severity.[14]

PAIN AND CO-MORBID PSYCHIATRIC CONDITIONS

Virtually all psychiatric conditions are treatable in patients with chronic pain, and the majority of patients who are provided with appropriate treatment improve significantly. Many physicians who treat pain patients often do not realize that this is the case. Of the disorders that most frequently afflict patients with chronic pain, major depression and anxiety disorders are the most common; moreover, they have the best response to medications. Whenever possible, medications that are effective for psychiatric illness and that have independent analgesic properties should be used. *Independent analgesia* refers to the efficacy of a pain medication such as a TCA or an SNRI for neuropathic pain, which is independent of its effect on mood.[15]

Regardless of the type of psychopathology present, improvement in psychiatric symptoms may result in reduction of pain levels, greater acceptance of the chronicity of pain, improved function, and an improved quality of life. Chronic pain may precipitate or worsen psychopathology and psychopathology may worsen pain. It is important for the physician who treats pain to recognize psychiatric illness early in the course of chronic pain and to treat both conditions. In general, as with most psychiatric illnesses, a combination of pharmacological and psychotherapeutic treatments is more effective in treating depression and anxiety in pain patients than is pharmacological treatment alone. There is good evidence that psychiatric co-morbidity can be successfully treated, even if pain does not improve.

Major Depression

The diagnosis and treatment of major depression in a patient with chronic pain is not significantly different from the approach to major depression in a patient with another medical illness. As in other patient groups, the combination of medications and cognitive-behavioral therapy (CBT) yields the best outcome.

Symptoms

Major depressive disorder (MDD) can be diagnosed by DSM-5 or similar research criteria in approximately 15% of those who suffer from chronic pain and in 50% of patients in chronic pain clinics. Recurrent affective illness, a family history of depression, and other psychiatric conditions (e.g., anxiety or substance use disorders) are often present. MDD can be distinguished from situational depression (also termed *demoralization* or an *adjustment disorder with depressed mood*) by the triad of persistently low mood, neurovegetative symptoms, and changes in self-attitude that last at least 2 weeks.[16] It may be important to distinguish which neurovegetative signs (such as sleep abnormalities) are the result of pain and which are the result of depression. However, given the high rate of co-morbid depression in chronic pain patients, it is prudent to err on the side of attributing neurovegetative symptoms to depression, particularly if they are accompanied by changes in mood or self-attitude. MDD is a serious complication of persistent pain; if not treated effectively it will reduce the effectiveness of all pain treatments. Even low levels of depression ("subthreshold depression") may worsen the physical impairment associated with chronic pain, and it should be treated.

Medication Treatment

There is some evidence that pain patients with MDD are more treatment-resistant, particularly when their pain is not effectively managed.[17] In general, the first-line agent for a patient in pain is an agent with independent analgesic properties. Among the antidepressants these include the TCAs and SNRIs (duloxetine and venlafaxine). Each has shown efficacy in a variety of neuropathic pain conditions. The details of prescribing a specific antidepressant are covered elsewhere in this text.

Selective Serotonin Reuptake Inhibitors. Since the introduction of fluoxetine (Prozac) in 1987, many selective serotonin reuptake inhibitors (SSRIs) have been developed. The antidepressant efficacy and low side-effect profile of SSRIs have made them the most widely prescribed class of antidepressants. Pain patients whose depression responds to an SSRI may have less pain, a finding that is attributable to

improvements in the affective components of their pain; there is little evidence to support the independent analgesic activity of SSRIs. SSRIs should not be prescribed in conjunction with tramadol, because of the heightened risk of seizures.

Other Antidepressants. Bupropion and mirtazapine are atypical antidepressants with unique mechanisms of action. Some preliminary evidence indicates that they have analgesic properties, but further study is required. Bupropion is particularly useful in pain patients because of its activating effects that lessen fatigue.

Coping and Psychotherapy

Improving coping skills is a mainstay of the treatment of any of the psychiatric conditions associated with chronic pain. In addition to improving psychological distress, use of active coping strategies improves pain and function (e.g., remaining active despite pain). Coping involves having adaptive defense mechanisms to negotiate maladaptive thoughts and feelings that arise in response to pain.

The psychodynamic aspects of coping involve conflicts over autonomy and care. Regression can be manifest as non-compliance, help-rejecting complaining, and behaviors akin to the metaphorical "cutting off your nose to spite your face." Pain may make both patients and physicians appear hateful; psychiatrists are well served by clarifying how these problems get played out in the physician–patient relationship. To help the patient cope, the psychiatrist must be sensitive to the unconscious feelings of the patient; in addition, denial must be managed, and family counseling, relaxation, exercise, physical rehabilitation, and pharmacotherapy should be considered.

CBT in conjunction with antidepressant therapy is the most efficacious treatment for MDD, including MDD that worsens in the setting of chronic pain. Typically, CBT improves coping skills and self-efficacy, and diminishes catastrophization. When CBT is used the patient must be properly motivated, have sufficient insight, and have the ego strength to tolerate challenges to his or her beliefs. CBT in pain patients focuses on the thoughts and cognitive distortions that surround chronic pain (such as fear of re-injury, the belief that the only meaningful life is one without pain, and thoughts that the patient's pain is not taken seriously by others).

Anxiety Disorders
Symptoms

Anxiety disorders encompass a broad spectrum of disorders (including generalized anxiety disorder [GAD], panic disorder, obsessive-compulsive disorder [OCD], and post-traumatic stress disorder [PTSD]). In addition, pain-related anxiety is the primary manner in which anxiety disorders are manifest in those with chronic pain.[12] Anxiety is prevalent in chronic pain clinics, with 30%–60% of the patients experiencing pathological anxiety.[18] Among the anxiety disorders, GAD is the condition that most often afflicts pain patients. More than 50% of patients with anxiety disorders also have a current or past history of MDD or another psychiatric disorder. Alcohol and substance abuse commonly accompany chronic pain; consequently, recognition and treatment of co-morbid depression and substance abuse are critical to long-term treatment outcome.

In pain patients, situational (state) anxiety may be centered on the pain itself and its negative consequences (pain-anxiety). Patients may have conditioned fear, believing that activities will cause uncontrollable pain, causing avoidance of those activities. Pain may also activate thoughts that a person is seriously ill.[12] Questions such as the following can be helpful:

"Does the pain make you panic? If you think about your pain, do you feel your heart beating fast? Do you have an overwhelming feeling of dread or doom? Do you experience a sense of sudden anxiety that overwhelms you?"

Anxiety amplifies both the perception and complaints of pain through several bio-psycho-social mechanisms (e.g., sympathetic arousal that lowers the nociceptive threshold, increased firing of ectopically active pain neurons, excessive focusing on pain symptoms, and implementation of poor coping skills). Patients with pathological anxiety are often restless, fatigued, irritable, and concentrate poorly. They may also have muscle tension and sleep disturbances.

Treatment

Overall, CBT demonstrates the best treatment outcomes for anxiety disorders, including pain-specific anxiety in chronic pain patients. Further improvement can be obtained with relaxation therapy, meditation, and biofeedback. Physical therapy by itself, with no other psychological treatment, is an effective therapy for addressing the fear of pain (termed *kinesiophobia*, the fear of movement because of pain). A flexibility program addresses muscle disuse (which by itself creates pain) and imparts several psychological insights: activity and function can be improved, despite high levels of pain; it is more meaningful to be active with pain than to remain inactive with pain; and fear of pain and re-injury can be diminished. Antidepressants are effective, but many need to be used at higher doses than are typically prescribed for depression. Anxiolytics (such as benzodiazepines and buspirone) are most useful in the initial stages of treatment. However, the side effects and potential for physiological dependency make them a poor choice for long-term treatment.

Antidepressants

Antidepressants may take 2 to 4 weeks until improvement is noted. To improve compliance, escalation of doses must be slow, because anxious patients tolerate side effects poorly. Antidepressants reduce the overall level of anxiety and prevent anxiety or panic attacks, but they have no role in the treatment of acute anxiety. Among antidepressants, the SSRIs are most effective. Effective doses are often higher than those used for depression. Of the SNRIs, both venlafaxine and duloxetine have demonstrated efficacy in GAD.[19,20]

Somatoform Disorders
Classification

The somatoform disorders comprise a group of disorders in which complaints and anxiety about physical symptoms are the dominant features. These complaints exist in the absence of sufficient organic findings to explain the extent of a person's pain. Most often there is a physical basis (including functional pathology, such as neuropathic pain) for at least a portion of the pain complaints, in which symptom-reporting is magnified by somatizing. Somatization is best thought of as a process. The spectrum of somatization includes amplification of symptoms, which entails "focusing upon the symptoms, racking with intense alarm and worry, extreme disability, and a reluctance to relinquish them."[21] Pain-related psychological symptoms amplify pain perception and disability. Hence, there is a tremendous overlap between the somatoform component of a chronic pain syndrome and other psychiatric co-morbidities. Four somatoform disorders may involve pain: somatization disorder, conversion disorder, hypochondriasis, and pain disorder (with or without a physical basis for pain). Somatoform disorders without any physical basis for pain are

estimated to occur in 5%–15% of patients with chronic pain who receive pain treatment.[22]

Symptom Presentation

Among somatizers, pains in the head or neck, epigastrium, and limbs predominate. Visceral pains from the esophagus, abdomen, and pelvis are associated with a high rate of psychiatric co-morbidity, particularly somatoform disorders, which can be challenging to diagnose.[23] Missed ovarian cancers, neuropathic pain following inflammatory disorders, and referred pain are often overlooked because of the non-specific presentations of visceral pain. Sufferers from somatoform disorders often have painful physical complaints and excessive anxiety about their physical illness. The most common co-morbid conditions among somatoform-disordered pain patients are MDD and anxiety disorders. Patients with somatization disorder consume health care resources at nine times the rate of the average person in the US.

Treatment Concepts

Among sufferers of somatoform disorders, most pain complaints are ill-defined, and a psychiatric diagnosis is often particularly difficult to establish. The treatment approach is similar across the spectrum of somatoform disorders, and the psychiatrist plays a key role in the coordination of care. First, the psychiatrist must work closely with the patient's other physicians to establish the physical basis or diagnosis for the pain, if any. The treatment team must agree on which symptoms, or to what degree the symptoms, are caused by structural or neuropathic pathology. This agreement involves a consensus among the providers not to aggressively pursue (with testing, medication, or procedural treatment) every pain or physical complaint. Other co-morbid psychiatric illnesses must be identified and treated. CBT is used to help the patient appreciate the connections between thoughts, emotions, perceived pain, and pain behaviors. This treatment involves a gradual escalation of activity, with continuous reassurance given that an increase in pain does not signal worsening of the patient's underlying physical condition (if any).

Conversion Disorder

Conversion disorder may be manifest as a pain syndrome with a significant loss of or alteration in physical function that mimics a physical disorder. Conversion symptoms may include paresthesia, numbness, dysphonia, dizziness, seizures, globus hystericus, limb weakness, sexual dysfunction, or pain. If pain or sexual symptoms are the sole complaints, the diagnosis is pain disorder or sexual pain disorder, rather than conversion disorder. Pain, numbness, and weakness often form a conversion triad.

Psychological factors are judged to be etiological for the pain when a temporal relationship between the symptoms and a psychosocial stressor exists; in addition, the person must not intentionally produce his or her symptom. A mechanism of primary or secondary gain needs to be evident before the diagnosis can be confirmed. Presence of *la belle indifférence* and histrionic personality traits has little value in making or excluding the diagnosis of conversion. A "conversion V" on the Minnesota Multiphasic Personality Inventory (MMPI) identifies the hypochondriacal traits and the relative absence of depression that often accompanies conversion.

Hypochondriasis

Hypochondriasis involves the persistent belief that one has a serious illness, despite extensive medical evaluation to the contrary. Head and orofacial pains, cardiac and gastrointestinal pains, and feelings of pressure, burning, and numbness are common hypochondriacal concerns. Care of the hypochondriac begins with a complete history and a comprehensive differential diagnosis. The persistence of vague complaints helps to rule out the most serious diseases, and to set the stage for an alliance with the patient by demonstrating an open mind. A pain drawing may help reveal psychotic somatic beliefs. The psychiatrist should reassure, and not reject, the patient.

Pain Disorder

Pain disorder is defined in DSM-IV as a syndrome in which the focus of the clinical presentation is pain that causes significant impairment in occupational or social function, induces marked distress, or both. Organic pathology, if present, does not explain the extent of pain complaints or the degree of associated social and occupational impairment. Pain disorder has three subtypes: psychological (in which psychological factors play the primary role in the onset, severity, exacerbation, or maintenance of the pain); non-psychiatric pain associated with a general medical condition; and combined type (pain associated with psychological factors and a general medical condition).

Pain disorder has been variously called *psychogenic pain disorder*, *somatoform pain disorder*, and *pain behavior*. When behavioral disability predominates, chronic pain syndrome is the behavioral description of this same syndrome. The meandering history of nomenclature is best understood as reflecting the mix of pain behaviors, as well as interpersonal and affective characteristics, that emphasize disability and entreat attention from others. Psychological antecedents of this syndrome may include a history of physical abuse, counterdependent personal relationships, a family history of alcoholism, and a personal developmental history of attachment problems. Co-morbid diagnoses (particularly depression, anxiety, and substance abuse) should be sought. Treatment must address the triad of self-defeating behavior, affective dysfunction, and psychodynamic conflicts, which causes poor coping, disability, and disrupted rehabilitation efforts.

Factitious Disorder with Physical Symptoms

Factitious disorder with physical symptoms involves the intentional production or feigning of physical symptoms. Onset is usually in early adulthood with successive hospitalizations forming a lifelong pattern. The cause is a psychological need to assume the sick role, and as such, the intentional production of painful symptoms distinguishes factitious disorder from somatoform disorders. Renal colic, orofacial pain, and abdominal pain are three of the common presentations for factitious disorder; of these, abdominal pain and a scarred belly herald the diagnosis most often. Despite the seeming irrationality of the behavior, those with factitious disorder are not psychotic.

Pain may be described as occurring anywhere in the body, and the patient often uses elaborate technical detail to intrigue the listener with *pseudologia fantastica*. Multiple hospitalizations under different names in different cities, inconclusive invasive investigations and surgery, lack of available family, and a truculent manner are characteristic features of this disorder. Unfortunately, there is no effective treatment.

GENERAL PRINCIPALS OF MULTIMODAL ANALGESIA

In the medication management of chronic pain, multimodal analgesia is the preferred method, since very commonly multiple receptor systems must be targeted to achieve optimal pain control. By logical extension, successful treatment of chronic pain typically involves the use of more than one medication, nerve blocks, physical therapy, and relaxation or biofeedback techniques (i.e., treatment is conducted by a multidisciplinary team or by an interdisciplinary pain medicine program). In general, treatment goals are reports of pain less than 5 out of 10 and an improvement in function. Typically, this corresponds to a 30%–50% long-term improvement in chronic pain and an improved quality of life. Studies have shown that at a level of 4 out of 10 or below, most patents are able to perform most of their activities of daily living with satisfaction. A 30% improvement in pain has been shown to be the level that is clinically meaningful, a level at which most patients will feel significantly better. Many of the nerve blocks (such as epidural steroid injections) are effective for acute exacerbations of chronic pain. But their relatively short duration of efficacy (2 to 6 weeks on average) makes them inadequate for the long-term management of chronic pain, if they are used as the only treatment modality. Interventional procedures with longer-term efficacy include spinal cord stimulation, radiofrequency lesioning, and intrathecal pump implantation.

Major Medication Classes
Non-steroidal Anti-inflammatory Drugs

Non-steroidal anti-inflammatory drugs (NSAIDs) are useful for acute and chronic pain (such as pain due to inflammation, muscle pain, vascular pain, or post-traumatic pain). NSAIDs are generally equally efficacious (whether they are non-selective or COX-2 inhibitors) and they have similar side effects, but there is great individual variability in response across the different NSAIDs (Table 17-2). Ketorolac (up to 30 mg every 6 hours) intramuscularly (IM) or intravenously (IV) followed by oral dosing has a rapid onset and a high potency, enabling it to be substituted for morphine (30 mg of ketorolac is equivalent to 10 mg of morphine). It should be used for no more than 5 days.

Side Effects. Most NSAIDs can cause bronchospasm in aspirin-sensitive patients, induce gastric ulcers, interact with angiotensin-converting enzyme (ACE) inhibitors (thereby contributing to renal failure), precipitate lithium toxicity, and impair renal function with long-term use. NSAIDs can elevate blood pressure in patients treated with β-blockers and diuretics. The COX-2 inhibitors (e.g., celecoxib) have a lower incidence than non-selective NSAIDs of ulcer disease in the first year of treatment, but not necessarily beyond this time frame.

Muscle Relaxants

These are useful for acute and chronic musculoskeletal pain. Their exact mechanism of action is unknown and mechanisms likely differ among the various compounds. In general, they are thought to enhance inhibition of descending pain pathways. Some of the most frequently prescribed include baclofen (an antispasticity agent), cyclobenzaprine, metaxalone, orphenadrine, and tizanidine.

Tricyclic Antidepressants

Tricyclic antidepressants (TCAs) are one of the primary medications used to treat neuropathic pain syndromes; TCAs have both independent analgesic properties and effects as adjuvant agents. A series of studies by Max and others[15] have illustrated the analgesic properties of TCAs, which are independent of their effects on improving depression. TCAs have been shown to be effective for the pain associated with diabetic neuropathy, for chronic regional pain syndromes, for chronic headache, for post-stroke pain, and for radicular pain. While

TABLE 17-2 Properties of Aspirin and Non-steroidal Anti-inflammatory Drugs

Drug	Dose (mg)	Dosage Interval (h)	Daily Dose (mg/day)	Peak Effect (h)	Half-life (h)
Aspirin	81–975	4	2,400	0.5–1	0.25
Celecoxib	100–200	12	400	1	11
Diclofenac	25–75	6–8	200	2	1–2
Diflunisal	250–500	12	1,500	1	13
Etodolac acid	200–400	6–8	1,200	1–2	7
Meloxicam	7.5–15	24	15	2	15–20
Flurbiprofen	50–100	6–8	300	1.5–3	3–4
Ibuprofen	200–800	6–8	2,400	1–2	2
Indomethacin	25–75	6–8	150	0.5–1	2–3
Ketoprofen	25–75	6–8	300	1–2	1.5–2.0
Ketorolac*					
Oral	10	6–8	40	0.5–1	6
Parenteral	60 load, then 30	6–8	120	0.5	6
Choline magnesium trisalicylate	500–1000	12	3,000	1	2–12
Nabumetone	1,000–2,000	12–24	2,000	3–5	22–30
Naproxen	500 load, then 250–375	6–8	1,000	2–4	12–15
Oxaprozin	60–1,200	24	1,200	2	3–3.5
Piroxicam	40 load, then 20	24	20	2–4	36–45
Sulindac	150–200	12	400	1–2	7–18
Tolmetin	200–600	8	1,800	4–6	2

*Use no longer than 5 days.
Adapted from Tarascon pocket pharmacopoeia, *California, 2006, Tarascon Publishers.*

the early studies were done with amitriptyline and desipramine, subsequent studies have confirmed that other TCAs also have equivalent analgesic properties. Of note, the typical doses for the analgesic benefit of TCAs (25–75 mg) are lower than the doses generally used for antidepressant effect (150–300 mg). Nevertheless, there is a dose–response relationship for analgesia, and some patients benefit from a TCA used in the traditional antidepressant dose range, in conjunction with blood level monitoring. A TCA and an antiepileptic drug (AED) are often combined for the treatment of chronic pain, and this combination facilitates treatment of mood disorders. Since pain patients are frequently on a variety of medications that may potentially increase TCA serum levels, the value of blood level monitoring, even at low doses, cannot be understated.

Serotonin-norepinephrine Reuptake Inhibitors

The serotonin-norepinephrine reuptake inhibitors (SNRIs) are a newer group of antidepressants, which, like the TCAs, act by inhibiting serotonin and norepinephrine reuptake. Venlafaxine and duloxetine are the most familiar drugs in this category; they have less alpha-1, cholinergic, or histamine inhibition than the TCAs. This results in fewer side effects than the TCAs, with equivalent antidepressant and potentially equal analgesic benefits. Placebo-controlled studies have demonstrated efficacy in neuropathic pain for both venlafaxine and duloxetine.

Structurally, venlafaxine is similar to tramadol, and in mice, venlafaxine demonstrates opioid-mediated analgesia that is reversed by naloxone. Duloxetine has a Food and Drug Administration indication for both diabetic peripheral neuropathic (DPN) pain and for MDD. Thus, it is an excellent choice for pain patients with psychiatric co-morbidity who have failed to respond to a TCA. It has also shown efficacy in fibromyalgia and GAD. It is started at 30 mg a day for a week (or 20 mg in the elderly), and then increased to 60 mg a day. Up to 120 mg a day can be prescribed for DPN. The most common side effects are nausea and sedation. Its metabolism is similar to that of venlafaxine. Many patients are unable to tolerate the side effects of TCAs, so both venlafaxine and duloxetine are promising agents in patients with co-morbid MDD and chronic pain.

Antiepileptic Drugs

Blocking abnormally high-frequency and spontaneous firing in afferent neurons, in the dorsal horn, and in the thalamus is the putative mechanism for the efficacy of anticonvulsants with regard to pain. The consequence of blocking the hyperexcitability of low-threshold mechanoreceptive neurons in the brain is pain relief. AEDs are used in this population primarily for treatment of neuropathic pain.

Opioids

Acute, severe, and unremitting pains in cancer patients, as well as non-cancer-related chronic pain, which have been refractory to other medication modalities typically requires treatment with opioids. At times, opioids are the most effective treatment for chronic, non-malignant pain, such as the pain associated with post-herpetic neuralgia, degenerative disorders, and vascular conditions. Nociceptive pain and absence of any co-morbid drug abuse have been associated with long-term opioid treatment efficacy. Morphine is often the initial opioid of choice for acute and chronic pain because it is well known to most physicians and has a good safety profile. Beyond these starting points, the basic principles of opioid treatment are outlined in Box 17-1 and Table 17-3.

Tramadol deserves special mention because it does have weak mu-opioid receptor activity, but it is not classified as a controlled substance in the US. It also has SNRI properties. Its analgesic mechanism is unknown, but it is thought to enhance descending pain inhibition. Tramadol should be prescribed cautiously concurrently with an SSRI or SNRI because of a unique interaction that results in an increased risk for seizure and development of serotonin syndrome. Caution should also be taken when prescribing it with other medications (such as bupropion, TCAs, and dopamine antagonists) that may also lower the seizure threshold.

Recent evidence suggests that patients should be screened for risk factors for opioid misuse or abuse (e.g., a current or past history of an SUD, a family history of an SUD, a significant legal history, and a significant mood disorder) before prescribing them, so that the physician can prescribe and monitor use of opiates appropriately. Once oral doses have

TABLE 17-3 Opioid Potencies and Special Features

Drug	Parenteral (mg equivalent)	Oral (mg)	Duration (h)	Special Features
Morphine	10	30	4	Morphine sulfate controlled release has 12-h duration
Codeine	120	200	4	Ceiling effect as dose increases, low lipophilic
Oxycodone	4.5	30	4	Every 12 h oxycontin (10, 20, 40 slow release mg)
Hydromorphone	2	8	5	Suppository 6 mg = 10 mg parenteral morphine
Levorphanol	2	4	4	Low nausea and vomiting, low lipophilic
Methadone	5	10	2–12	Cumulative effect; day 3–5 decrease respiration; equianalgesic ratio varies considerably
Meperidine	100	300	3	κ, proconvulsant metabolite, peristaltic slowing and sphincter of Oddi decrease
Fentanyl	0.1	25 μg SL	1 (patch 72 h)	50-μg patch = 30 mg/day morphine IM/IV
Sufentanil	Not recommended	15 μg SL	1	High potency with low volume of fluid
Propoxyphene	Not available	325	4	High dose leads to psychosis
Pentazocine	60	150	3	κ, σ agonist-antagonist, nasal 1 mg q1-2h
Butorphanol	2	Not available 3 (IM), 2 (NS)		μ, κ, σ, agonist-antagonist, nasal 1 mg q1-2h
Buprenorphine	0.3	4	4–6	Partial agonist
Tramadol	Not available	150	4	μ agonist, decreased reuptake 5-HT and NE, P450 metabolism
Nalbuphine	10	Not available	3	Agonist-antagonist

5-HT, 5-hydroxytryptamine; IM, intramuscular; IV, intravenous; NE, norepinephrine; NS, nasal; SL, sublingual.

BOX 17-1 Guidelines for Opioid Maintenance

- Maintenance opioids should be considered only after other methods of pain control have been proven unsuccessful. Alternative methods (which typically include use of NSAIDs, anticonvulsants, membrane-stabilizing drugs, monoaminergic agents, local nerve blocks, and physical therapy) vary from case to case.
- Opioids should be avoided for patients with addiction disorders unless there is a new major medical illness (e.g., cancer or trauma) accompanied by severe pain. In such cases, a second opinion from another physician (a pain medicine or addiction specialist) is suggested.
- If opioids are prescribed for longer than 3 months, the patient should have a second opinion, plus a follow-up consultation at least once per year. Monitoring with a urine toxicology screen, at least yearly, is also recommended.
- One pharmacy and one prescriber should be designated as exclusive agents.
- Dosages of opioids should be defined, as should expectations of what will happen if there are deviations from it. For example, abuse will lead to rapid tapering of the drug and entry into a detoxification program. There should be no doubt that the physician will stop prescribing the drug.
- Informed consent as to the rationale, risks, benefits, and alternatives should be documented.
- The course of treatment (in particular, the ongoing indications, changes in the disease process, efficacy, and the presence of abuse, tolerance, or addictive behavior) should be documented.

---

been initiated and titrated to a satisfactory level, the analgesic effect needs to be sustained by minimizing fluctuations in blood levels and the variable effects of dosing schedules. Long-acting or controlled-release formulations are ideal for this homeostasis, because they are released more slowly than are short-acting opioids.

For the treatment of chronic pain, dosing with short-acting medications only on an as-needed basis should be avoided when possible since this makes steady relief impossible. It also predisposes the patient to drug-respondent conditioning and to subsequent behavior problems. Typically, long-acting formulations are combined with short-acting agents for breakthrough pain. In those at risk for opioid misuse or with demonstrated aberrant drug behavior, longer-acting agents

(i.e., methadone, fentanyl patch) are preferred to avoid inappropriate self-medication. The most frequently reported side effects of opioid therapy are constipation, dry mouth, and sedation.

Treatment of Neuropathic Pain

Neuropathic pain is responsive to multiple medication classes, including TCAs, AEDs, and opioids, when used at higher doses than what is typically prescribed for chronic musculoskeletal pain. Multiple medications are often combined with physical therapy and with coping skills training for complete interdisciplinary care.

Sympathetically-Maintained Pain

Sympathetically-maintained pain is a type of neuropathic pain. Regardless of etiology (e.g., complex regional pain syndrome, inflammation, post-herpetic neuralgia, trauma, or facial pain) sympathetically-maintained or mediated pain can respond to sympathetic blockade. Medications often used in the sympathetic blockade are alpha-blocking drugs such as phentolamine, alpha-blocking antidepressants, and clonidine. Intrathecal, epidural, and systemic administration of a local anesthetic or clonidine also produces analgesia and may be useful in some types of vascular or neuropathic pain with a sympathetic component. β-Blockers are not efficacious in the treatment of sympathetically-maintained pain except in their use in the alleviation of migraine headaches. Guanethidine, bretylium, reserpine, and phentolamine have also been used to produce a chemical sympathectomy.

TREATMENT OF PAIN BEHAVIOR AND THE USE OF MULTIDISCIPLINARY PAIN CLINICS

Medicare guidelines offer a broad set of criteria to qualify for structured multidisciplinary pain management. The pain must last at least 6 months (and result in significant life disturbance and limited function), it must be attributable to a physical cause, and it must be unresponsive to the usual methods of treatment. Quality control guidelines developed by the Commission on Accreditation of Rehabilitation Facilities (CARF) have led to the certification of more than 100 multidisciplinary chronic pain management programs nationwide. Behavioral treatments are a key component of these programs and can be effective for the relief of pain and can help extinguish the behaviors associated with pain.

Inpatient or outpatient multidisciplinary pain treatment should be considered early in the course of chronic pain. This is particularly important when intensive observation is necessary (e.g., to rule out malingering); no single modality of outpatient treatment is likely to work; the patient has already obtained maximum benefit from outpatient treatments (such as NSAIDs, nerve blocks, antidepressants, and simple physical and behavioral rehabilitation); intensive daily interventions are required, usually with multiple concurrent types of therapy (such as nerve blocks, physical therapy, and behavior modification); and the patient exhibits abnormal pain behavior and agrees to the goals of improved coping, work rehabilitation, and psychiatric assessment.

REHABILITATION

Successful rehabilitation of patients who have chronic pain syndromes may require some combination of psychiatry, physiatry, and behavioral psychology. These treatments include exercise, gait training, spinal manipulation, orthoses, traction therapy, psychotherapy, and yoga. Successful rehabilitation aims to decrease symptoms, increase independence, and allow the patient to return to work. A positive, rapid return to light-normal activities and work is essential if disability is to be minimized. Psychologically, this is the key to coping with acute trauma. There is no evidence that a return to work adversely affects the course of the majority of chronic pain syndromes.

CONCLUSIONS

Pain is an exciting and burgeoning discipline for psychiatrists. Whether the psychiatrist is treating the pain or its psychological sequelae, it is critical to have a firm understanding of the physical basis for the pain complaints in conjunction with a thorough appreciation of how psychiatric co-morbidity interacts with the perceptions of pain. Patients who attend pain clinics have significant psychiatric pathology. This co-morbidity worsens their pain and disability, and this mental distress is an independent source of suffering, further reducing the quality of life. Fortunately, with the boom in psychotherapeutic medications over the past 15 years, and with more effective psychotherapies, significant improvement in pain treatment has been noted.

Access a list of MCQs for this chapter at https://expertconsult .inkling.com

REFERENCES

1. IASP Subcommittee on Taxonomy. Pain terms: a list with definitions and notes on usage. *Pain* 6(3):249–252, 1979.
2. Von Korff M, Crane P, Lane M, et al. Chronic spinal pain and physical-mental comorbidity in the United States: results from the National Comorbidity Survey Replication. *Pain* 113(3):331–339, 2005.
3. Teunissen SC, Wesker W, Kruitwagen C, et al. Symptom prevalence in patients with incurable cancer: a systematic review. *J Pain Symptom Manage* 34(1):94–104, 2007.
4. Walker EA, Keegan D, Gardner G, et al. Psychosocial factors in fibromyalgia compared with rheumatoid arthritis: II. Sexual, physical, and emotional abuse and neglect. *Psychosom Med* 59(6):572–577, 1997.
5. Fernandez E. Interactions between pain and affect. In *Anxiety, depression, and anger in pain*, Dallas, 2002, Advanced Psychological Resources.
6. Strain EC. Assessment and treatment of comorbid psychiatric disorders in opioid-dependent patients. *Clin J Pain* 18(4 Suppl.): S14–S27, 2002.
7. Sprenger T, Valet M, Boecker H, et al. Opioidergic activation in the medial pain system after heat pain. *Pain* 122:63–67, 2006.
8. Coghill RC, McHaffie JG, Yen YF. Neural correlates of interindividual differences in the subjective experience of pain. *Proc Natl Acad Sci* 100(14):8538–8542, 2003.
9. Gracely RH, Petzke F, Wolf JM, et al. Functional magnetic resonance imaging evidence of augmented pain processing in fibromyalgia. *Arthritis Rheum* 46(5):1333–1343, 2002.
10. Zubieta JK, Ketter TA, Bueller JA, et al. Regulation of human affective responses by anterior cingulate and limbic mu-opioid neurotransmission. *Arch Gen Psychiatry* 60(11):1145–1153, 2003.
11. Nelson D, Novy D. Self-report differentiation of anxiety and depression in chronic pain. *J Pers Assess* 69(2):392–407, 1997.
12. McCracken L, Gross RT, Aikens J, et al. The assessment of anxiety and fear in persons with chronic pain: a comparison of instruments. *Behav Res Ther* 34(11):927–933, 1996.
13. Keefe FJ, Rumble ME, Scipio CD, et al. Psychological aspects of persistent pain: current state of the science. *J Pain* 5(4):195–211, 2004.
14. Turk DC, Monarch ES. Biopsychosocial perspective on chronic pain. In Turk DC, Gatchel R, editors: *Psychological approaches to pain management*, New York, 2002, Guilford Press.
15. Max MB, Lynch SA, Muir J. Effects of desipramine, amitriptyline and fluoxetine on pain in diabetic neuropathy. *N Engl J Med* 326:1250–1256, 1992.
16. McHugh P, Slavney P. *The perspectives of psychiatry*, Baltimore, 1998, Johns Hopkins University Press.
17. Gallagher RM, Verma S. Managing pain and co-morbid depression: a public health challenge. *Semin Clin Neuropsych* 4(3):203–220, 1999.
18. Koenig T, Clark MR. Advances in comprehensive pain management. *Psychiatr Clin North Am* 19(3):589–611, 1996.
19. Thase ME, Entsuah AR, Rudolph RL. Remission rates during treatment with venlafaxine or selective serotonin reuptake inhibitors. *Br J Psychiatry* 178(3):234–241, 2001.
20. Goldstein DJ, Lu Y, Detke MJ, et al. Duloxetine vs. placebo in patients with painful diabetic neuropathy. *Pain* 116:109–118, 2005.
21. Barsky AJ. Patients who amplify bodily sensations. *Ann Intern Med* 91(1):63–70, 1979.
22. Sigvardsson S, von Knorring A, Bohman M. An adoption study of somatoform disorders. *Arch Gen Psychiatry* 41(9):853–859, 1984.
23. McDonald J. What are the causes of chronic gynecological pain disorders? *APS Bulletin* 5(6):20–23, 1995.

18 Neurotherapeutics

Joan A. Camprodon, MD, MPH, PhD, Navneet Kaur, BS, Scott L. Rauch, MD, and Darin D. Dougherty, MD, MSc

KEY POINTS

- Somatic therapies are a group of device-based techniques that modulate disease-relevant structures of the nervous system via surgical ablation or electrical stimulation with the goal of therapeutically modifying pathological patterns of brain activity and circuit connectivity.

- Ablative limbic system surgical procedures, such as anterior cingulotomy, sub-caudate tractotomy, limbic leucotomy, and anterior capsulotomy are viable treatment options for patients with treatment-refractory major depressive disorder (MDD) or obsessive-compulsive disorder (OCD).

- Deep brain stimulation (DBS) involves placing electrodes at target regions within the brain. It received approval by the United States Food and Drug Administration (FDA) for the treatment of refractory OCD in 2009 and clinical trials are underway for other disorders (particularly MDD) with promising results.

- Vagus nerve stimulation (VNS), approved by the FDA for treatment-resistant depression, involves intermittent stimulation of the left vagus nerve that results in electrical stimulation to brain regions involved in mood regulation.

- Repetitive transcranial magnetic stimulation (TMS) utilizes a magnetic field at the scalp surface to electrically stimulate the cortical surface. It received FDA approval for the treatment of MDD in 2008, and also in 2013 for the use of deep H-coils.

OVERVIEW

Therapeutic options for patients with affective, behavioral, or cognitive disorders include psychotherapy, pharmacotherapy, and somatic therapies. This chapter will focus on the latter.

Somatic therapies are also commonly known under the labels of *brain stimulation* or *neuromodulation*. They are a group of device-based techniques that target specific structures of the nervous systems via surgical ablation or electrical modulation with the goal of therapeutically modifying pathological patterns of brain activity and circuit connectivity. These therapies grow from a systems neuroscience paradigm that emphasizes the role of neural circuits and their processing strategies in healthy brain function, pathophysiology, and therapeutics.[1]

Somatic therapies can be divided into two general groups: invasive and non-invasive modalities. Invasive treatments require the surgical implantation of stimulating electrodes (or surgical ablative disconnection of aberrant pathways) and include ablative limbic system surgeries, deep brain stimulation (DBS), and vagus nerve stimulation (VNS). Non-invasive techniques are able to modulate brain activity transcranially without surgical intervention, and include transcranial magnetic stimulation (TMS) as its most paradigmatic modality.

Electroconvulsive therapy (ECT), the oldest of all somatic therapies, occupies a space in between the two categories, as it does not require surgical intervention but it does require general anesthesia; it is generally considered minimally invasive.

Many patients with psychiatric illness can be successfully treated with pharmacotherapy, psychotherapy, or both. However, a significant number of patients do not respond to these interventions. Studies have demonstrated that about 30% to 40% of patients with major depressive disorder (MDD) treated with pharmacotherapy achieve full remission, and 10% to 15% experience no symptom improvement.[2] In addition, the Sequenced Treatment Alternatives to Relieve Depression (STAR*D) study found that with each failed medication trial the remission rate decreased.[3] Clearly, alternative therapeutic interventions for patients with no response to these treatments are necessary. Nevertheless, while invasive neuromodulation should be reserved for the most refractory patients, non-invasive techniques (including ECT) are being considered in earlier phases of the therapeutic process and are not exclusively for severe treatment-resistant individuals, given their efficacy and relatively benign safety profile (which can be significantly better than certain pharmacological options).

ABLATIVE LIMBIC SYSTEM SURGERY

Concerns regarding ablative neurosurgery for psychiatric indications are understandable given the indiscriminate use of crude procedures, such as frontal lobotomy, in the middle of the twentieth century. These procedures were associated with severe adverse events, including frontal lobe symptoms (e.g., apathy) or even death. In the latter half of the twentieth century, neurosurgeons began to use much smaller lesions in well-targeted and specific brain regions. As a result, the incidence of adverse events dropped precipitously.[4] Currently used procedures include anterior cingulotomy, sub-caudate tractotomy, limbic leucotomy (which is a combination of an anterior cingulotomy and a sub-caudate tractotomy), and anterior capsulotomy (Figure 18-1). All of these procedures use craniotomy techniques. However, because of the small lesion volume required for an anterior capsulotomy, a gamma knife (a technique that uses focused gamma rays to create ablative lesions) can be used to perform this procedure. These procedures have been used in patients who suffer from intractable mood and anxiety disorders; modest response rates range from 30% to 70%.[5-9] Because patients eligible for these procedures have failed all other available treatments, a significant positive response to these interventions can be life-saving. While post-operative side effects may occur, they are almost always temporary. Inconvenient side effects include headache, nausea, and edema; more serious adverse events include infection, urinary difficulties, weight gain, seizures, cerebral hemorrhage or infarct, and cognitive deficits. Fortunately, these side effects are uncommon and typically transient.[6,8,9]

DEEP BRAIN STIMULATION

Deep brain stimulation (DBS) grew from the therapeutic tradition of ablative stereotaxic surgery and the technical

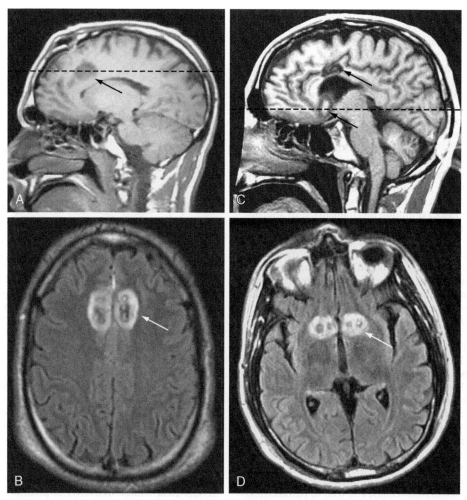

Figure 18-1. Ablative limbic system surgery. (A) Sagittal view of anterior cingulotomy lesions (*arrow*). (B) Axial view (at the level of the dotted line in panel A) of anterior cingulotomy lesions (*arrow*). (C) Sagittal view of anterior cingulotomy (*upper arrow*) and sub-caudate tractotomy (*lower arrow*) lesions. (D) Axial view (at the level of the dotted line in panel C) of sub-caudate tractotomy lesions (*arrow*).

developments that led to cardiac pacemakers.[4] It requires the surgical placement of stimulating electrodes in disease-specific deep brain structures via craniotomy and stereotaxic surgery. The intra-cranial electrodes are connected to an internal pulse generator (IPG), which consists of a battery and mini-processor able to generate electrical currents according to clinician-determined parameters. The IPG is surgically implanted in the pectoral region (although other sites are also possible) and connects to the intra-cranial electrodes via a wire that travels through the head and neck's subcutaneous tissue. Clinicians who employ DBS use control devices that communicate wirelessly with the IPG and are able to control and interrogate the system. Patients usually have a simpler version of this control device that allows them to turn the system on or off, and also to make limited changes when treaters allow it. Clinicians can change the voltage, frequency, and pulse width of the electrical pulses according to safety and efficacy criteria, and can also check the impedance of the system, battery status, and patterns of patient use. Most commercially available DBS systems have four contact positions in each stimulating electrode, which can be independently activated to provide positive or negative electrical charges. For example, patient A may have electrode 1 as an anode (positive) and electrode 2 as a cathode (negative), while patient B may have electrode 1 as a cathode (negative) and electrode 4 as an anode (positive), creating a wider electric field (i.e., able to recruit a larger number of fibers) with

opposite current direction. This flexibility allows clinicians a significant range of electrode combinations that increase the anatomical precision of stimulation, which can be individualized according to clinical response or biomarkers, such as MRI diffusion tractography.[10]

DBS is a surgical procedure and therefore invasive. Iatrogenic adverse events can be categorized in two primary groups: those related to the surgical procedures and those related to the stimulation of brain regions. Surgical adverse events have an incidence rate of 1% to 4% and include seizures, infection, and hemorrhage.[11] Effects related to stimulation vary depending on the anatomical location of the electrodes and include worsening depression, (hypo)mania, acute anxiety,[12] and gustatory or olfactory sensations.[13] Unlike ablative interventions, permanent cognitive deficits have not been reported in DBS patients. Nevertheless, reversible cognitive effects (such as diminished concentration) have been described, though these are stimulation-dependent and remit with re-adjustment of DBS parameters.[14]

The first US Food and Drug Administration (FDA)-approved indication for DBS was pain, although its approval was later withdrawn given doubts about its efficacy.[4] Today, the primary indication for this treatment modality is Parkinson's disease, and other movements disorders, such as dystonia and essential tremor.[15] The therapeutic approach for these condition requires the surgical modulation of key nodes in the motor circuitry: sub-thalamic nucleus for Parkinson's disease, globus pallidus pars interna for Parkinson's disease and dystonia, and ventral intermediate nucleus of the thalamus for essential tremor.[15] Over 80,000 patients with Parkinson's disease have had DBS electrodes implanted in these brain regions associated with the pathophysiology of the illness.[16]

Basic and clinical research studies investigated the use of DBS for refractory OCD using various brain targets that included the anterior limb of the internal capsule,[17-19] the ventral capsule/ventral striatum (VC/VS),[12,20] the nucleus accumbens (NAcc),[21-23] the sub-thalamic nucleus (STN)[24] and the inferior thalamic peduncle.[25] It should be noted that the first three anatomical targets are very similar, if not practically the same. In 2009, the FDA approved the use of DBS to the VC/VS for the treatment of treatment-resistant OCD (under the humanitarian device exemption mechanism), thus approving the first psychiatric indication and allowing DBS to enter clinical practice in psychiatry.[14]

Several open-label clinical trials have been published using DBS for the treatment of MDD stimulating three main regions: the VC/VS (the same as for OCD),[26,27] the sub-genual cingulate gyrus (SCG) or Brodmann area 25 (BA25/Cg25)[28-31] and the NAcc.[32,33] Response rates (from 50% to 60%) were similar for all regions.[34] Other brain regions, such as the medial forebrain bundle (MFB),[35,36] lateral habenula (LHb),[37] and inferior thalamic peduncle (ITP),[38] have also been used as DBS targets, but data are still limited to a small number of cases. While these initial results are encouraging, they stem primarily from prospective open-label trials (or case reports and series), and DBS for MDD remains an experimental procedure. Nevertheless, double-blind, placebo-controlled trials are currently underway seeking the necessary safety and efficacy evidence to expand the therapeutic options for patients with treatment refractory MDD.[34]

In addition to OCD and MDD, DBS is also being investigated as a treatment for other conditions that result from physiological changes in brain circuit and lead to pathological processing of affect, behavior, and cognition. A few examples under current active research include addiction, obesity, eating disorders, Tourette's syndrome (TS), Alzheimer's disease, and schizophrenia. Structures such as the ventral tegmental area (VTA) and the nucleus accumbens are targeted for addiction and schizophrenia and the hippocampal fornix is targeted for Alzheimer's disease.[39] As we improve our understanding of the mechanism of action of DBS and its effects on key targets, and we will be able to develop new technologies that increase its specificity, efficacy, and safety, DBS is likely to become a more commonly used treatment for the most refractory patients.

VAGUS NERVE STIMULATION

Vagus nerve stimulation (VNS) was approved for use in treatment-resistant epilepsy in 1994 in Europe and in 1997 in the US. VNS has been approved for treatment-refractory MDD and bipolar disorder in Europe and Canada since 2001. In July 2005, the FDA approved VNS for the treatment of MDD. Implantation of the VNS device involves surgical placement of electrodes around the left vagus nerve via an incision in the neck (only the left vagus nerve is used for VNS because the right vagus has a much higher percentage of parasympathetic branches to the heart) (Figure 18-2). A second incision is used to place an internal pulse generator (IPG) sub-cutaneously in the left sub-clavicular region, and the wire between the electrodes on the vagus nerve and the IPG is connected by means of sub-cutaneous tunneling between the two incision sites. After a 2-week post-operative recovery period, the IPG can be turned on and electrical stimulation of the left vagus nerve can be initiated.

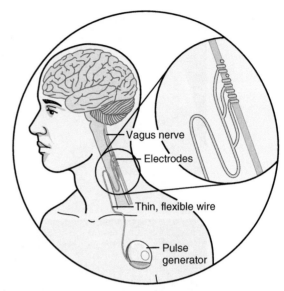

Figure 18-2. A schematic demonstrating the locations of the electrode lead on the left vagus nerve and the IPG following VNS device implantation. (Redrawn from Cyberonics, Inc. Physician's manual for the VNS Therapy™ Pulse Model 102 generator and VNS Therapy™ Pulse Duo Model 102R generator, Houston, TX, 2003.)

Interest in studying the efficacy of VNS for MDD arose from the clinical experience of treating over 40,000 patients with treatment-resistant epilepsy with VNS. Depression is more prevalent in patients with epilepsy than it is in the general population, and it was noted that many patients with treatment-resistant epilepsy being treated with VNS experienced improvement in symptoms of MDD.[40,41] Eighty percent of the fibers in the left vagus nerve are afferent, meaning that the electrical charge delivered is predominantly sent to the brain. The left vagus nerve enters the brain and first innervates the nucleus tractus solitarius (NTS). While the mechanism of action of VNS is not completely understood, we know that the NTS communicates with the parabrachial nucleus (PBN), the cerebellum, the dorsal raphe, the periaqueductal gray (PAG), the locus coeruleus, and ascending projections to limbic, paralimbic, and cortical regions.[42] Functional neuroimaging studies of subjects receiving VNS show increased cerebral blood flow in many of these brain regions that are implicated in the pathophysiology of MDD.[43,44] For instance, the locus coeruleus and dorsal raphe nuclei contain the cell bodies of noradrenergic and serotonergic neurons that then project throughout the central nervous system. Last, the PBN communicates with other brain regions (including the hypothalamus, thalamus, amygdala, and nucleus of the stria terminalis) implicated in the pathophysiology of MDD.[42]

The three pivotal trials submitted to the FDA for approval of VNS for MDD were conducted to assess efficacy and safety. The first clinical trial was a randomized, controlled, acute 8-week study that assessed adjunctive VNS therapy versus sham treatment.[45] It is important to stress that VNS was studied as an adjunctive treatment. Therefore, it is recommended that all patients who receive VNS should continue to receive pharmacotherapy, psychotherapy, or both (and even ECT, if necessary). For the purposes of the clinical trials, ongoing treatment other than VNS was referred to as *treatment-as-usual*. Therefore, during the acute 8-week clinical trial, all patients continued to receive treatment-as-usual in addition to active VNS or sham VNS treatment. There were 112 patients in the active VNS treatment group and 110 patients in the sham VNS treatment group. In this acute 8-week study, VNS therapy failed to exhibit statistically significant efficacy on the primary outcome measure, the Hamilton Depression Rating Scale (a clinician-administered scale). However, the VNS group did demonstrate statistically significant greater improvement on a secondary outcome measure, the Inventory of Depressive Symptomatology—Self-Report (a self-report scale). After the acute 8-week trial, patients in both groups (with a total of 205 patients) went on to receive open active adjunctive treatment (continuing treatment-as-usual) with VNS therapy for 1 year in the second clinical trial.[46] At the 1-year follow-up, 27.2% of patients receiving adjunctive VNS responded and 15.8% met criteria for remission. In addition, the rates of response and remission doubled from 3 months to 12 months, suggesting that longer-term treatment may be required with VNS. The third clinical trial compared the patients receiving adjunctive VNS therapy during the 1-year follow-up study to a matched group of 124 treatment-refractory MDD patients who received only treatment-as-usual.[47] Response rates between VNS plus treatment-as-usual (19.6%) versus treatment-as-usual only (12.1%) were not statistically significant. However, there was a statistically significant difference between remission rates with VNS therapy plus treatment-as-usual (13.2%) and treatment-as-usual alone (3.2%). Last, this study found that one-half of VNS plus treatment-as-usual responders at 3 months remained responders at 12 months, while only one treatment-as-usual only responder at 3 months remained a responder at 12 months.

Adjustment of the stimulation parameters is performed by using a device that communicates transcutaneously with the IPG. The dose parameters used by the clinician for VNS therapy include the magnitude of the electrical charge delivered to the left vagus nerve, the stimulation frequency, the stimulation pulse width, and the duration of stimulation. Settings used in the clinical trials submitted to the FDA for approval of the device for TRD included a median output of 0.75 mA (range 0 to 1.5 mA), a median signal frequency of 20 Hz, a median pulse width of 500 μS, a median on-time of 30 seconds, and a median off-time of 5 minutes.[45] In practice, many clinicians use higher-output currents; it should be noted that higher-output currents of 3 mA are routinely used in patients with treatment-resistant epilepsy. In patients who are not responding to VNS, many clinicians will increase the charge duty cycle. As described above, a 10% duty cycle (30 seconds on, 5 minutes off) was used in the clinical trials submitted for FDA approval. However, decreasing the off-time to 2 or 3 minutes or increasing the on-time to 60 seconds (or both) can increase the duty cycle to as high as 50%. Duty cycles higher than 50% should not be used, as animal studies suggest potential vagus nerve damage at duty cycles higher than 50%. Finally, decreasing the stimulation pulse width or stimulation frequency is often helpful for addressing potential side effects associated with VNS therapy.

Potential risks associated with VNS include standard risks associated with the surgical procedure itself. Most common side effects associated with active VNS therapy are likely due to the fact that the electrodes are attached to the left vagus nerve near the laryngeal and pharyngeal branches of the left vagus nerve. The most common side effect is voice alteration (seen in 54% to 60% of patients). Other side effects include cough, neck pain, paresthesias and dyspnea.[46] These side effects typically decrease or dissipate over time. Strategies such as decreasing the stimulation frequency or pulse width are often helpful for reducing these side effects as well. Despite these side effects, the device is well tolerated, with only seven patients withdrawing from the clinical trial due to adverse events. Patients also have the ability to turn off the device at any time by placing a magnet provided by the manufacturer over the IPG. The IPG will remain off (i.e., no stimulation will occur) as long as the magnet is in place. When the magnet is removed, the IPG returns to its previously set stimulation parameters.

In summary, the clinical trial data suggest that VNS plus treatment-as-usual is more efficacious than treatment-as-usual alone. In addition, the side effects are typically tolerable as demonstrated by the fact that only 7 of 205 patients in the 1-year clinical trial discontinued the trial due to adverse events. It is important to note that the FDA-approval language states that VNS is an adjunctive treatment for TRD and that it should be used in patients with severe, chronic, recurrent TRD who have failed at least four adequate antidepressant trials.

ELECTROCONVULSIVE THERAPY

Electroconvulsive therapy (ECT) is discussed in detail elsewhere in this book (see Chapter 19). ECT has been used to treat depression since the 1930s, and many consider it the "gold standard" of antidepressant treatment. ECT involves delivery of an electrical current to the brain through the scalp and skull in order to induce a generalized seizure. While the mechanism by which generalized seizures alleviate depressive symptoms is not fully understood, the efficacy of ECT for depression has been demonstrated in a large number of clinical trials. A recent meta-analysis that included most of these clinical trials found that active ECT was significantly more effective than sham ECT and more effective than pharmacotherapy.[48] However, many patients relapse unless they receive periodic maintenance treatments; there are common side effects, such as memory loss, that are associated with ECT.[49]

TRANSCRANIAL MAGNETIC STIMULATION

Transcranial magnetic stimulation (TMS) is a non-invasive neuromodulation modality that uses powerful and rapidly changing magnetic fields applied over the surface of the skull to generate targeted electrical currents in the brain, painlessly and without the need for surgery, anesthesia, or the induction of seizures. Since its development in the mid-1980s; it has become a widely used tool for neuroscience research and clinical applications (diagnostic and therapeutic). In 2008, the FDA approved the use of high-frequency repetitive TMS (rTMS) over the left dorsolateral prefrontal cortex (DLPFC) for the treatment of MDD, and in 2013 the use of deep TMS H-coils for the treatment of MDD was also approved.

One of the primary advantages of TMS is its non-invasive nature, which is made possible by the application of Faraday's principle of electromagnetic induction. Briefly (and overly simplified), this principle states that a changing electrical current flowing through a circular coil will generate a magnetic field tangential to the plane of the coil. If this magnetic field comes in contact with another conductive material (e.g., a pick-up coil) it will generate a secondary electrical current (Figure 18-3A). TMS systems use an electrical capacitor to generate a brief powerful current that flows through the TMS coil, which is a circular loop of wire (usually copper) connected to the capacitor and embedded in a protective plastic case. According to Faraday's principle, when the electrical current flows through the circular coil, a rapidly changing magnetic field is generated. If the TMS coil is placed on the surface of the skull, this magnetic field will travel towards the intra-cranial space unaltered by the different structures it will cross (e.g., soft tissue, bone, CSF), until it reaches the electrically conductive neurons of the cortex. These neurons will act as an organic pick-up coil, and a secondary electrical current will be generated able to trigger action potentials and force brain cells to fire (Figure 18-3B). It is important to note that the stimulation of neurons is actually electrical, not magnetic,

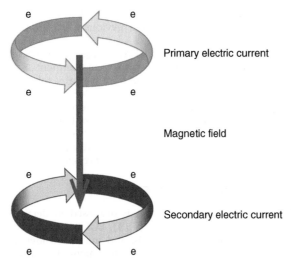

Figure 18-3. (A) This schematic illustrates the principle of electromagnetic induction, by which a primary electrical current generates a perpendicular magnetic field that, when in contact with a conductive material, leads to a secondary electrical current in the same plane, but opposite sense than the primary. (B) This drawing shows how this principle of physics is applied in TMS, placing a coil on the scalp surface leading to electrical stimulation of the cortex. (*Redrawn from Jalinous R. A guide to magnetic stimulation, Whitland, Carmarthenshire, Wales, UK, 1998, Magstim Company Ltd.*)

and the term "magnetic stimulation" is a misnomer. Magnetic pulses are used only as a vehicle to non-invasively transfer the electrical currents from the coil to the cortex. This avoids the need for surgical access to the intra-cranial space or the painful application of strong electrical currents on the skull.

Another important technical fact to take into account relates to the depth of TMS modulation. Although the magnetic field is practically unaltered by the various structures it finds on its path to the cortex, the strength of the field weakens as it moves away from its source in the TMS coil. As a result, the 1 to 2 Tesla magnetic pulse originated in the coil becomes too weak to generate neuronal action potentials 2–4 cm away from its origin on the surface of the skull. This sets a practical limitation to this technique, as only superficial cortical structures can be directly stimulated by TMS. Nevertheless, the effects of TMS are not only local but circuit-wide; once an action potential is generated in a cortical neuron, the volley of activation will travel through its axon and stimulate the post-synaptic neuron, leading to a cascade of events through the entire neural circuit (including deep cortical, sub-cortical and contralateral regions). This cascade of electrical events is specific to the brain circuit our target region is connected to, and not generalized like the effects of ECT. Therefore, although it is true that TMS can only directly modulate superficial cortical nodes, these nodes act as windows that provide modulatory access to an entire functional network of cortical and sub-cortical neurons.[50]

The effects of TMS are not only specific to the target of stimulation but also to the parameters used. This is important as we consider statements such as "TMS is (or is not) effective for a given condition", which lack meaning and are not informative. Alternatively, "TMS applied over a determined anatomical target at a specific frequency and dose for a particular condition" would be more clinically and neuroscientifically meaningful. Since the effects of TMS are specific to the stimulated region and the parameters used, we could certainly expect that stimulating prefrontal cortical areas that process

---

BOX 18-1 Transcranial Magnetic Stimulation Parameters

ANATOMICAL
1. Location (can be optimized with neuroimaging and neuronavigation).
2. Focality (depends primarily on coil architecture, also on intensity).
3. Depth (also depends primarily on coil architecture and partially on intensity).

PHYSIOLOGICAL
1. Frequency (can facilitate or inhibit a target region).
2. Intensity of stimulation (usually expressed as a percentage of the motor threshold).
3. Number of pulses per session (will also determine the duration of the session).
4. Number of sessions (treatment protocols require multiple sessions over weeks).

---

working memory or spatial attention would have little effect on mood, anhedonia, or neurovegetative symptoms of depression. Similarly, inhibiting a pathologically hypoactive region will most likely worsen a patient's condition, though its activation may prove therapeutic. Last, applying 2 weeks of stimulation when 6 or more weeks are needed should have minimal or no therapeutic impact. This highlights the need to have a basic understanding of the TMS parameters that clinicians and scientists are able to manipulate: the location or target of stimulation, the focality and depth, the frequency, and the dose of stimulation (which is a composite measure of stimulation intensity and duration) (Box 18-1). As mentioned above, the choice of the anatomical site of stimulation is crucial, as this will grant us access to modulate a specific functional network of interest. Recent developments in image-guided TMS using neuro-navigation have proved to increase the anatomical specificity and clinical efficacy of TMS,[51,52] but although this approach is common in cognitive neuroscience research it is still rare in clinical practice. Similarly, the focality of stimulation will be of relevance as the clinical impact and specificity won't be the same if one modulates a cortical area of 0.25 or 1 cm². Although the intensity of stimulation has an influence on the focality of its effects (the stronger the magnetic field, the deeper and less focal its effects),[53] focality is primarily controlled by the choice of TMS coil. Various types of coils are manufactured with differences in their internal architecture that allow varying degrees of focality and depth.[54] The most common types remain the circular coil (less focal) and the figure-of-eight or butterfly coil (more focal).[54,55] A new generation of deep TMS coils, such as the H-coil, have been developed in recent years and received FDA approval for the treatment of MDD in 2013.[56] Once these anatomical parameters are determined (location, focality, and depth), it is important to focus on physiological variables. Notably, TMS is able to either inhibit (down-regulate) or activate (up-regulate) populations of neurons, and these selective effects are primarily determined by the frequency of stimulation. With parameters similar to the ones leading to long-term depression (LTD) or long-term potentiation (LTP), low frequencies of 1 Hz are known to be inhibitory[57] while high frequencies of > 5 Hz (typically 10 or 20 Hz) are activating.[58] Newer TMS protocols with more complex patterns of stimulation (such as theta burst stimulation or TBS) have been developed in recent years.[59] Although the use of TBS in therapeutic settings has not been thoroughly tested, it is likely to have significant impact given its longer-lasting behavioral effects despite a significantly shorter stimulation time (a traditional therapeutic protocol for MDD lasts 37.5 minutes, while TBS can performed in 40 seconds). Once the target of stimulation and direction of modulation are set, the dose will be determined by deciding the strength of the magnetic field (pulse intensity) and the total number of pulses (duration). Duration also relates to the total number of sessions; typically, daily sessions over the course of weeks. Other more complex variables, such as the waveform of the electromagnetic current, are also relevant to define the dose.[60] As we improve our understanding of the mechanism of action of TMS, the parameter space available becomes more complex and rich, granting greater control and specificity to clinicians and scientists.[61]

The safety profile of TMS is notoriously benign, given its non-invasive nature. Nevertheless, it is an intervention and attention to safety and iatrogenic effects are important. The only contraindication considered to be absolute is the presence of metallic hardware in the area of stimulation, such as cochlear implants, brain stimulators, or medication pumps.[61] Still, the use of TMS on patients with DBS has been tested and considered relatively safe when the DBS system is off, although data are still very limited and extreme caution (in addition to an accurate risk/benefit analysis) should be used in these cases.[62] The primary safety concern with TMS remains the induction of seizures with repetitive trains, even if this is a very rare phenomenon; approximately 20 seizures have been reported out of the estimated 300,000 sessions (clinical or research) since its development in the early 1980s.[61] Since the 2008 FDA approval of the NeuroStar TMS Therapy® system (Neuronetics, Inc.), seven seizures have been reported in the USA from 250,000 treatment sessions in 8,000 patients.[63] This represents 1 case in 35,000 patients, which is similar or fewer than the seizure risk of most antidepressant medications. It should be noted that TMS may trigger a seizure but not cause epilepsy; seizures are always during (not after) rTMS, and do not lead to spontaneous events afterwards. Nevertheless, one should screen patients for a personal history of epilepsy and possible risk factors that increase their seizure risk (such as brain lesions or medications that lower the seizure threshold). Other less severe but more common side effects include headaches, local discomfort in the area of stimulation, facial twitching, tinnitus, anxiety, and vasovagal syncope.[61]

TMS is routinely used for diagnostic applications, primarily in clinical neurophysiology.[64] Therapeutic applications for various neurological and psychiatric conditions have been investigated since the development of repetitive TMS. In this chapter we will focus on therapeutic studies for MDD, since it is the most widely used indication and the only one with FDA approval in the US (although in other countries TMS is approved for other neuropsychiatric indications as well). The evidence for the use of high-frequency rTMS to the left DLPFC or low-frequency rTMS to the right DLPFC is supported by multiple clinical studies including over 2,000 patients and summarized in more than 10 meta-analyses and critical reviews.[65-78] Although conclusions from these analyses confirm the clinical efficacy of TMS, early trials used highly heterogeneous study designs and stimulation parameters, which in retrospect were often sub-therapeutic (e.g., only 2 weeks of stimulation or less than 1,000 pulses per session). This is to be expected in the early phases of any treatment development because the limits of safety are not well defined, but it was particular in TMS as most seizures occurred in the initial years, increasing the caution of researchers in the field. As a result, meta-analyses that included early studies were often burdened with excessive variability that compromised the capacity to extract clinically meaningful conclusions. Indeed, Gross and colleagues compared the efficacy of clinical trials published in

2007 against all previously published studies, and demonstrated the therapeutic superiority of recent studies.[69] Naturally, as the field developed, the use of more effective protocols became more consistent, and larger studies with more appropriate parameters were conducted.

In 2007, O'Reardon and colleagues published the first large multi-center, randomized clinical trial (RCT).[79] This trial was industry-sponsored and its data led to the FDA approval of the Neurostar TMS Therapy ® system (Neuronetics Inc.). Similarly, large RCTs, initiated by academic researchers and sponsored by the National Institutes of Health, have subsequently been conducted with similar results.[80] The Neurostar TMS trial conducted by O'Reardon and colleagues,[79] enrolled 325 patients with moderate to severe MDD who had failed at least one, but no more than four antidepressant treatments in the current episode. Patients started with a 1-week washout period in which medications were discontinued, as the study aimed to determine the effects of TMS monotherapy. Sessions occurred Monday to Friday over the course of 6 weeks, and were followed by a 3-week taper period. The parameters of stimulation were 10 Hz rTMS over the left DLPFC at 120% of the motor threshold, using 3,000 pulses per session. The left DLPFC was identified as the point 5 cm anterior to the primary motor cortex (where the motor threshold was calculated). Using this TMS regimen, which was much more aggressive than previously tested parameters, they proved this intervention to be very safe, not causing any seizures and only minimum-risk side effects, such as discomfort under the site of stimulation or headaches. Most importantly, TMS proved to be an effective antidepressant with response rates of 23.9%–24.5% (compared to 12.3%–15.1% for placebo) and remission rates of 14.2%–17.4% (compared to 5.5%–8.2% for placebo) after 6 weeks of treatment. It is significant to note that remission rates doubled from week 4 to week 6, and outcomes continued to improve during the taper phase, with response rates increasing from 23.9% to 27.7% and remission rates from 14.2% to 20.6% using the primary outcome (Montgomery-Asberg Depression Rating Scale or MADRS).

From a safety perspective, these data demonstrated how conservative TMS protocols in previous studies had been, as the upper limit of tolerable risks seems to be far even from this more aggressive regimen. In terms of efficacy, these results provided robust evidence for the dose-dependent antidepressant effects of TMS, as stimulation over weeks 4, 6, and the taper period continued to improve response and remission rates, and further separated active from placebo arms.

While RCTs are imperative to prove the efficacy of any treatment compared to placebo in a very controlled manner, the generalizability of these studies is usually limited by their strict inclusion and exclusion criteria that do not reflect the prototypical patient in standard clinical settings (e.g., suffering from multiple medical and psychiatric co-morbidities, undergoing concomitant treatments). This is why naturalistic effectiveness studies are needed to complement RCTs. Carpenter and colleagues[81] conducted a multi-site open label naturalistic trial in which they enrolled 339 patients who, on average, were more refractory, had a longer duration for the current episode and presented with more complex co-morbidities than the cohort in the Neurostar TMS trial[79]; i.e., they were sicker and more representative of the average patient. All participants were naïve to TMS but were allowed to continue with their ongoing pharmacological and psychotherapeutic treatments in addition to TMS. They received the same TMS protocol as reported by O'Reardon, consisting of 6 weeks of daily left prefrontal 10Hz TMS.[79] After 6 weeks of treatment, response rate for the primary outcome (Clinical Global Impressions—Severity or CGI-S) was 58% and remission rate 37.1%. Secondary outcome measures showed a range of response and remission rates of 41.5%–58% and 26.5%–37.1%, respectively. Age and severity of the current episode were negative predictors of response, but unlike patient in the Neurostar TMS trial, the number of previously failed medication trials did not negatively predict therapeutic response, as both mild and severely refractory patients presented with very similar outcomes. Other naturalistic studies have reported similar results.[82] These studies present effectiveness data in less controlled but more realistic settings, which better describe the outcomes expected for patients treated in clinics and hospitals with current standard protocols.

As TMS has entered clinical practice with more homogeneous protocols leading to greater effects sizes and decreased variability, researchers have explored what variables may predict the antidepressant response of TMS. Fregni and colleagues analyzed the pooled data for 195 patients from six independent studies.[83] They reported that age and the number of previously failed medication trials were negative predictors of response, i.e., younger and less refractory patients had better outcomes. Lisanby and colleagues analyzed the data from the Neurostar TMS trial and also identified the number of previously failed trials as a predictor of poor response, in addition to the duration of the current episode and the presence of co-morbid anxiety.[84] Interestingly, these clinical variables are not specific to TMS, but they seem to predict antidepressant response across treatment modalities including pharmacological and psychotherapeutic interventions. As the field moves towards identifying not only clinical or demographic variables but also biological markers that predict response to treatment, the hope is that the biomarkers linked to the therapeutics targets specifically modulated by the different treatment modalities will help stratify patients and individually select the most effective treatments.[85]

In summary, TMS is a powerful research and clinical tool with FDA approval for diagnostic applications in clinical neurophysiology and antidepressant therapy in the USA, although therapeutic indications are wider in other countries. Its non-invasive nature and benign safety profile, added to its proven antidepressant efficacy, have contributed to its introduction in community and academic clinics as standard of care. Future developments should advance our understanding of the efficacy of different parameters and present new stimulation protocols that expand the indications to other disorders and increase the cost-effectiveness of this consolidated treatment.

CONCLUSION

In this chapter, we have provided an overview of neurotherapeutic interventions for psychiatric disorders that are currently available or are being studied in clinical trials. Some of these treatments have been available for many years (e.g., ECT and ablative limbic system surgery), some (such as VNS, DBS or TMS) have only recently been approved by the FDA for psychiatric indications. Systems neuroscience and translational neuropsychiatry research are in the path to expand our therapeutic armamentarium even further with new indications and protocols for these treatments and novel technologies. These innovations will change how we practice, maximizing safety and efficacy and allowing us to individualize treatment decisions in the near future.

Access the complete reference list and multiple choice questions (MCQs) online at https://expertconsult.inkling.com

KEY REFERENCES

5. Dalgleish T, Yiend J, Bramham J, et al. Neuropsychological processing associated with recovery from depression after stereotactic subcaudate tetractomy. *Am J Psychiatry* 161:1913–1916, 2004.

6. Dougherty DD, Baer L, Cosgrove GR, et al. Prospective long-term follow-up of 44 patients who received cingulotomy for treatment-refractory obsessive-compulsive disorder. *Am J Psychiatry* 159:269–275, 2002.

11. Hardesty DE, Sackeim HA. Deep brain stimulation in movement and psychiatric disorders. *Biol Psychiatry* 61(7):831–835, 2007.

14. Corse D, Chou T, Arulpragasam AR, et al. Deep brain stimulation for obsessive-compulsive disorder. *Psychiatr Ann* 43(8):351–357, 2013.

26. Malone DA Jr, Dougherty DD, Rezai AR, et al. Deep brain stimulation of the ventral capsule/ventral striatum for treatment-resistant depression. *Biol Psychiatry* 65(4):267–275, 2009.

28. Mayberg HS, Lozano AM, Voon V, et al. Deep brain stimulation for treatment-resistant depression. *Neuron* 45(5):651–660, 2005.

29. Lozano AM, Mayberg HS, Giacobbe P, et al. Subcallosal cingulate gyrus deep brain stimulation for treatment-resistant depression. *Biol Psychiatry* 64(6):461–467, 2008.

31. Holtzheimer PE, Kelley ME, Gross RE, et al. Subcallosal cingulate deep brain stimulation for treatment-resistant unipolar and bipolar depression. *Arch Gen Psychiatry* 69(2):150–158, 2012.

32. Schlaepfer TE, Cohen MX, Frick C, et al. Deep brain stimulation to reward circuitry alleviates anhedonia in refractory major depression. *Neuropsychopharmacology* 33(2):368–377, 2008.

34. Kaur N, Chou T, Corse AK, et al. Deep brain stimulation for treatment-resistant depression. *Psychiatr Ann* 43(8):358–365, 2013.

39. Arulpragasam AR, Chou T, Kaur N, et al. Future directions of deep brain stimulation: current disorders, new technologies. *Psychiatr Ann* 43(8):366–373, 2013.

42. Nemeroff CB, Mayberg HS, Krahl SE, et al. VNS therapy in treatment-resistant depression: clinical evidence and putative neurobiological mechanisms. *Neuropsychopharmacology* 31:1345–1355, 2006.

47. George MS, Rush AJ, Marangell LB, et al. A one-year comparison of vagus nerve stimulation with treatment as usual for treatment-resistant depression. *Biol Psychiatry* 58:364–373, 2005.

48. The UK ECT Review Group. Efficacy and safety of electroconvulsive therapy in depressive disorders: a systematic review and meta-analysis. *Lancet* 361:799–808, 2003.

78. Slotema CW, Blom JD, Hoek HW, et al. Should we expand the toolbox of psychiatric treatment methods to include repetitive transcranial magnetic stimulation (rTMS)? A meta-analysis of the efficacy of rTMS in psychiatric disorders. *J Clin Psychiatry* 71(7):873–884, 2010.

19

Electroconvulsive Therapy

Charles A. Welch, MD

KEY POINTS

- Remission rates of 70%–90% have been reported in clinical trials of electroconvulsive therapy (ECT) and ECT is currently the most promising prospect for addressing the unmet worldwide need for effective treatment of individuals suffering from depression.

- The symptoms that predict a good response to ECT are those of major depression (e.g., anorexia, weight loss, early morning awakening, impaired concentration, pessimistic mood, motor restlessness, increased speech latency, constipation, and somatic or self-deprecatory delusions).

- Psychotic illness is the second most common indication for ECT; ECT is effective in up to 75% of patients with catatonia, regardless of the underlying cause, and is the treatment of choice as a primary treatment for most patients with catatonia.

- The greatest challenge facing ECT patients is the high rate of relapse after a successful index course of ECT. There is an urgent need to improve on current strategies of continuation ECT and continuation pharmacotherapy.

- The use of ultra-brief pulse waveform (0.3 ms) is becoming the standard of practice worldwide because of its extremely low side-effect profile. Nevertheless, some patients still require standard waveform (1.0 ms) to achieve full remission of symptoms.

OVERVIEW

Electroconvulsive therapy (ECT) remains an indispensable treatment because of the large number of depressed patients who are unresponsive to drugs or who are intolerant to their side effects. In the largest clinical trial of antidepressant medication, only 50% of depressed patients achieved a full remission, while an equal percentage were non-responders or achieved only partial remission.[1] On the other hand, remission rates of 70%–90% have been reported in clinical trials of ECT with response rates as high as 95% in delusional depression.[2,3] Depression requires effective treatment because it is associated with increased mortality (mainly due to cardiovascular events or suicide).[4] Furthermore, among all diseases, depression currently ranks fourth in global disease burden, and is projected to rank second by the year 2020.[5] ECT is currently the most promising prospect for addressing the unmet worldwide need for effective treatment of individuals suffering from medication-resistant depression.

INDICATIONS FOR ELECTROCONVULSIVE THERAPY

Major depression is the most common indication for ECT. The symptoms that predict a good response to ECT are those of major depression (e.g., anorexia, weight loss, early morning awakening, impaired concentration, pessimistic mood, motor restlessness, increased speech latency, constipation, and delusions).[6,7] The cardinal symptom is the acute loss of interest in

activities that formerly gave pleasure. These are exactly the same symptoms that constitute the indication for antidepressant drugs, and at the present time there is no way to predict which patients will ultimately be drug-resistant. There is currently little consensus on the definition of drug-resistant depression,[8] and the designation of drug failure varies with the adequacy of prior treatment.[9] Medical co-morbidities are also important to this definition. Young, healthy patients can safely receive four or more different drug regimens before moving to ECT, whereas older depressed patients may be unable to tolerate more than one drug trial without developing serious medical complications.

Other factors also affect the threshold for moving from drug therapy to ECT. Suicidal ideation and intent respond to ECT 80% of the time,[10] and are an indication for an early transition from drug therapy.[11] Lower response rates to ECT have been reported in depressed patients with a co-morbid personality disorder,[12] and a longer duration of depression,[13] but there is conflicting evidence in the literature as to whether a history of medication-resistance is associated with a lower response rate to ECT. However, none of these factors constitute a reason to avoid ECT if neurovegetative signs are present.

Psychotic illness is the second most common indication for ECT. Although it is not a routine treatment for schizophrenia, ECT, in combination with a neuroleptic, may result in sustained improvement in up to 80% of drug-resistant patients with chronic schizophrenia.[14,15] Young patients with psychosis conforming to the schizophreniform profile (i.e., with acute onset, positive psychotic symptoms, affective intactness, and medication-resistance) are more responsive to ECT than are those with chronic schizophrenia, and they may have a full and enduring remission of their illness with treatment.[16–18]

Bipolar depression has over a 50% remission rate with ECT. Mania also responds well to ECT,[19,20] but drug treatment remains the first-line therapy. Nevertheless, in controlled trials, ECT is as effective as lithium (or more so), and in drug-refractory mania, more than 50% of cases have remitted with ECT.[21] ECT is highly effective in the treatment of medication-resistant mixed affective states[22] and refractory bipolar disorder in adolescents.[23]

Although most patients initially receive a trial of medication regardless of their diagnosis, several groups of patients (see below) are appropriate for ECT as a primary treatment. These include: patients who are severely malnourished, dehydrated, and exhausted due to protracted depressive illness (they should be treated promptly after careful re-hydration); patients with complicating medical illness (such as cardiac arrhythmia or coronary artery disease) because these individuals are often more safely treated with ECT than with antidepressants; patients with delusional depression (as they are often resistant to antidepressant therapy,[24] but respond to ECT 80%–90% of the time)[25–27]; patients who have been unresponsive to medications during previous episodes (because they are often better served by proceeding directly to ECT); and, the majority of patients with catatonia (as they respond promptly to ECT).[28–30] Although the catatonic syndrome is most often associated with an affective disorder, catatonia may also be a manifestation of schizophrenia, metabolic disorders, structural brain lesions, anti-NMDA receptor encephalitis, or systemic lupus erythematosus. Prompt treatment is essential because the mortality of untreated catatonia is as high as 50%,

217

and even its non-fatal complications (including pneumonia, venous embolus, limb contracture, and decubitus ulcer) are serious. ECT is effective in up to 75% of patients with catatonia, regardless of the underlying cause, and is the treatment of choice as a primary treatment for most patients with catatonia.[31] Lorazepam has also been effective for short-term treatment of catatonia,[32] but its long-term efficacy has not been confirmed. While neuroleptic malignant syndrome (NMS) may be clinically indistinguishable from catatonia,[33] high fever, opisthotonos, and rigidity are more common in the former. ECT has been reported effective in NMS,[34] but intensive supportive medical treatment, discontinuation of neuroleptic therapy, use of dantrolene, and use of bromocriptine are still the essential steps of management.

RISK FACTORS ASSOCIATED WITH ELECTROCONVULSIVE THERAPY

As the technical conduct of ECT has improved, factors that were formerly considered absolute contraindications to ECT have become relative risk factors. The patient is best served by weighing the risk of treatment against the morbidity or lethality of remaining depressed. The prevailing view is that there are no longer any absolute contraindications to ECT, but the following conditions warrant careful work-up and management.

The heart is physiologically stressed during ECT.[35] Cardiac work increases abruptly at the onset of the seizure initially because of sympathetic outflow from the diencephalon, through the spinal sympathetic tract, to the heart (Figure 19-1). This outflow persists for the duration of the seizure and is augmented by a rise in circulating catecholamine levels that peak about 3 minutes after the onset of seizure activity (Figure 19-2A).[36,37] After the seizure ends, parasympathetic tone remains strong, often causing transient bradycardia and hypotension, with a return to baseline function in 5–10 minutes (see Figure 19-2B).

The cardiac conditions that most often worsen under this autonomic stimulus are ischemic heart disease, hypertension, congestive heart failure (CHF), and cardiac arrhythmias. These conditions, if properly managed, have proved to be surprisingly tolerant to ECT. The idea that general anesthesia is contraindicated within 6 months of a myocardial infarction (MI) has acquired a certain sanctity, which is surprising considering the ambiguity of the original data.[38] A more rational approach involves careful assessment of the cardiac reserve, a reserve that is needed as cardiac work increases during ECT.[39] Vascular aneurysms should be repaired before ECT if possible, but in practice, they have proved surprisingly durable during treatment.[40,41] Critical aortic stenosis should be surgically corrected before ECT to avoid ventricular overload during the seizure. Patients with cardiac pacemakers generally tolerate ECT uneventfully, although proper pacer function should be ascertained before treatment. Implantable cardioverter defibrillators should be converted from demand mode to fixed mode by placing a magnet over the device during ECT.[42] Patients with compensated CHF generally tolerate ECT well, although a transient decompensation into pulmonary edema for 5–10 minutes may occur in patients with a baseline ejection fraction below 20%. It is unclear whether the underlying cause is a neurogenic stimulus to the lung parenchyma or a reduction in cardiac output because of increased heart rate and blood pressure.

The brain is also physiologically stressed during ECT. Cerebral oxygen consumption approximately doubles, and cerebral blood flow increases several-fold. Increases in intracranial pressure and the permeability of the blood–brain barrier also develop. These acute changes may increase the risk of ECT in patients with a variety of neurological conditions.[43]

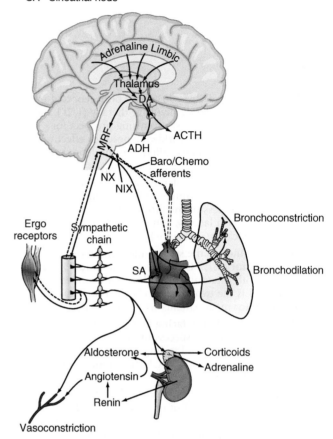

DA - Defense area in hypothalamus
MRF - Medullary reticular formation
SA - Sinoatrial node

Figure 19-1. Schematic of sympathetic outflow from the diencephalon to the heart and other organs.

Space-occupying brain lesions were previously considered an absolute contraindication to ECT, and earlier case reports described clinical deterioration when ECT was given to patients with brain tumors.[44] However, more recent reports indicate that with careful management patients with brain tumor or chronic subdural hematomas may be safely treated.[45–48] Recent cerebral infarction probably represents the most common intracranial risk factor. Case reports of ECT after recent cerebral infarction indicate that the complication rate is low,[43] and consequently ECT is often the treatment of choice for post-stroke depression.[49] The interval between infarction and time of ECT should be determined by the urgency of treatment for depression.

ECT has been safe and efficacious in patients with hydrocephalus, arteriovenous malformations, cerebral hemorrhage, multiple sclerosis, systemic lupus erythematosus, Huntington's disease, and mental retardation. Patients with depression and Parkinson's disease experience improvement of both disorders with ECT, and Parkinson's disease alone may constitute an indication for ECT.[50] Depressed patients with pre-existing dementia are likely to develop especially severe cognitive deficits secondary to ECT, but most return to their baseline after treatment, and many actually improve.[51,52]

The pregnant mother who is severely depressed may require ECT to prevent malnutrition or suicide. Although reports of ECT during pregnancy are reassuring,[53] fetal monitoring is recommended during treatment. The fetus may be protected from the physiological stress of ECT by nature of its lack of

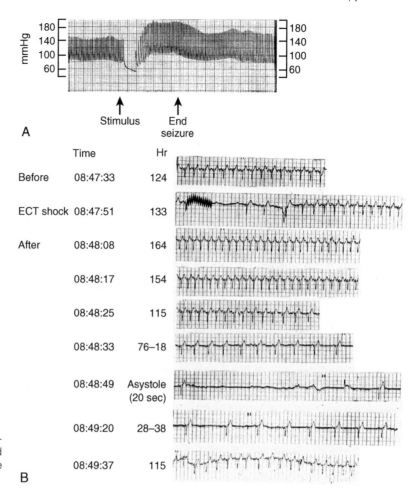

Figure 19-2. (A) Graphic of the impact of electroconvulsive therapy (ECT) on catecholamine levels and blood pressure following a seizure. (B) Graphic of the effects of ECT on cardiac rhythm.

direct neuronal connection to the maternal diencephalon, which spares it the intense autonomic stimulus experienced by maternal end organs during the ictus.

TECHNIQUE FOR CONDUCTING ELECTROCONVULSIVE THERAPY

The routine pre-ECT work-up usually includes a thorough medical history and physical examination, along with: a chest film; an electrocardiogram (EKG); a urinalysis; a complete blood count; and determination of blood glucose, blood urea nitrogen, and electrolytes. Additional studies may be necessary, at the clinician's discretion. In a patient with cognitive deficits, it is sometimes difficult to decide whether a CNS work-up is indicated because depression itself is usually the cause of this deficit. A metabolic screen, computed tomography (CT) scan, and magnetic resonance imaging (MRI) are often useful to rule out causes of impaired cognition unrelated to depression. Whenever a question of primary dementia arises, neurological consultation should be requested. Neuropsychological testing may be diagnostically helpful in making the distinction between primary dementia and depressive pseudomentia.[54,55]

It is essential that the patient's medical condition be optimized before starting treatment. Elderly patients often arrive at the hospital severely malnourished and dehydrated, and ECT should be delayed until they have had several days of re-hydration, with alimentation via feeding tube, if necessary. Antihypertensive regimens should be optimized before treatment to reduce the chance of a severe hypertensive reaction during treatment. Most diabetic patients are more stable if the

morning dose of insulin is held until after their treatment. The insulin requirement usually decreases as a diabetic patient recovers from depression, and blood glucose levels must be monitored frequently during the course of ECT.

Antidepressant medications do not necessarily have to be discontinued prior to ECT, since there is little evidence of a harmful interaction. Indeed, there is preliminary evidence that neuroleptics, tricyclic antidepressants (TCAs), selective serotonin re-uptake inhibitors (SSRIs), and mirtazapine are not only safe to prescribe during a course of ECT, but also may enhance the therapeutic effectiveness of the treatment.[56] Monoamine oxidase inhibitors (MAOIs) may be safely given during a course of ECT, as long as sympathomimetic drugs are not administered.[57] Early case reports described excessive cognitive disturbance and prolonged apnea in a small percentage of patients receiving lithium during ECT, but more recent data indicate that this is a rare complication, and that concurrent administration of lithium is usually safe.[58] Benzodiazepines are antagonistic to the ictal process and should be discontinued.[59] Even short-acting benzodiazepines may have a long half-life in a sick, elderly person and make effective treatment less likely. For sedation, patients receiving ECT usually do well with a sedating atypical antipsychotic, such as quetiapine, or a non-benzodiazepine hypnotic, such as hydroxyzine. Anticonvulsants, prescribed as mood stabilizers, are usually discontinued prior to ECT, but in a recent series of bipolar patients the concurrent administration of lamotrigine did not interfere with treatment, and facilitated transition to maintenance pharmacotherapy.[60] In the patient with a pre-existing seizure disorder, the anticonvulsant regimen should be continued for patient safety. The elevated seizure threshold can almost always be over-ridden with an ECT stimulus, and patients managed in this manner usually have the same clinical response as patients not taking anticonvulsants.[61]

Because of the profound systemic physiological responses unique to this treatment, anesthesia for ECT should be performed by an anesthesiologist familiar with it. ECT presents special challenges in anesthetic management, and a careful reading of the pertinent literature is essential preparation for the anesthesiologist.[62] The use of cardiac monitoring and pulse oximetry on all patients undergoing general anesthesia has been endorsed by the American Society of Anesthesiologists. Most existing ECT machines record the EKG only during the treatment itself, but recording of baseline and post-ictal rhythms is essential, and a separate operating room monitor with paper recording capability is therefore necessary to monitor the EKG adequately.

Prior to induction, atropine or glycopyrrolate may be administered routinely to all patients, but in many treatment centers their use is reserved for patients who are prone to bradycardia. Atropine does not reduce oral secretions in ECT.[63]

The four most commonly used induction agents are methohexital, propofol, etomidate, and ketamine, and each has its pros and cons.[64] Methohexital does not affect the seizure threshold, and has been extensively studied. Propofol increases seizure threshold, and is associated with shorter seizures, a higher intensity of the stimulus, and a higher number of treatments.[65] Nevertheless, overall therapeutic response rates with propofol are no worse than with the other agents, and it has a uniquely smooth emergence syndrome. Etomidate lowers seizure threshold and is associated with longer seizures,[66] but has the disadvantage of causing adrenal suppression, even in single doses. Ketamine also lowers the seizure threshold, and is associated with less memory disturbance than etomidate.[67] Both methohexital and propofol cause a significant drop in blood pressure on induction, while etomidate and ketamine do not. In most treatment centers, either methohexital or propofol is used as the routine induction agent, while etomidate or ketamine is reserved for patients with high seizure thresholds or a fragile cardiovascular status.

Sevoflurane, an inhaled anesthetic, is a proven ECT-induction agent for patients with severe needle phobia, agitation, or poor tolerance of intravenous (IV) induction agents.[68] For children it is often the least traumatic induction method. It can be used as the only induction agent, or it can be augmented with IV agents once the patient is unconscious.

Paralytic drugs are essential to the safe conduct of ECT. Prior to the use of paralytic agents, over 30% of ECT patients suffered compression fractures of the spine. The standard agent is succinylcholine, which is a depolarizing muscle relaxant. Depolarizing drugs cause a rise in serum potassium, which is usually well tolerated, but may be exaggerated in patients who are inactive or bed-ridden, paretic secondary to stroke or injury, or who have the suffered recent major burns. In these patients, a non-depolarizing muscle relaxant offers important advantages, since it does not cause a rise in serum potassium.[69] Cisatrocurium and rocuronium are the two shortest acting non-depolarizing agents currently available, but both have a duration of action of 10–20 minutes, which is several-fold longer than succinylcholine.

Short-acting IV β-blockers effectively reduce stress on the heart. These agents attenuate hypertension, tachycardia, ectopy, and cardiac ischemia, and with proper use they rarely result in hypotension or bradycardia. Esmolol (2–4 mg/kg) or labetalol (0.2–0.4 kg/mg) given IV immediately before the anesthetic induction is usually sufficient, but higher doses may be necessary in individual patients.[70] Esmolol has the advantage of being much shorter-acting than labetalol. Although theoretically these drugs may result in decompensa-tion of CHF, this has not been reported in practice. Nitroglycerine (infused at 0.5 to 3.0 mg/kg/minute) may be used to blunt the hypertensive response of patients who are already receiving β-blockers or calcium channel blockers and who require additional antihypertensives. For patients refractory to these approaches, nitroprusside delivered by slow IV infusion is highly effective, but requires blood pressure monitoring with an intra-arterial line to avoid overshooting the blood pressure target.

Treating hypertension adequately before a course of ECT usually reduces the hypertensive response during the treatment itself. Maintenance β-blockers (such as atenolol 25–50 mg orally every day) may render the use of a short-acting antihypertensive during treatment unnecessary.

Conduction system abnormalities during treatment have been reported in 20% to 80% of ECT patients,[71] but such abnormalities are usually transient. Persistent or severe arrhythmias occasionally require treatment, and the approach depends on the type of arrhythmia. Supraventricular tachycardias generally are best treated with calcium channel blockers, whereas ventricular ectopy is most rapidly stabilized with IV lidocaine. Many arrhythmias can be prevented by pre-treatment with a short-acting IV β-blocker before subsequent treatments.

Decompensation of CHF is usually treatable with oxygen and with elevation of the head. Occasionally, IV furosemide and morphine become necessary, but this is extremely rare. Most patients re-compensate within 10 to 15 minutes of the treatment without aggressive intervention.

Cardiac arrest is a rare complication of ECT. The majority of patients have some degree of sinus pause after the ECT stimulus that may last up to eight seconds, and this may be mistaken for a true arrest.[35] Patients who receive non-convulsive stimuli may be especially at risk for extended sinus pauses. Because the intense parasympathetic outflow caused by the stimulus is not counteracted by the sympathetic outflow of the seizure itself, severe bradycardia or arrest may ensue. Immediately following the cessation of ictal activity, parasympathetic tone is predominant and bradycardia is common. However, a full cardiac arrest may also occur during the immediate post-ictal interval.

The relative efficacy of unilateral and bilateral electrode placement remains unclear, but for most patients, a unilateral stimulus, when performed under optimal conditions, is as effective as a bilateral stimulus.[72,73] Ineffective unilateral ECT is associated with use of threshold stimulus intensity.[74] Consequently, a unilateral stimulus should be well over threshold with the electrodes placed in the d'Elia position (Figure 19-3A and 19-3B). Recent studies report equal efficacy as long as unilateral ECT is performed with a stimulus intensity well above seizure threshold.[75] Bifrontal electrode placement has not been extensively studied, but evidence thus far indicates that it has equal effectiveness when compared to bitemporal and right unilateral electrode placement.[76,77]

Use of brief pulse waveform has become standard practice in the US (Figure 19-4). Brief pulse waveform is efficient at inducing seizure activity and is associated with little post-treatment confusion and amnesia.[78] Recently, modification of brief pulse waveform, by reducing pulse width and extending the stimulus duration, has resulted in a stimulus referred to as ultra-brief pulse.[79-81]

Generalization of the seizure to the entire brain is essential for efficacy.[82] The standard way to monitor seizure generalization is to inflate a blood pressure cuff on an arm or ankle above systolic pressure, just before injection of succinylcholine. The convulsion can then be observed in the unparalyzed extremity. In unilateral ECT, the cuff is placed on the limb ipsilateral to the stimulus. Most ECT instruments have a built-in single-channel electroencephalographic monitor, but this is not always a reliable indicator of full seizure generalization because partial seizures may also generate a typical seizure tracing.

Following ECT, patients should not be left in the supine position but should be turned on their side to allow better drainage of secretions. Patients should be monitored carefully by a recovery nurse; vital signs should be taken regularly and pulse oximetry employed. Some patients, typically young, healthy individuals, may develop an agitated delirium with a vacant stare, disorientation, and automatisms immediately

following treatment. This clinical picture is usually due to tardive seizures; it clears promptly with midazolam (2–5 mg IV), diazepam (5–10 mg IV) or propofol (20–40 mg IV). Post-treatment agitation may be preemptively treated with propofol 30–50 mg intravenously immediately after cessation of the seizure. Post-treatment nausea may be effectively treated with droperidol (1.25–2.5 mg IV), and prevented in subsequent treatments with pre-medication using ondansetron (4 mg IV).

The average number of ECT procedures necessary to treat major depression is consistently reported to be between 6 and 12 treatments, but occasional patients may require up to 30. The customary timing is three sessions per week with one full seizure per session. The use of more than one seizure per session (multiple monitored ECT) has no proven advantages. The most objective comparison of single and multiple ECT was performed by Fink,[83] who concluded, "Multiple ECT carried more risks and fewer benefits than conventional ECT for our patients."

ADVERSE EFFECTS OF ELECTROCONVULSIVE THERAPY

Survey data indicate a mortality rate of 0.03% in patients who undergo ECT.[84] Although there is no evidence for structural brain damage as a result of ECT,[85] there are important effects on cognition. Memory impairment varies greatly in severity and is associated with bilateral electrode placement, high stimulus intensity, inadequate oxygenation, prolonged seizure activity, advanced age, alcohol abuse, and lower premorbid cognitive function.[86] Difficulty recalling new information (anterograde amnesia) is usually experienced during the ECT series, but it normally resolves within a month after the last treatment. Difficulty remembering events before ECT (retrograde amnesia) is usually more severe for events closer to the time of treatment. Bilateral ECT causes more memory disturbance than does unilateral, and this is true for both retrograde and anterograde memory function and for both verbal and non-verbal recall.[87]

A meta-analysis of cognitive function testing in 2,981 patients in 84 studies[88] found significant decreases in cognitive performance scores 0 to 3 days after completion of a series of ECT. However, within 15 days of the last ECT treatment, almost all mean test scores were at or above pre-ECT levels. After 15 days, improvements compared to baseline were observed in processing speed, working memory, anterograde memory, and aspects of executive function.

Severe encephalopathy associated with ECT may require discontinuation of treatment. Usually, substantial improvement occurs within 48 hours after the last treatment. If symptoms become more severe with time after cessation of treatment, a full neurological work-up is indicated to assess whether there is an underlying cause other than ECT.

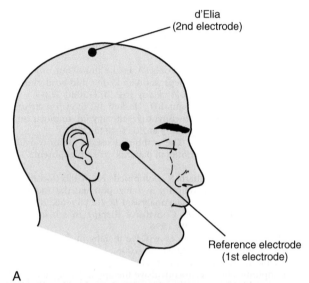
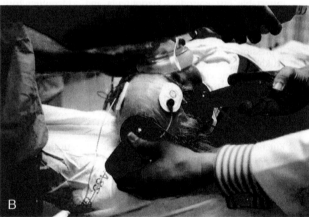

Figure 19-3. (A) Schematic of electrode placements during electroconvulsive therapy (ECT). (B) Photograph of electrodes being placed during ECT.

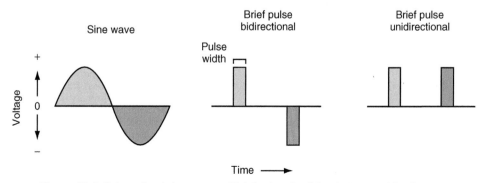

Figure 19-4. Schematic of sine wave and brief pulse stimuli for electroconvulsive therapy.

MAINTENANCE ELECTROCONVULSIVE THERAPY TREATMENT

Following successful treatment with ECT, without any continuation therapy the risk of depressive relapse is greater than 80% at 6 months.[89] Continuation therapy with nortriptyline plus lithium is associated with a relapse rate of about 50% at 6 months.[89-91] Continuation therapy with venlafaxine plus lithium is associated with a relapse rate of approximately 40% at 6 months.[91] In a recent comparison of pharmacotherapy alone versus ECT plus pharmacotherapy, relapse rates at 1 year were 61% with pharmacotherapy alone and 32% with pharmacotherapy plus maintenance ECT.[92] Continuation ECT alone (weekly for 4 weeks, biweekly for 8 weeks, and monthly for 3 months) lowers the relapse rate at 6 months to below 40%.[90] Large controlled trials of other antidepressant drugs after ECT have not yet been conducted. Although questions remain about the relative effectiveness of continuation ECT and continuation pharmacotherapy, the cumulative evidence over the last decade indicates that continuation ECT is a valuable and effective strategy for most patients.

ELECTROCONVULSIVE THERAPY IN CHILDREN

The first meta-analysis of published reports of ECT in children, published in 1997, reported response rates of 63% in depression, 80% in mania, 42% in schizophrenia, and 80% in catatonia.[93] In 2004, the American Academy of Child and Adolescent Psychiatry published its *Practice Parameter for Use of Electroconvulsive Therapy with Adolescents*,[94] in which it recognized the high effectiveness of ECT in children, set forth guidelines for safe administration of ECT in adolescents, and addressed the ethical and legal issues involved with ECT in this age group. Recent published reviews have addressed ECT for children with catatonia,[95] autism,[96] schizophrenia,[97] and maintenance ECT.[98] There is a rapidly growing body of evidence that ECT in children and adolescents is safe, effective, well tolerated, and long lasting.[99,100]

CONCLUSION

ECT continues to undergo reduction in side effects, improved effectiveness, more exact indications, and enhanced safety. Although the mechanism of action remains unknown, current research into these issues will ultimately produce important insights into the pathophysiology of mood disorders. In view of its unique effectiveness in patients unresponsive to other therapies, it is likely that the technique of ECT will continue to be refined, and its indications expanded. It is likely that ECT will not only be a cornerstone of psychiatric treatment for the foreseeable future but also an important window on the pathophysiology of mood disorders and psychosis.

Access a list of MCQs for this chapter at https://expertconsult .inkling.com

REFERENCES

1. Rush A. STAR*D: what have we learned? *Am J Psychiatry* 164:201–204, 2007.
2. Petrides G, Fink M, Husain MM, et al. ECT remission rates in psychotic versus non-psychotic depressed patients: a report from CORE. *J ECT* 17:244–253, 2001.
3. Koh KH, van Vreeswijk MA, Simpson S, et al. A meta-analysis of electroconvulsive therapy efficacy in depression. *J ECT* 19:139–147, 2003.
4. Angst F, Stassen HH, Clayton PJ, et al. Mortality of patients with mood disorders: follow-up over 34–38 years. *J Affect Disorders* 68:167–181, 2002.
5. Murray CJL, Lopez AD. Alternative projections of mortality and disability by cause 1990–2020: Global Burden of Disease Study. *Lancet* 349:1498–1504, 1997.
6. Carney MWP, Roth M, Garside RF. The diagnosis of depressive syndromes and the prediction of ECT response. *Br J Psychiatry* 3:659–674, 1965.
7. Swartz CM, editor: *Electroconvulsive and neuromodulation therapies*, Cambridge, 2009, Cambridge University Press.
8. Souery D, Papakostas GI, Trivedi MH. Treatment-resistant depression. *J Clin Psychiatry* 67(Suppl. 6):16–26, 2006.
9. Sackeim HA. The definition and meaning of treatment-resistant depression. *J Clin Psychiatry* 62(Suppl. 16):10–17, 2001.
10. Kellner CH, Fink M, Knapp R, et al. Relief of expressed suicidal intent by ECT: a consortium for research in ECT study. *Am J Psychiatry* 162:977–982, 2005.
11. Patel M, Patel S, Hardy DW, et al. Should electroconvulsive therapy be an early consideration for suicidal patients? *J ECT* 22:113–115, 2006.
12. Feske U, Mulsant BH, Pilkonis PA, et al. Clinical outcome of ECT inpatients with major depression and comorbid borderline personality disorder. *Am J Psychiatry* 161:2073–2080, 2004.
13. Dombrovski AY, Mulsant BH, Haskett RF, et al. Predictors of remission after electroconvulsive therapy in unipolar major depression. *J Clin Psychiatry* 66:1043–1049, 2005.
14. Braga RJ, Petrides G. The combined use of electroconvulsive therapy and antipsychotics in patients with schizophrenia. *J ECT* 21:75–83, 2005.
15. Painuly N, Chakrabarti S. Combined use of electroconvulsive therapy and antipsychotics in schizophrenia: the Indian evidence. A review and meta analysis. *J ECT* 22:59–66, 2006.
16. Fink M, Sackeim HA. Convulsive therapy in schizophrenia? *Schizophr Bull* 22:27–39, 1996.
17. Ucok A, Cakir S. Electroconvulsive therapy in the first-episode schizophrenia. *J ECT* 22:22–38, 2006.
18. Suzuki K, Atawa S, Takano T, et al. Improvement of psychiatric symptoms after electroconvulsive therapy in young adults with intractable first episode schizophrenia and schizophreniform disorder. *Tohoku J Exp Med* 210:213–220, 2006.
19. Dierckx B, Heijnen WT, van den Broek WW, et al. Efficacy of electroconvulsive therapy in bipolar versus unipolar major depression: a meta-analysis. *Bipolar Disord* 14:146–150, 2012.
20. Mukherjee S, Sackeim HA, Schnur DB. Electroconvulsive therapy of acute manic episodes: a review of 50 years experience. *Am J Psychiatry* 151:169–176, 1994.
21. Mukherjee S, Sackeim HA, Lee C. Unilateral ECT in the treatment of manic episodes. *Convuls Ther* 4:74–80, 1988.
22. Devanand DP, Polanco P, Cruz R, et al. The efficacy of ECT in mixed affective states. *J ECT* 16:32–37, 2000.
23. Kutcher S, Robertson HA. Electroconvulsive therapy in treatment-resistant bipolar youth. *J Child Adolesc Psychopharmacol* 5:167–175, 1995.
24. Wheeler Vega JA, Mortimer AM, Tyson PJ. Somatic treatment of psychotic depression: review and recommendations for practice. *J Clin Psychopharmacol* 20:504–519, 2000.
25. Kroessler D. Relative efficacy rates for therapies of delusional depression. *Convuls Ther* 1:173–182, 1985.
26. Janicak PG, Easton M, Comaty JE, et al. Efficacy of ECT in psychotic and nonpsychotic depression. *Convuls Ther* 5:314–320, 1989.
27. Spiker DG, Stein J, Rich CL. Delusional depression and electroconvulsive therapy: one year later. *Convuls Ther* 1:167–172, 1985.
28. Mann SC, Caroff SN, Bleier HR, et al. Lethal catatonia. *Am J Psychiatry* 143:1374–1381, 1986.
29. Mann SC, Caroff SN, Bleier HR, et al. Electroconvulsive therapy of the lethal catatonia syndrome. *Convuls Ther* 6:239–247, 1990.
30. Rohland BM, Carroll BT, Jacoby RG. ECT in the treatment of the catatonic syndrome. *J Affect Disord* 29:255–261, 1993.
31. Fink M. Is catatonia a primary indication for ECT? *Convuls Ther* 6:1–4, 1990.
32. Rosebush PI, Hildebrand AM, Furlong BG, et al. Catatonic syndrome in a general psychiatric inpatient population: frequency, clinical presentation, and response to lorazepam. *J Clin Psychiatry* 51:357–362, 1990.
33. Fink M. Neuroleptic malignant syndrome and catatonia: one entity or two? *Biol Psychiatry* 39:1–4, 1996.

34. Davis JM, Janicak PG, Sakkas P, et al. Electroconvulsive therapy in the treatment of the neuroleptic malignant syndrome. *Convuls Ther* 7:111–120, 1991.
35. Welch CA, Drop LJ. Cardiovascular effects of ECT. *Convuls Ther* 5:35–43, 1989.
36. Khan A, Nies A, Johnson G, et al. Plasma catecholamines and ECT. *Biol Psychiatry* 20:799–804, 1985.
37. Liston EH, Salk JD. Hemodynamic responses to ECT after bilateral adrenalectomy. *Convuls Ther* 6:160–164, 1990.
38. Goldman L. Multifactorial index of cardiac risk of non-cardiac surgical procedures. *N Engl J Med* 297:845–850, 1977.
39. Drop JD, Welch CA. Anesthesia for electroconvulsive therapy in patients with major cardiovascular risk factors. *Convuls Ther* 5:88–101, 1989.
40. Drop LJ, Bouckoms AJ, Welch CA. Arterial hypertension and multiple cerebral aneurysms in a patient treated with electroconvulsive therapy. *J Clin Psychiatry* 49:280–282, 1988.
41. Viguera A, Rordorf G, Schouten R, et al. Intracranial hemodynamics during attenuated responses to electroconvulsive therapy in the presence of an intracerebral aneurysm. *J Neurol Neurosurg Psychiatry* 64:802–805, 1998.
42. Dolenc TJ, Barnes RD, Hayes DL. Electroconvulsive therapy in patients with cardiac pacemakers and implantable cardioverter defibrillators. *Pace* 27:1257–1263, 2004.
43. Hsiao JK, Messenheimer JA, Evans DL. ECT and neurological disorders. *Convuls Ther* 3:121–136, 1987.
44. Maltbie AA, Wingfield MS, Volow MR, et al. Electroconvulsive therapy in the presence of brain tumor: case reports and an evaluation of risk. *J Nerv Ment Dis* 168:400–405, 1980.
45. Fried D, Mann JJ. Electroconvulsive treatment of a patient with known intracranial tumor. *Biol Psychiatry* 23:176–180, 1988.
46. Malek-Ahmadi P, Beceiro JR, McNeil BW, et al. Electroconvulsive therapy and chronic subdural hematoma. *Convuls Ther* 6:38–41, 1990.
47. Zwil AS, Bowring MA, Price TRP, et al. Prospective electroconvulsive therapy in the presence of intracranial tumor. *Convuls Ther* 6:299–307, 1990.
48. Patkar AA, Hill KP, Weinstein SP, et al. ECT in the presence of brain tumor and increased intracranial pressure: evaluation and reduction of risk. *J ECT* 16:187–189, 2000.
49. Currier MB, Murray GB, Welch CA. Electroconvulsive therapy for post-stroke depressed geriatric patients. *J Neuropsychiatry Clin Neurosci* 4:140–144, 1992.
50. Fink M. ECT for Parkinson's disease? *Convuls Ther* 4:189–191, 1988.
51. Steif BL, Sackeim HA, Portnoy S, et al. Effects of depression and ECT on anterograde memory. *Biol Psychiatry* 21:921–930, 1986.
52. Nelson JP, Rosenberg DR. ECT treatment of demented elderly patients with major depression: a retrospective study of efficacy and safety. *Convuls Ther* 7:157–165, 1991.
53. Ferrill MJ, Kehoe WA, Jacisin JJ. ECT during pregnancy: physiologic and pharmacologic considerations. *Convuls Ther* 8:186–200, 1992.
54. Austin MP, Mitchell K, Wilhelm G, et al. Cognitive function in depression: a distinct pattern of frontal impairment in melancholia? *Psychol Med* 29:73–85, 1999.
55. Austin MP, Mitchell P, Goodwin GM. Cognitive deficits in depression: possible implications for functional neuropathology. *Br J Psychiatry* 178:200–206, 2001.
56. Baghi TC, Marcuse A, Brosch M, et al. The influence of concomitant antidepressant medication on safety, tolerability, and clinical effectiveness of electroconvulsive therapy. *World J Biol Psychiatry* 7:82–90, 2006.
57. Dolenc TJ, Habl SS, Barnes RD, et al. Electroconvulsive therapy in patients taking monoamine oxidase inhibitors. *J ECT* 20:258–261, 2004.
58. Dolenc TJ, Rasmussen KG. The safety of electroconvulsive therapy and lithium in combination. A case series and review of the literature. *J ECT* 21:165–170, 2005.
59. Greenberg RM, Pettinati HM. Benzodiazepines and electroconvulsive therapy. *Convuls Ther* 9:262–273, 1993.
60. Penland HR, Ostroff RB. Combined use of lamotrigine and electroconvulsive therapy in bipolar depression: a case series. *J ECT* 22:142–147, 2006.
61. Lunde ME, Lee EK, Rasmussen KG. Electroconvulsive therapy in patients with epilepsy. *Epilepsy & Behavior* 9:355–359, 2006.

62. Ding Z, White PF. Anesthesia for electroconvulsive therapy. *Anesth Analg* 94:1351–1364, 2002.
63. Bouckoms AJ, Welch CA, Drop LJ, et al. Atropine in electroconvulsive therapy. *Convuls Ther* 5:48–55, 1989.
64. Avramov MN, Husain MM, White PF. The comparative effects of methohexital, propofol, and etomidate for electroconvulsive therapy. *Anesth Analg* 81:596–602, 1995.
65. Vaidya P, Anderson E, Bobb A, et al. A within-subject comparison of propofol and methohexital anesthesia for electroconvulsive therapy. *J ECT* 28(1):14–19, 2010.
66. Khalid N, Atkins M, Kirov G. The effects of etomidate on seizure duration and electrical stimulus dose in seizure-resistant patients during electroconvulsive therapy. *J ECT* 22:184–188, 2006.
67. McDaniel WW, Sahota AK, Vyas BV, et al. Ketamine appears associated with better word recall than etomidate after a course of 6 electroconvulsive therapies. *J ECT* 22:103–106, 2006.
68. Rasmussen KG, Spackman TN, Hooten MW. The clinical utility of inhalational anesthesia with sevoflurane in electroconvulsive therapy. *J ECT* 21:239–242, 2005.
69. Mirzakhani H, Welch C, Eikermann M, et al. Neuromuscular blocking agents for electroconvulsive therapy: a systematic review. *Acta Anaesthesiol Scand* 56(1):3–16, 2012.
70. Castelli I, Steiner A, Kaufmann MA, et al. Comparative effects of esmolol and labetolol to attenuate hyperdynamic states after electroconvulsive therapy. *Anesth Analg* 80:557–561, 1995.
71. Gerring JP, Shields HM. The identification and management of patients with a high risk for cardiac arrhythmias during modified ECT. *J Clin Psychiatry* 43:140–143, 1982.
72. Ottoson JO. Is unilateral nondominant ECT as efficient as bilateral ECT? A new look at the evidence. *Convuls Ther* 7:190–200, 1991.
73. Sackeim HA, Prudic J, Devanand DP, et al. A prospective, randomized, double-blind comparison of bilateral and right unilateral electroconvulsive therapy at different stimulus intensities. *Arch Gen Psychiatry* 57:425–434, 2000.
74. Sackeim H, Decina P, Prohovnik I, et al. Seizure threshold in electroconvulsive therapy: effects of sex, age, electrode placement, and number of treatments. *Arch Gen Psychiatry* 44:355–360, 1987.
75. McCall WV, Dunn BA, Rosenquist PB, et al. Markedly suprathreshold right unilateral ECT versus minimally suprathreshold bilateral ECT: antidepressant and memory affects. *J ECT* 18:126–129, 2002.
76. Delva NJ, Brunet D, Hawken ER, et al. Electrical dose and seizure threshold: relations to clinical outcome and cognitive effects in bifrontal, bitemporal, and right unilateral ECT. *J ECT* 16:361–369, 2000.
77. Rankesh F, Barekatian M, Kuchakian S. Bifrontal versus right unilateral and bitemporal electroconvulsive therapy in major depressive disorder. *J ECT* 21:207–210, 2005.
78. Squire LR, Zouzounis JA. ECT and memory: brief pulse versus sine wave. *Am J Psychiatry* 143:596, 1986.
79. Sackeim H, Prudic J, Nobler M, et al. Effects of pulse width and electrode placement on the efficacy and cognitive effects of electroconvulsive therapy. *Brain Stimul* 1:71–83, 2008.
80. Sienaert P, Vansteelandt K, Demyttenaere K, et al. Absence of cognitive side effects after ultrabrief electroconvulsive therapy. *J ECT* 24:44–49, 2008.
81. Loo C, Sheehan P, Pigot M, et al. A comparison of right unilateral ultra-brief pulse (0.3ms) ECT and standard right unilateral ECT. *J ECT* 24:51–55, 2008.
82. Ottoson JO. Experimental studies on the mode of action of electroconvulsive therapy. *Acta Psychiatr Neural Scand* 35(Suppl. 145):1–141, 1960.
83. Fink M. *Convulsive therapy: theory and practice*, New York, 1979, Raven Press.
84. Kramer B. Use of ECT in California, 1977–1983. *Am J Psychiatry* 142:1190–1192, 1985.
85. Devanand DP, Dwork AJ, Hutchinson ER, et al. Does ECT alter brain structure? *Am J Psychiatry* 151:957–970, 1994.
86. Sackeim HA, Prudic J, Fuller R. The cognitive effects of electroconvulsive therapy in community settings. *Neuropsychopharmacology* 32:244–254, 2007.
87. Daniel WF, Crovitz HP. Acute memory impairment following electroconvulsive therapy: 2. effects of electrode placement. *Acta Psychiatr Scand* 67:57–68, 1983.

88. Semkovska M, McLoughlin DM. Objective cognitive performance associated with electroconvulsive therapy for depression: a systematic review and meta analysis. *Biol Psychiatry* 68:568–577, 2010.

89. Sackeim HA, Haskett RF, Mulsant BH, et al. Continuation pharmacotherapy in the prevention of relapse following electroconvulsive therapy: a randomized controlled trial. *JAMA* 285:1299–1307, 2001.

90. Kellner CH, Knapp RG, Petrides G, et al. Continuation electroconvulsive therapy versus pharmacotherapy for relapse prevention in major depression. *Arch Gen Psychiatry* 63:1337–1344, 2006.

91. Prudic J, Haskett R, McCall V. Pharmacological strategies in the prevention of relapse after electroconvulsive therapy. *J ECT* 28:3–12, 2013.

92. Nordenskjold A, von Knorring L, Ljung T, et al. Continuation electroconvulsive therapy with pharmacotherapy versus pharmacotherapy alone for prevention of relapse of depression. *J ECT* 29:86–92, 2013.

93. Rey JM, Walter G. Half a century of ECT use in young people. *Am J Psychiatry* 154:595–602, 1997.

94. Ghaziuddin N, Kutcher S, Knapp P, et al. Practice parameter for use of electroconvulsive therapy with adolescents. *J Am Acad Child Adolesc Psychiatry* 43:1521–1539, 2004.

95. Consoli A, Benmiloud M, Wachtel L, et al. Electroconvulsive therapy in adolescents with the catatonia syndrome: efficacy and ethics. *J ECT* 26:259–265, 2010.

96. Wachtel L, Hermida A, Dhossche D. Maintenance electroconvulsive therapy in autistic catatonia: a case series review. *Prog Neuro-Psychopharmacol Biol Psychiatry* 34(4):581–587, 2010.

97. Cohen D, Olivier T, Flament M, et al. Absence of cognitive impairment at long-term follow-up in adolescents treated with ECT for severe mood disorder. *Am J Psychiatry* 157:460–462, 2000.

98. Baeza I, Flamarique I, Garrido J, et al. Clinical experience using electroconvulsive therapy in adolescents with schizophrenia spectrum disorders. *J Child Adolesc Psychopharm* 20:205–209, 2010.

99. Ghaziuddin N, Dumas S, Hodges E. Use of continuation or maintenance electroconvulsive therapy in adolescents with severe treatment resistant depression. *J ECT* 27:168–174, 2011.

100. Wachtel L, Dhossche D, Kellner C. Is electroconvulsive therapy appropriate for children and adolescents? *Med Hypotheses* 76:395–399, 2011.

Index

Page numbers followed by "f" indicate figures, "t" indicate tables, and "b" indicate boxes.